Atlas of
GASTROINTESTINAL IMAGING
Radiologic-Endoscopic Correlation

Atlas of GASTROINTESTINAL IMAGING
Radiologic-Endoscopic Correlation

Perry J. Pickhardt, MD
Department of Radiology
University of Wisconsin Medical School
Madison, Wisconsin
Department of Radiology
Uniformed Services University
of the Health Sciences
Bethesda, Maryland

Glen M. Arluk, MD
Department of Gastroenterology
Naval Medical Center Portsmouth
Portsmouth, Virginia
Department of Medicine
Uniformed Services University
of the Health Sciences
Bethesda, Maryland

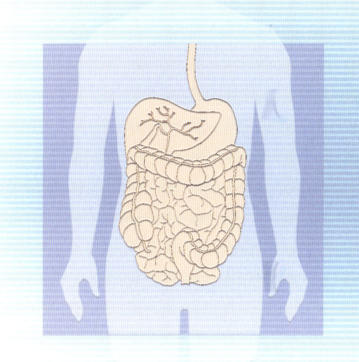

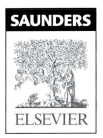

SAUNDERS

ELSEVIER

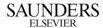

1600 John F. Kennedy Boulevard
Ste 1800
Philadelphia, Pennsylvania 19103-2899

ATLAS OF GASTROINTESTINAL IMAGING: Radiologic-Endoscopic Correlation
ISBN: 978-14160-3202-1

Copyright © 2007 by Saunders, an imprint of Elsevier Inc.

All rights reserved. No part of this publication may be reproduced or transmitted in any form or by any means, electronic or mechanical, including photocopying, recording, or any information storage and retrieval system, without permission in writing from the publisher. Permissions may be sought directly from Elsevier's Health Sciences Rights Department in Philadelphia, PA, USA: phone: (+1) 215 239 3804, fax: (+1) 215 239 3805, e-mail: healthpermissions@elsevier.com. You may also complete your request on-line via the Elsevier homepage (http://www.elsevier.com), by selecting 'Customer Support' and then 'Obtaining Permissions'.

The opinions expressed herein are solely those of the authors and do not reflect those of the United States Navy, the Department of Defense, or the United States Government.

Notice

Knowledge and best practice in this field are constantly changing. As new research and experience broaden our knowledge, changes in practice, treatment and drug therapy may become necessary or appropriate. Readers are advised to check the most current information provided (i) on procedures featured or (ii) by the manufacturer of each product to be administered, to verify the recommended dose or formula, the method and duration of administration, and contraindications. It is the responsibility of the practitioner, relying on his or her own experience and knowledge of the patient, to make diagnoses, to determine dosages and the best treatment for each individual patient, and to take all appropriate safety precautions. To the fullest extent of the law, neither the Publisher nor the Authors assume any liability for any injury and/or damage to persons or property arising out of or related to any use of the material contained in this book.

The Publisher

Library of Congress Cataloging-in-Publication Data
Atlas of gastrointestinal imaging: radiologic-endoscopic correlation/[edited by] Perry J. Pickhardt, Glen M. Arluk.
  p. ; cm.
  ISBN 978-1-4160-3202-1
  1. Digestive organs—Imaging—Atlases. 2. Laparoscopy—Atlases. I. Pickhardt, Perry J.
II. Arluk, Glen M.
  [DNLM: 1. Digestive System Diseases—diagnosis—Atlases. 2. Diagnostic Imaging—Atlases.
3. Endoscopy, Digestive System. WI 17 A87918 2007]

RC804.D52A85 2007
616.3'075400222—dc22
                                                                                              2007003001

Acquisitions Editor: Rebecca Schmidt-Gaertner
Developmental Editor: Martha Limbach
Publishing Services Manager: Tina Rebane
Design Direction: Ellen Zanolle

Working together to grow
libraries in developing countries

www.elsevier.com | www.bookaid.org | www.sabre.org

ELSEVIER   BOOK AID International   Sabre Foundation

Printed in China

Last digit is the print number: 9 8 7 6 5 4 3 2 1

*To Bethney,
my wife and love of my life*
PJP

*To my wife, Shaye,
and my children, Brianna,
Madison, and Dylan,
for their love and support*
GMA

CONTRIBUTORS

Andrew D. Lee, MD
Department of Radiology
University of Wisconsin Medical School
Madison, Wisconsin
The Duodenum; The Pancreas

David H. Kim, MD
Department of Radiology
University of Wisconsin Medical School
Madison, Wisconsin
The Stomach; The Mesenteric Small Bowel; The Liver

Peter J. Chase, MD
Department of Radiology
University of Wisconsin Medical School
Madison, Wisconsin
The Biliary System

PREFACE

The primary motivation for this work was to help bridge the perceived gap between radiology and gastroenterology practice by way of a digestible atlas of correlative imaging. With regard to imaging of gastrointestinal diseases, continued advances in both fields have actually blurred the once clear distinction between these two medical subspecialties. Gastroenterologists have not only incorporated fluoroscopic and sonographic techniques into endoscopic procedures, but there is also an ever-increasing need for clinicians to appreciate the radiologic imaging manifestations of abdominal pathology. On the other hand, radiologists have a growing need to appreciate the endoscopic appearance of gastrointestinal disease, particularly as 3D volume rendering and virtual endoscopic radiologic imaging techniques continue to emerge. Although both radiologic-pathologic and endoscopic-pathologic correlations have been extensively covered, the same cannot be said for radiologic-endoscopic correlation. The complementary nature of radiologic and endoscopic evaluation should become apparent in the pages of this atlas. To underscore their common diagnostic bonds, the radiologic and endoscopic findings of disease are discussed together as "imaging features." Gastrointestinal imaging will continue to evolve as a complex but perhaps unifying field that combines both radiologic and endoscopic approaches to bring about better care of our patients.

It should be noted that a basic working knowledge of abdominal radiology and gastroenterology is assumed herein, as there is no formal review of normal imaging findings. Furthermore, the supporting text material is not intended to represent an exhaustive review of the various disease entities. For more detailed information, the reader is encouraged to consult reference works such as the *Textbook of Gastrointestinal Radiology,* edited by Drs. Richard M. Gore and Marc S. Levine, and *Sleisenger & Fordtran's Gastrointestinal and Liver Disease,* edited by Mark Feldman, Lawrence S. Friedman, and Marvin H. Sleisenger, both of which were invaluable resources for this atlas. Instead, we sought to maximize our ability to demonstrate the radiologic and endoscopic imaging appearance of gastrointestinal pathology. Some diseases have no real radiologic correlate, whereas other diseases have no endoscopic correlate, but these entities have been largely retained to facilitate "cross pollination" and collaborative appreciation (the liver chapter is a prime example of this). Not all side-by-side examples of radiologic-endoscopic comparison will be of the same patient; rather, we chose to include examples that were most representative to optimize comparison. The chapters are organized along a journey through the gastrointestinal tract, followed by a trip through the hepatopancreatobiliary system. Enjoy!

Perry J. Pickhardt, MD

ACKNOWLEDGMENTS

This atlas represents the collective output from many fine clinical radiologists and gastroenterologists who have consistently provided wonderful patient care over many years and have graciously shared their handiwork with us. Although we could not possibly list all deserving individuals, we extend a special note of gratitude to the following physicians for their invaluable input: Sanjeev Bhalla, Cooky Menias, Dennis Balfe, and Marilyn Siegel from the Mallinckrodt Institute of Radiology at Washington University: Andrew Taylor, Jesus Bianco, Deepak Gopal, Tom Winter, and Scott Perlman from the University of Wisconsin; Bruce Greenwald, Peter Darwin, and Eric Goldberg from the University of Maryland; Frank Moses, Kent Holtzmuller, and Eric Frizzell from Walter Reed Army Medical Center; John Smith, Richard Dobhan, and Theodore Schafer from the Naval Medical Center, Portsmouth; Amy Hara from the Mayo Clinic, Scottsdale; Bill Thompson from Duke University; Julien Puylaert from MCH Westeinde Hospital, The Hague, The Netherlands; Alvaro Huete from Pontificia Universidad Catolica, Santiago, Chile; and Walter Coyle from the Naval Medical Center, San Diego. Special thanks also to Bethney Pickhardt for her invaluable administrative support. Finally, we would also like to express our appreciation to past residents and fellows at the University of Wisconsin, the Mallinckrodt Institute, and the National Capital Consortium for their dedication and involvement in obtaining many of the images displayed herein.

PJP
GMA

LIST OF ABBREVIATIONS

AFP   α-fetoprotein
AIDS   acquired immunodeficiency syndrome
BE   barium enema
CMV   cytomegalovirus
CT   computed tomography
CTC   computed tomographic colonography
DSA   digital subtraction angiography
EGD   esophagogastroduodenoscopy
EHE   epithelioid hemangioendothelioma
ERCP   endoscopic retrograde cholangiopancreatography
EUS   endoscopic ultrasound
FAP   familial adenomatous polyposis
FNH   focal nodular hyperplasia
GAVE   gastric antral vascular ectasia
GERD   gastroesophageal reflux disease
GI   gastrointestinal
GIST   gastrointestinal stromal tumor
HCC   hepatocellular carcinoma
HIV   human immunodeficiency virus
HSP   Henoch-Schönlein purpura
HSV   herpes simplex virus
HU   Hounsfield units (for CT)
IPMN   intraductal papillary mucinous tumor
IV   intravenous
IVC   inferior vena cava
IBD   inflammatory bowel disease
IBS   irritable bowel syndrome
LES   lower esophageal sphincter
MAI   *Mycobacterium avium-intracellulare*
MALT   mucosa-associated lymphoid tissue

MCN   mucinous cystic neoplasm
MEN   multiple endocrine neoplasia
MR   magnetic resonance
MRCP   magnetic resonance cholangiopancreatography
MRI   magnetic resonance imaging
NASH   nonalcoholic steatohepatitis
NSAIDs   nonsteroidal antiinflammatory drugs
PEG   percutaneous endoscopic gastrostomy
PET   positron emission tomography
PSC   primary sclerosing cholangitis
PTC   percutaneous transhepatic cholangiography
PTLD   post-transplantation lymphoproliferative disorder
PUD   peptic ulcer disease
RPC   recurrent pyogenic cholangitis
SBFT   small bowel follow-through
SBO   small bowel obstruction
SGE   spoiled gradient echo (for MRI)
SLE   systemic lupus erythematosus
SMA   superior mesenteric artery
SMV   superior mesenteric vein
SSFSE   single-shot fast spin-echo (for MRI)
SVC   superior vena cava
TB   tuberculosis
THAD   transient hepatic attenuation difference (for CT)
THID   transient hepatic intensity difference (for MR)
TRUS   transrectal ultrasound
UGI   upper gastrointestinal series
UC   ulcerative colitis
US   ultrasound

CONTENTS

CHAPTER 1
THE ESOPHAGUS, 1
Perry J. Pickhardt

- 1.1 ESOPHAGEAL TUMORS, 1
  - Adenocarcinoma, 1
  - Squamous Cell Carcinoma, 6
  - Mesenchymal Tumors, 10
  - Other Esophageal Neoplasms, 13
  - Non-neoplastic Lesions, 16
- 1.2 GASTROESOPHAGEAL REFLUX DISEASE (GERD), 18
  - Reflux Esophagitis, 18
  - Peptic Strictures, 21
  - Barrett's Esophagus, 23
- 1.3 ESOPHAGITIS (NON-GERD), 24
  - Infectious Esophagitis, 24
  - Drug-Induced, Caustic, and Radiation Injury, 28
  - Other Esophagitides, 31
- 1.4 ESOPHAGEAL DYSMOTILITY DISORDERS, 33
  - Achalasia, 33
  - Diffuse Esophageal Spasm, 36
  - Scleroderma (Progressive Systemic Sclerosis), 36
- 1.5 OTHER ESOPHAGEAL CONDITIONS, 38
  - Vascular Lesions, 38
  - Pharyngoesophageal Diverticula, 40
  - Duplication Cysts, 43
  - Mechanical Injury, 44
  - Foreign Body Impaction, 47
  - Esophageal Fistulas, 49
  - Intramural Pseudodiverticulosis, 51
  - Rings, Webs, and Stenosis, 53
  - Vascular Rings and Slings, 55
  - Hypopharyngeal Disease, 57

CHAPTER 2
THE STOMACH, 61
David H. Kim, MD • Perry J. Pickhardt, MD

- 2.1 GASTRIC TUMORS, 61
  - Mucosal Polyps, 61
  - Adenocarcinoma, 65
  - Lymphoma, 70
  - Mesenchymal Tumors, 73
  - Other Submucosal Tumors, 78
- 2.2 GASTRITIS AND GASTROPATHY, 81
  - Peptic Ulcer Disease, 81
  - Reactive Gastropathies, 84
  - Zollinger-Ellison Syndrome, 87
  - Infectious Gastritis, 88
  - Granulomatous Diseases, 91
  - Ménétrier's Disease, 93
  - Other Inflammatory Conditions, 94
- 2.3 OTHER GASTRIC CONDITIONS, 97
  - Vascular Lesions, 97
  - Gastric Hernias, 101
  - Gastric Fistulas, 104
  - Heterotopic Pancreatic Rest, 106
  - Duplication Cysts, 107
  - Gastric Bezoars, 108
  - Gastric Volvulus, 109
  - Gastric Diverticula, 110
  - Complications of Percutaneous Endoscopic Gastrostomy, 111

CHAPTER 3
THE DUODENUM, 113
Andrew D. Lee, MD • Perry J. Pickhardt, MD

- 3.1. DUODENAL TUMORS, 113
  - Mucosal Neoplasms, 113
  - Submucosal Tumors, 117
  - Non-neoplastic Lesions, 122
- 3.2 INFLAMMATORY CONDITIONS, 126
  - Peptic Ulcer Disease, 126
  - Duodenitis, 129
- 3.3 OTHER DUODENAL CONDITIONS, 133
  - Vascular Lesions, 133
  - Aortoduodenal Fistula, 136
  - Duodenal Diverticula, 137
  - Duodenal Duplication Cyst, 140
  - Infiltrative Diseases, 140

CHAPTER 4
THE MESENTERIC SMALL BOWEL, 143
David H. Kim, MD • Perry J. Pickhardt, MD

- 4.1 SMALL BOWEL TUMORS, 143
  - Adenocarcinoma, 143
  - Carcinoid Tumor, 145
  - Lymphoma, 149
  - Mesenchymal Tumors, 151
  - Metastatic Disease, 158
- 4.2 ENTERITIS, 160
  - Crohn's Disease, 160
  - Infectious Enteritis, 166
  - Other Inflammatory Conditions, 171
- 4.3 OTHER SMALL BOWEL CONDITIONS, 175
  - Small Bowel Obstruction, 175
  - Mesenteric Ischemia, 182
  - Small Bowel Herniation, 188
  - Celiac Disease, 192
  - Small Bowel Diverticula, 195
  - Malrotation, 200
  - Small Bowel Wall Thickening, 203
  - Small Bowel Perforation, 205
  - Vascular Ectasia, 208

CHAPTER 5
THE COLON AND RECTUM, 211
Perry J. Pickhardt, MD

- 5.1 COLORECTAL POLYPS AND MASSES, 211
  - Benign Mucosal Neoplasms, 212
  - Non-neoplastic Mucosal Lesions, 218
  - Submucosal Lesions, 222
  - Colonic Adenocarcinoma, 229
  - Rectal Adenocarcinoma, 234
  - Other Colorectal Tumors, 238

CTC Diagnostic Tools, 242
CTC Pitfalls, 253
5.2 COLITIS, 261
Ulcerative Colitis, 261
Crohn's Disease, 266
Infection, 271
Ischemia, 275
Other Colitides, 279
5.3 COLONIC DIVERTICULAR DISEASE, 283
Diverticulosis, 283
Acute Diverticulitis, 286
Diverticular Fistulas and Strictures, 289
Diverticular Hemorrhage, 292
Giant Sigmoid Diverticulum, 293
5.4 THE APPENDIX, 294
Appendicitis, 294
Appendiceal Tumors, 297
5.5 OTHER COLORECTAL CONDITIONS, 301
Anorectal Disease, 301
Intussusception, 307
Vascular Lesions, 310
Colonic Volvulus, 314
Endometriosis, 317
Pneumatosis Coli, 318
Colonic Hernias, 320
Complications of Colonoscopy, 323
Epiploic Appendagitis, 326
Melanosis Coli, 327

CHAPTER 6

THE BILIARY SYSTEM, 329

Peter J. Chase, MD • Perry J. Pickhardt, MD

6.1 BILIARY TUMORS, 329
Cholangiocarcinoma, 329
Gallbladder Carcinoma, 333
Periampullary Tumors, 335
Metastatic Disease, 338
Other Biliary Tumors, 341
6.2 BILIARY CALCULI, 344
Cholelithiasis, 344
Choledocholithiasis, 347
Mirizzi's Syndrome, 351
Biliary-Enteric Fistulas, 352
6.3 INFLAMMATORY DISEASES, 355
Cholecystitis, 355
Primary Sclerosing Cholangitis (PSC), 359
Ascending Cholangitis, 362
Recurrent Pyogenic Cholangitis, 364
AIDS Cholangiopathy, 365
6.4 OTHER BILIARY CONDITIONS, 366
Choledochal Cysts, 366
Caroli's Disease, 368
Adenomyomatosis, 370
Porcelain Gallbladder, 372

Biliary Leak, 373
Other Causes of Stricture and Obstruction, 375
Hemobilia, 378

CHAPTER 7

THE PANCREAS, 381

Andrew D. Lee, MD • Perry J. Pickhardt, MD

7.1 PANCREATIC NEOPLASMS, 381
Ductal Adenocarcinoma, 381
Mucinous Cystic Neoplasms, 386
Intraductal Papillary Mucinous Neoplasm, 387
Serous Cystadenoma, 390
Islet Cell Tumors, 393
Solid-Pseudopapillary Tumor, 397
Metastatic Disease, 399
Other Pancreatic Neoplasms, 401
7.2 PANCREATITIS, 403
Acute Pancreatitis, 403
Chronic Pancreatitis, 408
Pancreatic Pseudocysts, 410
Autoimmune Pancreatitis, 415
7.3 OTHER PANCREATIC CONDITIONS, 417
Pancreas Divisum, 417
Annular Pancreas, 418
Simple Pancreatic Cysts, 420
Pancreatic Trauma, 422

CHAPTER 8

THE LIVER, 423

David H. Kim, MD • Perry J. Pickhardt, MD

8.1 NEOPLASTIC LESIONS, 423
Hepatocellular Carcinoma, 423
Metastatic Disease, 428
Cavernous Hemangioma, 432
Hepatocellular Adenoma, 436
Intrahepatic (Peripheral) Cholangiocarcinoma, 438
Other Hepatic Tumors, 440
8.2 NON-NEOPLASTIC LESIONS, 445
Focal Nodular Hyperplasia, 445
Benign Hepatic Cysts, 448
Hepatic Abscess, 450
Vascular Findings, 453
8.3 OTHER HEPATIC CONDITIONS, 459
Cirrhosis and Portal Hypertension, 459
Budd-Chiari Syndrome, 463
Fatty Liver Disease (Hepatic Steatosis), 466
Hemochromatosis, 469
The Hyperdense Liver on CT, 471
Post-transplant Complications, 473

INDEX, 477

CHAPTER 1

THE ESOPHAGUS

Perry J. Pickhardt, MD

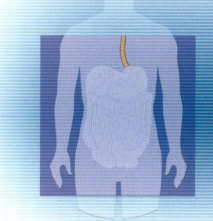

1. **ESOPHAGEAL TUMORS**
   1.1 Adenocarcinoma
   1.2 Squamous Cell Carcinoma
   1.3 Mesenchymal Tumors
   1.4 Other Esophageal Neoplasms
   1.5 Non-neoplastic Lesions
2. **GASTROESOPHAGEAL REFLUX DISEASE (GERD)**
   2.1 Reflux Esophagitis
   2.2 Peptic Strictures
   2.3 Barrett's Esophagus
3. **ESOPHAGITIS (NON-GERD)**
   3.1 Infectious Esophagitis
   3.2 Drug-induced, Caustic, and Radiation Injury
   3.3 Other Esophagitides
4. **DYSMOTILITY DISORDERS**
   4.1 Achalasia
   4.2 Diffuse Esophageal Spasm
   4.3 Scleroderma (Progressive Systemic Sclerosis)
5. **OTHER ESOPHAGEAL CONDITIONS**
   5.1 Vascular Lesions
   5.2 Pharyngoesophageal Diverticula
   5.3 Duplication Cysts
   5.4 Mechanical Injury
   5.5 Foreign Body Impaction
   5.6 Esophageal Fistulas
   5.7 Intramural Pseudodiverticulosis
   5.8 Rings, Webs, and Stenosis
   5.9 Vascular Rings and Slings
   5.10 Hypopharyngeal Disease

Although the role of fluoroscopic barium examination in the gut continues to diminish as other advanced imaging techniques evolve, it remains a valuable, noninvasive tool for initial evaluation of dysphagia and other disorders of the hypopharynx and esophagus. Endoscopic, fluoroscopic, and cross-sectional studies all provide complementary anatomic and physiologic information. The broad topics of esophageal tumors, gastroesophageal reflux disease (GERD), non-reflux causes of esophagitis, esophageal dysmotility disorders, and a variety of other esophageal conditions are discussed in this chapter.

1. ESOPHAGEAL TUMORS

Adenocarcinoma and squamous cell carcinoma account for the vast majority of epithelial esophageal malignancies. The prognosis of esophageal cancer remains dismal, with overall 5-year survival less than 10%. Although squamous cell carcinoma remains the most common form of esophageal cancer worldwide, adenocarcinoma, once relatively uncommon, is now the most common form in the United States. Despite their different risk factor profiles, the diagnostic workup and treatment approaches are fairly similar. Other focal esophageal tumors, both neoplastic and non-neoplastic, are also discussed.

1.1 Adenocarcinoma
(Figures 1.1.1-1.1.10)

CLINICAL FEATURES

- Adenocarcinoma is strongly associated with reflux disease; most if not all adenocarcinomas arise in Barrett's metaplasia.
- High-grade dysplasia in Barrett's esophagus is a major risk factor.
- Many adenocarcinomas involving the gastroesophageal junction that have been previously classified as gastric primaries are, in fact, esophageal cancers arising in Barrett's metaplasia.
- Dysphagia, odynophagia, and weight loss are common presenting features; a history of long-standing reflux disease is typical.
- Endoscopy is the imaging modality of choice when the clinical suspicion for cancer is high.
- Most cases are advanced at presentation, in part because the esophagus has a rich lymphovascular supply and lacks a serosal coating.
- Neoadjuvant chemoradiotherapy is often performed prior to surgical resection in patients with lymph node metastasis or tumors extending through the muscularis propria.

- Endoscopic treatment options for T1 lesions in patients who are poor surgical candidates include cap-assisted endoscopic mucosal resection, photodynamic therapy, and tumor ablation with argon plasma coagulation.
- Endoscopic stenting can be performed for palliative care for inoperable obstructing lesions.

IMAGING FEATURES

- Growth patterns can consist of various combinations of infiltrative, polypoid, and ulcerative features.
- Most adenocarcinomas are advanced and have an infiltrative component with irregular luminal narrowing.
- Most of these tumors arise in the distal third, followed by the middle third of the esophagus; subdiaphragmatic spread to the gastric cardia is common.
- Long-segment involvement from submucosal spread can have a varicoid appearance on imaging.
- CT, EUS, and PET all play important and complementary roles in staging.
- Common routes of spread include local invasion, lymphatic (including subdiaphragmatic nodes), and hematogenous (especially liver).

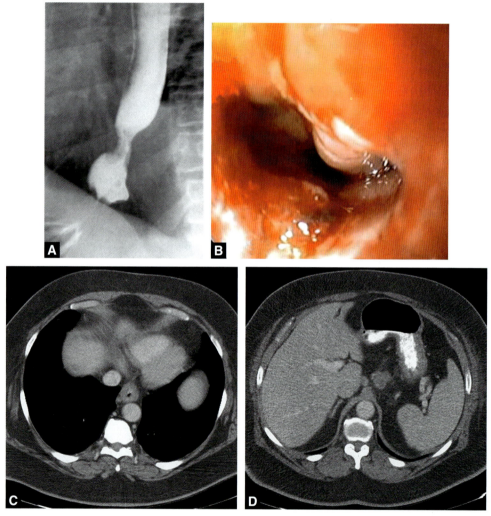

FIGURE 1.1.1 Esophageal adenocarcinoma. Barium esophagram **(A)** in a patient with solid food dysphagia and subsequent EGD **(B)** show focal mucosal irregularity with annular narrowing. CT image **(C)** shows circumferential esophageal soft tissue thickening causing luminal narrowing. CT image below the diaphragm **(D)** shows gastrohepatic lymphadenopathy. Subdiaphragmatic spread is relatively common.

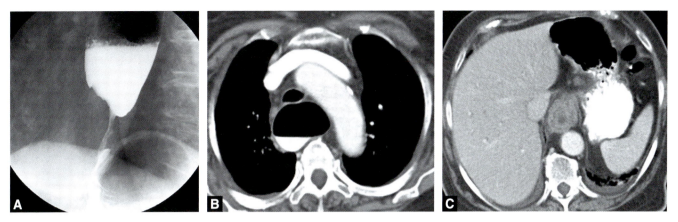

FIGURE 1.1.2 Esophageal adenocarcinoma with luminal obstruction. Barium esophagram (A) in a patient with severe dysphagia shows high-grade luminal narrowing of the distal esophagus with proximal dilatation. CT images (A and B) show the proximal dilatation (B) and distal circumferential wall thickening (C). Note adjacent gastrohepatic lymphadenopathy.

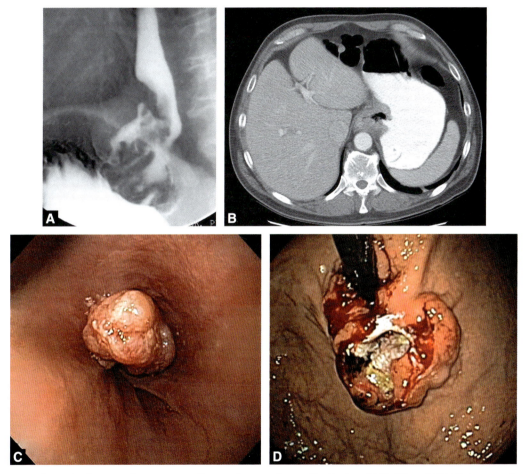

FIGURE 1.1.3 Esophageal adenocarcinoma extending to the gastric cardia. Barium UGI (A) and CT (B) images show a large ulcerated mass at the gastroesophageal junction. Subsequent images from EGD show a polypoid intraluminal component in the distal esophagus (C) and an irregular ulcerated mass extending into the gastric cardia (D).

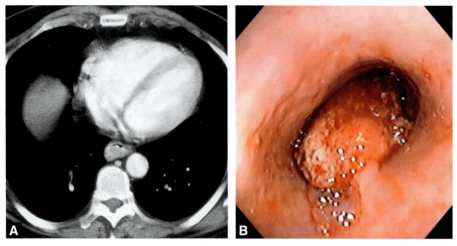

FIGURE 1.1.4 Adenocarcinoma involving the mid-esophagus. CT image **(A)** shows eccentric soft tissue causing esophageal luminal narrowing. Image from EGD **(B)** also shows the luminal narrowing from the eccentric soft tissue mass.

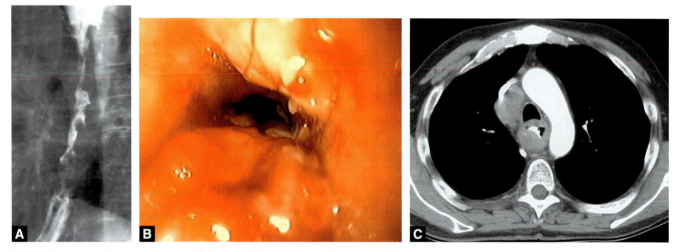

FIGURE 1.1.5 Adenocarcinoma with "varicoid" appearance. Barium esophagram **(A)** shows a long segment of irregular luminal narrowing that simulates varices. A small hiatal hernia is present. EGD image **(B)** shows diffuse irregular luminal narrowing with friability of the mucosa. CT image **(C)** shows both the primary esophageal mass and bulky right paratracheal metastatic lymphadenopathy.

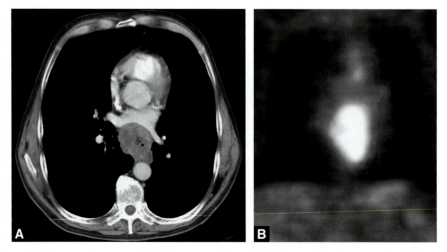

FIGURE 1.1.6 Esophageal adenocarcinoma on PET. Contrast-enhanced CT image **(A)** shows marked circumferential esophageal wall thickening, with mass effect on the left atrium. Coronal image from whole-body FDG PET **(B)** shows significant uptake within the primary tumor. No other hypermetabolic foci were seen. The use of PET scanning in the preoperative workup of esophageal carcinoma is now the standard of care for identifying early nodal metastasis and helping to guide endosonographic fine-needle aspiration.

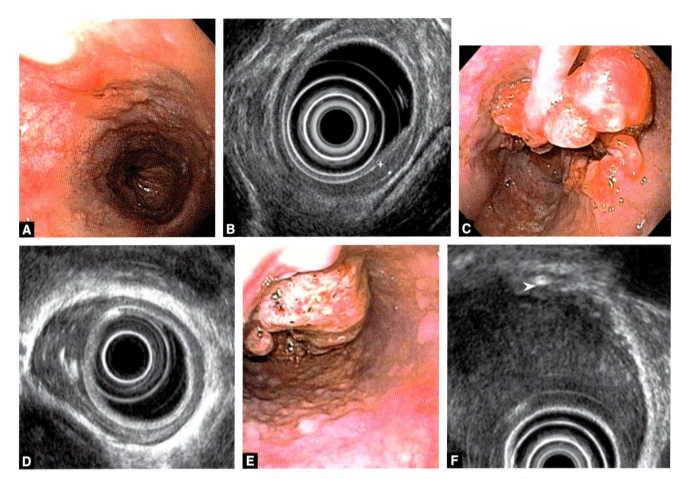

FIGURE 1.1.7 T staging of esophageal adenocarcinoma with EUS. EGD image **(A)** shows an area of nodularity in a segment of Barrett's esophagus that was biopsy-proven adenocarcinoma. At EUS **(B)**, a hypoechoic lesion is seen originating from the mucosal layer and infiltrating the middle hyperechoic layer (submucosa) without involvement of the outer hypoechoic layer (muscularis propria), consistent with a T1 lesion. EGD image from a different patient **(C)** shows a large fungating intraluminal mass. Corresponding EUS image **(D)** shows a hypoechoic, heterogeneous lesion with invasion into but not through the muscularis propria (T2 lesion). EGD image from a third patient **(E)** shows an irregular eccentric mucosal mass that nearly obstructs the esophageal lumen. Corresponding EUS image **(F)** shows a large hypoechoic mass extending through the muscularis propria and into the tunica adventitia consistent with a T3 lesion. Note the irregular external margins (*arrowhead*). A T4 lesion (not shown) is defined as infiltrating neighboring organs such as the aorta.

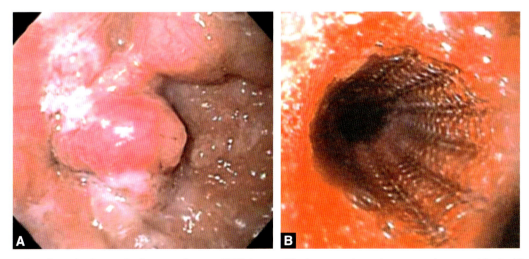

FIGURE 1.1.8 Stenting of advanced adenocarcinoma. EGD image **(A)** shows an irregular mucosal mass with significant luminal compromise. Esophageal stenting **(B)** with an endoscopically placed expandable metal stent was performed for palliative care.

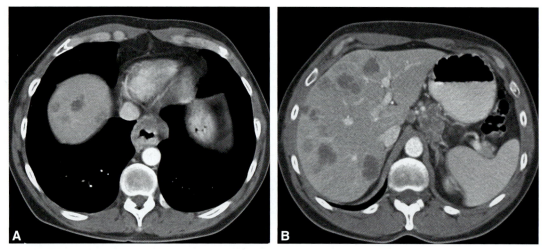

FIGURE 1.1.9 **Esophageal adenocarcinoma with metastatic disease.** Contrast-enhanced CT image **(A)** at the level of the esophageal primary (note circumferential soft tissue) shows low-attenuation metastases at the liver dome. A more caudal CT image **(B)** shows extensive hepatic metastatic disease and bulky gastrohepatic lymphadenopathy.

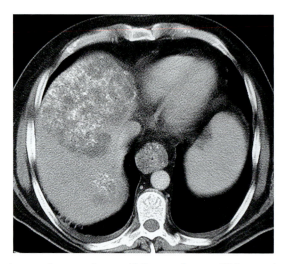

FIGURE 1.1.10 **Mucinous adenocarcinoma of the esophagus.** CT image shows stippled calcification involving both the primary esophageal mass and liver metastases, suggestive of mucinous histology. This CT appearance is rare.

1.2 Squamous Cell Carcinoma
(Figures 1.2.1-1.2.6)

CLINICAL FEATURES

- A variety of risk factors have been identified, including alcohol, tobacco, particular carcinogens, dietary habits, geographic location, and certain predisposing conditions (e.g., achalasia, lye stricture, tylosis).
- Squamous cell carcinoma of the esophagus is now less common than adenocarcinoma in the United States.
- Dysphagia, odynophagia, and weight loss are common presenting features.
- As seen in adenocarcinoma, a majority of cases are advanced at presentation, including lymph node metastases and local tumor invasion into adjacent structures.
- Endoscopy is indicated when the clinical suspicion for cancer is high.
- Screening of high-risk populations for dysplastic epithelium or early carcinoma is controversial.
- Endoscopic treatment options for T1 lesions in patients who are poor surgical candidates include cap-assisted endoscopic mucosal resection, photodynamic therapy, and tumor ablation with argon plasma coagulation.
- Endoscopic stenting can be performed for palliative care in inoperable candidates with obstructing lesions.

IMAGING FEATURES

- Growth patterns include infiltrating, polypoid, ulcerating, and superficial spreading lesions.
- The lesions may be eccentric or circumferential.
- In contrast to adenocarcinoma, most arise in the middle and upper thirds of the esophagus.
- Superficial spreading carcinomas can manifest as multifocal nodules or plaques.

- Chromoendoscopy utilizing Lugol's solution often helps detect early squamous cell carcinoma or dysplasia; dysplastic tissue does not take up the solution and remains unstained.
- As with adenocarcinomas, long-segment submucosal spread can appear varicoid.
- CT, EUS, and PET all play important and complementary roles in staging.
- Metastatic spread to gastrohepatic and celiac nodes can manifest as a large, ulcerating submucosal fundal mass.

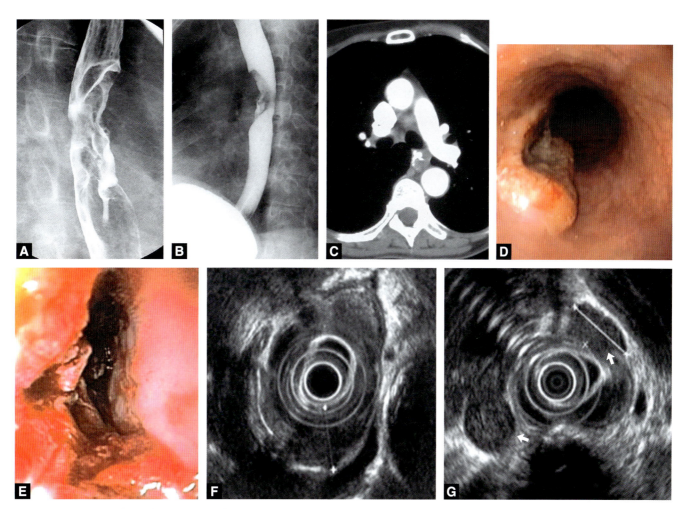

FIGURE 1.2.1 **Esophageal squamous cell carcinoma.** Double-contrast (**A**) and single-contrast (**B**) views from barium esophagram show an irregular eccentric lesion with shouldering in the mid-esophagus. CT (**C**) and EGD (**D**) images from a second patient show an eccentric ulcerated mass in the mid-esophagus. EGD image (**E**) from a third patient shows mucosal irregularity and luminal narrowing. Note the friability of the mucosa. Corresponding EUS image (**F**) shows the primary tumor as a hypoechoic, heterogeneous lesion (*calipers*) with invasion through the outer hypoechoic layer (muscularis propria) and into the tunica adventitia, consistent with a T3 lesion. Endosonographic examination proximal to the tumor (**G**) reveals two enlarged hypoechoic lymph nodes (*arrows*). Fine-needle aspiration confirmed metastatic disease.

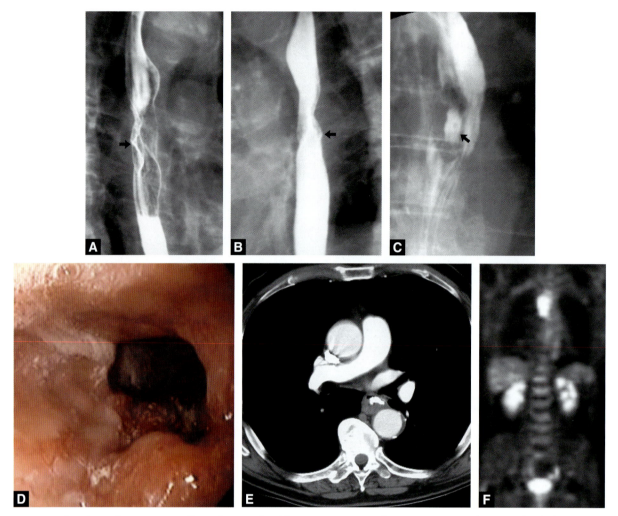

FIGURE 1.2.2 **Esophageal squamous cell carcinoma.** Double-contrast **(A)**, single-contrast **(B)**, and mucosal relief **(C)** views from barium esophagram show a persistent posterior defect with central ulceration (*arrows*). Subsequent EGD **(D)** confirms the ulcerated mass. Contrast-enhanced CT image **(E)** to evaluate for metastatic disease shows the posterior esophageal mass with ulceration. Coronal image from whole-body FDG PET **(F)** shows hypermetabolic uptake in the primary esophageal tumor.

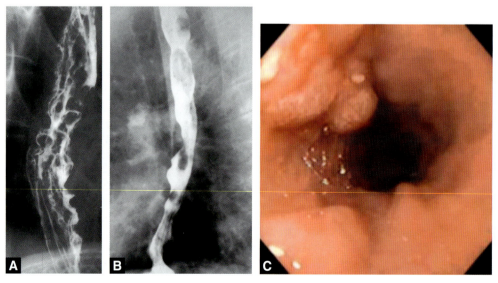

FIGURE 1.2.3 **"Varicoid" squamous cell carcinoma.** Barium esophagram **(A** and **B)** and EGD **(C)** images show infiltrating tumors with a nodular longitudinal appearance that roughly simulate esophageal varices.

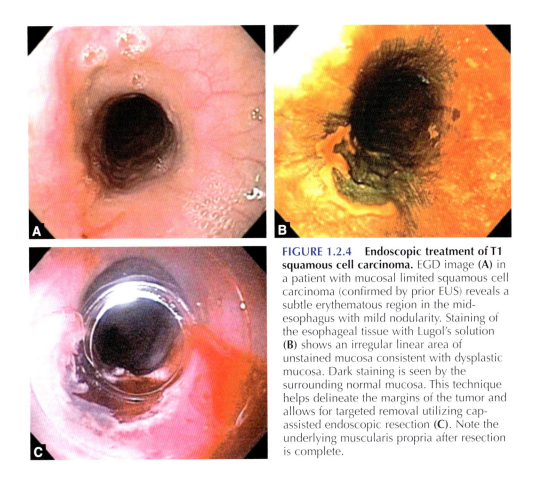

FIGURE 1.2.4 **Endoscopic treatment of T1 squamous cell carcinoma.** EGD image (A) in a patient with mucosal limited squamous cell carcinoma (confirmed by prior EUS) reveals a subtle erythematous region in the mid-esophagus with mild nodularity. Staining of the esophageal tissue with Lugol's solution (B) shows an irregular linear area of unstained mucosa consistent with dysplastic mucosa. Dark staining is seen by the surrounding normal mucosa. This technique helps delineate the margins of the tumor and allows for targeted removal utilizing cap-assisted endoscopic resection (C). Note the underlying muscularis propria after resection is complete.

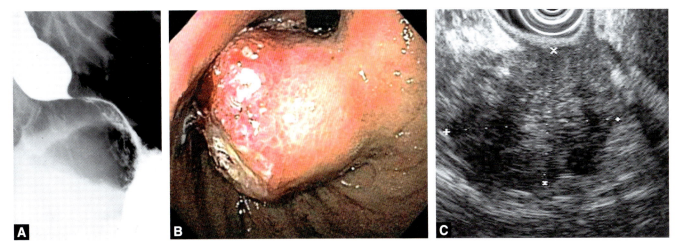

FIGURE 1.2.5 **Upper abdominal nodal metastases presenting as a fundal mass.** Barium esophagram (A) in a patient with squamous cell carcinoma shows extrinsic mass effect related to massive gastrohepatic lymphadenopathy. EGD image (B) from a different patient shows a large ulcerating fundal mass. EUS image (C) shows a large heterogeneous mass with poorly defined margins in the celiac axis region. Fine-needle aspiration confirmed celiac node metastasis.

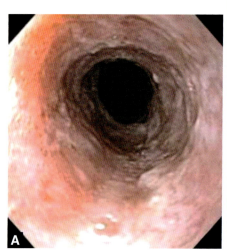 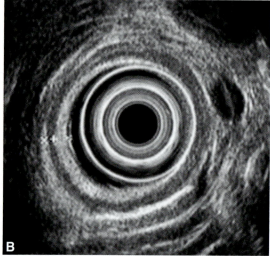

FIGURE 1.2.6 Severe squamous dysplasia. EGD image **(A)** shows diffusely abnormal esophageal mucosa with nodularity and plaque-like lesions. No mucosal uptake was seen with chromoendoscopy utilizing Lugol's solution (not shown). Biopsies and mucosal brushings revealed severe dysplasia without carcinoma. EUS image **(B)** shows circumferential thickening of the inner hyperechoic layer, which represents both the mucosa and submucosa in this case. The inability to differentiate the two layers is due to associated inflammation from the dysplastic process.

1.3 Mesenchymal Tumors
(Figures 1.3.1-1.3.5)

CLINICAL FEATURES

- Leiomyomas are the most common benign tumors of the esophagus; GI stromal tumors (GISTs), which are generally more common than leiomyomas elsewhere in the GI tract, are relatively rare in the esophagus.
- Esophageal leiomyosarcomas arise from the distal two thirds of the esophagus; although bulky at presentation, these tumors have a better overall prognosis than esophageal carcinoma.
- Fibrovascular polyps, also known as pedunculated lipomas, typically arise from the cervical esophagus and are composed of loose fibrovascular stroma and adipocytes.
- Fibrovascular polyps often lead to progressive dysphagia, but regurgitation and even asphyxiation have been reported.

IMAGING FEATURES

- Leiomyomas most often present as solitary submucosal lesions; calcification is uncommon but strongly suggests the diagnosis when present.
- Leiomyosarcomas are typically large, heterogeneous, exoenteric masses, often with luminal cavitation.
- Esophageal GISTs appear similar to GISTs elsewhere in the GI tract.
- Fine-needle aspiration under EUS guidance with immunohistochemical staining can help differentiate leiomyomas, leiomyosarcomas, and GISTs, which can all have a similar endosonographic appearance.
- Fibrovascular polyps are typically large, expansile pedunculated lesions arising from the cervical esophagus; fatty composition can be demonstrated at CT or EUS.
- Smaller sessile esophageal lipomas are rare.

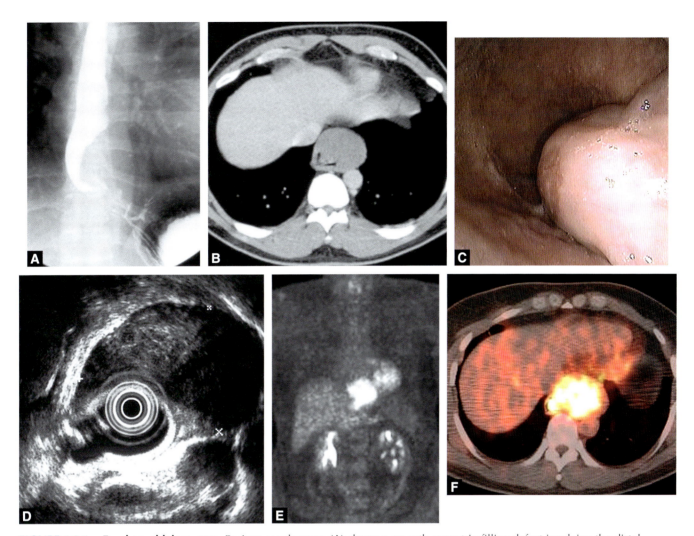

FIGURE 1.3.1 **Esophageal leiomyoma.** Barium esophagram (**A**) shows a smooth eccentric filling defect involving the distal esophagus. Contrast-enhanced CT image (**B**) shows a large intramural esophageal mass with a small projection into the lumen. EGD (**C**) shows this relatively minor intraluminal component, whereas EUS (**D**) demonstrates the larger hypoechoic exophytic component originating from the muscularis propria. Note the smooth outer border of the tumor. Coronal image from whole-body FDG PET (**E**) shows marked uptake in the lesion, but fused PET-CT image (**F**) more clearly shows the hypermetabolic activity within the leiomyoma. A benign leiomyoma was confirmed by histology.

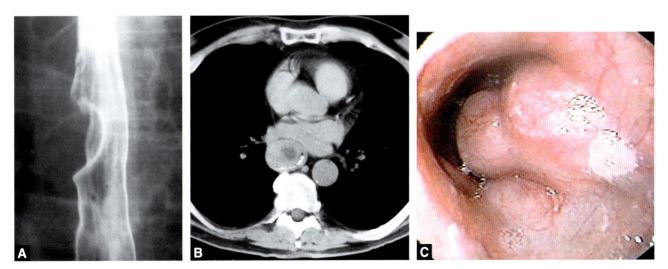

FIGURE 1.3.2 **Esophageal leiomyoma.** Images from barium esophagram (**A**), contrast-enhanced CT (**B**), and EGD (**C**) from three different patients show typical leiomyomas, with a predominantly intramural location and smooth submucosal impression into the lumen.

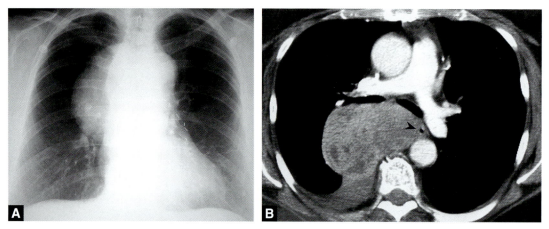

FIGURE 1.3.3 Esophageal leiomyosarcoma. Frontal chest radiograph **(A)** shows a large lobulated mediastinal mass. Contrast-enhanced CT image **(B)** shows a large heterogeneous soft tissue mass located within the middle mediastinum. Gas is seen within the esophageal lumen (*arrowhead*), which seems so peripheral to this exoenteric mass that the primary intramural esophageal nature is obscured.

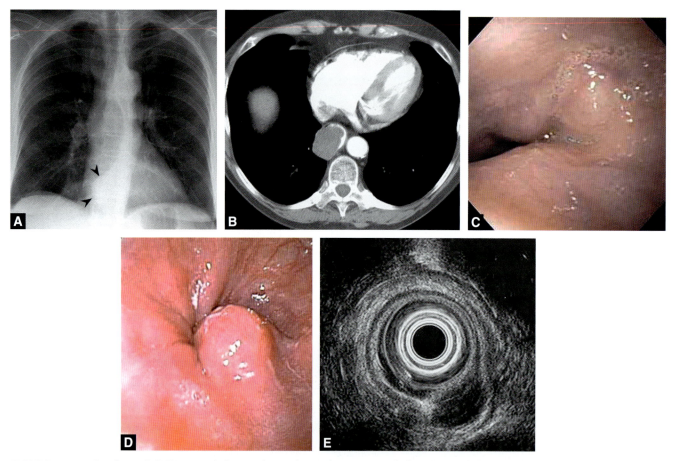

FIGURE 1.3.4 Esophageal GIST. Frontal chest radiograph **(A)** shows a rounded mediastinal contour deformity (*arrowheads*). Contrast-enhanced CT image **(B)** shows a rounded intramural soft tissue mass with smooth impression that displaces the luminal contrast. EGD image **(C)** shows only narrowing of the lumen by the intramural lesion. EGD image **(D)** from a different patient shows a smooth rounded lesion located deep to the normal overlying mucosa. Corresponding EUS image **(E)** shows a hypoechoic lesion with smooth outer borders originating from the muscularis propria.

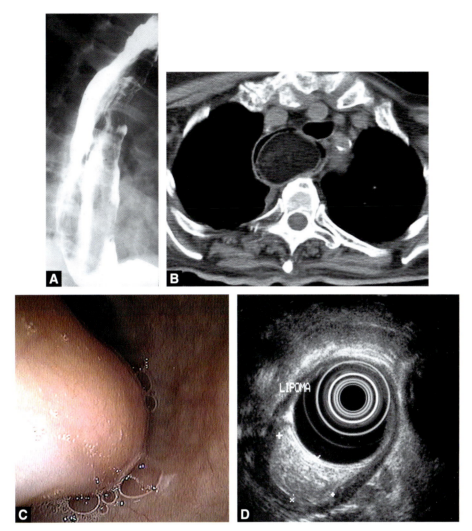

FIGURE 1.3.5 **Fibrovascular polyp (pedunculated esophageal lipoma).** Image from barium esophagram (**A**) shows a large, smooth, elongated filling defect originating in the cervical esophagus. CT image (**B**) from a different patient shows a large luminal mass composed of fat attenuation that expands the esophageal lumen. EGD image (**C**) from a third patient shows a large, smooth pedunculated mass within the esophageal lumen. Corresponding EUS image (**D**) shows that the mass (*calipers*) originates from the submucosal layer and is homogenously hyperechoic, consistent with fatty composition.

1.4 Other Esophageal Neoplasms
(Figures 1.4.1-1.4.5)

CLINICAL FEATURES

- Granular cell tumor is a benign submucosal lesion believed to be of neural derivation.
- Squamous papillomas are uncommon benign tumors often associated with chronic reflux; they are usually small and solitary but can rarely present with innumerable foci (esophageal papillomatosis).
- The esophagus is the least common GI site for lymphoma; most cases represent secondary involvement.
- Metastatic disease to the esophagus is typically from direct extension; hematogenous spread is rare.
- Rare primary esophageal malignancies include spindle cell carcinoma (carcinosarcoma), small cell carcinoma, Kaposi's sarcoma, and primary esophageal melanoma.

IMAGING FEATURES

- Granular cell tumors often appear as yellowish-white submucosal lesions up to 2 cm in size; they are typically solitary and most often involve the mid- to distal esophagus.
- Papillomas often have a lobulated appearance at imaging.
- Primary esophageal lymphoma manifests with a variety of submucosal appearances.
- Spindle cell carcinoma usually appears as a large, expansile intraluminal polypoid lesion.
- Primary small cell carcinoma commonly presents as a bulky, often ulcerated, polypoid mass.
- Primary esophageal melanoma usually manifests as a bulky, nonobstructive intraluminal mass.

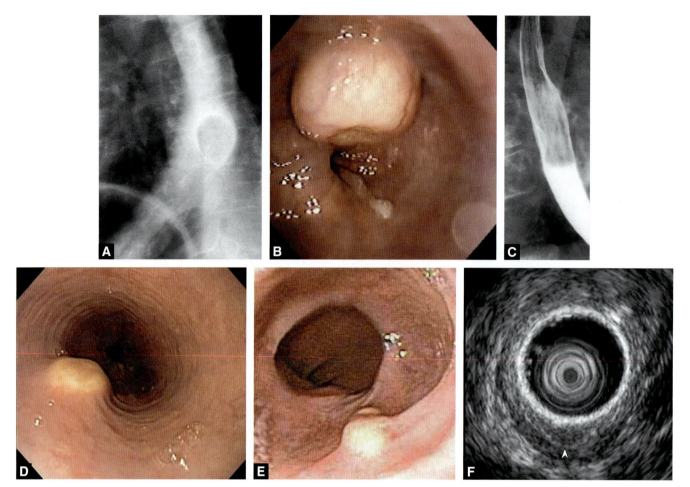

FIGURE 1.4.1 Granular cell tumor. Image from barium esophagram **(A)** shows a smooth, rounded filling defect, which corresponds to a submucosal lesion at EGD **(B)**. Barium **(C)** and EGD **(D)** images from two different patients show smooth submucosal lesions. Note the yellowish appearance at endoscopy. EGD **(E)** image from a final patient shows a smooth, yellowish lesion, which at EUS **(F)** appears as a small hypoechoic lesion within the submucosal layer (*arrowhead*).

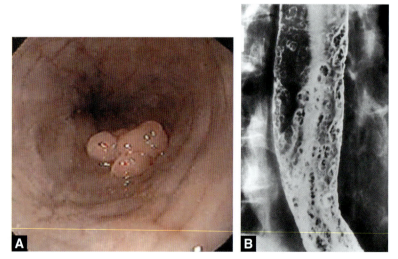

FIGURE 1.4.2 Squamous papilloma and papillomatosis. EGD image **(A)** shows a polypoid, lobulated mucosal lesion. Barium esophagram image **(B)** from a different patient shows multiple small lobulated filling defects carpeting the esophageal lumen.

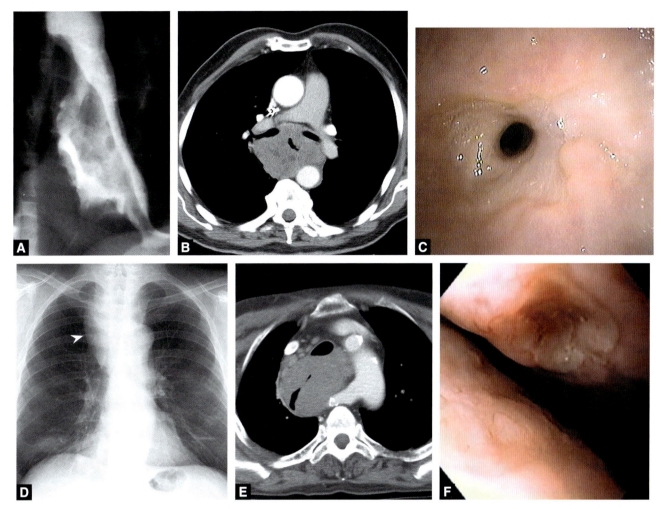

FIGURE 1.4.3 **Primary esophageal lymphoma.** Barium esophagram (**A**) shows a large ulcerated mass that grossly distorts the esophageal lumen. CT (**B**) from a second patient shows marked circumferential soft tissue thickening of the mid-esophagus, with luminal narrowing at EGD (**C**). Frontal chest radiograph (**D**) from a third patient shows smooth fullness of the mediastinum (*arrowhead*), which on CT (**E**) is shown to be due to massive soft tissue enlargement of the esophagus. The esophageal lumen is stretched and distorted but not obstructed. Note also multiple sub-centimeter mediastinal lymph nodes and aberrant right subclavian artery. EGD image (**F**) shows mucosal ulceration and luminal distortion.

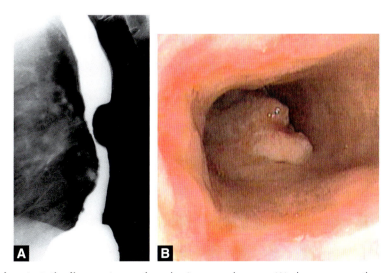

FIGURE 1.4.4 **Esophageal metastatic disease.** Image from barium esophagram (**A**) shows a smooth, rounded filling defect from submucosal metastasis from cervical cancer. EGD image (**B**) from a patient with bronchogenic carcinoma shows an irregular submucosal metastasis.

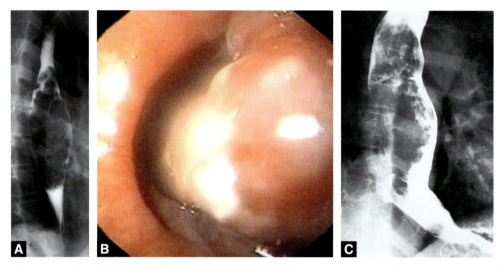

FIGURE 1.4.5 Rare primary esophageal malignancies. Barium esophagram (**A**) from a patient with primary spindle cell carcinoma (carcinosarcoma) shows a large intraluminal mass that causes fusiform dilatation of the esophagus. EGD image (**B**) from a patient with esophageal small cell carcinoma shows a large mass occupying the esophageal lumen. Barium esophagram (**C**) from a patient with primary esophageal melanoma shows a large irregular filling defect that expands the esophagus.

1.5 Non-neoplastic Lesions
(Figures 1.5.1-1.5.4)

CLINICAL FEATURES

- Glycogenic acanthosis is a common benign condition characterized by cytoplasmic glycogen accumulation within the squamous epithelium; prevalence increases with age.
- Esophageal hamartomas are rare; even with Cowden's disease, esophageal lesions are usually due to severe glycogenic acanthosis.
- Ectopic gastric mucosa in the cervical esophagus (so-called "inlet patch") is generally an incidental finding not related to GERD or Barrett's metaplasia.
- Inflammatory fibroid polyps are a non-neoplastic sequela of GERD.

IMAGING FEATURES

- On the double-contrast esophagram, glycogenic acanthosis manifests as multiple small (usually <5 mm) subtle rounded lesions; at endoscopy, the lesions appear as white mucosal nodules.
- Esophageal involvement in Cowden's disease is characterized by severe glycogenic acanthosis.
- On endoscopy, inlet patches manifest as well-circumscribed foci of salmon-colored mucosa in the upper esophagus; a subtle depression can sometimes be seen on barium examination.
- Inflammatory fibroid polyps are generally located at or near the gastroesophageal junction in patients with GERD; "inflammatory esophagogastric folds" are a closely related condition (see section 2.1).

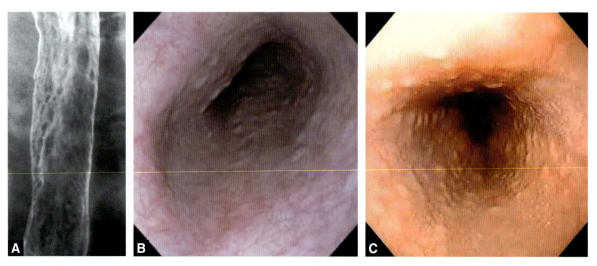

FIGURE 1.5.1 Glycogenic acanthosis. Double-contrast barium esophagram (**A**) and EGD images (**B** and **C**) from three different patients show multiple tiny polypoid lesions.

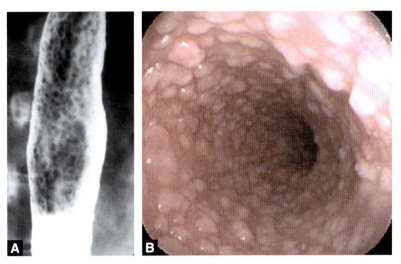

FIGURE 1.5.2 **Severe glycogenic acanthosis in Cowden's disease.** Barium esophagram (**A**) and EGD image (**B**) from two different patients with Cowden's disease show innumerable uniform polypoid lesions carpeting the esophagus, which should not be mistaken for hamartomatous polyps.

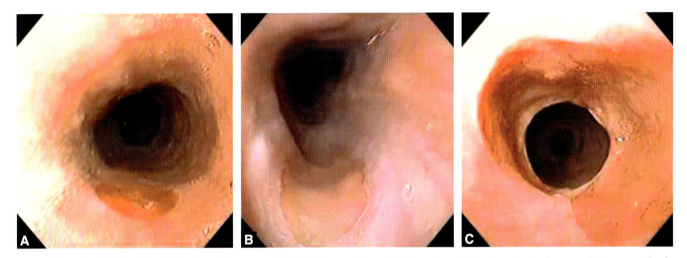

FIGURE 1.5.3 **Inlet patch (ectopic gastric mucosa).** EGD images (**A** and **B**) from two different patients show well-circumscribed foci of salmon-colored mucosa involving the proximal esophagus. EGD image from a third patient (**C**) with dysphagia shows a peptic stricture 3 cm distal to the upper esophageal sphincter caused by acid secretion from an adjacent circumferential inlet patch. This is a rare but well-documented complication of this entity.

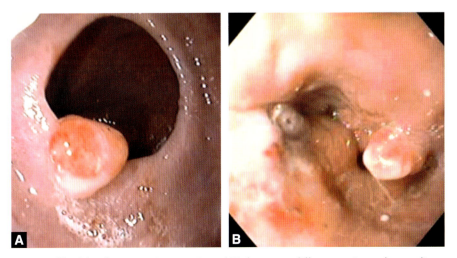

FIGURE 1.5.4 **Inflammatory fibroid polyp.** EGD images (**A** and **B**) from two different patients show solitary erythematous polyps located just proximal to the gastroesophageal junction. In **A** the polyp is situated on a Schatzki's ring.

2. GASTROESOPHAGEAL REFLUX DISEASE (GERD)

Gastroesophageal reflux disease (GERD) is a very common condition, but prevalence estimates vary widely depending on the reference standard and how the disease is defined. The significance of gastroesophageal reflux depends on a variety of factors, such as the frequency, rate of clearance, contents of refluxate, and mucosal resistance. Noted complications of untreated GERD include reflux esophagitis, peptic stricture, Barrett's esophagus, and adenocarcinoma.

2.1 Reflux Esophagitis
(Figures 2.1.1-2.1.5)

CLINICAL FEATURES

- Typical GERD symptoms include heartburn (pyrosis), regurgitation, and dysphagia; more atypical symptoms include laryngitis, asthma, cough, chest pain, and odynophagia.
- Development of reflux esophagitis is multifactorial and relates to frequency and duration of reflux, acid content of the refluxate, and the intrinsic mucosal resistance; degree of mucosal injury is difficult to predict.
- Hiatal hernia likely has a permissive role in the development of reflux esophagitis, but its mere presence is a poor predictor.
- A subset of symptomatic patients will have nonerosive GERD.
- Predisposing conditions include scleroderma, Zollinger-Ellison syndrome, and pregnancy.
- Initial treatment targets symptom relief and can include lifestyle modifications and acid suppressive medication; antireflux surgery (e.g., fundoplication) can be considered in cases where medical therapy fails.

IMAGING FEATURES

- Spontaneous GERD can be identified by fluoroscopy, scintigraphy, and pH monitoring, but its presence is neither sensitive nor specific for clinically significant GERD or reflux esophagitis.
- Barium findings of reflux esophagitis include abnormal motility at fluoroscopy, mucosal irregularity, fold thickening, transient transverse folds, and ulceration; an associated hiatal hernia is a common finding.
- Endoscopic findings include erythema, friability, exudates, erosions, and ulcers; however, a significant number of patients with symptomatic reflux have endoscopically normal-appearing esophageal mucosa.
- Endoscopic classification systems have been developed for more objective assessment (e.g., the modified Los Angeles classification).
- Barium examination can evaluate for complications of stricture or adenocarcinoma but, unlike endoscopy, is insensitive to Barrett's metaplasia; endoscopy also allows for mucosal biopsy.
- Inflammatory esophagogastric polyps or folds have a characteristic appearance and represent a benign finding at imaging.
- Fluoroscopic examination can be useful after fundoplication to assess the status of the wrap.

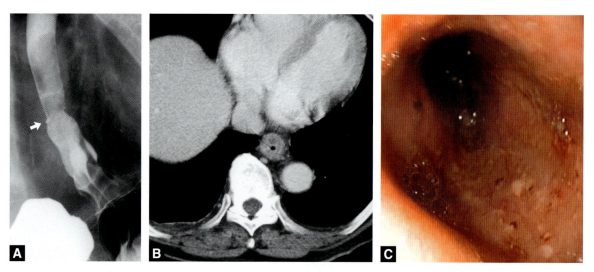

FIGURE 2.1.1 Gastroesophageal reflux disease (GERD). Barium esophagram **(A)** shows a small focal ulceration (*arrow*) associated with a small sliding hiatal hernia. Spontaneous reflux was seen during real-time examination. Contrast-enhanced CT image **(B)** shows circumferential inflammatory esophageal wall thickening related to reflux esophagitis. EGD image **(C)** shows diffuse mucosal inflammation with multiple small erosions involving the distal esophagus.

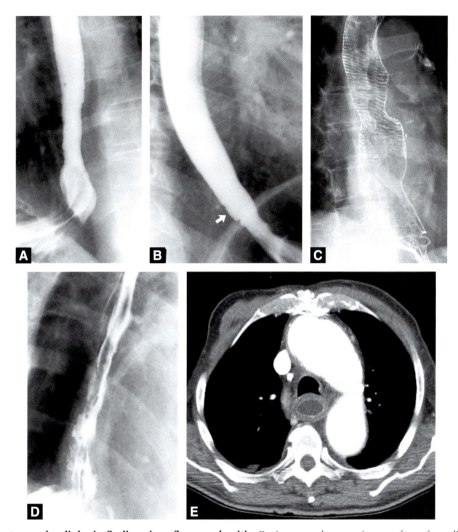

FIGURE 2.1.2 **Spectrum of radiologic findings in reflux esophagitis.** Barium esophagram images from four different patients show mucosal irregularity from erosive esophagitis (**A**), focal shallow ulceration (**B**, *arrow*), transient transverse esophageal folds (**C**), and diffuse irregular fold thickening from severe inflammation (**D**). A small sliding hiatal hernia is present in **A**. The transient, closely spaced transverse folds in **C** should not be confused with the fixed rings seen in eosinophilic esophagitis. CT image (**E**) from a different patient shows marked circumferential esophageal wall thickening in a patient with profound inflammation from reflux.

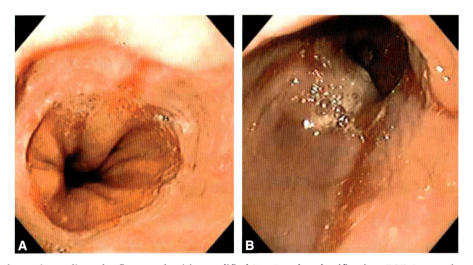

FIGURE 2.1.3 **Endoscopic grading of reflux esophagitis: modified Los Angeles classification.** EGD images from four different patients show examples of the different grades of reflux esophagitis. Grade A (**A**) is classified as one or more mucosal breaks <5 mm and not extending between two folds. Grade B (**B**) is classified as one or more mucosal breaks >5 mm and not extending between two folds.

Illustration continued on following page

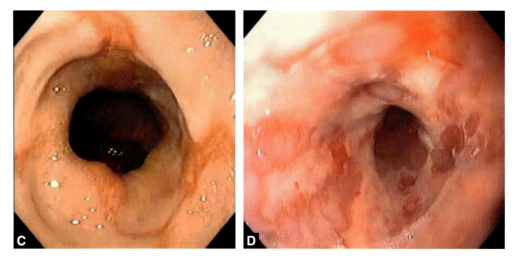

FIGURE 2.1.3 (Continued)   **Endoscopic grading of reflux esophagitis: modified Los Angeles classification.** Grade C **(C)** is classified as one or more mucosal breaks continuous between the tops of two or more mucosal folds, but with involvement of <75% of the esophageal circumference. Grade D **(D)** is classified as one or more mucosal breaks involving >75% of the circumference.

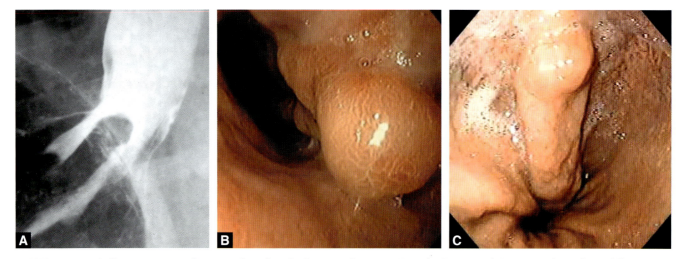

FIGURE 2.1.4   **Inflammatory esophagogastric polyp.** Barium esophagram **(A)** and EGD **(B and C)** images from three different patients show a thickened polypoid fold extending from the gastric cardia into the distal esophagus.

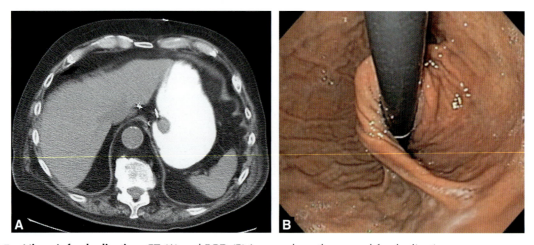

FIGURE 2.1.5   **Nissen's fundoplication.** CT **(A)** and EGD **(B)** images show the normal fundoplication appearance.

Illustration continued on following page

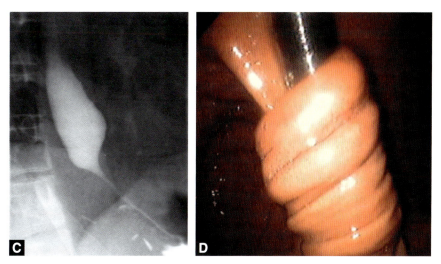

FIGURE 2.1.5 (Continued)   Nissen's fundoplication. Barium esophagram (C) in a patient with dysphagia shows a long segment of narrowing resulting from an excessively tight wrap. EGD image (D) taken in retroflexion from another symptomatic patient shows the endoscope traversing a tight fundoplication wrap.

2.2 Peptic Strictures
(Figures 2.2.1-2.2.3)

CLINICAL FEATURES

- The prevalence of peptic strictures in patients with reflux esophagitis is about 10% to 25%.
- Endoscopic dilatation is effective but repeat dilatation may be necessary in 50% or more of cases.
- Many investigators believe that Schatzki's rings (symptomatic lower esophageal rings) are caused by reflux.

IMAGING FEATURES

- The vast majority of peptic strictures involve the distal esophagus above a hiatal hernia.

- Barium esophagography is very sensitive for detection; smooth concentric tapering is classic but asymmetry from eccentric scarring is also relatively common.
- Endoscopy is generally indicated to exclude more significant pathology and to effect treatment.
- Long-segment strictures are more common in the setting of Zollinger-Ellison syndrome and intramural pseudodiverticulosis (see section 5.7); peptic strictures are also a common complication of scleroderma.
- Findings of reflux esophagitis may accompany a Schatzki's ring.

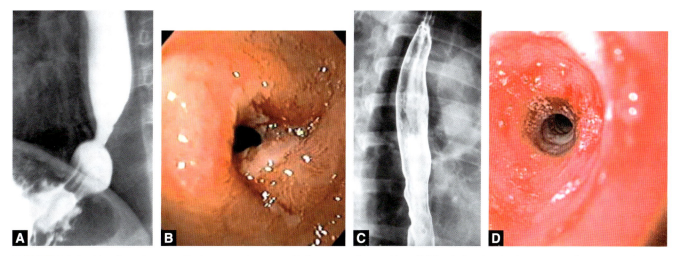

FIGURE 2.2.1   Peptic strictures. Barium esophagram (A) from a patient with solid-food dysphagia shows smooth segmental narrowing of the distal esophagus above a small hiatal hernia. EGD image (B) from a different patient shows a similar distal peptic stricture. Barium esophagram (C) from a third patient shows fixed eccentric narrowing of the mid-distal esophagus. EGD image (D) from a fourth patient shows a long-segment stenosis from chronic reflux esophagitis.

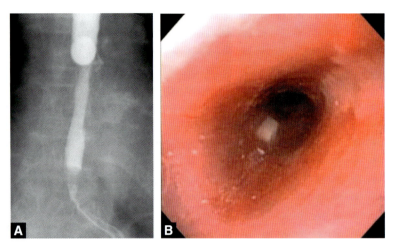

FIGURE 2.2.2 **Long-segment peptic stricture in Zollinger-Ellison syndrome.** Barium esophagram (A) shows a barium tablet lodged above a long-segment stricture that extends to the gastroesophageal junction. EGD image (B) re-demonstrates the stricture.

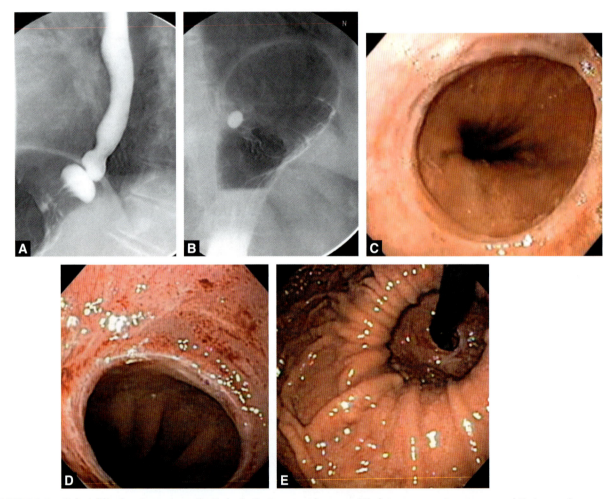

FIGURE 2.2.3 **Schatzki's ring (symptomatic B ring).** Barium esophagram (A) shows a prominent mucosal B ring at the gastroesophageal junction above a small hiatal hernia. Passage of a barium tablet (B) was held up at this level, which reproduced the patient's dysphagia complaints. EGD image (C) from a second patient shows the typical endoscopic appearance of a Schatzki's ring as a fibrous band at the gastroesophageal junction. Note the small hiatal hernia just distal to the ring. EGD images from a third patient taken above (D) and below (E) a Schatzki's ring show associated mucosal inflammation from reflux esophagitis and a sliding hiatal hernia.

2.3 Barrett's Esophagus
(Figures 2.3.1-2.3.2)

CLINICAL FEATURES

- Barrett's esophagus is a condition of progressive columnar metaplasia related to long-standing GERD.
- It is considered a premalignant condition due to a greatly increased risk for adenocarcinoma.
- Long-segment Barrett's esophagus (>3 cm) has a higher risk of developing adenocarcinoma.
- Of patients with high-grade dysplasia in Barrett's esophagus, 10% to 30% may develop adenocarcinoma within 5 years.
- Surveillance and management strategies are controversial because many patients are asymptomatic and most cases will not progress to cancer; management centers on treating GERD and surveillance for cancer.
- Strong male and Caucasian prevalence (approximately 10:1 for each); obesity is also a risk factor.

IMAGING FEATURES

- Generally, there are no direct radiographic findings, although a reticular mucosal pattern is rarely appreciated.
- At endoscopy, salmon-colored mucosa extends proximally from the gastroesophageal junction, which can appear circumferential, tongue-like, or as islands standing out against the normal, whitish squamous epithelium.
- Definitive diagnosis requires biopsy; surveillance strategy depends on the presence of dysplasia.
- Barrett's esophagus is suggested at barium evaluation in the setting of a high (mid-esophageal) stricture or ulcer.
- The presence of a mass lesion generally signifies adenocarcinoma.

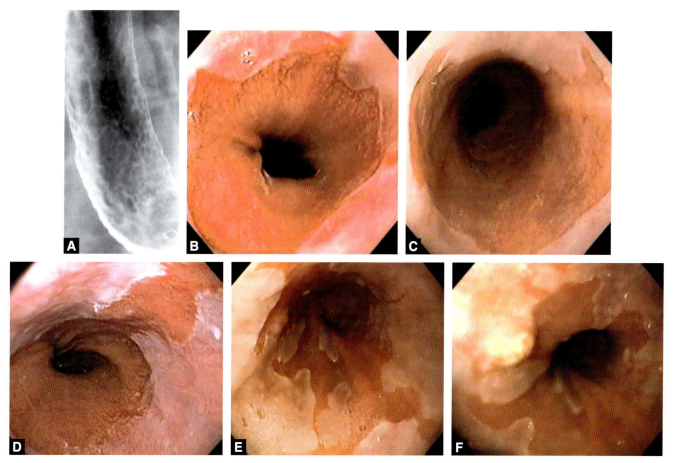

FIGURE 2.3.1 Barrett's esophagus. Double-contrast barium esophagram (**A**) in a patient with Barrett's metaplasia shows a reticular mucosal pattern, which can be demonstrated in only a small minority of cases. EGD images (**B to F**) show a spectrum of endoscopic findings in Barrett's esophagus, including an irregular Z line (**B**), long-segment Barrett's extending 5 cm proximal from the gastroesophageal junction (**C**), predominantly short-segment involvement with a tongue of metaplasia extending along one side (**D**), and Barrett's metaplasia surrounding multiple squamous islands (**E**). The nodule seen at the 9 o'clock position in **E** is shown to have grown one year later (**F**) and represented a focus of high-grade dysplasia.

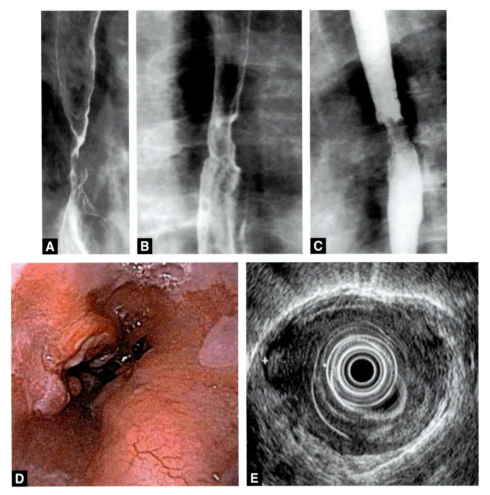

FIGURE 2.3.2 Barrett's esophagus complicated by stricture and adenocarcinoma. Barium esophagram (**A**) shows an irregular but benign stricture in the setting of long-segment Barrett's esophagus. A subtle reticular appearance in the mucosa above the stricture is suggested. Double- (**B**) and single- (**C**) contrast images from barium esophagography in a different patient with long-segment Barrett's esophagus shows irregular narrowing with shouldering in the mid-esophagus from adenocarcinoma. EGD image (**D**) from a third patient shows an irregular mucosal mass from adenocarcinoma in the setting of Barrett's metaplasia. Corresponding EUS image (**E**) shows a hypoechoic lesion extending through the muscularis propria and into the tunica adventitia consistent with a T3 lesion.

3. ESOPHAGITIS (NON-GERD)

Most esophageal infections are opportunistic, predominantly affecting patients with varying degrees of immunodeficiency. Noninfectious causes of esophagitis include recognizable insults, such as GERD (covered in the previous section), radiation, and certain ingested substances, as well as idiopathic conditions such as Crohn's disease, eosinophilic esophagitis, and certain dermatologic disorders.

3.1 Infectious Esophagitis
(Figures 3.1.1-3.1.5)

CLINICAL FEATURES

- Distinguishing fungal from viral infection on clinical grounds can be difficult.
- Candidiasis (usually *C. albicans*) is the most common cause of infectious esophagitis; dysphagia, odynophagia, and oral thrush are typical features.
- Although herpes simplex virus (HSV) esophagitis most often affects immunocompromised patients, it is somewhat unique in that it can also affect immunocompetent individuals; severe odynophagia is common.
- Cytomegalovirus (CMV) esophagitis is generally seen only in immunocompromised patients.
- HIV infection itself has been associated with esophageal ulceration in patients with AIDS.
- Esophageal involvement by tuberculosis is almost always due to extension of mediastinal disease.

IMAGING FEATURES

- Candidiasis usually manifests on the double-contrast barium esophagram as multiple plaque-like lesions, often with a longitudinal orientation; with severe disease, a "shaggy" appearance is typical.
- At endoscopy, candidiasis appears as white or yellow plaques; erythematous, friable mucosa can be seen when lesions are lifted off.
- HSV esophagitis typically appears as multiple, small, superficial ulcers on double-contrast esophagram.

- At endoscopy, the earliest finding of HSV esophagitis is small vesicles, which rupture to form discrete ulcers; the endoscopic appearance of more advanced disease overlaps with that of candidiasis.
- At imaging, CMV esophagitis may begin as superficial erosions similar to HSV but often progresses to large shallow or deep ulcers; endoscopic biopsy is necessary to confirm the diagnosis.
- HIV-associated idiopathic ulcers most often manifest as large lesions that mimic CMV ulcers.
- Imaging features of tuberculous esophagitis include strictures, sinus tracts, and fistulas.

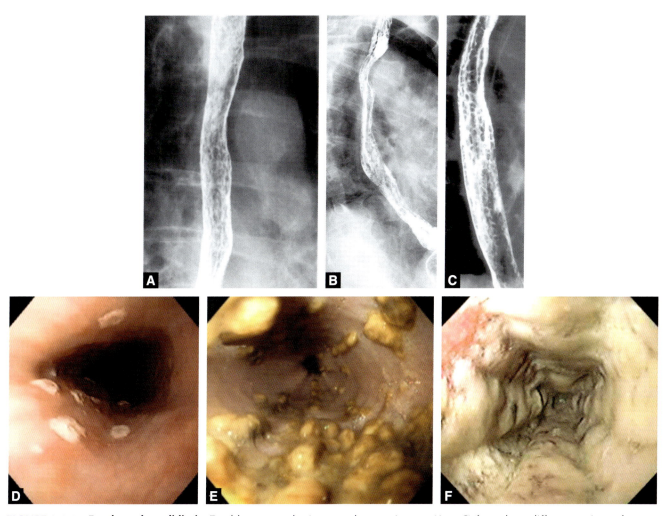

FIGURE 3.1.1 Esophageal candidiasis. Double-contrast barium esophagram images **(A to C)** from three different patients show innumerable plaque-like filling defects carpeting the esophageal mucosa. EGD images **(D to F)** from three patients with candidiasis of increasing severity show the characteristic white or yellow plaques, which have a roughly longitudinal orientation in **E** and largely coalesce in **F**.

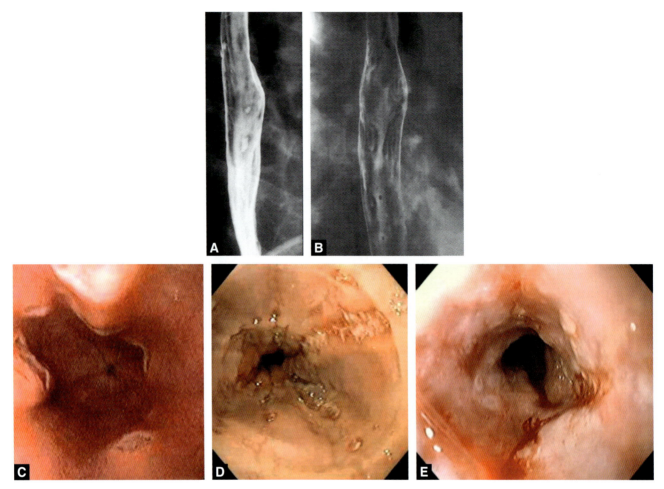

FIGURE 3.1.2 **HSV esophagitis.** Barium esophagram images (**A** and **B**) from two patients show multiple shallow barium-coated ulcers with a thin surrounding halo of edema. EGD images (**C** and **D**) from two patients with HSV esophagitis of increasing severity show the characteristic punched-out "volcano lesions" (**C**) or stellate ulcers (**D**) with variable mounds of edema. EGD image (**E**) from a final patient shows circumferential inflammation.

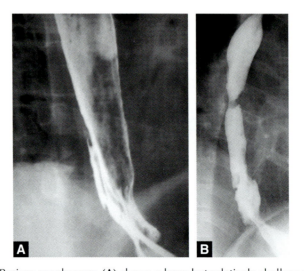

FIGURE 3.1.3 **CMV esophagitis.** Barium esophagram (**A**) shows a large but relatively shallow ulcer in profile involving the distal esophagus. Barium esophagram (**B**) from a different patient shows an even larger and more irregular CMV ulcer involving the entire mid-distal esophagus.

Illustration continued on following page

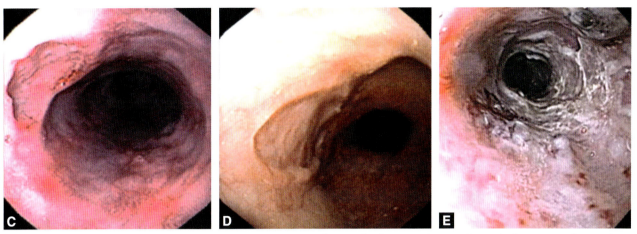

FIGURE 3.1.3 (Continued) **CMV esophagitis.** EGD image **(C)** from a third patient shows a large shallow CMV ulcer with irregular borders. Follow-up EGD image after treatment **(D)** shows healing with residual deformity. EGD image **(E)** from a final patient with CMV esophagitis shows circumferential mucosal ulceration.

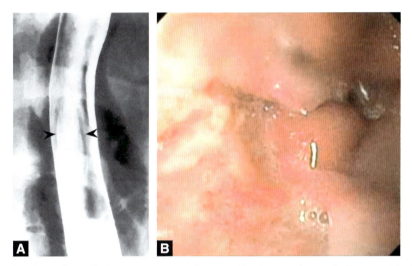

FIGURE 3.1.4 **HIV-associated esophageal ulcer.** Barium esophagram **(A)** shows a large, shallow ovoid ulcer (*arrowheads*) from HIV that resembles the appearance of CMV. EGD image **(B)** from a different patient shows mucosal ulceration related to HIV. Multiple biopsies and serologic studies revealed no evidence of CMV or HSV.

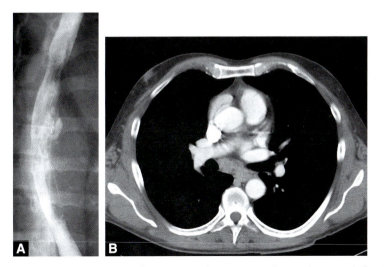

FIGURE 3.1.5 **Esophageal tuberculosis.** Barium esophagram **(A)** shows mucosal irregularity with focal ulceration in the midesophagus from tuberculosis. Contrast-enhanced CT image **(B)** from a different patient with tuberculosis shows mediastinal lymphadenopathy. The small focus of lower attenuation may represent caseous necrosis.

Illustration continued on following page

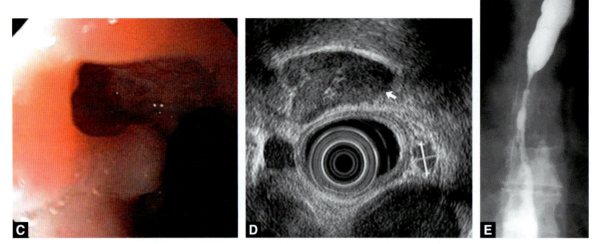

FIGURE 3.1.5 (Continued)   Esophageal tuberculosis. EGD image (C) shows a deep ulceration located in the mid-esophagus. Corresponding EUS image (D) obtained from just proximal to the ulcer reveals a large hypoechoic, heterogeneous subcarinal lymph node (*arrow*). A smaller abnormal-appearing lymph node is also present (*calipers*). Barium esophagram (E) from a third patient shows a long-segment tubercular stricture involving the mid-esophagus.

3.2 Drug-Induced, Caustic, and Radiation Injury

(Figures 3.2.1.-3.2.5)

CLINICAL FEATURES

- Doxycycline is the most common cause of pill esophagitis; other causes include bisphosphonates, potassium chloride, quinidine, NSAIDs, and ascorbic acid.
- Bisphosphonates (e.g., alendronate), used for osteoporosis, can result in severe ulcerative esophagitis
- Ingestion of lye (concentrated sodium hydroxide) is the most common cause of severe caustic esophagitis in the United States.
- Phases of caustic injury include acute necrosis (1-4 days), subacute ulceration and granulation (3-5 days), and chronic stricture formation (1-3 months).
- Photodynamic therapy for superficial esophageal neoplasia represents an iatrogenic form of caustic esophagitis.
- Acute, self-limited radiation esophagitis is common and usually does not require imaging evaluation.
- Chronic radiation strictures typically develop months after cessation of therapy.

IMAGING FEATURES

- Ulceration from the tetracycline antibiotics and certain other medications are typically shallow; single or multiple ulcers are classically clustered at the level of the aortic arch or left main bronchus.
- Esophagitis associated with the bisphosphonates, sodium chloride, and quinidine often manifests as more severe ulcerative disease; stricture formation may ensue.
- If caustic ingestion is suspected in the acute or subacute phase, endoscopy is warranted (in the absence of perforation and mediastinitis); delayed endoscopy can evaluate for stricture formation.
- Barium esophagography is more useful in the chronic phase for assessing the degree and extent of caustic strictures.
- Erosions usually develop about two weeks after commencement of radiation therapy.
- Radiation strictures can be documented at barium evaluation or endoscopy; fistula formation with the airway (most often left main bronchus) can de detected at fluoroscopy, CT, or endoscopy.

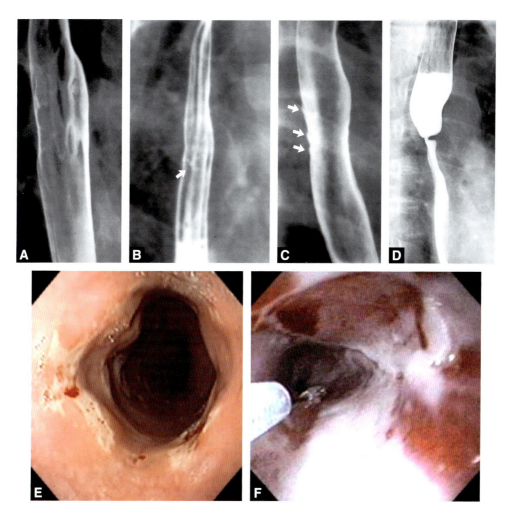

FIGURE 3.2.1 Drug-induced injury. Barium esophagram images from three patients with pill esophagitis show multiple ulcers from tetracycline (**A**), a single stellate ulcer from doxycycline (**B,** *arrow*), and small, subtle ulcers from ascorbic acid (**C,** *arrows*). Barium esophagram (**D**) from a different patient shows a short-segment diaphragm-like stricture related to chronic NSAID use (aspirin). EGD image (**E**) shows shallow stellate ulcers from doxycycline. EGD image (**F**) from a sixth patient shows severe ulcerative esophagitis related to alendronate.

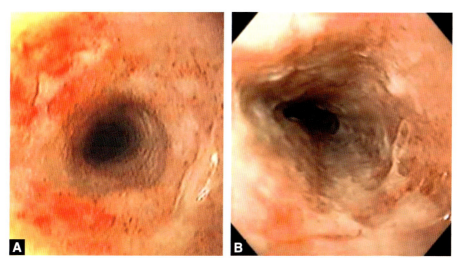

FIGURE 3.2.2 Caustic injury (alkali agents). EGD images from two patients show caustic esophagitis related to sodium hydroxide (**A**) and sodium hypochlorite (**B**) ingestion.

Illustration continued on following page

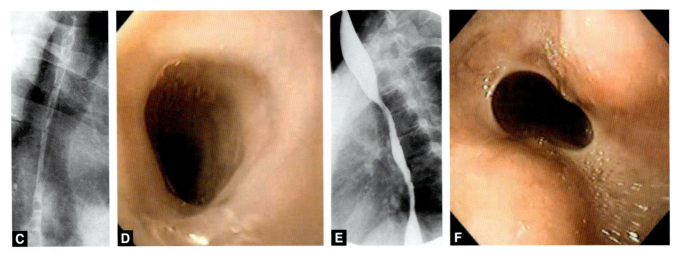

FIGURE 3.2.2 (Continued) **Caustic injury (alkali agents).** Barium esophagram **(C)** and EGD **(D)** images from two different patients show diffuse luminal narrowing related to lye (sodium hydroxide) strictures. Barium esophagram **(E)** from another patient with previous lye ingestion shows a long-segment stricture with mild dilation of the proximal esophagus. Corresponding EGD image **(F)** from above the stricture demonstrates the scarred mucosa from the previous chemical insult.

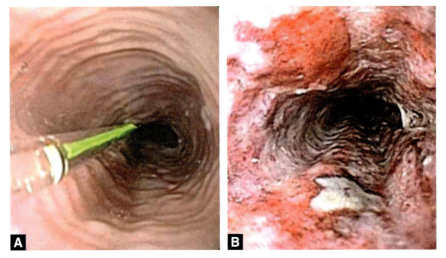

FIGURE 3.2.3 **Injury from photodynamic therapy.** EGD images during **(A)** and two days after **(B)** photodynamic therapy for T1 squamous cell carcinoma show the caustic effect of this therapy, which resulted in severe ulcerative esophagitis.

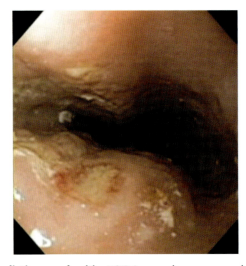

FIGURE 3.2.4 **Acute radiation esophagitis.** EGD image shows mucosal ulcerations related to ongoing radiation therapy.

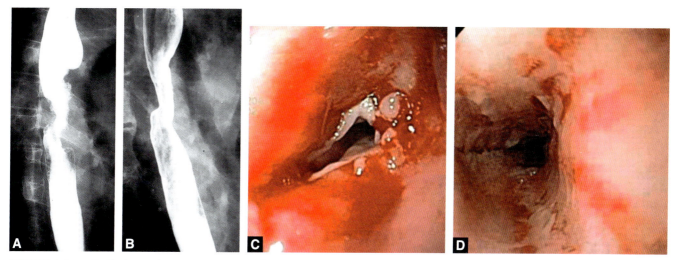

FIGURE 3.2.5 Radiation strictures. Barium esophagram **(A)** shows marked radiation esophagitis with irregular luminal narrowing and ulceration. Follow-up barium esophagram **(B)** shows healing with a smooth stricture. EGD image **(C)** from a different patient shows a tight radiation stricture. Note friability of the fibrous tissue related to the stricture. EGD image **(D)** from a third patient shows another radiation-induced stricture in the mid-esophagus that is approximately 5 cm in length.

3.3 Other Esophagitides
(Figures 3.3.1-3.3.4)

CLINICAL FEATURES

- The esophagus is the least common GI site for involvement by Crohn's disease; preexisting or concurrent bowel disease is almost always present.
- Eosinophilic esophagitis usually presents with solid-food dysphagia in a young patient; a history of concurrent atopy may also be present.
- Dermatologic conditions that can affect the esophagus include epidermolysis bullosa (the dystrophica form), pemphigoid (the benign mucous membrane form), and pemphigus.

IMAGING FEATURES

- Esophageal Crohn's disease can result in the same spectrum of imaging features seen with bowel involvement, including aphthoid ulcers, thickened folds, deeper ulcers, fistulas, and strictures.
- Eosinophic esophagitis can manifest with upper to mid-esophageal strictures and a rigid ringed appearance on barium evaluation.
- Suggestive endoscopic features of eosinophilic esophagitis include a narrowed luminal caliber, mucosal fragility, ringed appearance, and white exudate; biopsy will reveal mucosal eosinophilia.
- Epidermolysis bullosa and pemphigoid often result in cervical esophageal webs or strictures, which can be demonstrated on barium examination; endoscopy should generally be avoided in this setting.

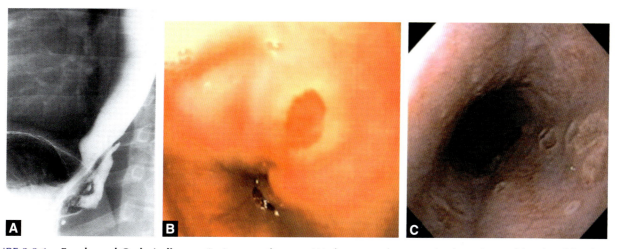

FIGURE 3.3.1 Esophageal Crohn's disease. Barium esophagram **(A)** shows esophagogastric ulceration and localized fistula formation. EGD image **(B)** from a different patient shows an aphthoid ulcer in the distal esophagus representing early Crohn's involvement. EGD image **(C)** from a third patient shows multiple well-defined mucosal ulcerations in a patient with known ileal Crohn's disease.

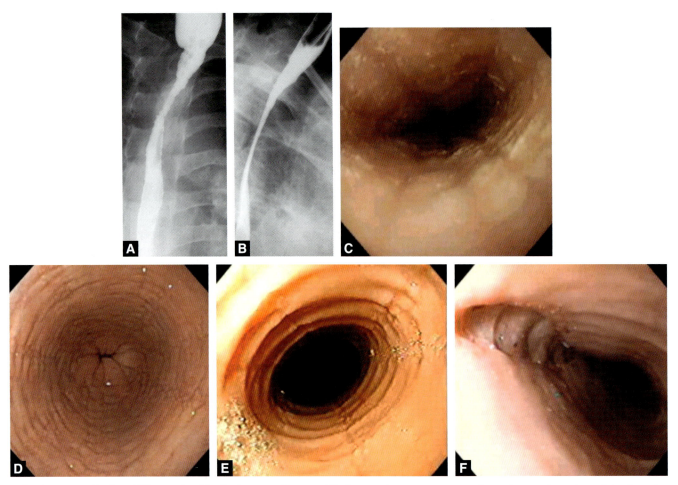

FIGURE 3.3.2 **Eosinophilic esophagitis.** Barium esophagram (**A**) shows a long-segment esophageal stenosis and a subtle ringed appearance, which is generally more conspicuous at endoscopy. Barium esophagram (**B**) from a different patient shows severe esophageal stenosis without a ringed appearance. EGD image (**C**) from a third patient shows mild granularity of the mucosa associated with pinpoint whitish exudates. EGD image (**D**) from a different patient shows the linear furrowing pattern that is sometimes seen. EGD image (**E**) from a final patient shows the characteristic fixed-ring appearance, associated with luminal narrowing. EGD image (**F**) after dilatation shows a large iatrogenic mucosal rent, which is a relatively common complication due to mucosal fragility.

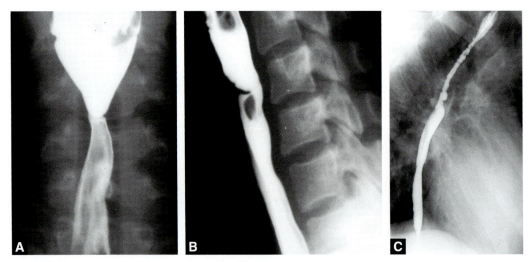

FIGURE 3.3.3 **Epidermolysis bullosa.** Frontal (**A**) and lateral (**B**) projections from a barium esophagram study show a cervical esophageal web with proximal dilatation. Barium esophagram (**C**) from a different patient shows long-segment esophageal stenosis punctuated by multiple focal strictures.

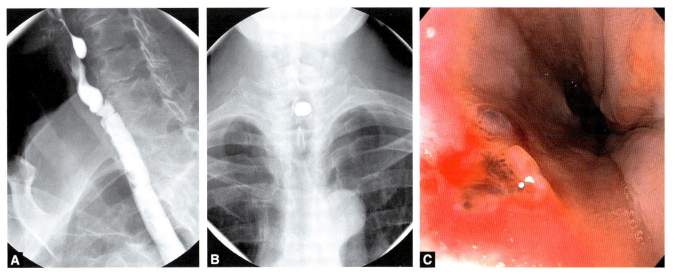

FIGURE 3.3.4 Pemphigoid and pemphigus. Barium esophagram (**A**) from a patient with long-standing pemphigoid shows two discrete, web-like strictures involving the cervical esophagus. The remainder of the esophagus was normal. Passage of a barium tablet was impeded at this level (**B**), which reproduced the patient's dysphagia. EGD image (**C**) from a patient with bullous pemphigus and hematemesis shows a small circular erosion with oozing and a small adjacent bulla.

4. ESOPHAGEAL DYSMOTILITY DISORDERS

This section covers the primary motility disorders of achalasia and diffuse esophageal spasm, as well as scleroderma, an important secondary cause of esophageal dysmotility. Both fluoroscopic and endoscopic evaluation play useful roles in evaluating motor disorders of the esophagus.

4.1 Achalasia
(Figures 4.1.1-4.1.5)

CLINICAL FEATURES

- Achalasia is characterized by incomplete relaxation of the lower esophageal sphincter (LES) that results in functional obstruction, which is further compounded by aperistalsis of the esophageal body.
- The cause of disease remains uncertain, but ganglion cells in the LES region are decreased.
- Common presenting symptoms include dysphagia, regurgitation, chest discomfort, and weight loss.
- Fluoroscopic barium examination is a useful first test to screen for possible achalasia.
- It is important to exclude potential causes of secondary achalasia (pseudoachalasia), particularly tumors.
- Infection caused by the protozoan *Trypanosoma cruzi* (Chagas' disease) can result in esophageal findings that are identical to primary achalasia.
- Long-standing achalasia is associated with an increased risk of squamous cell carcinoma; chronic mucosal inflammation from stasis of esophageal contents may be the precipitating factor.
- Treatment options to relieve LES pressure include pneumatic dilatation, esophagomyotomy, and injection of botulinum toxin.

IMAGING FEATURES

- At barium fluoroscopy, primary peristalsis is absent and the esophagus ends in a tapered, beak-like manner.
- Intermittent LES opening confirms functional nature and excludes stricture; exposure to amyl nitrate relaxes the LES.
- At endoscopy, the LES often appears puckered but the scope can easily pass into the stomach.
- Esophageal dilatation and retained luminal food or fluid are common features as the disease progresses.
- Classic manometric findings consist of absent primary peristalsis, elevated resting LES pressures, and incomplete or absent LES relaxation.
- The imaging appearance of Chagas' disease is similar to that of primary achalasia.

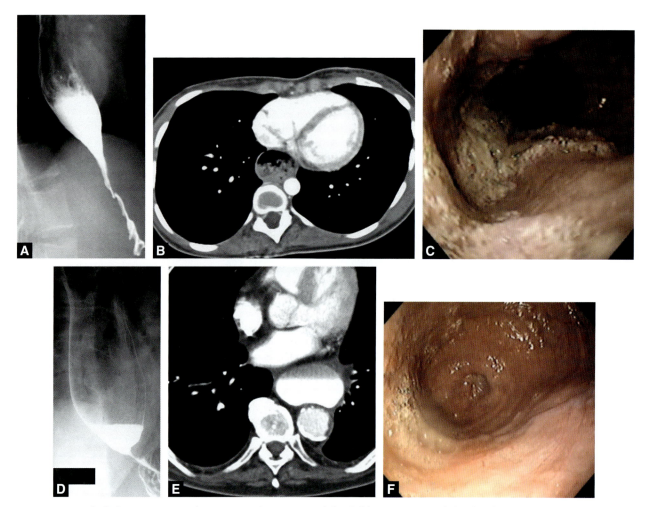

FIGURE 4.1.1 Achalasia. Barium esophagram (**A**) shows tapered, beak-like narrowing of the distal esophagus. CT (**B**) and EGD (**C**) images show luminal debris and mild dilatation. Barium esophagram (**D**) from a different patient shows beak-like narrowing of the LES with more advanced luminal dilatation. CT (**E**) and EGD (**F**) images show the dilated esophageal lumen, as well as a puckered appearance of the LES at endoscopy.

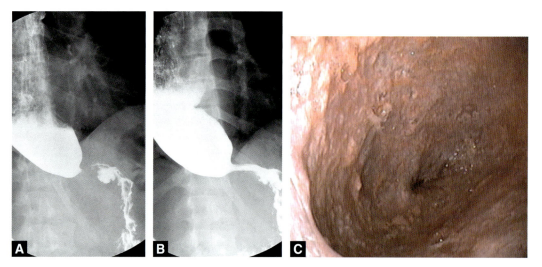

FIGURE 4.1.2 Achalasia: effect of amyl nitrate. Barium esophagram (**A**) before exposure to amyl nitrate shows characteristic findings of long-standing achalasia, including a dilated, debris-filled lumen and tight LES. Image obtained immediately after exposure to amyl nitrate (**B**) shows LES relaxation with passage of barium into the stomach. EGD image (**C**) shows tonic LES contraction, dilated esophageal lumen, and mucosal irregularity. Esophagitis caused by irritation from static luminal contents is a common finding at endoscopy.

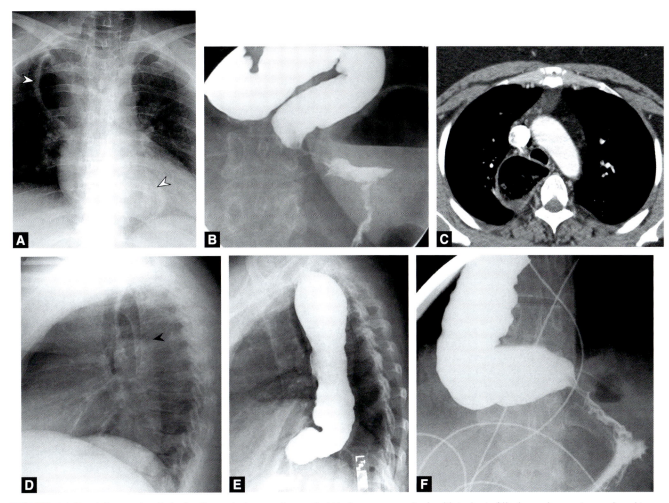

FIGURE 4.1.3 Advanced achalasia. Frontal chest radiograph (**A**) shows a massively dilated, air-filled esophagus (*arrowheads*). Barium esophagram (**B**) shows marked esophageal dilatation and tortuosity, associated with functional LES narrowing. CT image (**C**) from a different patient shows a similar configuration to the dilated and tortuous esophagus. Note the residual luminal debris. Lateral chest radiograph (**D**) shows tubular soft-tissue fullness along the mediastinum, with an air-fluid level (*arrowhead*). Subsequent images from barium esophagram (**E** and **F**) show massive esophageal dilatation with beak-like narrowing at the LES.

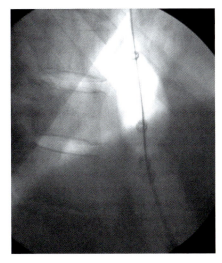

FIGURE 4.1.4 Pneumatic dilatation in achalasia. Fluoroscopic image from a 3-cm pneumatic balloon dilatation shows waist-like narrowing at the LES. The balloon is inflated until the waist is obliterated. Due to an approximately 3% iatrogenic perforation rate, a post-dilation barium esophagram is recommended.

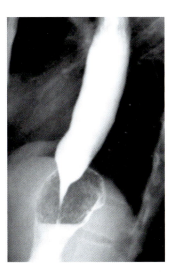

FIGURE 4.1.5 Chagas' disease. Barium esophagram shows moderate esophageal dilatation with distal beak-like narrowing. The imaging appearance is indistinguishable from primary achalasia.

4.2 Diffuse Esophageal Spasm

(Figure 4.2.1)

CLINICAL FEATURES

- Diffuse esophageal spasm is characterized by repetitive, nonpropulsive, simultaneous smooth muscle contractions, associated with retrosternal chest pain and often dysphagia.
- It is part of a spectrum of spastic disorders of unknown etiology.
- The LES usually functions normally, and swallowing is not affected.

IMAGING FEATURES

- At fluoroscopy, simultaneous nonperistaltic contractions involve the smooth muscle portion of the esophagus; trapping of barium between contractions can have a "corkscrew" or "rosary bead" appearance.
- There is no anatomic correlate for spastic disorders of the esophagus at endoscopy.
- The manometric features mirror the esophagram findings; simultaneous waves are seen on more than 30% of wet swallows; normal peristaltic waves are seen intermittently.

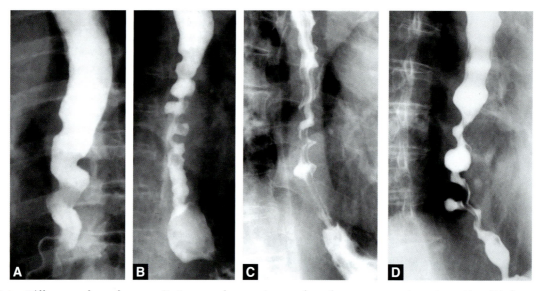

FIGURE 4.2.1 Diffuse esophageal spasm. Barium esophagram images from four symptomatic patients (**A** to **D**) show varying degrees of diffuse nonperistaltic tertiary contractions, which give rise to "corkscrew" or "rosary bead" appearance.

4.3 Scleroderma (Progressive Systemic Sclerosis)

(Figure 4.3.1)

CLINICAL FEATURES

- Scleroderma is a systemic connective tissue disease characterized by smooth muscle fibrosis and atrophy.
- The esophagus is involved in the vast majority of cases.
- Smooth muscle atrophy and fibrosis result in decreased or absent peristalsis in the distal two thirds of the esophagus and a patulous, incompetent LES, which predisposes to prominent gastroesophageal reflux.

IMAGING FEATURES

- Barium esophagram findings include a combination of dysmotility, dilatation, reflux esophagitis, and peptic strictures; rarely, wide-mouth diverticula or sacculations from asymmetrical fibrosis are seen.
- At endoscopy, the dilated atonic appearance can simulate achalasia, but any distal narrowing is fixed (peptic stricture) and not functional.
- At CT, the combination of esophageal dilatation and lower lobe pulmonary fibrosis is highly suggestive of a connective tissue disorder.

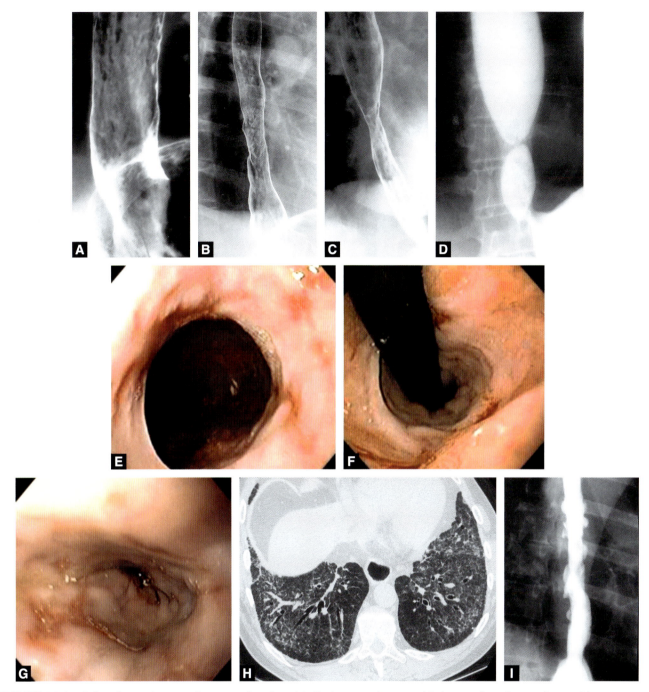

FIGURE 4.3.1 Scleroderma (progressive systemic sclerosis). Barium esophagographic images from four patients with scleroderma show a patulous, incompetent LES with mucosal irregularity from reflux esophagitis (**A** and **B**) and fixed areas of narrowing due to peptic strictures (**B** to **D**). EGD image (**E**) from a different patient shows reflux esophagitis and a stricture. Retroflexed view (**F**) from the same patient as in **E** demonstrates a patulous LES just below the stricture. EGD image (**G**) from another patient shows mild reflux esophagitis and a distal stricture. CT image (**H**) from a different patient shows bibasilar interstitial fibrosis and bronchiectasis, associated with a mildly dilated, air-filled esophagus. Barium esophagram (**I**) from a final patient shows multiple wide-mouth diverticula, a rare but distinctive imaging appearance in scleroderma.

5. OTHER ESOPHAGEAL CONDITIONS

5.1 Vascular Lesions
(Figures 5.1.1-5.1.6)

CLINICAL FEATURES

- Esophageal varices usually represent portosystemic collaterals in a patient with cirrhosis and portal hypertension (so-called "uphill" varices).
- "Downhill" varices are uncommon and related to obstruction of the superior vena cava.
- The importance of varices in the esophageal submucosa is the risk of rupture and GI hemorrhage; hemorrhage is usually severe with hemodynamic instability and a mortality rate of approximately 50%.
- Endoscopic treatment options include ligation (banding) and, less commonly, sclerotherapy; continued hemorrhage may require balloon tamponade and ultimately TIPS placement to lower portal pressures.
- Primary vascular lesions, such as cavernous hemangioma or angiodysplasia, are uncommon outside of a predisposing condition.
- Pyogenic granulomas (or capillary hemangiomas) usually involve the skin and oral cavity, but rarely can be found in the GI tract as a cause of bleeding.

IMAGING FEATURES

- Varices appear as tortuous or serpiginous filling defects on barium studies and are best seen in the recumbent position; their appearance can rapidly change if effaced or emptied.
- On CT, findings of cirrhosis and portal hypertension are evident, often with other portosystemic collaterals; varices are best evaluated on the portal venous phase as they are generally unopacified on earlier phases.
- On CT, paraesophageal varices are generally much more apparent than submucosal esophageal varices, which appear relatively small in size.
- At endoscopy, submucosal varices are quite evident, often demonstrating a bluish hue; the "red wale" and "white nipple" signs are suggestive of recent or impending variceal hemorrhage.
- Long-segment submucosal spread of carcinoma can rarely mimic varices on barium studies (so-called "varicoid" appearance — see Figures 1.1.5 and 1.2.3).
- The presence of calcified phleboliths can suggest the rare diagnosis of esophageal cavernous hemangioma.
- Pyogenic granulomas are usually pedunculated or polypoid and appear red due to the rich blood supply; overlying whitish material from superficial erosions may be present.

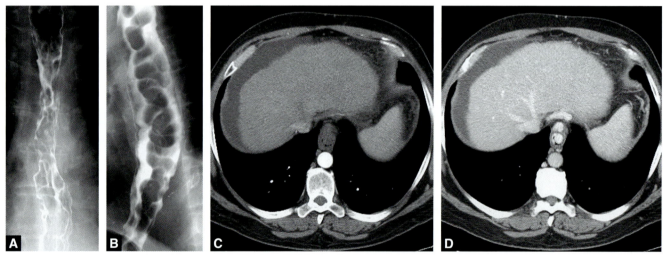

FIGURE 5.1.1 Radiologic evaluation of esophageal varices. Image from double-contrast esophagram (**A**) shows extensive irregular filling defects. The appearance could be difficult to distinguish from an infiltrating "varicoid" carcinoma. Subsequent image obtained with the patient in a recumbent position (**B**) shows smooth tubular filling defects that are easily recognized as varices. Arterial-phase CT image (**C**) from a different patient shows soft tissue fullness in the esophageal region, which is shown to represent enhancing esophageal and paraesophageal varices on portal venous phase (**D**). Note CT findings of cirrhosis.

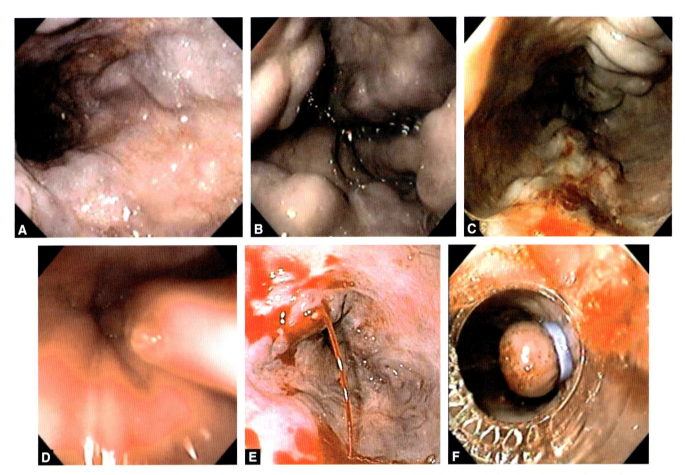

FIGURE 5.1.2 Endoscopic evaluation of esophageal varices. EGD images (**A** to **F**) from six different patients with portal hypertension show submucosal esophageal varices of varying severity. The "red wale" sign with evidence of recent bleeding is seen in **C**, the "white nipple" sign is seen in **D**, and active bleeding is seen in **E**. With the banding device situated on the endoscope, after band placement a varix is seen in **F**.

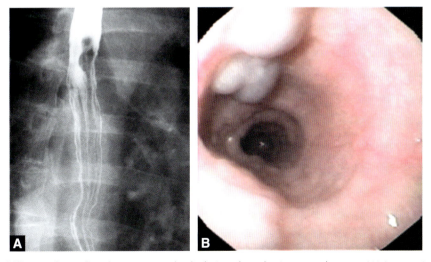

FIGURE 5.1.3 "Downhill" esophageal varices. Mucosal relief view from barium esophagram (**A**) in a patient with superior vena cava obstruction shows a lobulated filling defect involving the upper esophagus, which is confirmed to represent submucosal varices at EGD (**B**).

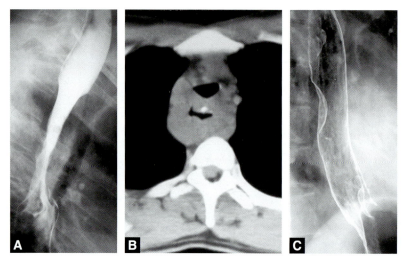

FIGURE 5.1.4 **Esophageal hemangiomas.** Barium esophagram **(A)** and CT **(B)** images show marked circumferential soft tissue thickening on CT with only mild luminal narrowing involving the entire mid-esophagus. The presence of calcified phleboliths is specific for hemangioma. Double-contrast barium esophagram **(C)** from a patient with blue rubber bleb nevus syndrome shows multiple smooth, broad-based filling defects from hemangiomas.

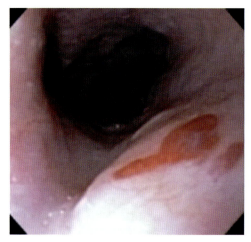

FIGURE 5.1.5 **Esophageal angioectasia.** EGD image shows a well-defined cherry-red vascular lesion.

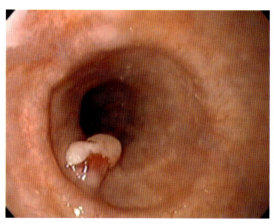

FIGURE 5.1.6 **Pyogenic granuloma (capillary hemangioma).** EGD image shows a pedunculated lesion with a bright red stalk and overlying whitish material in the mid-esophagus. The red stalk is indicative of its rich blood supply, and endoscopic resection must be performed with caution.

5.2 Pharyngoesophageal Diverticula
(Figures 5.2.1-5.2.4)

CLINICAL FEATURES

- These diverticula are generally classified by their location: pharyngoesophageal (Zenker and Killian-Jamieson diverticula), mid-esophageal, and distal esophageal (epiphrenic diverticula).
- Most diverticula are pulsion type; traction diverticula related to mediastinal fibrosis are uncommon.
- Zenker's diverticulum is a common acquired herniation at the level of the cricopharyngeus muscle (Killian's dehiscence); symptoms may be seen in the elderly, such as dysphagia, regurgitation, aspiration, and fetid breath.
- Incomplete relaxation of the upper esophageal sphincter (UES) is felt to contribute to the development of Zenker's diverticula.
- Killian-Jamieson diverticula are generally of no clinical significance.
- Diverticula involving the esophageal body are usually asymptomatic but are often associated with dysmotility disorders; dysphagia and regurgitation are typical of large symptomatic diverticula.

IMAGING FEATURES

- Diverticula are readily diagnosed at barium examination due to preferential filling.
- Zenker's diverticula may present problems at endoscopy and care must be taken to avoid false passage.
- Killian-Jamieson diverticula may be mistaken for a Zenker's diverticulum but are more inferior and lateral in location.
- Large diverticula of the mid-distal esophagus often retain swallowed contents; an air-fluid level may be noted on chest radiography and mistaken for a hiatal hernia.

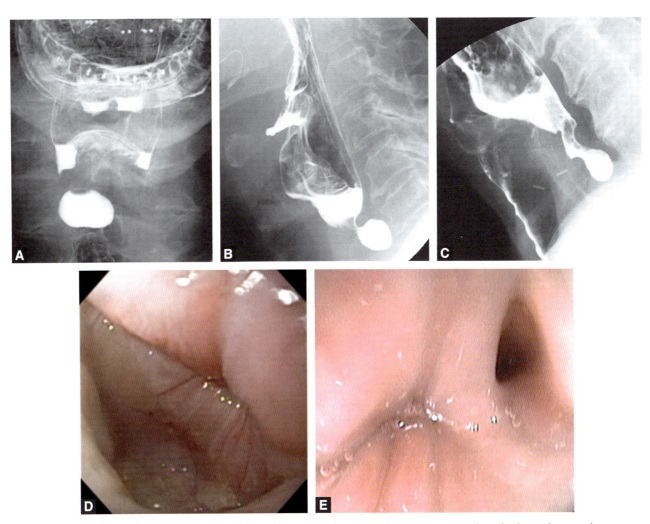

FIGURE 5.2.1 **Zenker's diverticulum.** Frontal (**A**) and lateral (**B**) fluoroscopic images centered on the hypopharynx show a barium-filled diverticulum extending posteriorly near the junction with the cervical esophagus. Lateral fluoroscopic image (**C**) from a different patient shows a barium-filled Zenker's diverticulum, which appeared to be the cause of delayed aspiration after swallowing. Note barium coating the anterior aspect of the trachea. EGD images (**D** and **E**) from two different patients show Zenker's diverticula. Note the upper esophageal sphincter and its proximity to the diverticulum in each image.

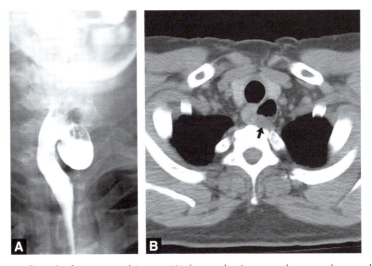

FIGURE 5.2.2 **Killian-Jamieson diverticulum.** Frontal image (**A**) from a barium esophagram shows a barium-filled diverticulum extending laterally off the cervical esophagus. The location is inferior and lateral to the more common Zenker's diverticulum. CT image (**B**) shows the same Killian-Jamieson diverticulum (*arrow*), which contains fluid or debris and is adjacent to the collapsed cervical esophagus.

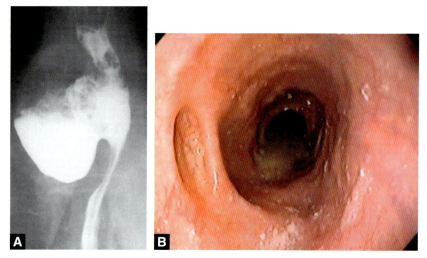

FIGURE 5.2.3 Mid-esophageal diverticulum. Images from barium esophagram **(A)** and EGD **(B)** show a relatively large diverticulum arising from the mid-esophagus. The true size is not fully appreciated on this endoscopic view.

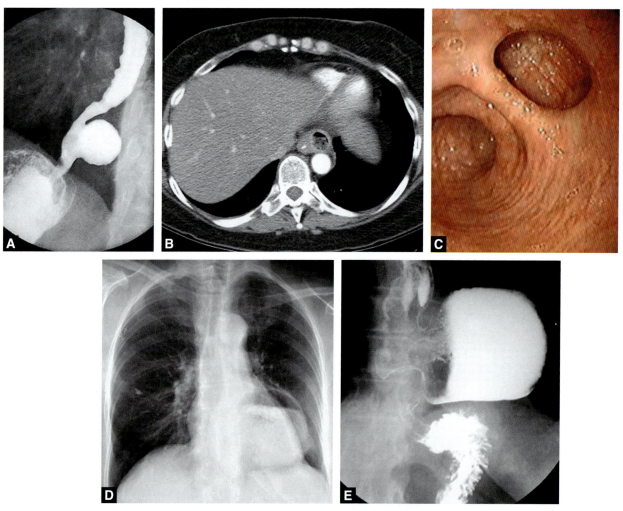

FIGURE 5.2.4 Epiphrenic diverticulum. Barium esophagram **(A)** shows a rounded barium-filled epiphrenic diverticulum. CT image **(B)** from a different patient shows an air- and debris-filled epiphrenic diverticulum. Oral contrast is seen within the true esophageal lumen. EGD image **(C)** from a third patient shows a typical epiphrenic diverticulum. Frontal chest radiograph **(D)** from a final patient shows a large rounded structure in the left hemithorax that contains an air-fluid level. Although the appearance is most suggestive of a large hiatal hernia, barium evaluation **(E)** shows that this represents a large epiphrenic diverticulum.

5.3 Duplication Cysts

(Figures 5.3.1-5.3.2)

CLINICAL FEATURES

- Esophageal duplication cysts represent about 20% of all congenital GI tract duplication cysts.
- They often involve the mid-distal esophagus and tend to be right-sided.
- Typically they are rounded or ovoid cystic lesions that rarely communicate with the esophageal lumen.
- Rarely symptomatic, they are most often incidentally discovered on imaging.
- Bleeding or perforation are more common in cysts containing gastric mucosa.
- Distinction from bronchogenic cysts, another type of foregut duplication cyst, may be difficult on imaging.

IMAGING FEATURES

- The cysts generally appear as nonspecific, smooth, broad-based submucosal masses on luminal studies such as barium evaluation and endoscopy; the findings may be quite subtle in some cases.
- CT, MR, and EUS can all demonstrate the simple cystic nature of these lesions.
- In selected cases, ^{99m}Tc pertechnetate scintigraphy can demonstrate ectopic gastric mucosa.
- Duplication cysts are often anechoic in nature, whereas bronchogenic cysts may appear more complex and hypoechoic at EUS examination.

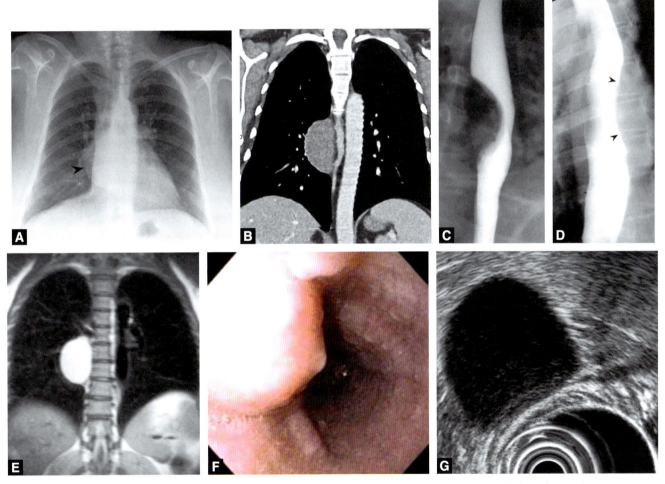

FIGURE 5.3.1 Esophageal duplication cysts. Frontal chest radiograph (**A**) shows an abnormal rounded mediastinal contour (*arrowhead*), which has a cystic appearance on the coronal contrast-enhanced CT image (**B**). The close relationship of this cyst with the esophagus was demonstrated better on other images (not shown). Barium esophagram (**C**) shows a smooth, broad-based filling defect suggestive of an intramural or extrinsic lesion. Barium esophagram (**D**) from a different patient shows a more subtle impression (*arrowheads*) that corresponds to a cystic lesion on coronal T2-weighted SSFSE MR image (**E**). EGD image (**F**) from a final patient shows a smooth submucosal lesion, which appears well-defined and anechoic at EUS (**G**), consistent with a cyst. Note the contiguity of the esophageal muscularis propria to the cyst wall.

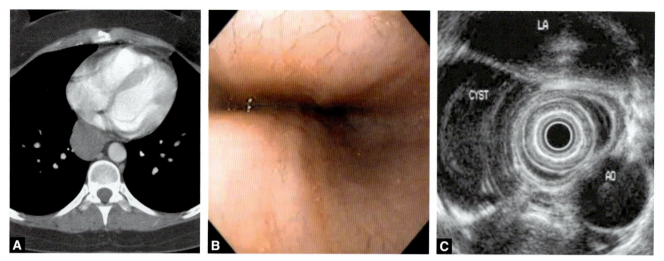

FIGURE 5.3.2 **Bronchogenic foregut duplication cyst.** Contrast-enhanced CT image **(A)** shows a cystic lesion in the middle mediastinum that resembles the esophageal duplication cysts in the preceding figure. EGD image **(B)** shows nonspecific bulging from an intramural or extrinsic process, but EUS **(C)** shows the cystic lesion ("cyst") in the same orientation as the CT image (AO = aorta; LA = left atrium). The increased echogenicity of this hypoechoic lesion and location external to the esophageal muscularis propria favor a bronchogenic origin. A bronchogenic cyst was confirmed after surgical resection.

5.4 Mechanical Injury
(Figures 5.4.1-5.4.5)

CLINICAL FEATURES

- Focal esophageal injury may be "spontaneous" (e.g., retching or ingested substance) or due to iatrogenic trauma (e.g., esophageal instrumentation).
- Mallory-Weiss tears are a relatively common cause of upper GI bleeding but are typically self-limited; a history of retching preceding hematemesis or melena may be elicited.
- Nonspontaneous esophageal mucosal tears and perforation are most often related to medical instrumentation; ingested foreign bodies and penetrating trauma are less common causes.
- Boerhaave's syndrome describes spontaneous full-thickness perforation, usually related to violent retching or vomiting.
- The prognosis is much worse for full-thickness tears than for partial-thickness tears, given the risk of mediastinitis.

IMAGING FEATURES

- Mallory-Weiss tears are superficial lacerations at or near the gastroesophageal junction and are diagnosed at endoscopy (rarely seen at barium examination).
- Mucosal tears can remain localized or lead to intramural hematoma or dissection; contrast fluoroscopy is useful for documenting the extent of injury and excluding frank perforation.
- Pneumomediastinum seen on radiologic studies generally signifies perforation; CT may be useful in conjunction with contrast fluoroscopy to evaluate the mediastinum.

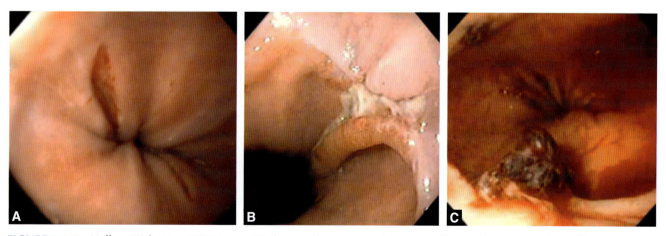

FIGURE 5.4.1 **Mallory-Weiss tear.** EGD image **(A)** shows a linear mucosal tear extending to the gastroesophageal junction. EGD image **(B)** from a different patient shows a clean-based, irregular mucosal defect extending from the cardia to the distal esophagus. EGD image **(C)** from a third patient shows an adherent clot with oozing from an underlying Mallory-Weiss tear that required epinephrine injection for hemostasis. Spontaneous cessation of bleeding is seen with the majority of these injuries, which usually obviates the need for endoscopic therapy.

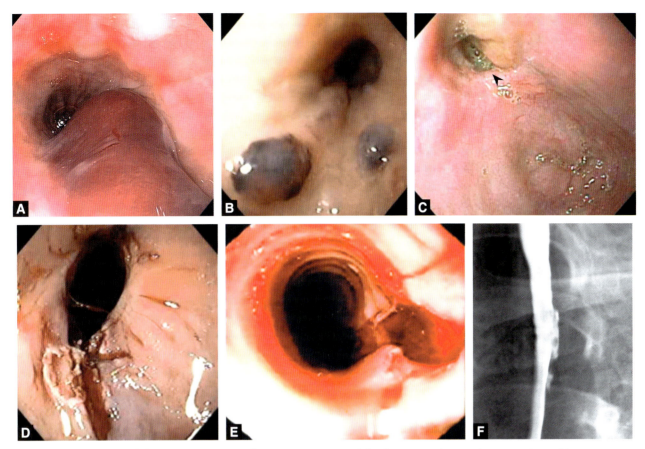

FIGURE 5.4.2 Iatrogenic injury. EGD image **(A)** from a patient on antiplatelet agents shows a large esophageal hematoma seen on withdrawal of the endoscope. Note the small mucosal tear, which was likely the nidus for hematoma formation. EGD image **(B)** from a patient with a malpositioned nasogastric tube shows two submucosal hematomas from suction trauma on the esophageal mucosa. EGD image **(C)** from a third patient shows a small perforation (*arrowhead*) after complicated endoscopic placement of a Savary guidewire. EGD image **(D)** from a fourth patient after balloon dilatation of an anastomotic stricture shows a large tear with bleeding that required endoscopic treatment to achieve hemostasis. EGD image **(E)** from a fifth patient status post bougie dilatation shows a linear mucosal rent with evidence of bleeding. Corresponding barium esophagram **(F)** shows the linear tear but excludes frank perforation. Note the narrow luminal caliber and ringed appearance in this case, suggestive of eosinophilic esophagitis.

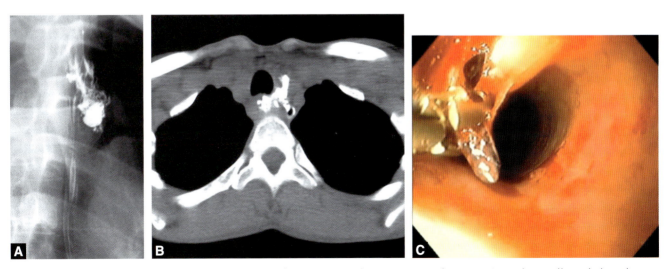

FIGURE 5.4.3 Injury from foreign body. Barium esophagram **(A)** and CT **(B)** images from a patient who swallowed glass show a contained perforation involving the cervical esophagus. EGD image **(C)** shows endoscopic removal of a glass shard that had pierced the esophageal wall.

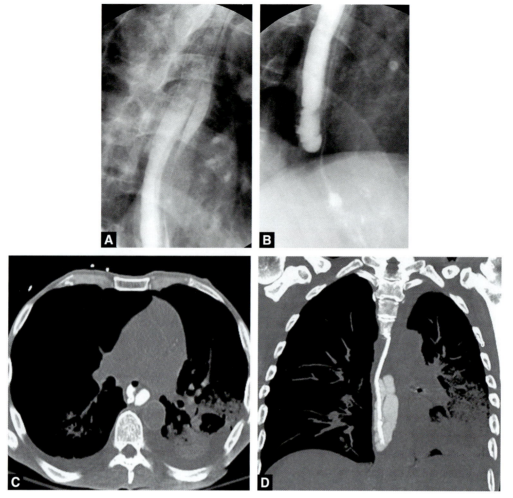

FIGURE 5.4.4 **Intramural esophageal dissection.** Images from a barium esophagram (**A** and **B**) following endoscopy show an intramural dissection that creates a "double-barrel" appearance. The larger-caliber channel represents the false lumen, which ends blindly above the diaphragm. Transverse (**C**) and coronal (**D**) CT images with enteric contrast from a patient status post esophageal dilatation procedure, show another double-barrel appearance to the esophagus. The denser linear structure is a nasogastric tube within the true lumen. Pulmanary disease is also present.

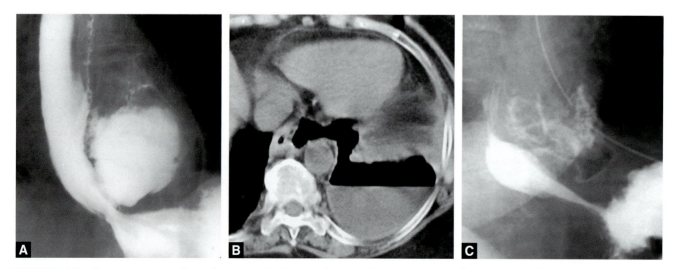

FIGURE 5.4.5 **Spontaneous esophageal rupture.** Barium esophagram (**A**) in a patient with severe pain after vomiting shows an extraluminal barium collection due to a full-thickness tear (Boerhaave's syndrome). CT image (**B**) from a different patient shows a large left pleural or extrapleural collection adjacent to the esophagus but of unproven origin. Subsequent fluoroscopic contrast study (**C**) shows communication with the distal esophagus, diagnostic of rupture.

Illustration continued on following page

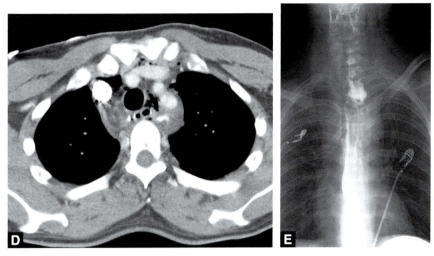

FIGURE 5.4.5 *(Continued)* **Spontaneous esophageal rupture.** CT image **(D)** from another patient with spontaneous esophageal rupture shows pneumomediastinum. Subsequent fluoroscopic contrast study **(E)** shows an irregular collection of extraluminal contrast from a cervical esophageal rupture. Linear gas collections originating from the pneumomediastinum extend into the soft tissues of the neck. *(B and C, from Pickhardt PJ, Bhalla S, Balfe DM: Acquired gastrointestinal fistulas: Classification, etiologies, and imaging evaluation [review]. Radiology 2002;224:9-23.)*

5.5 Foreign Body Impaction
(Figures 5.5.1-5.5.2)

CLINICAL FEATURES

- Most pharyngoesophageal foreign body impactions involve accidental ingestions in children.
- Distal esophageal food impactions in adults are often associated with an underlying stricture or ring.
- Dysphagia symptoms of distal impaction are often referred to the hypopharynx or proximal esophagus.
- Most foreign bodies impacted in the esophagus require endoscopic removal; impaction for greater than 24 hours leads to an increased risk of tissue necrosis and subsequent perforation.

IMAGING FEATURES

- Barium studies are useful in cases of low clinical suspicion; food impaction can simulate a mass lesion.
- Endoscopy is generally indicated for dislodging food impactions; radiologic techniques also exist.
- Exclusion of underlying pathology (stricture or ring) is best performed after removal of the impacted bolus.
- Contrast fluoroscopy is useful for excluding perforation in selected cases.

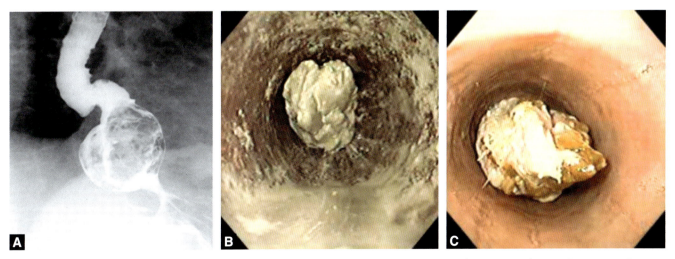

FIGURE 5.5.1 **Distal esophageal meat impaction ("steakhouse syndrome").** Barium esophagram **(A)** shows a large, irregular, rounded filling defect lodged at the distal esophagus. EGD image **(B)** from another patient with a meat impaction shows barium coating the impacted bolus and esophageal mucosa.

Illustration continued on following page

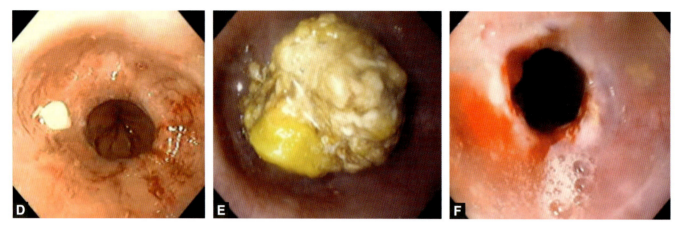

FIGURE 5.5.1 (Continued) Distal esophageal meat impaction. EGD images before (C) and after (D) endoscopic disimpaction show an underlying Schatzki's ring that contributed to the obstruction. EGD images from a different patient (E and F) show another impaction secondary to a reflux-induced stricture.

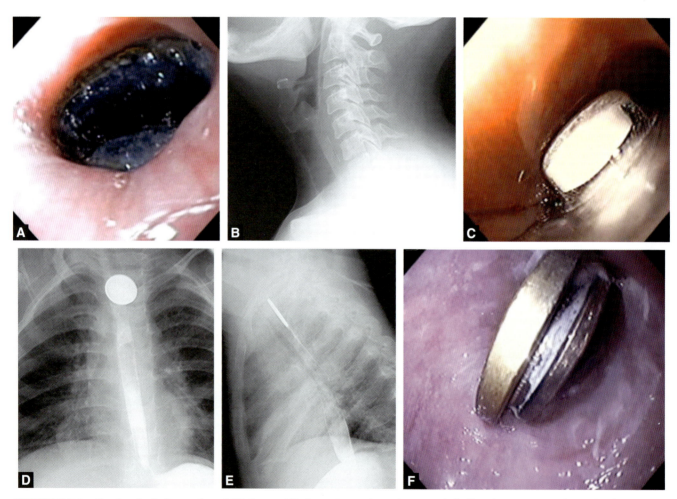

FIGURE 5.5.2 Foreign body impaction. EGD image (A) shows impaction of a mussel shell at the upper esophageal sphincter. Lateral neck radiograph (B) from a patient who swallowed a pill still in its foil wrapper shows a thin linear density posterior to the trachea. EGD image (C) from the same patient shows the packaged pill lodged in the upper esophagus. Frontal (D) and lateral (E) views from fluoroscopic barium evaluation show a metallic coin impacted at the proximal esophagus. This was a child who had previously undergone repair for esophageal atresia. Airway narrowing is present from associated tracheomalacia. EGD image (F) from an adult patient shows several coins lodged in the esophageal lumen.

5.6 Esophageal Fistulas
(Figures 5.6.1-5.6.4)

CLINICAL FEATURES

- Congenital esophagorespiratory fistulas include tracheoesophageal and esophagobronchial types; most patients present with symptoms early in life.
- Acquired esophagorespiratory fistulas are most often malignant from either esophageal or bronchogenic carcinoma; they usually present after radiation therapy with dysphagia and aspiration-type symptoms.
- Benign causes of esophagorespiratory fistulas include instrumentation, trauma, and infections from fungal, mycobacterial, and viral organisms.
- Aortoesophageal fistulas are rare and most often represent a complication of thoracic aortic aneurysm.
- Esophagopericardial fistulas are also rare and are most often associated with esophageal cancer, surgery, or both.

IMAGING FEATURES

- The lateral projection at contrast fluoroscopy is best for documenting tracheoesophageal fistulas; high-osmolar aqueous contrast should be avoided due to the risk of significant pulmonary edema.
- CT is useful in evaluating for tumor and defining fistula extent in the setting of malignancy.
- Contrast esophagography is typically the initial study for suspected aortoesophageal fistula; CT is useful for detecting extraluminal gas, contrast, or fluid.
- The presence of pneumopericardium suggests the possibility of GI fistula, which can be confirmed on fluoroscopy with water-soluble contrast.

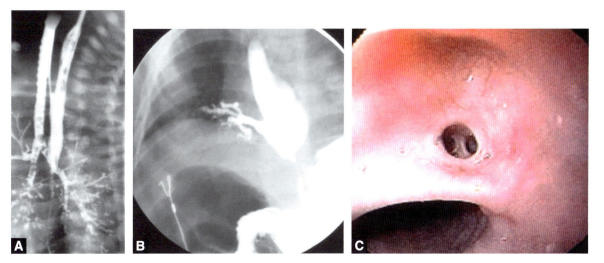

FIGURE 5.6.1 **Congenital esophagorespiratory fistulas.** Lateral projection from a tube esophagram (**A**) in a neonate shows a tracheoesophageal fistula without esophageal atresia. Fluoroscopic contrast study (**B**) from an infant shows a congenital esophagobronchial connection. EGD image (**C**) from an adult patient shows an esophagobronchial fistula that was assumed to be congenital in nature. The bronchial tree is visible through the fistula.

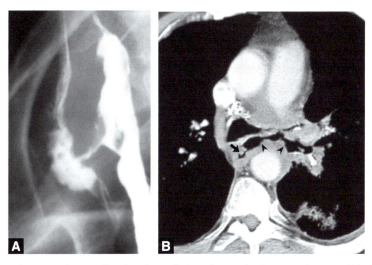

FIGURE 5.6.2 **Malignant esophagorespiratory fistulas.** Lateral view from a barium esophagram (**A**) shows a fistulous tract extending from the esophagus to the trachea, which is anteriorly displaced by a large infiltrative esophageal carcinoma. Oblique transverse CT image (**B**) from a patient with bronchogenic carcinoma shows an irregular fistulous tract (*arrowheads*) extending from the esophageal lumen (*arrow*) to the left bronchial tree. Oral contrast is seen in the left bronchial airway.

Illustration continued on following page

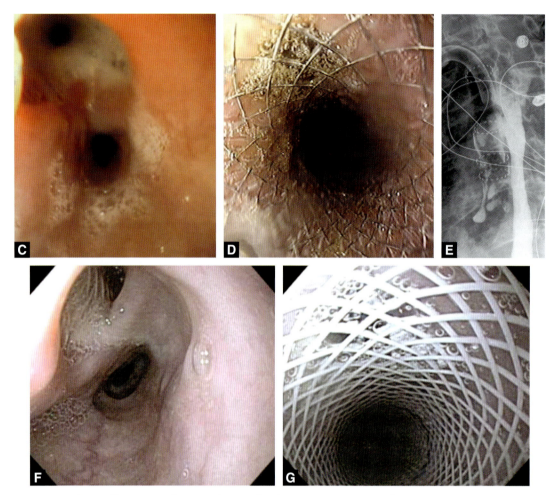

FIGURE 5.6.2 (Continued) **Malignant esophagorespiratory fistulas.** EGD image (C) redemonstrates the esophagobronchial fistula, which was treated by endoscopic stenting (D). Image from contrast fluoroscopy (E) from a patient status post radiation therapy for laryngeal carcinoma shows contrast within the previously stented trachea. EGD image (F) directly shows the fistula and tracheal stent. A covered silicone stent was placed endoscopically that sealed the fistula (G). (A and B, from Pickhardt PJ, Bhalla S, Balfe DM: Acquired gastrointestinal fistulas: Classification, etiologies, and imaging evaluation [review]. Radiology 2002;224:9-23.)

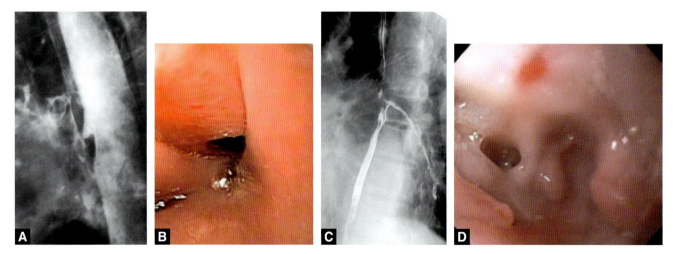

FIGURE 5.6.3 **Esophageal fistulas resulting from infection.** Lateral view from barium esophagram (A) shows an esophagorespiratory fistula due to granulomatous infection (histoplasmosis). EGD image (B) from a patient with CMV esophagitis shows severe ulceration of the proximal esophagus that penetrated into the trachea. Note the bubbles that were seen during examination. Barium esophagram (C) from a patient with idiopathic HIV esophageal ulcers shows an esophagorespiratory fistula originating from the mid-esophagus. EGD image (D) shows markedly denuded and ulcerated mucosa with the presence of a fistula. (A, from Pickhardt PJ, Bhalla S, Balfe DM: Acquired gastrointestinal fistulas: Classification, etiologies, and imaging evaluation [review]. Radiology 2002;224:9-23.)

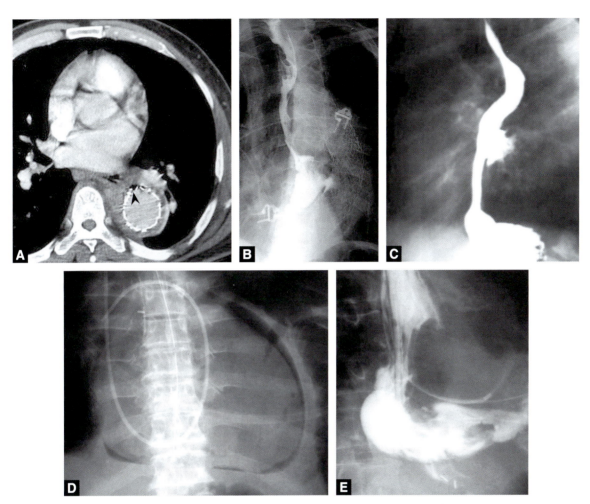

FIGURE 5.6.4 Other benign acquired esophageal fistulas. Contrast-enhanced CT image **(A)** from a patient status post stent repair of a thoracic aortic aneurysm shows air within the mediastinum and adjacent to the aortic stent (*arrowhead*). Subsequent contrast esophagram **(B)** shows extraluminal contrast extending to the aortic stent, diagnostic of an aortoesophageal fistula. Barium esophagram **(C)** from a different patient shows an irregular collection of extraluminal contrast in the mid-esophagus related to fistula formation with a large thoracic aortic aneurysm. Frontal radiograph **(D)** from a patient status post distal esophagectomy for cancer shows pneumopericardium. Subsequent contrast study **(E)** demonstrates an esophagopericardial fistula. (*A, B, and E, from Pickhardt PJ, Bhalla S, Balfe DM: Acquired gastrointestinal fistulas: Classification, etiologies, and imaging evaluation [review]. Radiology 2002;224:9-23.*)

5.7 Intramural Pseudodiverticulosis
(Figure 5.7.1)

CLINICAL FEATURES

- In this uncommon entity, the pseudodiverticula represent dilated ducts of submucosal glands.
- It is likely a sequela of reflux esophagitis, given the high association with benign strictures, but precise etiology and pathogenesis remain unknown.
- Incidental colonization with *Candida* is likely of no clinical significance.
- Main clinical significance centers on the presence or absence of stricture.

IMAGING FEATURES

- The small pseudodiverticula can be identified on both barium and endoscopic evaluation.
- The imaging findings are virtually pathognomonic.
- Associated esophageal strictures are present in the majority of cases.
- Distribution of outpouchings may be diffuse or segmental and are not always centered around the stricture.

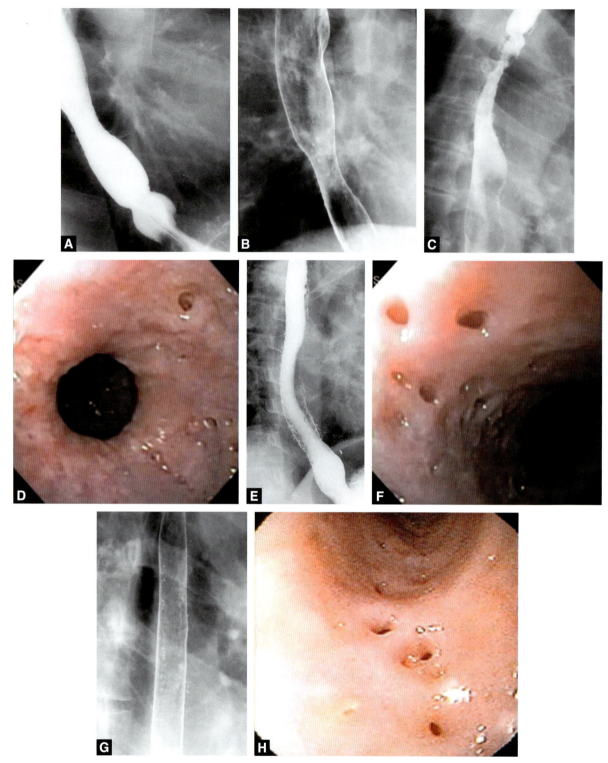

FIGURE 5.7.1 Intramural pseudodiverticulosis. Images from barium esophagography (**A** and **B**) show a persistent smooth stricture in the mid-distal esophagus, associated with multiple small, subtle, additional intramural collections of barium. Barium esophagram (**C**) and EGD image (**D**) from a different patient show an irregular stricture in the proximal esophagus associated with "flask-shaped" outpouchings. Barium esophagrams (**E** and **G**) and EGD images (**F** and **H**) from two additional patients show findings of intramural pseudodiverticulosis without associated stricture.

5.8 Rings, Webs, and Stenosis

(Figures 5.8.1-5.8.5)

CLINICAL FEATURES

- A symptomatic lower esophageal B ring (at the esophagogastric junction) is termed a *Schatzki's ring*; its etiology is uncertain but many believe reflux esophagitis is a primary cause.
- Schatzki's ring often presents with solid food dysphagia.
- Webs are congenital or acquired thin eccentric folds most often found in the cervical esophagus; most are asymptomatic, but some may cause dysphagia.
- A "ringed esophagus" has been attributed to various causes, but the majority of cases may be due to eosinophilic esophagitis (see section 3.3); endoscopic dilatation should be performed with care given the risk for linear tears.
- Congenital esophageal stenosis is rare and of unknown etiology; patients with a relatively mild stenosis may go undetected for years unless dysphagia worsens.

IMAGING FEATURES

- At barium evaluation, a Schatzki's ring appears as a thin concentric constriction above a hiatal hernia; visualization generally requires recumbent positioning with adequate distention.
- B rings resulting in a diameter less than 13 mm are typically symptomatic, whereas those greater than 20 mm rarely cause symptoms; endoscopic dilatation is effective but may need to be repeated if symptoms recur.
- Cervical esophageal webs are best demonstrated on lateral projection at barium evaluation.
- The ringed esophagus is more often identified at endoscopy and often is associated with a narrowed lumen.
- Congenital esophageal stenosis typically manifests as long-segment narrowing; other potential causes such as eosinophilic esophagitis, iatrogenic or caustic stricture, and bullous skin conditions should be excluded.
- The appearance of acquired esophageal stenosis depends on the underlying cause.
- Postsurgical anastomotic strictures after esophagectomy are common due to the development of fibrosis after healing; serial dilations may be required to maintain luminal patency and symptom relief.

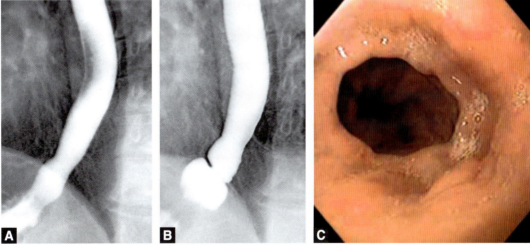

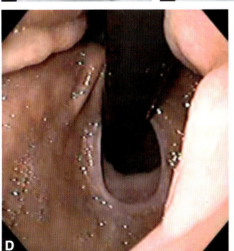

FIGURE 5.8.1 Schatzki's ring (symptomatic B ring). Barium esophagram images obtained without (**A**) and with (**B**) Valsalva's maneuver show a thin concentric ring at the esophagogastric junction above a sliding hiatal hernia, both of which in this case are seen only as the patient bears down. EGD images from above (**C**) and retroflexed view from below (**D**) the esophagogastric junction show another Schatzki's ring above a hiatal hernia.

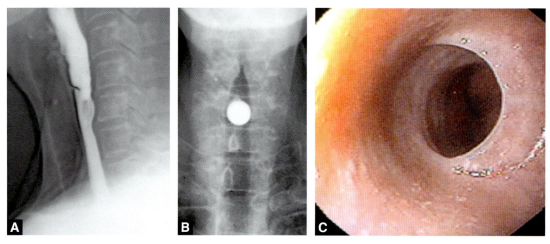

FIGURE 5.8.2 **Cervical esophageal web.** Lateral view **(A)** from barium esophagram in a patient with dysphagia shows a thin eccentric fold off the anterior aspect of the cervical esophagus. A barium tablet is lodged at this level, which is better seen on the frontal view **(B)** after the liquid barium has passed. EGD image **(C)** from a different patient shows a similar eccentric mucosal fold.

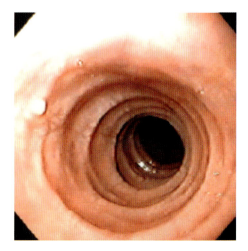

FIGURE 5.8.3 **Multiple esophageal rings.** EGD image shows multiple thin uniform concentric rings. Although some cases have been attributed to congenital stenosis or even GERD, eosinophilic esophagitis now appears to be the leading cause for this appearance.

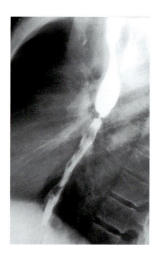

FIGURE 5.8.4 **Congenital esophageal stenosis.** Barium esophagram shows long-segment narrowing of the mid-distal esophagus that was presumed to be congenital in nature, possibly related to tracheobronchial remnants as suggested by the focal ring-like stenosis in the mid-esophagus.

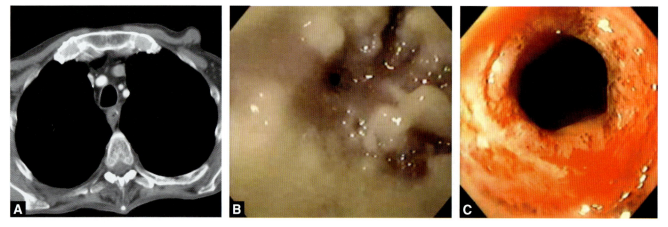

FIGURE 5.8.5 **Anastomotic stricture.** CT image **(A)** of a patient previously treated for esophageal adenocarcinoma via partial esophagectomy shows concentric thickening at the esophagogastric anastomosis, suspicious for local recurrence of tumor. EGD image **(B)** shows a pinpoint lumen at the anastomosis. Note the surrounding candidiasis caused by stasis of luminal contents. Mucosal biopsies revealed only chronic inflammation without malignancy. Serial wire-guided balloon dilatation treatments led to gradual widening of the lumen **(C)** and symptom relief.

5.9 Vascular Rings and Slings
(Figures 5.9.1-5.9.4)

CLINICAL FEATURES

- Vascular ring anomalies include double aortic arch and right aortic arch with aberrant left subclavian artery.
- Most vascular rings present early in life with stridor, but a significant percentage present later with dysphagia.
- Aberrant right subclavian artery does not represent a vascular ring but may rarely present with mild dysphagia ("dysphagia lusoria") or aneurysm.
- Due to their diverticular origin, aberrant subclavian arteries are more prone to aneurysm formation.
- "Pulmonary sling" refers to an aberrant left pulmonary artery arising from the right pulmonary artery.

IMAGING FEATURES

- All of the above entities result in extrinsic impression on the esophagus at barium esophagography.
- Double aortic arch and aberrant subclavian artery anomalies cause a posterior impression, whereas the pulmonary sling (aberrant left pulmonary artery) causes an anterior esophageal impression.
- CT or MR allows for confirmation and preoperative planning.
- Extrinsic impression from an anomalous artery is often very difficult to diagnose at endoscopy.

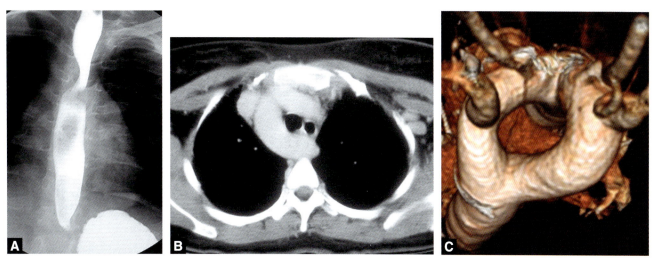

FIGURE 5.9.1 Double aortic arch (vascular ring). Barium esophagram (**A**) from a child with dysphagia shows smooth bilateral impressions on the proximal esophagus, associated with a right-sided aortic arch. Diagnosis of a vascular ring can be made, but distinction between a double aortic arch and right arch with aberrant left subclavian artery is not possible on this study. Transverse (**B**) and volume-rendered (**C**) CT images show a double aortic arch encircling the trachea and esophagus.

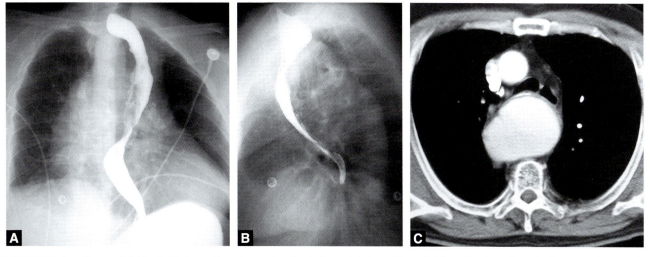

FIGURE 5.9.2 Aberrant left subclavian artery (vascular ring). Frontal (**A**) and lateral (**B**) projections from barium esophagram in an elderly patient with progressive dysphagia show a right-sided aortic arch and significant anterolateral displacement of the barium-filled esophagus. CT (**C**) confirms a right arch and shows massive aneurysmal dilation of the aberrant left subclavian artery, which courses posterior to the trachea and gives rise to the radiographic findings.

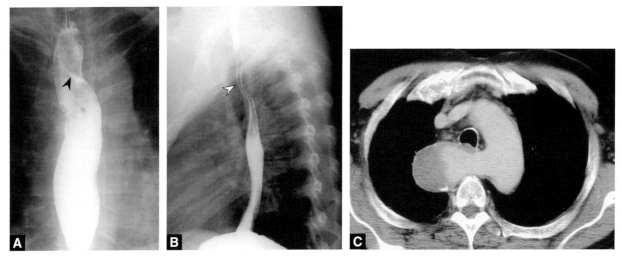

FIGURE 5.9.3 **Aberrant right subclavian artery (not a vascular ring).** Frontal (**A**) and lateral (**B**) projections from barium esophagram show a subtle smooth oblique posterior impression upon the esophagus (*arrowheads*) due to an aberrant right subclavian artery coursing posteriorly. This is typically an incidental finding of no clinical concern. Contrast-enhanced CT image (**C**) from a different patient shows marked aneurysmal dilation of an aberrant right subclavian artery, which can be seen originating from the distal arch and extending to the right, posterior to the trachea and esophagus. Low-attenuation luminal thrombus is present within the aneurysm.

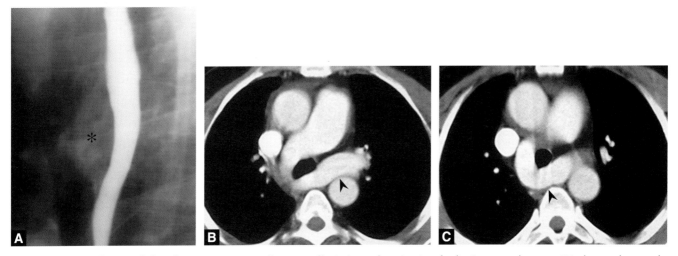

FIGURE 5.9.4 **Aberrant left pulmonary artery (pulmonary sling).** Lateral projection for barium esophagram (**A**) shows abnormal soft tissue (*asterisk*) between the trachea and esophagus, which causes a subtle anterior impression upon the latter. Contrast-enhanced CT images (**B** and **C**) show an aberrant left pulmonary artery (*arrowheads*) arising from the right pulmonary artery. The esophagus is displaced posteriorly.

5.10 Hypopharyngeal Disease
(Figures 5.10.1-5.10.5)

CLINICAL FEATURES

- Anatomic division between the oropharynx and hypopharynx is somewhat arbitrary because some use the hyoid bone and others use the pharyngoepiglottic fold; the hypopharynx lies both posterior and lateral to the larynx.
- The main components of the hypopharynx are the piriform sinuses and the midline post-cricoid space.
- Squamous cell carcinoma is the predominant cancer of the hypopharynx; prognosis is generally poor since most patients present late with cervical nodal metastases.

IMAGING FEATURES

- Videofluoroscopic evaluation of the swallowing mechanism is commonly performed in the setting of dysphagia.
- Barium examination is also useful for excluding hypopharyngeal masses.
- CT and MR are used for staging of hypopharyngeal malignancy, as well as for assessing response to therapy.
- The hypopharynx can be a relative blind spot at EGD, but this area can generally be inspected on withdrawal.
- Hypopharyngeal inflammation seen at endoscopy may occasionally be an important indication of clinical disease; radiologic imaging can evaluate for suspected retropharyngeal abscesses.
- Conventional radiography has been traditionally used to evaluate for radiopaque pharyngoesophageal foreign bodies, such as chicken and fish bones and metallic objects; CT may be used as well.

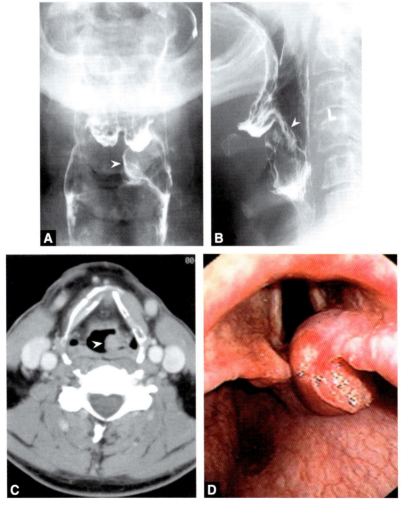

FIGURE 5.10.1 Hypopharyngeal carcinoma (piriform sinus). Frontal **(A)** and lateral **(B)** fluoroscopic views of the hypopharynx show a barium-coated filling defect (*arrowheads*) occupying the left piriform sinus. Hypopharyngeal soft tissue mass from squamous cell carcinoma is confirmed on subsequent contrast-enhanced CT **(C**, *arrowhead*). Endoscopic image **(D)** from a different patient shows a similar piriform sinus mass from squamous cell carcinoma.

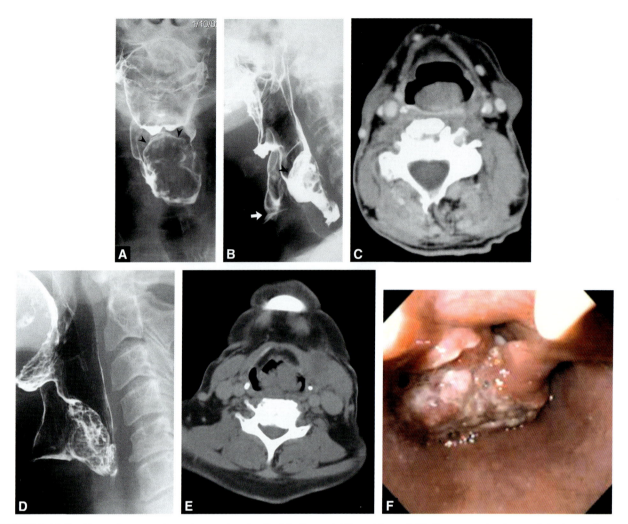

FIGURE 5.10.2 **Hypopharyngeal carcinoma (post-cricoid).** Frontal (**A**) and lateral (**B**) fluoroscopic views of the hypopharynx show a large barium-coated, midline mass (*arrowheads*) in the post-cricoid region, which was causing gross aspiration (*arrow*) due to its size and location. The midline hypopharyngeal mass was confirmed on contrast-enhanced CT (**C**). Lateral view of the hypopharynx (**D**) from a different patient shows an irregular mass from squamous cell carcinoma that also resulted in aspiration. CT image (**E**) from another patient shows a central post-cricoid mass, which on EGD appears to almost completely obstruct the lumen (**F**).

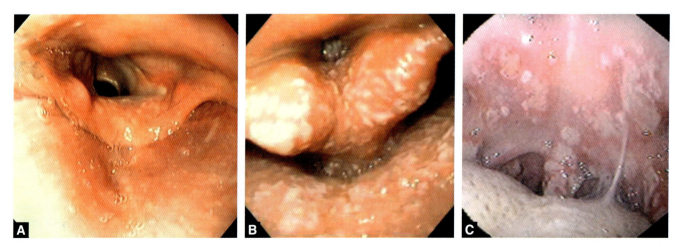

FIGURE 5.10.3 **Hypopharyngeal inflammatory conditions.** Endoscopic images from three different patients show erythematous and edematous aryepiglottic folds resulting from GERD (**A**), multiple white plaques overlying the hypopharyngeal mucosa from oral candidiasis (thrush) (**B**), and multiple aphthous ulcerations involving the hard palate from oral involvement with Crohn's disease (**C**).

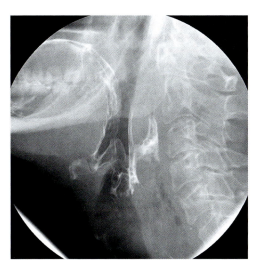

FIGURE 5.10.4 Retropharyngeal abscess. Lateral radiograph from a swallowing study in a patient who developed dysphagia after swallowing a "hard noodle" shows marked soft tissue thickening and gas tracking within the retropharyngeal space. Oral contrast is seen communicating with this space via a large persistent fistulous communication.

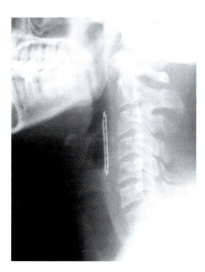

FIGURE 5.10.5 Hypopharyngeal foreign body. Lateral radiograph of the neck with soft tissue technique shows a razor blade posterior to the epiglottis within the hypopharynx.

CHAPTER 2

THE STOMACH

David H. Kim, MD • Perry J. Pickhardt, MD

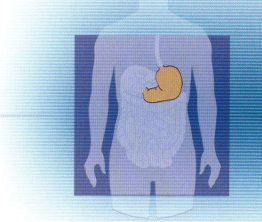

1. **GASTRIC TUMORS**
   1.1 Mucosal Polyps
   1.2 Adenocarcinoma
   1.3 Lymphoma
   1.4 Mesenchymal Tumors
   1.5 Other Submucosal Tumors
2. **GASTRITIS AND GASTROPATHY**
   2.1 Peptic Ulcer Disease
   2.2 Reactive Gastropathies
   2.3 Zollinger-Ellison Syndrome
   2.4 Infectious Gastritis
   2.5 Granulomatous Diseases
   2.6 Ménétrier's Disease
   2.7 Other Inflammatory Conditions
3. **OTHER GASTRIC CONDITIONS**
   3.1 Vascular Lesions
   3.2 Gastric Hernias
   3.3 Gastric Fistulas
   3.4 Heterotopic Pancreatic Rest
   3.5 Duplication Cysts
   3.6 Gastric Bezoars
   3.7 Gastric Volvulus
   3.8 Gastric Diverticula
   3.9 Complications of Percutaneous Endoscopic Gastrostomy

Fluoroscopic and endoscopic studies are an excellent means for examining the mucosa and luminal contour of the stomach. Cross-sectional imaging modalities such as CT and EUS provide additional information with regard to submucosal and intramural evaluation, as well as for evaluation of adjacent structures. Gastric tumors, inflammatory disorders, and a number of miscellaneous conditions are discussed in this chapter. The complementary nature of the various radiologic and endoscopic imaging modalities for gastric evaluation should become apparent.

1. GASTRIC TUMORS

Gastric tumors are composed of a diverse group of entities ranging from benign mucosal-based polyps to intramural mesenchymal tumors to malignant neoplasms such as adenocarcinoma, lymphoma, and metastatic disease.

1.1 Mucosal Polyps
(Figures 1.1.1-1.1.11)

CLINICAL FEATURES

- Mucosal-based lesions include fundic gland polyps, hyperplastic polyps, adenomas, and hamartomas.
- Sporadic fundic gland polyps are most common and comprise nearly 50% of all gastric polyps; they are often associated with the use of acid suppression therapy.
- Fundic gland polyposis (>10 polyps) can be seen sporadically or with underlying familial adenomatous polyposis (FAP) (often hundreds of polyps).
- Hyperplastic polyps, although not premalignant, are associated with a slight increase in risk for gastric adenocarcinoma owing to the common association with atrophic gastritis.
- Adenomas comprise <20% of gastric polyps; the majority are tubular or tubulovillous.
- Although the adenoma-carcinoma sequence may rarely apply to gastric adenomas, the majority of gastric adenocarcinomas are believed to develop de novo.
- Gastric hamartomas may occur in isolation or with a variety of polyposis syndromes, such as Peutz-Jeghers syndrome, Cowden's disease, and Cronkhite-Canada syndrome.
- Other rare gastric polyps include inflammatory polyps and xanthelasmas.

IMAGING FEATURES

- Mucosal polyps typically present as smooth sessile projections at barium UGI and EGD evaluations; some polyps may become lobulated or pedunculated.
- CT is poor at evaluating for mucosal polyps if the lumen is not optimally distended.
- Fundic gland polyps are located in the fundus and body and are typically diminutive, are sessile, and characteristically "chunk" off when sampled.

- Hyperplastic polyps are usually <1 cm but can be large and multiple; large hyperplastic polyps are often friable and prone to bleeding.
- Adenomas tend to be solitary (in the absence of polyposis syndromes) and of variable size.
- Multiple polyps may suggest a polyposis syndrome.
- Size remains a surrogate for histology; biopsy of large or dominant lesions is required to exclude significant neoplasia.

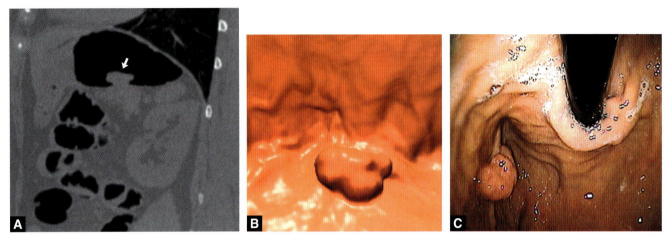

FIGURE 1.1.1 Fundic gland polyp. 2D sagittal image (**A**) and 3D endoluminal image (**B**) from CTC show a polypoid gastric lesion (**A**, *arrow*) that was incidentally detected at colorectal cancer screening. Retroflexed view from subsequent EGD (**C**) shows the same lesion, which proved to be a fundic gland polyp.

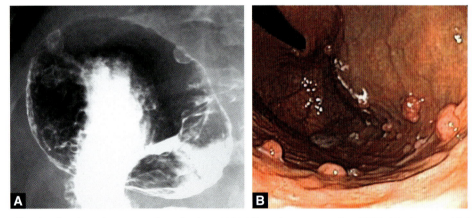

FIGURE 1.1.2 Fundic gland polyposis. Images from barium UGI (**A**) and corresponding EGD (**B**) show multiple fundal polyps, representing isolated fundic gland polyposis without underlying FAP.

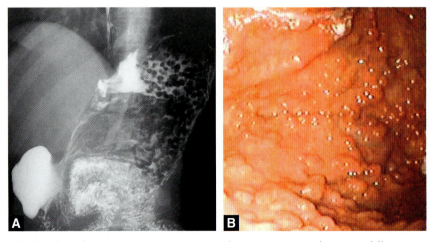

FIGURE 1.1.3 Fundic gland polyposis in FAP. Barium UGI (**A**) and EGD (**B**) images from two different patients with FAP show innumerable subcentimeter polyps carpeting the mucosa within the fundus and proximal stomach.

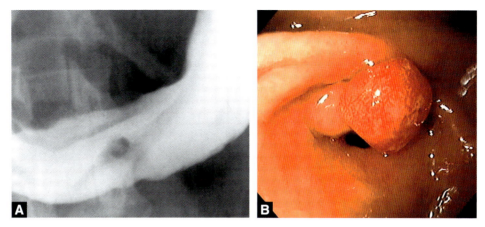

FIGURE 1.1.4 Hyperplastic polyps. Images from barium UGI (**A**) and EGD (**B**) from two different patients show solitary hyperplastic polyps. The lesion on endoscopy appears friable and nearly obstructs the pylorus.

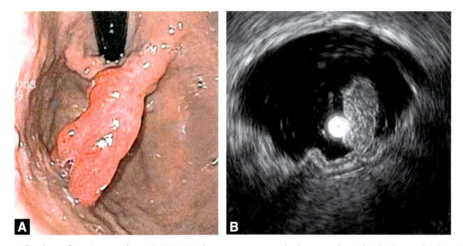

FIGURE 1.1.5 Hyperplastic polyp. Image from EGD (**A**) shows an unusual elongated cardia lesion, which originates from the mucosal layer and has a homogeneous echotexture at EUS (**B**).

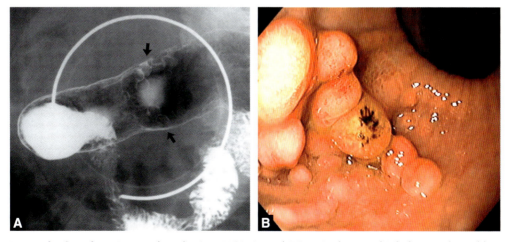

FIGURE 1.1.6 Hyperplastic polyps. Images from barium UGI (**A**) and EGD (**B**) show multiple large polypoid lesions in the gastric body (**A**, *arrows*).

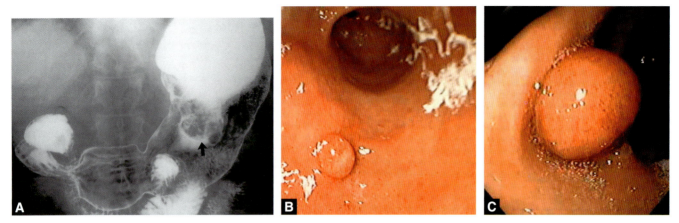

FIGURE 1.1.7   Adenomatous polyps. Three different patients with gastric adenomas. Image from barium UGI **(A)** shows a large lobulated mass (*arrow*) in the gastric body. Images from EGD show a small **(B)** and a large **(C)** gastric adenoma.

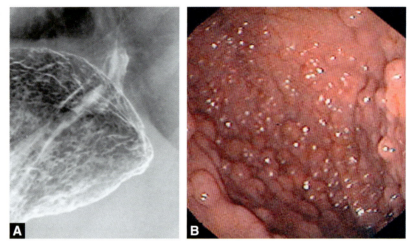

FIGURE 1.1.8   Peutz-Jeghers syndrome. Images from barium UGI **(A)** and EGD **(B)** from two different patients show innumerable small hamartomatous polyps in the gastric fundus and proximal body. The appearance is similar to that of fundic gland polyposis.

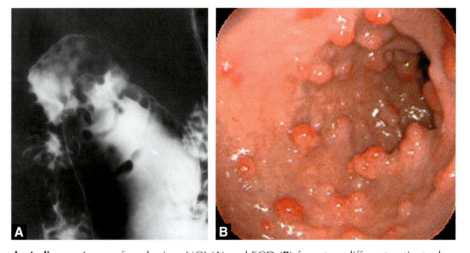

FIGURE 1.1.9   Cowden's disease. Images from barium UGI **(A)** and EGD **(B)** from two different patients show multiple small gastric hamartomas.

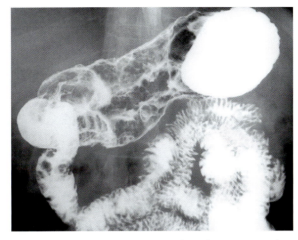

FIGURE 1.1.10 **Cronkhite-Canada syndrome.** Image from barium UGI shows irregular polypoid fold thickening of the stomach and duodenum. Mild uniform jejunal fold thickening is also present.

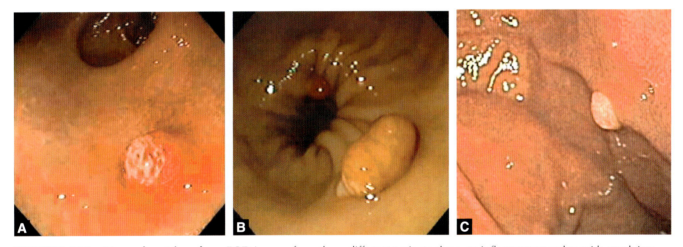

FIGURE 1.1.11 **Unusual gastric polyps.** EGD images from three different patients show an inflammatory polyp with overlying surface erosion (**A**), an inflammatory fibroid polyp (**B**), and a yellowish polypoid lesion representing a xanthelasma (**C**).

1.2 Adenocarcinoma
(Figures 1.2.1-1.2.13)

CLINICAL FEATURES

- Most adenocarcinomas present as advanced tumors with a dismal prognosis (overall 5-year survival < 20%).
- Early cancers (limited to mucosa or submucosa) have a favorable 5-year survival (>90%) but are uncommon.
- Marked variation in incidence is seen related to geography (highest in Japan).
- *Helicobacter pylori*, diet, and atrophic gastritis are major risk factors.
- Gastric stump cancers after Billroth II procedures may present 10 to 15 years later.
- Routes of spread include direct extension to adjacent organs (including the esophagus), lymphatic, peritoneal seeding, and hematogenous (particularly the liver).

IMAGING FEATURES

- An adenocarcinoma may manifest as a plaque-like, lobulated, fungating, annular constricting, or ulcerated mass.
- EGD is the imaging study of choice for diagnosis, with the ability to perform biopsies at time of discovery.
- An adenocarcinoma may also present as an infiltrating submucosal process with rigid luminal narrowing (linitis plastica).
- On barium UGI, "malignant ulcers" manifest with thick, irregular folds at the edge of the ulcer crater; the ulcer generally projects within the gastric lumen.
- Gaseous distention of the gastric lumen greatly improves CT evaluation and allows for virtual endoscopic views; pseudomasses are common with inadequate luminal distention.
- CT aids in evaluating for extragastric involvement for staging purposes.
- Low-attenuation wall thickening with calcification at CT can suggest mucinous histology.
- EUS with fine-needle aspiration (FNA) is the most accurate imaging modality for determining local tumor extension and local nodal involvement.

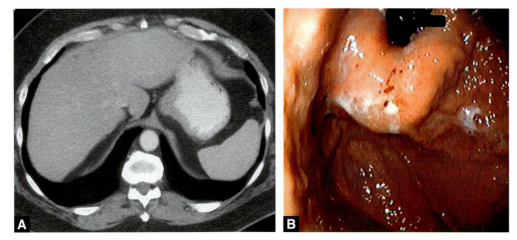

FIGURE 1.2.1   Gastric adenocarcinoma. CT **(A)** and corresponding EGD **(B)** images show localized fullness at the gastric cardia. The CT appearance is relatively nonspecific since this is a common location for a pseudomass due to incomplete distention (see Fig 1.2.13).

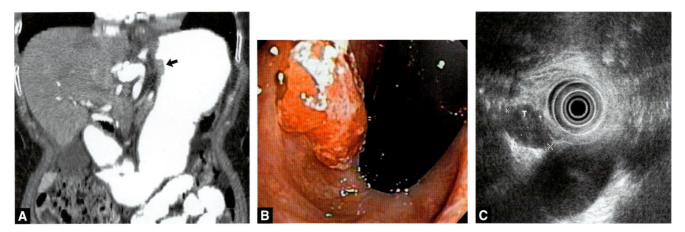

FIGURE 1.2.2   Gastric adenocarcinoma. Curved reformatted coronal CT image **(A)** and corresponding images from EGD **(B)** and EUS **(C)** show a small polypoid lesion (**A**, *arrow*) near the gastric cardia, which was incidentally detected at CT. At EUS, the hypoechoic lesion (T) demonstrates irregular margins that penetrate into the outer hypoechoic layer (muscularis propria).

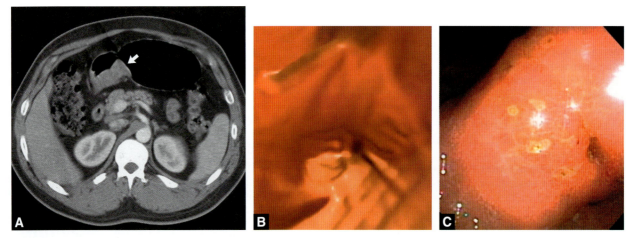

FIGURE 1.2.3   Gastric adenocarcinoma. 2D transverse **(A)** and 3D endoluminal **(B)** CT images obtained with a gas-filled stomach show massive eccentric thickening of the posterior antrum (**A**, *arrow*). Note the thin appearance of normal distended gastric wall on 2D CT. Corresponding EGD image **(C)** shows the mass, with induration and erosions related to tumor infiltration.

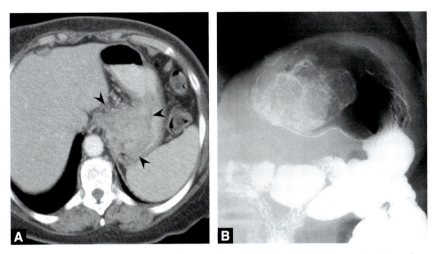

FIGURE 1.2.4 Gastric adenocarcinoma. CT image (**A**) shows a large soft tissue mass (*arrowheads*) at the gastric fundus, which is not well evaluated due to incomplete distention. Corresponding image from barium UGI (**B**) more clearly depicts the large lobulated mucosal mass.

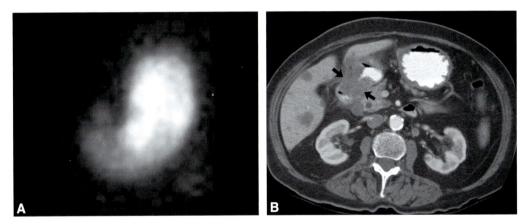

FIGURE 1.2.5 Adenocarcinoma with gastric outlet obstruction. Delayed image from nuclear medicine gastric emptying study (**A**) shows essentially no evidence of emptying, related to either severe gastroparesis or obstructing mass. Image from subsequent CT study (**B**) shows an annular mass (*arrows*) involving the distal antrum as the cause for gastric outlet obstruction. Note the multiple liver metastases.

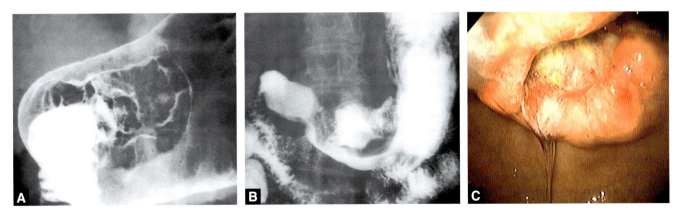

FIGURE 1.2.6 Gastric adenocarcinoma (ulcerating masses). Barium UGI images from two patients (**A** and **B**) show large ulcerating masses along the lesser curvature. Note the thick tumor rind. In the second case (**B**), barium is trapped within the malignant ulcer, which projects within the expected gastric lumen. EGD image from a third patient (**C**) shows a similar ulcerated mass with heaped-up edges.

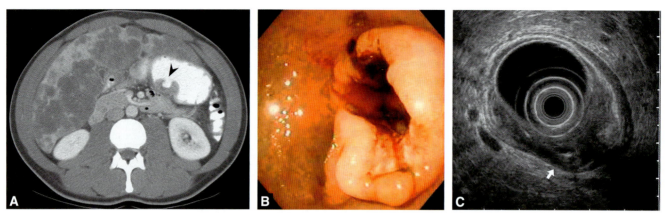

FIGURE 1.2.7 Gastric adenocarcinoma (ulcerating masses). CT image **(A)** shows an ulcerated gastric mass (*arrowhead*) and extensive hepatic metastatic disease. EGD **(B)** and EUS **(C)** images from a different patient show a similar lesion, with large heaped-up edges and oozing from the central crater. Note the invasion of the tumor into but not through the muscularis propria consistent with a T2 lesion (**C**, *arrow*).

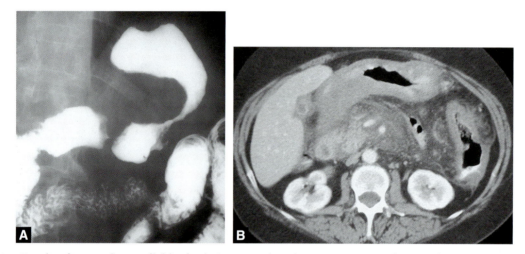

FIGURE 1.2.8 Gastric adenocarcinoma (linitis plastica). Images from barium UGI **(A)** and CT **(B)** from two patients show circumferential luminal narrowing from submucosal tumor infiltration. Note how CT directly demonstrates the wall thickening and extension into the perigastric fat.

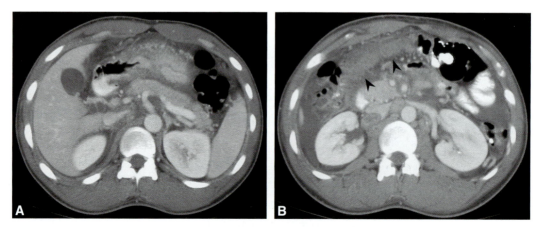

FIGURE 1.2.9 Gastric adenocarcinoma (linitis plastica). CT images **(A and B)** show gastric wall thickening, as well as diffuse perigastric soft tissue infiltration, thickening of the transverse colon (*arrowheads*), retroperitoneal lymphadenopathy, and ascites.

Illustration continued on following page

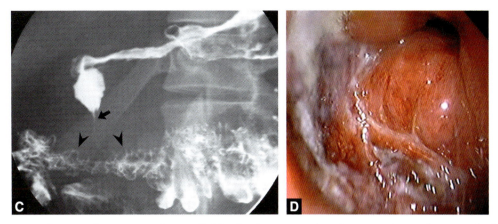

FIGURE 1.2.9 (Continued) **Gastric adenocarcinoma (linitis plastica).** Image from barium UGI **(C)** shows marked luminal narrowing of the distal stomach, with poor distensibility. Extrinsic narrowing of the postbulbar duodenum (*arrow*) and proximal transverse colon (*arrowheads*) is related to direct retroperitoneal and gastrocolic ligamentous extension of tumor, respectively. Corresponding EGD image **(D)** shows rigid luminal narrowing secondary to diffuse tumor infiltration.

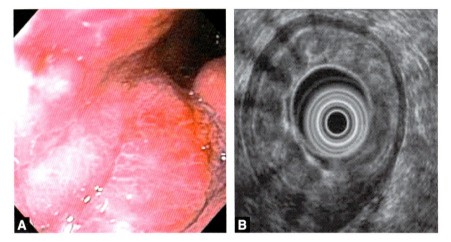

FIGURE 1.2.10 **Gastric adenocarcinoma (linitis plastica).** EGD image **(A)** shows fixed irregular fold thickening with luminal narrowing. Insufflation of the stomach with air shows poor distensibility. Diffuse mucosal and submucosal wall thickening from tumor infiltration is demonstrated on EUS **(B)**. Note the loss of distinctive mucosal and submucosal layers.

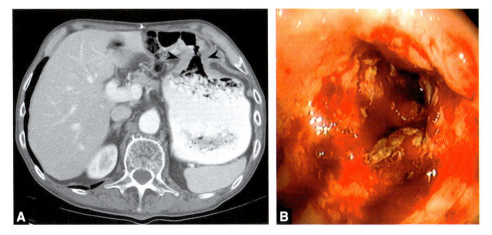

FIGURE 1.2.11 **Recurrent adenocarcinoma after partial gastrectomy.** CT **(A)** and EGD **(B)** images show an annular constricting mass at the gastrojejunal anastomosis (*arrowheads*) in a patient with Billroth II anatomy.

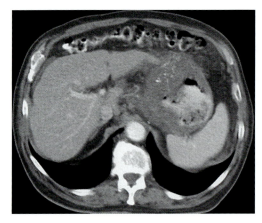

FIGURE 1.2.12 Gastric mucinous adenocarcinoma. CT image shows prominent low-attenuation wall thickening of the gastric wall, associated with stippled calcifications, both of which are suggestive of mucinous histology.

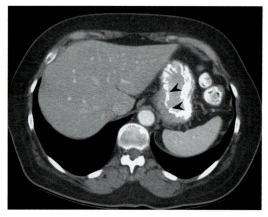

FIGURE 1.2.13 Gastric wall pseudothickening. CT image shows apparent wall thickening (*arrowheads*) at the gastric cardia related to incomplete distention. Note the similarity to cancer in Figure 1.2.1. The distal antrum is another common location for pseudothickening.

1.3 Lymphoma
(Figures 1.3.1-1.3.9)

CLINICAL FEATURES

- The stomach is the most frequently involved segment of the GI tract (50% of all GI lymphomas).
- The majority are of non-Hodgkin's histology and of high grade (usually B-cell origin).
- Low-grade lymphomas from mucosa-associated lymphoid tissue (MALT) represent 30% to 40% of primary gastric lymphomas; *H. pylori*, which causes chronic gastritis, is considered an etiologic agent.
- MALT lymphomas are generally more indolent and have a better prognosis.
- In contrast to adenocarcinoma, lymphomas are more often symptomatic early in disease course, with nausea, vomiting, and dyspepsia as common presenting symptoms.
- Overall, prognosis of gastric lymphoma is favorable compared with adenocarcinoma (50%-60% 5-year survival).

IMAGING FEATURES

- Gastric lymphomas may manifest as nodular fold thickening, ulcerating lesions, or polypoid masses; *H. pylori* gastritis can mimic the more subtle nodular form of MALT lymphoma.
- High-grade lymphomas more often present as an infiltrative process with extensive fold thickening.
- Degree of fold thickening at barium UGI and wall thickening at CT are usually greater than seen with adenocarcinoma.
- Transpyloric spread to the duodenum is reportedly more common with lymphoma than adenocarcinoma.
- CT is useful in assessing for extent of mural involvement and for nodal disease.

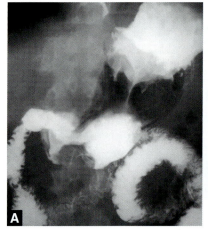
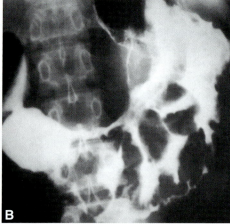

FIGURE 1.3.1 Gastric lymphoma. Barium UGI images (**A** and **B**) from two patients show multifocal fold thickening with irregular masses.

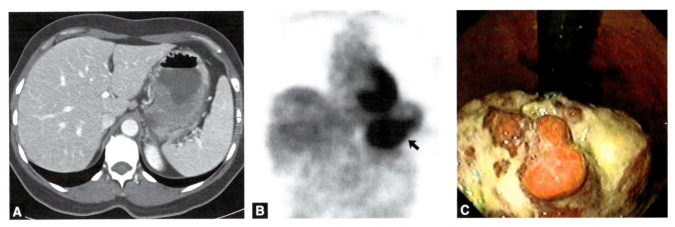

FIGURE 1.3.2 Gastric lymphoma. CT (**A**) and PET (**B**) images show a focal hypermetabolic fundal mass (*arrow*). EGD image (**C**) from a second patient shows a large lobulated polypoid mass in the fundal region.

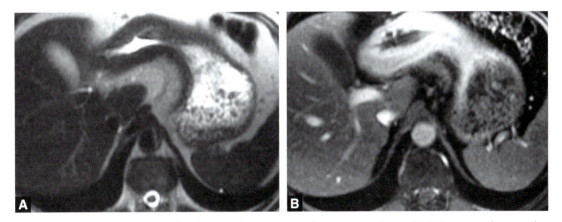

FIGURE 1.3.3 Gastric lymphoma. T2-weighted (**A**) and post-contrast fat-suppressed SGE (**B**) MR images show uniform wall thickening of the distal stomach with marked contrast enhancement.

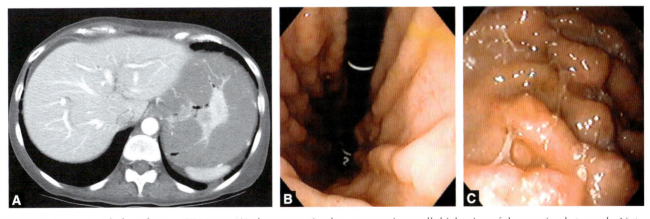

FIGURE 1.3.4 Gastric lymphoma. CT image (**A**) shows massive low-attenuation wall thickening of the proximal stomach. Note how contrast extends between enlarged folds. Corresponding EGD images (**B** and **C**) show diffuse nodular fold thickening.

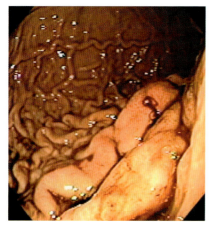

FIGURE 1.3.5 **Low-grade MALT lymphoma.** EGD image shows diffuse gastric fold thickening.

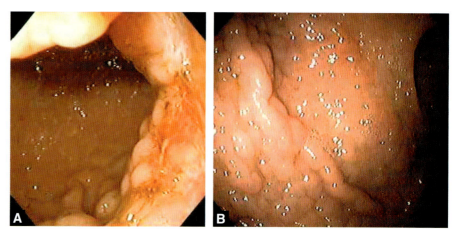

FIGURE 1.3.6 **MALT lymphoma versus nodular *H. pylori* gastritis.** EGD images from two patients show a multinodular appearance of MALT lymphoma in one (**A**) and the nodular form of *H. pylori* infection in the other (**B**).

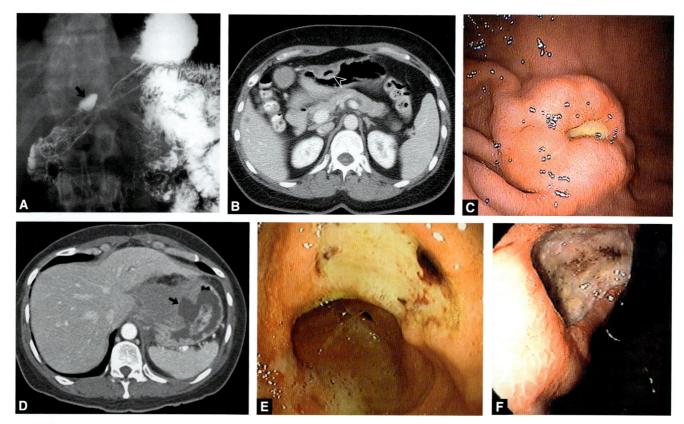

FIGURE 1.3.7 **Gastric lymphoma (ulcerating masses).** Barium UGI image (**A**) shows diffuse luminal narrowing and a focal barium-filled cavity from ulceration (*arrow*). Contrast-enhanced CT (**B**) and EGD (**C**) images from a second patient show an ulcerated mass (*arrowhead*) along the anterior wall of the stomach. Contrast-enhanced CT image (**D**) from a third patient shows a bulky fundal mass with a large fluid-filled ulceration. EGD images (**E** and **F**) from two additional patients show large malignant ulcers.

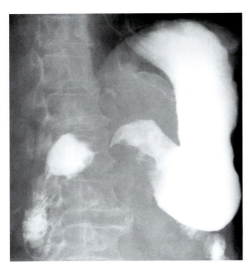

FIGURE 1.3.8 **Transpyloric spread of gastric lymphoma.** Image from barium UGI shows a nodular mass lesion in the distal antrum, with severe narrowing of the pyloric channel related to lymphomatous spread. Transpyloric spread can also be seen with adenocarcinoma but at a relatively lower frequency.

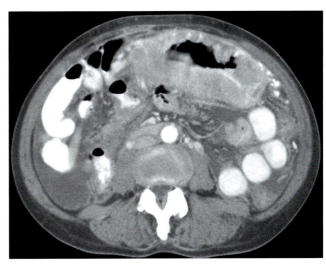

FIGURE 1.3.9 **T-cell lymphoma.** CT image shows diffuse gastric wall thickening and peritoneal lymphomatosis. T-cell lymphoma less commonly involves the stomach, but the imaging appearance cannot be distinguished from B-cell disease.

1.4 Mesenchymal Tumors
(Figures 1.4.1-1.4.10)

CLINICAL FEATURES

- These tumors are intramural lesions that arise deep to the gastric mucosa and often grow in an exoenteric fashion.
- GI stromal tumors (GISTs) account for the majority of solid gastric mesenchymal tumors; others include leiomyomas, schwannomas, lipomas, and hemangiomas.
- GISTs arise from interstitial cells of Cajal (GI pacemaker cells) and were previously misclassified as smooth muscle tumors; express KIT, a receptor tyrosine kinase protein encoded by the *c-KIT* gene.
- Mesenchymal tumors may present with UGI hemorrhage secondary to ulceration of the overlying mucosa.
- Malignant mesenchymal tumor spread is most often via direct local extension, intraperitoneal seeding, or hematogenous (to liver).
- Most nerve sheath tumors (e.g., schwannomas, neurofibromas) are benign.
- Gastric lipomas are generally benign incidental findings.

IMAGING FEATURES

- Mesenchymal tumors are submucosal (intramural) masses that typically manifest as smooth, broad-based impressions on barium UGI and EGD studies; they may be difficult to distinguish from extrinsic lesions.
- The overlying mucosa is intact unless the lesion has ulcerated (more common with malignant tumors).
- CT and EUS are useful for demonstrating the extent of exoenteric growth, which is typically much more prominent than the endoluminal component.
- EUS allows for identification of the tissue layer of origin, which can select lesions that may be amenable to endoscopic resection (i.e., those originating from the muscularis mucosa or submucosal layers).
- CT can evaluate for metastatic disease and monitor response to therapy.
- A densely calcified lesion is suggestive of leiomyoma.
- CT and EUS can provide an image-specific diagnosis for lipomas, obviating tissue sampling.
- Hemangiomas are rare and manifest as nonspecific submucosal lesions; the presence of calcified phleboliths may allow for a specific imaging diagnosis.
- Extrinsic impression from extragastric structures can simulate a submucosal mass on luminal imaging studies.

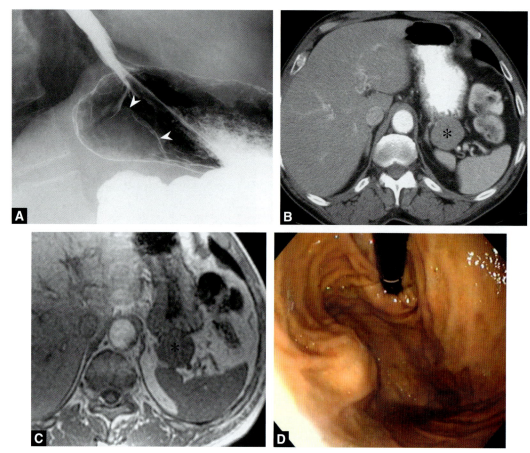

FIGURE 1.4.1 GI stromal tumor. Image from barium UGI **(A)** shows a nonspecific smooth broad-based impression (*arrowheads*), suggesting an intramural or extrinsic process. CT **(B)** and T1-weighted SGE MR **(C)** images show the full extent of the rounded exoenteric soft tissue mass arising from the gastric wall (*asterisk*). Image from EGD **(D)** shows luminal impression from the mass. Note how endoluminal images (**A** and **D**) depict only the "tip of the iceberg."

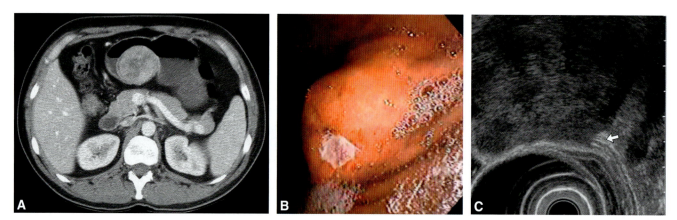

FIGURE 1.4.2 GI stromal tumor. CT image **(A)** shows brisk heterogeneous contrast enhancement of a GIST involving the gastric antrum. Note how the displaced submucosal layer is well defined in areas, demonstrating its intramural location. EGD **(B)** and corresponding EUS **(C)** images from another patient show a submucosal mass with central ulceration. The EUS image shows the lesion originating from the muscularis propria (*arrow*). The large size (>4 cm), cystic spaces within the tumor, and irregular borders suggest malignant potential.

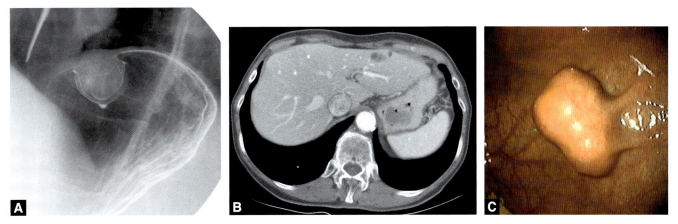

FIGURE 1.4.3 GI stromal tumor. Images from barium UGI **(A)**, CT **(B)**, and EGD **(C)** show a gastric GIST that is predominately submucosal in location, without an exoenteric component.

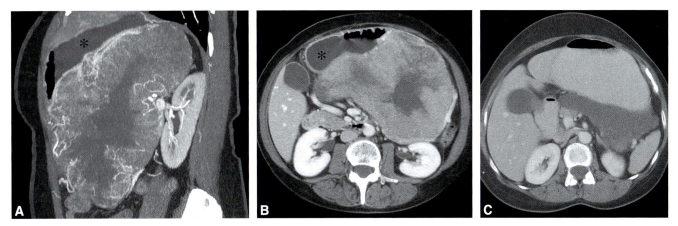

FIGURE 1.4.4 GI stromal tumor with response to treatment. Sagittal contrast-enhanced CT image during the arterial phase **(A)** and transverse CT image from portal venous phase **(B)** show a massive GIST extending inferiorly off the displaced stomach (*asterisks*). Note prominent tumor vessels and central low attenuation. Follow-up CT image **(C)** after treatment with imatinib shows marked reduction in tumor size and characteristic nonenhancing cystic appearance to the lesion.

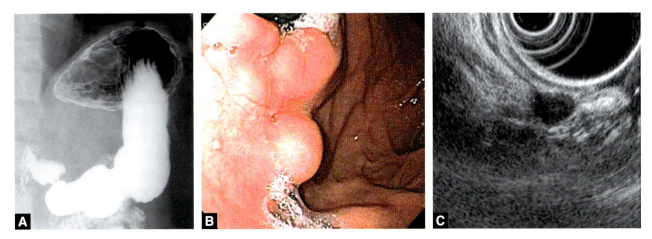

FIGURE 1.4.5 Gastric leiomyoma. Image from barium UGI **(A)** shows a smooth lobulated filling defect from a gastric leiomyoma. EGD **(B)** and EUS **(C)** images from a different patient show a similar lobulated lesion that appears hypoechoic at EUS and arises from the muscularis propria. The endosonographic appearance is indistinguishable from a small GIST. Immunohistochemical analysis of obtained tissue can help differentiate the two lesions.

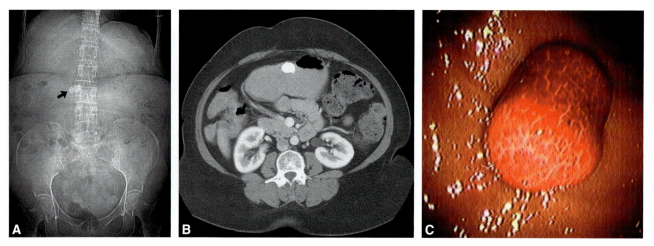

FIGURE 1.4.6 Calcified leiomyoma. Scout image from CT **(A)** shows an incidental calcific focus (*arrow*) overlying the mid-abdomen. CT image **(B)** shows that calcified lesion involves the anterior gastric wall. Subsequent EGD **(C)** demonstrates a firm polypoid lesion that proved to be a densely calcified leiomyoma after surgical resection.

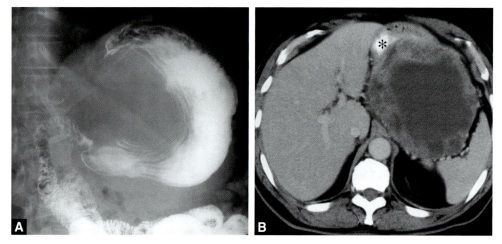

FIGURE 1.4.7 Gastric leiomyosarcoma. Image from barium UGI **(A)** shows significant mass effect on the stomach, with preservation of the mucosal folds. The appearance suggests an extrinsic process (e.g., lesser sac pseudocyst or large extragastric tumor) or an intramural mesenchymal lesion. CT image **(B)** shows a large heterogeneous mass displacing the contrast-filled gastric lumen anteriorly (*asterisk*). Low-attenuation cystic areas likely represent central necrosis.

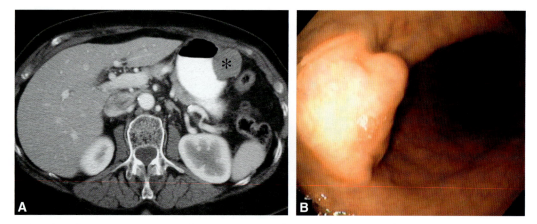

FIGURE 1.4.8 Gastric schwannoma. CT **(A)** and EGD **(B)** images show a submucosal soft tissue mass (*asterisk*) associated with the gastric wall, suggestive of a mesenchymal tumor. Pathologic evaluation after surgical resection revealed a gastric schwannoma.

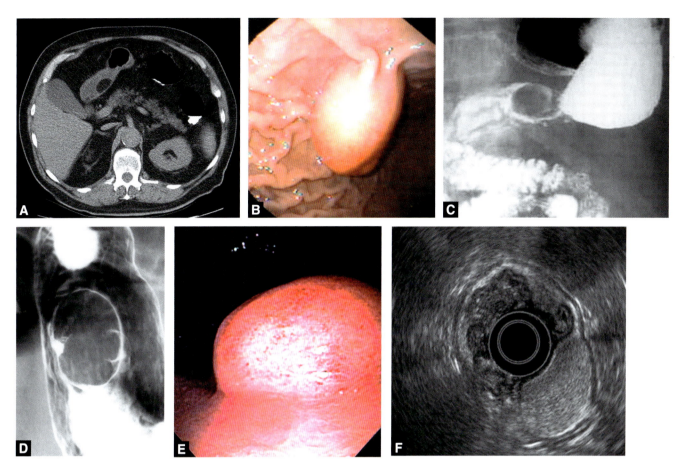

FIGURE 1.4.9 **Gastric lipomas.** Noncontrast CT image from CTC **(A)** shows an ovoid fat-attenuation lesion within the gastric antrum, diagnostic of lipoma. EGD image **(B)** from a second patient shows a similar smooth ovoid yellowish lesion, which was pliable at endoscopy with a positive "pillow sign." Barium UGI images **(C** and **D)** show well-defined ovoid filling defects; contrast fluoroscopy is less specific for the diagnosis. EGD **(E)** and EUS **(F)** images from a final patient show a homogeneously hyperechoic lesion originating from the submucosal layer, which is diagnostic for lipoma.

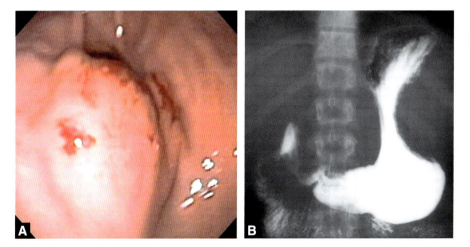

FIGURE 1.4.10 **Extrinsic impression.** EGD **(A)** and barium UGI **(B)** images from two patients show smooth broad-based impressions that are both caused by the adjacent spleen. The appearance of extrinsic impression may mimic an intramural lesion on luminal studies, but this distinction is clear on cross-sectional imaging such as CT.

1.5 Other Submucosal Tumors

(Figures 1.5.1-1.5.7)

CLINICAL FEATURES

- Beyond mesenchymal tumors, other tumors arising deep to the mucosa include hematogenous metastases, Kaposi's sarcoma, and carcinoid tumor.
- Common primary sites resulting in hematogenous metastases include melanoma, breast, and lung.
- Hematogenous tumor emboli seed the submucosa layer; ulcerated lesions may present with GI bleeding.
- Gastric Kaposi's sarcoma is almost always associated with AIDS; small bowel involvement is common.
- Carcinoid tumors are usually asymptomatic and can be sporadic or associated with atrophic gastritis or multiple endocrine neoplasia type 1 (MEN-1) syndrome; clinical carcinoid syndrome is rare and generally requires hepatic metastases.

IMAGING FEATURES

- Hematogenous metastases generally manifest as nonspecific submucosal masses; central ulceration gives rise to a "target" appearance at contrast fluoroscopy.
- Metastatic disease with submucosal infiltration can mimic linitis plastica (most often from breast cancer).
- Peritoneal carcinomatosis can secondarily involve the stomach.
- The differential diagnosis for ulcerating submucosal lesions includes hematogenous metastases, mesenchymal tumors (e.g., GIST), Kaposi's sarcoma, lymphoma, and carcinoid tumor.
- Kaposi's sarcoma can manifest as discrete submucosal lesions or irregular fold thickening from submucosal infiltration; at EGD, the lesions often have a purplish or reddish appearance.
- Sporadic carcinoid tumors are usually solitary and larger than those associated with atrophic gastritis, which are usually small and may be numerous.

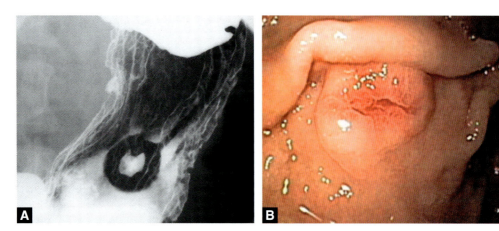

FIGURE 1.5.1 Hematogenous metastases. Image from barium UGI in a patient with lung cancer (**A**) shows a classic "target" or "bull's eye" submucosal metastasis with barium caught in the central ulcer crater. EGD image in a patient with renal cell carcinoma (**B**) shows a submucosal metastasis with early signs of central ulceration.

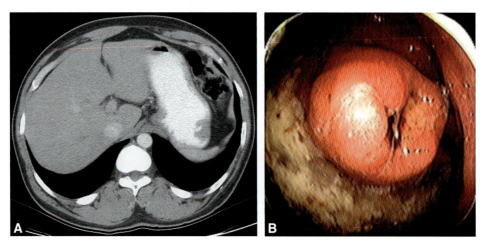

FIGURE 1.5.2 Metastatic melanoma. CT (**A**) and EGD (**B**) images show a typical ulcerated submucosal lesion in the gastric fundus.

OTHER SUBMUCOSAL TUMORS

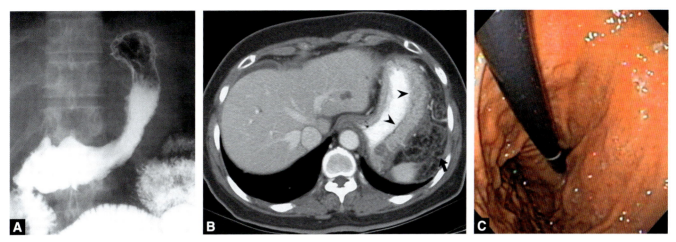

FIGURE 1.5.3   Linitis plastica appearance from metastatic breast cancer. Image from barium UGI (**A**) shows fixed luminal narrowing of the gastric fundus and body due to submucosal infiltration of tumor. CT image (**B**) in another patient shows gastric wall thickening (*arrowheads*) and perigastric soft tissue infiltration (*arrow*), reflecting peritoneal carcinomatosis. The corresponding EGD image in this patient (**C**) shows normal gastric mucosa; assessment for wall thickening at endoscopy would require EUS. Note the similarity to linitis plastica from primary gastric adenocarcinoma in these cases.

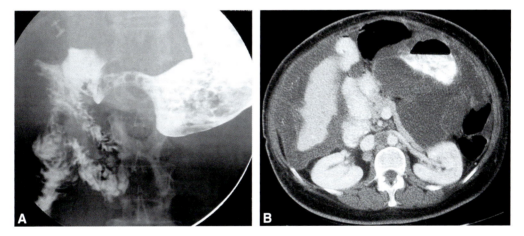

FIGURE 1.5.4   Extrinsic involvement by peritoneal carcinomatosis. Barium UGI (**A**) and CT (**B**) images in a patient with pseudomyxoma peritonei from mucinous adenocarcinoma of the appendix show antral narrowing related to extrinsic peritoneal disease. Solid intraluminal debris is present due to poor gastric emptying. Note also the unsuspected intestinal malrotation. *(From Pickhardt PJ, Bhalla S: Intestinal malrotation in adolescents and adults: Spectrum of clinical and imaging features. AJR 2002;179:1429-1435.)*

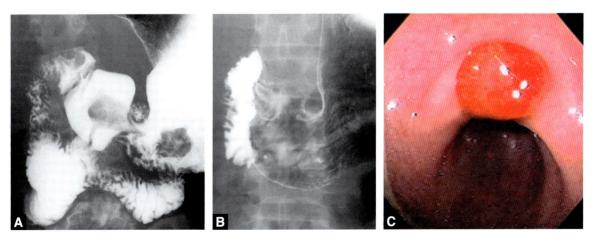

FIGURE 1.5.5   Kaposi's sarcoma. Single-contrast (**A**) and double-contrast (**B**) images from barium UGI in a patient with AIDS show multiple submucosal lesions, some of which have a target appearance from central ulceration. EGD image in a different AIDS patient (**C**) shows a polypoid lesion with a cherry-red appearance often seen with Kaposi's sarcoma.

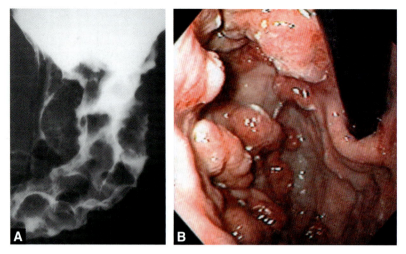

FIGURE 1.5.6 **Kaposi's sarcoma.** Images from barium UGI **(A)** and EGD **(B)** from two different patients show the more diffuse form of gastric Kaposi's sarcoma, manifesting as irregular lobulated fold thickening. Note the surface erosions and friable mucosa seen on the endoscopy image.

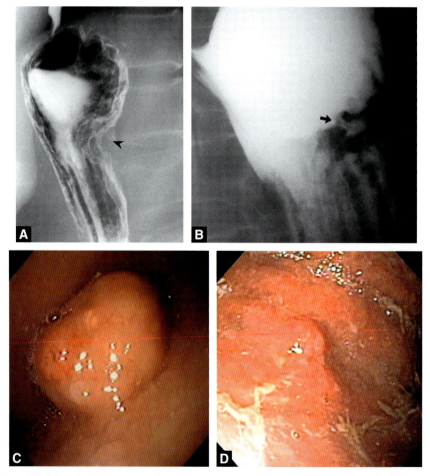

FIGURE 1.5.7 **Gastric carcinoid tumor.** Image from barium UGI **(A)** shows a submucosal filling defect (*arrowhead*). Barium UGI from a second patient **(B)** shows an ulcerated gastric lesion that traps barium (*arrow*). EGD image from a third patient **(C)** shows a large submucosal mass from carcinoid tumor. EGD image from a patient with autoimmune atrophic gastritis **(D)** shows a small erythematous nodule surrounded by mottled mucosa; other similar lesions were present.

2. GASTRITIS AND GASTROPATHY

Gastritis and gastropathies have a variety of imaging appearances, ranging from erythematous and thickened folds to large ulcerations and nodular, friable mucosa. Because these conditions are primarily superficial processes, luminal studies such as EGD and barium UGI remain the most effective means for evaluation. Differentiating between gastritis (with a significant mucosal inflammatory infiltrate) and gastropathy (without such inflammation) requires a good clinical history and histologic evaluation of the mucosa. In this section the imaging characteristics of these varied disease processes are reviewed, which may help differentiate among the broad list of possible diagnoses.

2.1 Peptic Ulcer Disease
(Figures 2.1.1-2.1.6)

CLINICAL FEATURES

- Peptic ulcer disease (PUD) is defined as ulceration related to injury from prolonged exposure to acid and pepsin.
- *H. pylori* and non-steroidal anti-inflammatory drugs (NSAIDs) are the major risk factors for PUD; eradication of *H. pylori*, if present, is important to facilitate healing.
- The majority of gastric ulcers are benign and related to PUD; however, follow-up EGD 6 to 8 weeks after therapy is standard to exclude an ulcerated malignancy.
- Peptic ulcers may present with epigastric pain, nausea, bleeding, iron deficiency, or gastric outlet obstruction; however, many ulcers are asymptomatic and may be found incidentally.

IMAGING FEATURES

- Frank ulcers extend past the muscularis mucosa into the submucosa and deeper layers; gastric erosions are epithelial defects confined to the mucosa.
- On barium UGI, benign gastric ulcers tend to retain contrast and project beyond the expected lumen in profile.
- En face, ulcers on UGI are typically surrounded by a smooth mound of edema, often with symmetrical folds radiating to the crater without interruption (compare with malignant ulcers earlier).
- Gastric ulcers may be initially detected at CT in patients with unexplained abdominal symptoms; perforated ulcers will manifest with free intraperitoneal air and/or fluid.
- Ulcers at EGD are readily identifiable as well-defined craters of mucosal breach with smooth regular edges.
- In the setting of acute blood loss, clean-based ulcers are at the lowest risk for re-bleeding (2%), as compared with those showing a pigmented spot (7%), adherent clot (33%), or visible vessel (50%).
- Ulcer size and location generally have no relevance to potential malignant cause.

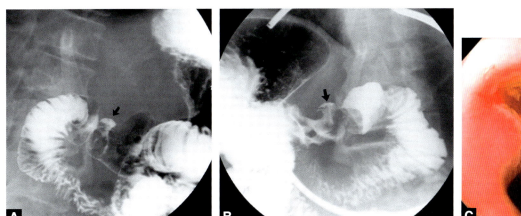
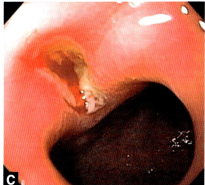

FIGURE 2.1.1 Benign gastric ulcers. Barium UGI images with double-contrast (**A**) and mucosal relief (**B**) techniques show a benign-appearing barium-filled ulcer (*arrows*) along the lesser curvature near the pyloric channel. EGD image (**C**) from a different patient shows a similar benign gastric ulcer with evidence of bleeding.

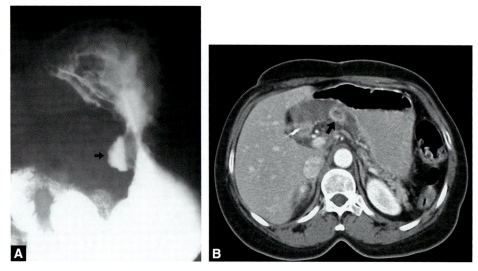

FIGURE 2.1.2 Benign ulcers in profile. Images from barium UGI **(A)** and CT **(B)** in two patients show benign gastric ulcers in profile (*arrows*). Note how the ulcer projects beyond the expected luminal contour at fluoroscopy and the prominent low-attenuation submucosal edema at CT.

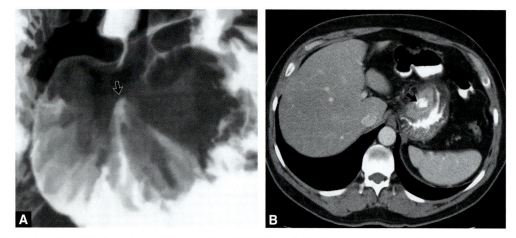

FIGURE 2.1.3 Benign ulcers en face. Images from barium UGI **(A)** and CT **(B)** in two patients show benign gastric ulcers seen en face (*arrows*). Note how the smooth gastric folds extend up to the ulcer crater at fluoroscopy and the surrounding mound of edema at CT.

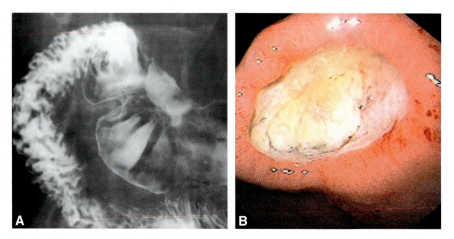

FIGURE 2.1.4 Large benign ulcers. Images from barium UGI **(A)** and EGD **(B)** in two patients show large benign ulcers involving the lesser curvature. Note the uniform folds extending to the ulcer crater at fluoroscopy and the clean base and smooth margins at endoscopy.

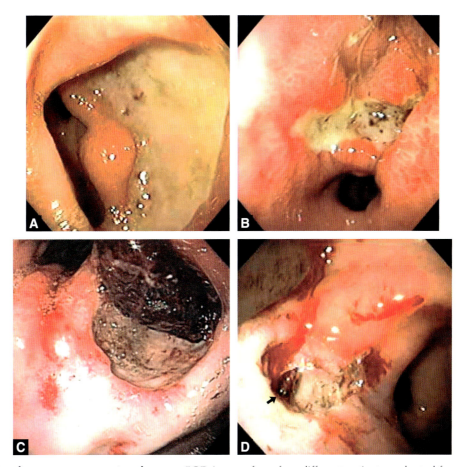

FIGURE 2.1.5 Ulcer base appearances at endoscopy. EGD images from four different patients evaluated for upper GI tract bleeding. The first case (**A**) shows a clean white ulcer base. The second case (**B**) shows multiple pigmented spots within a prepyloric ulcer. The third case (**C**) shows a large cratered ulcer with an adherent clot. The fourth case (**D**) shows a visible vessel (*arrows*) with active bleeding. Endoscopic therapy is indicated for ulcers with high-risk stigmata of re-bleeding (i.e., adherent clot, visible vessel, and active bleeding) because such treatment decreases the re-bleed rate by up to two thirds.

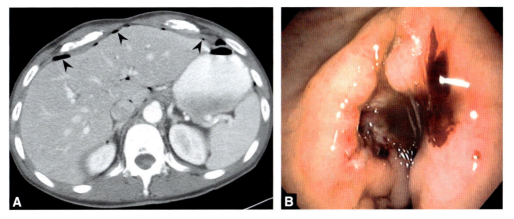

FIGURE 2.1.6 Complications from gastric ulcers. CT image (**A**) shows multiple gas bubbles (*arrowheads*) free within the peritoneal cavity (pneumoperitoneum) from a perforated gastric ulcer. EGD image (**B**) from a different patient shows a pyloric channel ulcer causing acute gastric outlet obstruction.

Illustration continued on following page

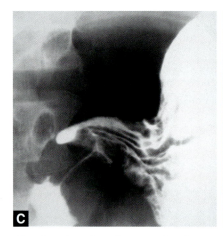
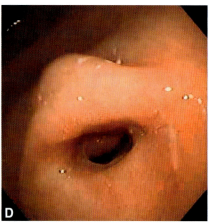

FIGURE 2.1.6 (Continued) **Complications from gastric ulcers.** Barium UGI (**C**) and EGD (**D**) images from two different patients show fixed pyloric thickening and luminal narrowing related to previous peptic ulcer disease. This has been referred to as "adult hypertrophic pyloric stenosis."

2.2 Reactive Gastropathies
(Figures 2.2.1-2.2.6)

CLINICAL FEATURES

- This is termed *gastropathy* secondary to the paucity of mucosal inflammatory infiltrate (seen at histology).
- A wide variety of causes include NSAIDs, alcohol use, radiation, bile acid reflux, trauma, and portal hypertensive gastropathy.
- Most patients are asymptomatic, but they can present with dyspepsia, occult blood loss, or acute hemorrhage.
- NSAIDs are the most common cause of gastropathy.
- Chronic radiation changes may present as frank ulceration or the development of mucosal angioectasia.
- Bile acid gastropathy is most common in post-antrectomy patients but may also occur post cholecystectomy.
- Forceful vomiting with gastric prolapse or nasogastric tube trauma may lead to focal subepithelial hemorrhage.
- Portal hypertensive gastropathy is due to chronic portal venous hypertension with the development of capillary and venous ectasias; it is an important cause of blood loss in cirrhotics.

IMAGING FEATURES

- A large spectrum of endoscopic characteristics can be seen based on the etiology.
- NSAID-induced erosions typically manifest on UGI as punctate barium collections with mild surrounding edema; they can be difficult to distinguish from innocuous barium precipitates if edema is absent.
- NSAID gastropathy is most often seen in the distal stomach, and the erosions are typically multiple and of similar size.
- Radiation changes to the mucosa include erythema, thickening, and visible angioectasias.
- Bile acid gastropathy is usually most severe in the distal stomach where the highest bile acid exposure is present.
- Traumatic gastropathy manifests as subepithelial hemorrhage and is usually localized based on the etiology.
- Portal hypertensive gastropathy has a wide range of appearances based on severity, from mild mucosal changes ("snakeskin pattern") to friable, edematous folds with spontaneous oozing.

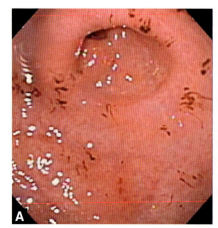
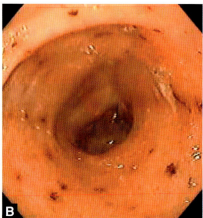

FIGURE 2.2.1 **NSAID gastropathy.** EGD images from two patients (**A** and **B**) show multiple punctate regions of recent bleeding without subepithelial hemorrhage.

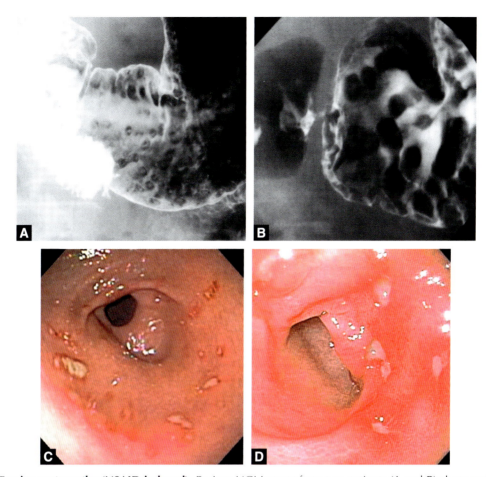

FIGURE 2.2.2 **Erosive gastropathy (NSAID induced).** Barium UGI images from two patients (**A** and **B**) show multiple punctate barium collections surrounded by a radiolucent rim of edema. The degree of inflammation present in the second case (**B**) is atypical. EGD images from two more patients (**C** and **D**) show multiple superficial erosions and ulcerations, respectively. Note relative uniformity of lesions and distribution within the antrum in all cases. NSAID gastropathy was the underlying cause in all four cases.

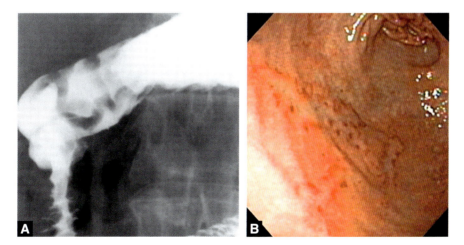

FIGURE 2.2.3 **Chronic radiation gastropathy.** Barium UGI image (**A**) shows gastric and duodenal fold thickening related to radiation therapy. EGD image (**B**) shows antral erythema with mucosal thickening and angioectasias from previous radiation therapy involving the upper abdomen.

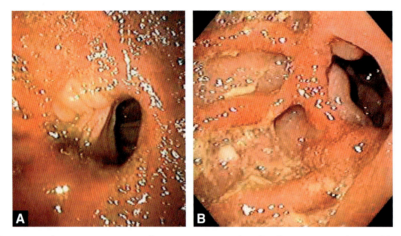

FIGURE 2.2.4 **Bile acid gastropathy.** EGD image **(A)** from a patient with Billroth I anatomy shows diffuse erythematous mucosa proximal to the anastomosis secondary to chronic bile exposure from duodenal reflux. Note the bile staining of the mucosa. EGD image **(B)** from a second patient status post Billroth I surgery shows thickened, erythematous folds just proximal to the anastomosis.

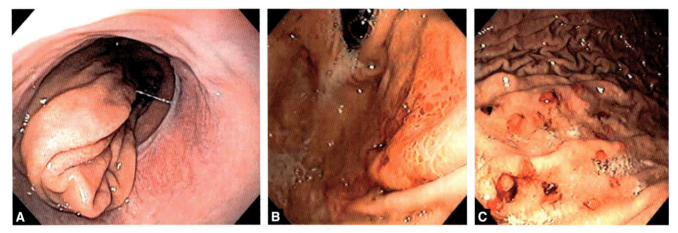

FIGURE 2.2.5 **Gastropathy related to repetitive trauma.** Repeated episodes of gastric mucosal prolapse **(A)** from repetitive retching and vomiting can lead to well-circumscribed areas of erythema and erosions due to subepithelial hemorrhage **(B)**. Subepithelial hemorrhage can also be seen from nasogastric tube suction trauma **(C)**, where the erythematous foci are circular and roughly the expected size of the tube.

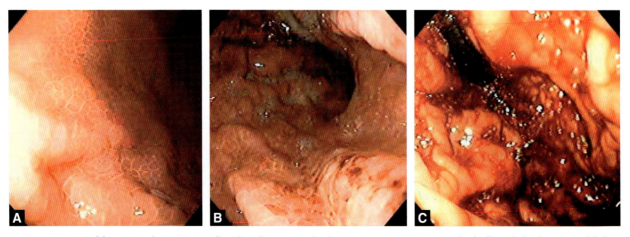

FIGURE 2.2.6 **Portal hypertensive gastropathy.** The classic "snakeskin" or mosaic pattern is the hallmark finding in mild disease **(A)**. Chronic *H. pylori* infection can have a similar appearance (see Fig. 2.4.1C). More advanced disease can lead to punctate erythema and submucosal hemorrhage **(B)** or diffuse mucosal oozing with significant blood loss **(C)**.

2.3 Zollinger-Ellison Syndrome
(Figures 2.3.1-2.3.2)

CLINICAL FEATURES
- This syndrome is secondary to a functioning gastrinoma (pancreatic > duodenal primary) that results in hypergastrinemia, increased acid production, and, ultimately, formation of multiple ulcers.
- It often presents as epigastric discomfort similar to PUD and/or chronic malabsorptive diarrhea due to the effect on pancreatic enzymes and intestinal mucosa.
- The majority of cases occur in isolation, but some are associated with MEN-1.
- Gastrin level >1000 pg/mL not in the setting of achlorhydria is highly specific for Zollinger-Ellison syndrome.

IMAGING FEATURES
- Imaging features include diffuse gastric fold thickening and multiple ulcers involving the stomach and duodenum.
- The presence of postbulbar duodenal ulcers should suggest the possibility of this syndrome (see Chapter 3).
- Evidence of severe erosive esophagitis may also be seen at imaging (see Chapter 1).
- CT or MR may demonstrate the underlying gastrinoma and evaluate for possible hepatic metastases.
- EUS can often identify small (<1 cm) tumors in the pancreas or duodenum not seen by noninvasive imaging.
- Octreotide scintigraphy can help to localize the lesion and assess for metastatic disease (see Chapter 7).

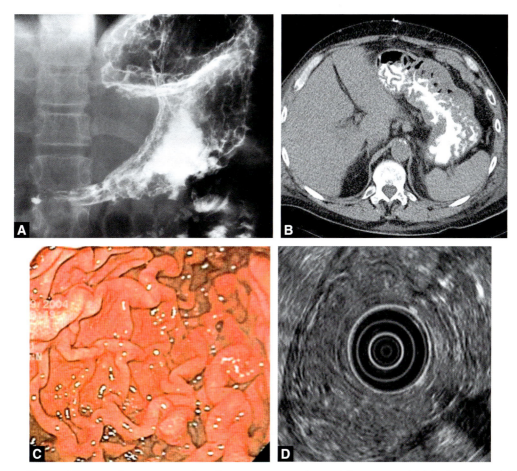

FIGURE 2.3.1 Zollinger-Ellison syndrome. Image from barium UGI (**A**) shows diffuse gastric fold thickening and focal ulceration. CT image (**B**) in a second patient shows prominent thickening of the gastric folds and gastric wall. EGD (**C**) and EUS (**D**) images from a third patient show enlarged rugae caused by significant hypertrophy of the mucosal layer of the stomach wall.

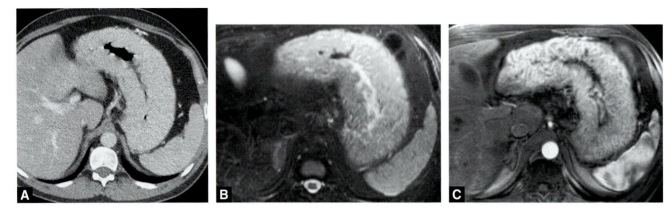

FIGURE 2.3.2 Zollinger-Ellison syndrome. CT image (A) shows massive diffuse gastric wall thickening with prominent contrast enhancement. Fat-suppressed T2-weighted MR image (B) shows increased signal throughout the thickened gastric wall. Fat-suppressed post-contrast T1-weighted SGE image (C) shows prominent contrast enhancement of the gastric wall. A gastrinoma was present within the "gastrinoma triangle" region (not shown).

2.4 Infectious Gastritis
(Figures 2.4.1-2.4.5)

CLINICAL FEATURES

- *H. pylori* is the most common gastric infection worldwide; gastritis and ulcer disease are common manifestations, but chronic infection is also associated with adenocarcinoma and MALT lymphoma.
- Cytomegalovirus (CMV) gastritis is usually seen in the setting of immunocompromise; presentation can include severe pain and bleeding.
- Emphysematous gastritis is typically caused by significant injury with subsequent infection from a gas-forming organism; it is associated with a high mortality.
- Other atypical gastric infections include various bacterial, fungal, viral, and parasitic diseases (mycobacterial infection is covered in the following section).

IMAGING FEATURES

- *H. pylori* gastritis typically presents as nonspecific inflammation involving the gastric corpus; varied appearances at EGD also include follicular and mosaic forms, with or without associated ulcers.
- CMV gastritis manifests on imaging with prominent mucosal nodularity, fold thickening, and ulcers; the severity of findings can range from focal and mild to diffuse and severe.
- Secondary syphilis may present as erosions, irregular ulcers, or mucosal nodules; tertiary syphilis can result in scarring with antral narrowing that is indistinguishable from lesions of other causes.
- Emphysematous gastritis is diagnosed by intramural gas seen on radiologic imaging; CT is more sensitive for detection than conventional radiography.
- EGD can be useful for both diagnosis and treatment of some gastric roundworm infestations.

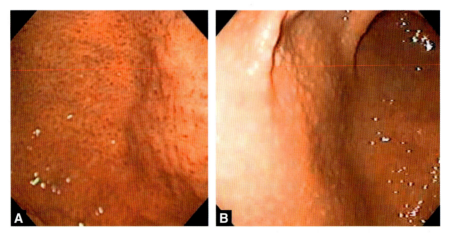

FIGURE 2.4.1 Spectrum of endoscopic findings in *H. pylori* gastritis. EGD images from two patients with *H. pylori* gastritis show nonspecific red-mottled inflammation (A) and a nodular or follicular appearance (B).

Illustration continued on following page

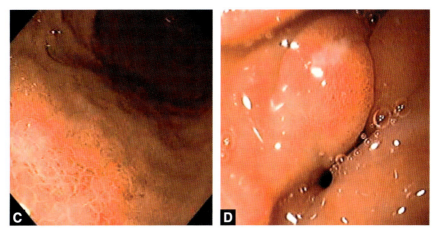

FIGURE 2.4.1 (Continued)   **Spectrum of endoscopic findings in *H. pylori* gastritis.** EGD images from two additional patients with *H. pylori* gastritis show a mosaic appearance (**C**) and inflammation with ulceration (**D**).

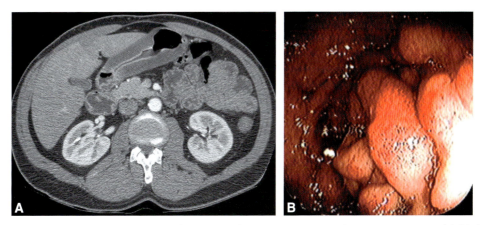

FIGURE 2.4.2   ***H. pylori* gastritis.** CT image (**A**) and corresponding EGD image (**B**) show extensive antral fold thickening, which demonstrates submucosal low attenuation at CT.

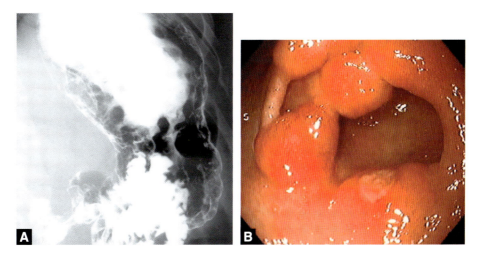

FIGURE 2.4.3   **CMV gastritis.** Barium UGI (**A**) and EGD (**B**) images from two immunocompromised patients show prominent inflammatory fold thickening from CMV. Ulceration is apparent at EGD.

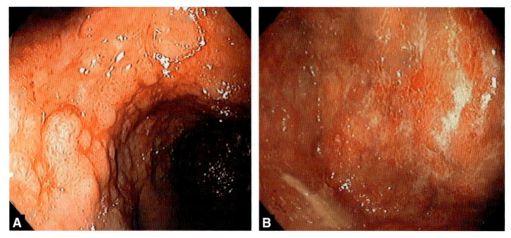

FIGURE 2.4.4 **Gastric syphilis.** EGD images (**A** and **B**) in a patient with tertiary syphilis show diffuse mucosal inflammation with erythema, friability, and nodularity. Inflammation involves the entire stomach in this case, but can also manifest as focal ulceration.

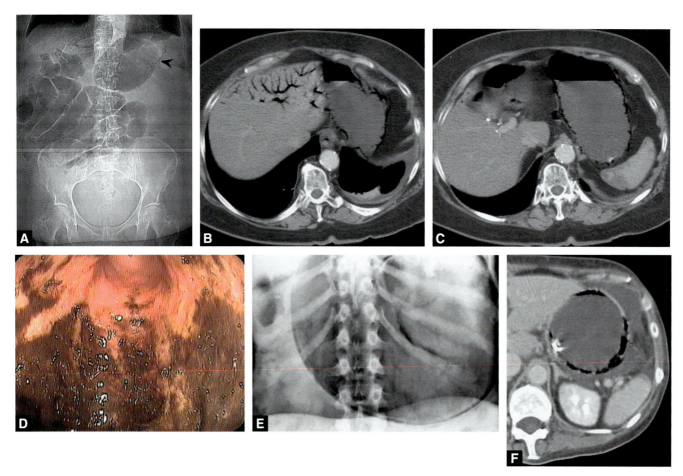

FIGURE 2.4.5 **Emphysematous gastritis.** CT scout radiograph (**A**) shows subtle linear air tracking along the gastric wall (*arrowhead*), as well as portal venous gas. However, these findings are much more apparent on the transverse CT images (**B** and **C**). Subsequent EGD image (**D**) shows extensive mucosal necrosis and ulceration. The patient did well with conservative medical treatment. Conventional radiograph (**E**) and CT image (**F**) show gastric pneumatosis from two additional patients.

2.5 Granulomatous Diseases

(Figures 2.5.1-2.5.4)

CLINICAL FEATURES

- Granulomatous diseases affecting the stomach include Crohn's disease, sarcoidosis, and tuberculosis.
- Gastric Crohn's disease usually occurs in patients with known ileocolonic disease and is usually not symptomatic until its later stages; gastrocolic fistulas may result (see section 3.3).
- Gastric sarcoidosis is typically asymptomatic unless advanced; although uncommon, the stomach is the most frequent GI site of involvement.
- Tuberculous gastritis is rare and usually associated with generalized disease.

IMAGING FEATURES

- Granulomatous diseases have a general predilection for the distal gastric body and antrum.
- As with other sites, aphthoid ulcers are the earliest manifestation of Crohn's disease, followed by deeper ulcers, nodular fold thickening, and fistula formation; antroduodenal scarring may have a "ram's horn" configuration.
- Sarcoidosis may present with irregular fold thickening and luminal narrowing.
- Tuberculosis can present with ulcers of the antrum and pylorus, which may lead to scarring and outlet obstruction; as with Crohn's disease, fistula formation is possible.

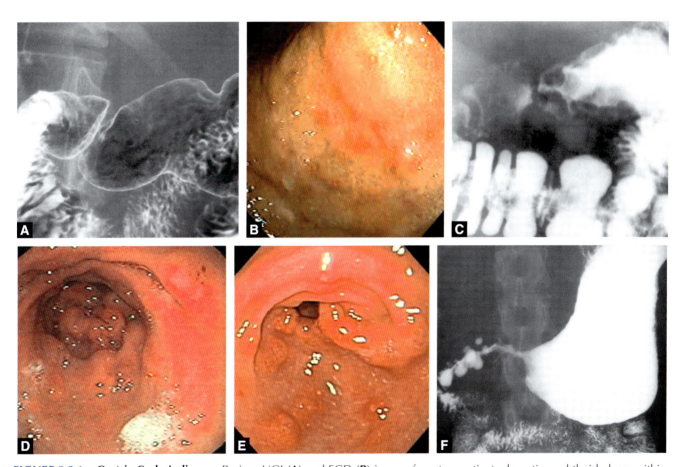

FIGURE 2.5.1 Gastric Crohn's disease. Barium UGI (**A**) and EGD (**B**) images from two patients show tiny aphthoid ulcers within the gastric antrum representing early findings. Barium UGI (**C**) and EGD (**D**) images from a third patient and EGD image from a fourth patient (**E**) show nodular antral inflammation and ulceration. Barium UGI from a fifth patient (**F**) shows severe antroduodenal scarring with luminal narrowing and diverticular outpouchings from long-standing Crohn's disease.

Illustration continued on following page

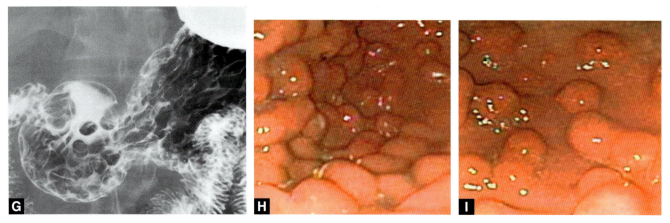

FIGURE 2.5.1 (Continued)   **Gastric Crohn's disease.** Barium UGI (**G**) and EGD (**H** and **I**) images from a final patient show innumerable polypoid lesions believed to represent postinflammatory polyposis from long-standing disease.

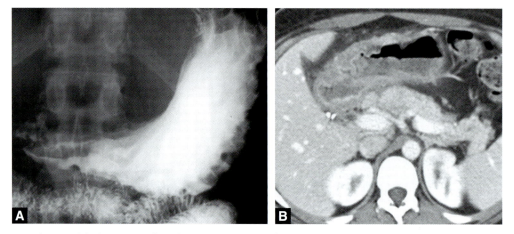

FIGURE 2.5.2   **Gastric sarcoidosis.** Images from barium UGI (**A**) and CT (**B**) from two different patients show gastric fold thickening and low-attenuation wall thickening, respectively.

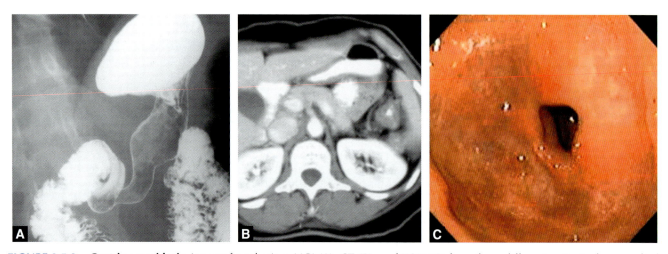

FIGURE 2.5.3   **Gastric sarcoidosis.** Images from barium UGI (**A**), CT (**B**), and EGD (**C**) from three different patients show marked narrowing of the distal stomach with a relatively featureless appearance on barium and CT, likely indicative of long-standing disease. Endoscopically, the mucosa appears diffusely erythematous and mottled.

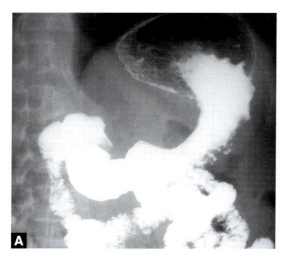
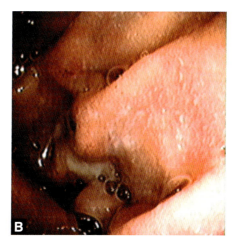

FIGURE 2.5.4 **Gastric tuberculosis.** Barium UGI image (**A**) shows fixed narrowing and irregularity of the gastric body and antrum. EGD image (**B**) from a second patient shows mucosal inflammation and multiple small erosions from gastroduodenal tuberculosis.

2.6 Ménétrier's Disease
(Figures 2.6.1-2.6.3)

CLINICAL FEATURES

- This disease is also classically referred to as hypertrophic gastropathy.
- It is a rare entity characterized by giant hypertrophied gastric folds with epithelial/foveolar hyperplasia.
- Clinical features include a protein-losing gastropathy with hypochlorhydria.
- Presenting symptoms may include epigastric pain, nausea, vomiting, diarrhea, and weight loss.

IMAGING FEATURES

- Marked thickening of folds occurs predominantly in the gastric fundus and body, often with relative sparing of the antrum; the disease rarely presents as a more focal lesion simulating a polypoid carcinoma.
- Massively enlarged folds can have a "cerebriform" appearance at imaging.
- Although the diagnosis may be suggested based on the imaging appearance, biopsy is necessary to exclude neoplastic infiltration.

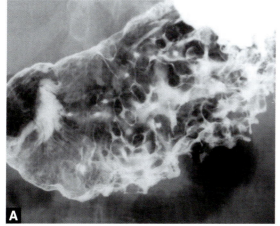
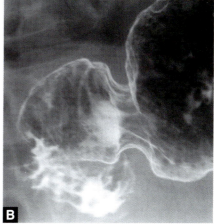

FIGURE 2.6.1 Barium UGI images show massive fold thickening of the proximal stomach (**A**) with sparing of the antrum (**B**).

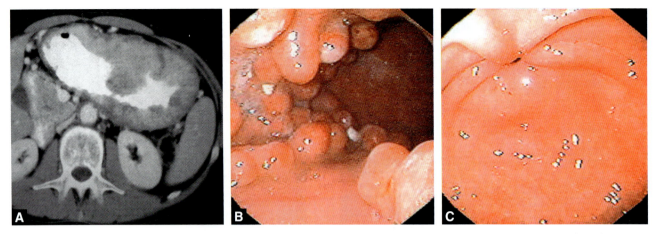

FIGURE 2.6.2 **Ménétrier's disease.** CT **(A)** and EGD **(B** and **C)** images from two different patients show massive fold thickening of the proximal stomach with relative sparing of the antrum.

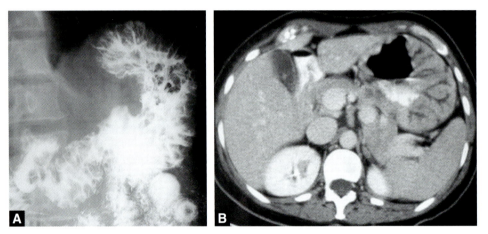

FIGURE 2.6.3 **Ménétrier's disease.** Barium UGI **(A)** and CT **(B)** images from two different patients show prominent "cerebriform" thickening of the gastric folds.

2.7 Other Inflammatory Conditions
(Figures 2.7.1-2.7.8)

CLINICAL FEATURES

- Atrophic gastritis may be due to an autoimmune process (type A) or various insults, including chronic *H. pylori* infection (type B); it is associated with an increased risk for gastric adenocarcinoma.
- Antibodies to parietal cells in autoimmune atrophic gastritis lead to pernicious anemia and achlorhydria, which predisposes to an increased risk of developing carcinoid tumors.
- Eosinophilic gastritis is characterized by eosinophilic infiltration of the gastric wall, with or without peripheral eosinophilia; response to corticosteroid therapy is typical, but relapses can occur.
- Caustic ingestion of either an alkali or acid substance may lead to extensive injury; acids affect the distal stomach and duodenum, whereas alkaline substances tend to affect the esophagus more.
- Additional causes of gastric inflammation include pancreatitis, vasculitis, and graft-versus-host disease.

IMAGING FEATURES

- Type A atrophic gastritis (diffuse corporal atrophic gastritis) typically involves the fundus and body whereas type B (multifocal atrophic gastritis) is antral predominant but may also involve the corpus.
- EGD findings of atrophic gastritis include a pale or shiny mucosa, loss of folds, and prominence of the submucosal vessels.
- Imaging features of eosinophilic gastritis range from mild erosions and mucosal nodularity to wall thickening and ascites; primary muscle layer involvement may cause pyloric obstruction.
- The acute phase of caustic ingestion may demonstrate ulceration, thickened folds, hemorrhage, or frank necrosis; scarring with luminal narrowing and outlet obstruction marks the reparative and chronic phases.
- Extrinsic inflammation from acute pancreatitis primarily involves the posterior stomach, which contacts the lesser sac.

OTHER INFLAMMATORY CONDITIONS

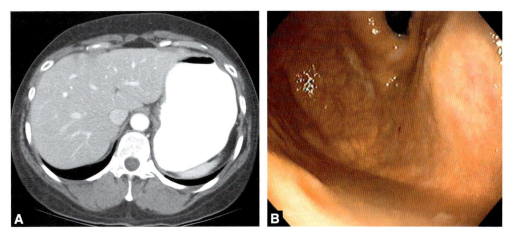

FIGURE 2.7.1 **Atrophic gastritis (type A).** CT image **(A)** in a patient with pernicious anemia shows featureless thinning of the gastric wall. Corresponding EGD image **(B)** shows mucosal pallor with loss of the normal rugal fold pattern.

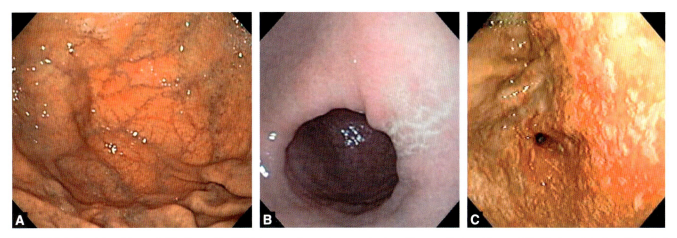

FIGURE 2.7.2 **Atrophic gastritis (type B).** EGD images from three patients with type B atrophic gastritis likely related to *H. pylori* show thin fundal mucosa with prominence of the submucosal vessels **(A)**, loss of rugal folds with a mottled appearance to the antral mucosa **(B)**, and antral erythema punctuated by pale raised areas representing foci of intestinal metaplasia **(C)**.

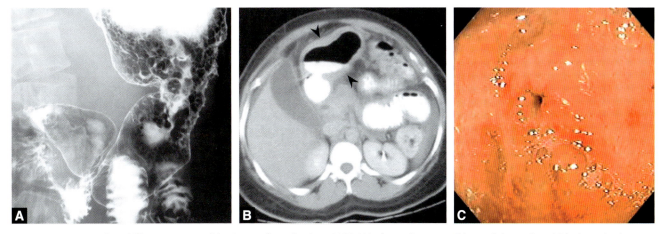

FIGURE 2.7.3 **Eosinophilic gastroenteritis.** Image from barium UGI **(A)** shows innumerable nodular polypoid lesions in the proximal stomach. CT image from a second patient **(B)** shows gastric wall thickening (*arrowheads*), as well as small bowel wall thickening and peritoneal disease from extensive eosinophilic gastroenteritis. EGD image from a third patient **(C)** shows mucosal inflammation and mild nodularity.

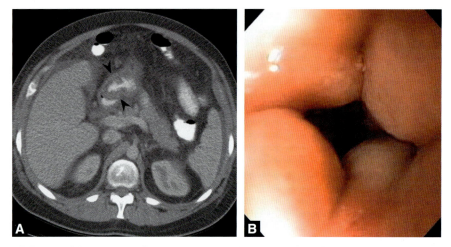

FIGURE 2.7.4 **Eosinophilic gastritis.** CT **(A)** and EGD **(B)** images show antral fold thickening (**A**, *arrowheads*) without mucosal abnormality due to submucosal involvement by eosinophilic gastritis.

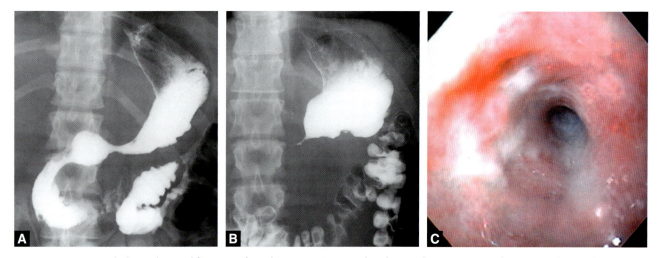

FIGURE 2.7.5 **Caustic ingestion (acid).** Image from barium UGI 2 weeks after acid ingestion **(A)** shows antral irregularity and narrowing. Repeat barium **(B)** and EGD **(C)** evaluation at 3 weeks show significant progression of antral scarring with high-grade gastric outlet obstruction.

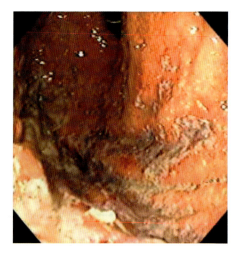

FIGURE 2.7.6 **Caustic ingestion (alkali).** EGD image in a patient after ingestion of bleach shows severe inflammation and mucosal sloughing in the gastric fundus and proximal body.

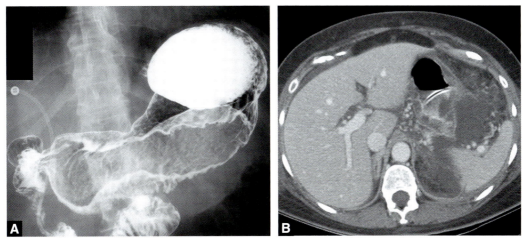

FIGURE 2.7.7 Gastric inflammation secondary to pancreatitis. Barium UGI (**A**) and CT (**B**) images from two different patients show secondary involvement of the posterior stomach with mass effect at fluoroscopy (**A**) and low-attenuation wall thickening with perigastric inflammation at CT (**B**).

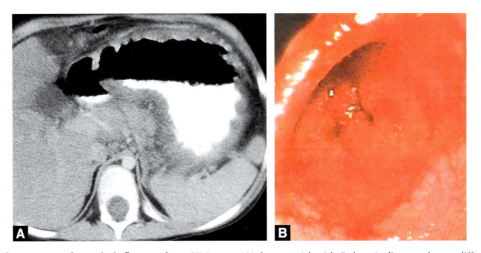

FIGURE 2.7.8 Other causes of gastric inflammation. CT image (**A**) from a girl with Behçet's disease shows diffuse gastric wall thickening related to underlying vasculitis. EGD image (**B**) in a patient with graft-versus-host disease shows severe antral inflammation with diffuse mucosal sloughing.

3. OTHER GASTRIC CONDITIONS

3.1 Vascular Lesions
(Figures 3.1.1-3.1.6)

CLINICAL FEATURES

- Vascular lesions of the stomach include a variety of arterial and venous entities.
- Gastric telangiectasias or arteriovenous malformations may occur sporadically or in the setting of Osler-Weber-Rendu syndrome (hereditary hemorrhagic telangiectasia).
- Dieulafoy's lesion (exulceratio simplex) consists of an abnormally large-caliber artery in the submucosa, often with an overlying mucosal defect; this is a rare but serious cause of massive spontaneous GI hemorrhage.
- Blue rubber bleb nevus syndrome is a rare entity characterized by multiple cutaneous and GI venous hemangiomas.
- Gastric varices can occur in isolation with splenic vein thrombosis or in conjunction with esophageal varices in the setting of portal hypertension.
- Gastric antral vascular ectasia (GAVE) is characterized by tortuous vascular channels radiating from the pylorus and may present as either acute or chronic blood loss.
- Gastric wall hematomas may result from iatrogenic or other traumatic injury, tumor, or underlying bleeding diathesis.

IMAGING FEATURES

- Telangiectasias are readily visible at EGD as focal cherry-red lesions but generally have no radiologic correlate.
- Dieulafoy's lesion is most often located 6 cm distal to the gastroesophageal junction; active arterial "spurting" may be identified at EGD.
- Gastric venous hemangiomas in blue rubber bleb nevus syndrome appear as smooth submucosal lesions with a bluish hue at EGD.

- Gastric varices appear as lobulated tubular or even mass-like structures involving the fundus and proximal body at barium UGI; venous enhancement and the underlying cause are usually evident at CT.
- Dilated submucosal veins at EGD can generally be distinguished from actual fold thickening.
- A characteristic "watermelon" appearance of the antrum at EGD typifies GAVE.
- Gastric hematomas are submucosal in location and may compromise the lumen if they are large.

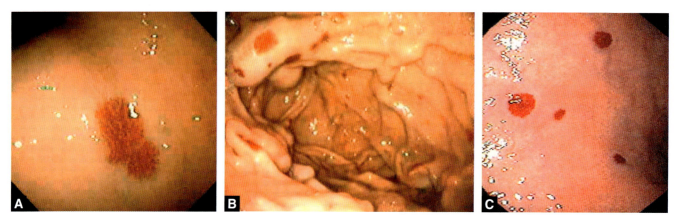

FIGURE 3.1.1 Gastric telangiectasias. Image from EGD **(A)** shows a typical solitary cherry-red telangiectasia. EGD images **(B and C)** from two patients with hereditary hemorrhagic telangiectasia (Osler-Weber-Rendu syndrome) show multiple gastric telangiectasias.

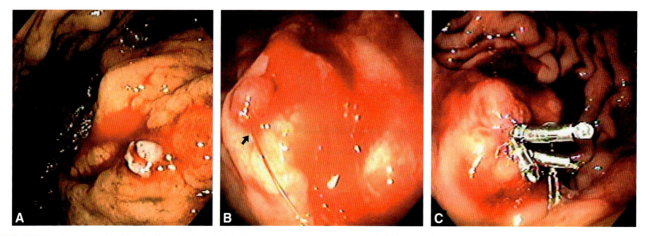

FIGURE 3.1.2 Gastric Dieulafoy's lesion. EGD image **(A)** shows a mucosal defect without surrounding ulceration that contains a visible vessel with evidence of recent bleeding. Initial EGD image from a second patient **(B)** shows active bleeding (*arrow*) from a Dieulafoy's lesion, which was successfully controlled by endoscopic clipping **(C)**.

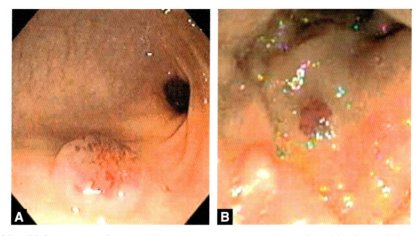

FIGURE 3.1.3 Blue rubber bleb nevus syndrome. EGD images from two patients show bluish-purplish submucosal nodules, including a large classic-appearing lesion with a wrinkled surface (**A**) and a smaller one with an almost macular appearance (**B**).

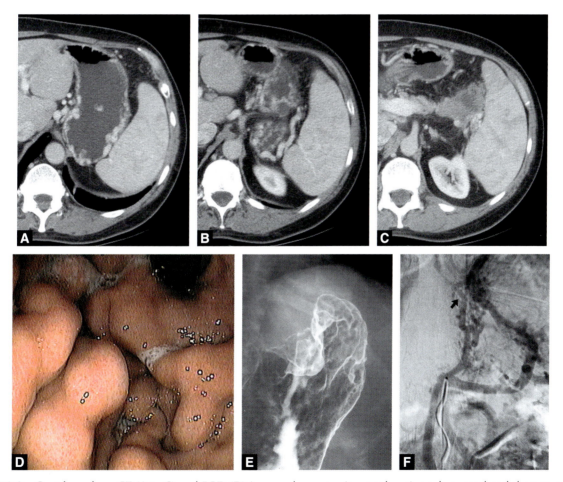

FIGURE 3.1.4 Gastric varices. CT (**A** to **C**) and EGD (**D**) images show prominent enhancing submucosal and short gastric varices resulting from splenic vein thrombosis due to a pancreatic-tail mucinous cystadenocarcinoma. Barium UGI image (**E**) from a different patient with splenic vein thrombosis shows a large lobulated fundal filling defect due to gastric varices. Delayed venous phase from digital subtraction angiography (**F**) from another patient with splenic vein thrombosis shows prominent gastric varices (*arrow*).

Illustration continued on following page

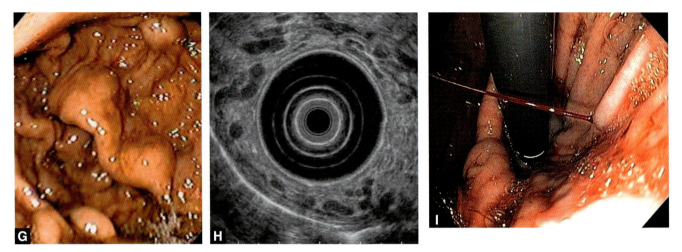

FIGURE 3.1.4 (Continued) **Gastric varices.** EGD (**G**) and EUS (**H**) images show submucosal gastric varices, which appear sonographically as tortuous hypoechoic channels. Retroflexed EGD image (**I**) from a final patient with a history of alcohol abuse and hematemesis shows a briskly bleeding gastric varix. Hemostasis was achieved via endoscopic banding (not shown).

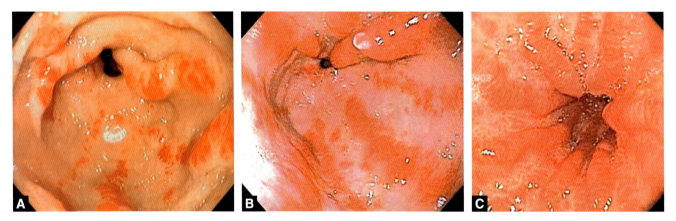

FIGURE 3.1.5 **Gastric antral vascular ectasia (GAVE).** EGD images (**A** to **C**) from three patients show multiple vascular lesions in a linear array of varying degrees of severity.

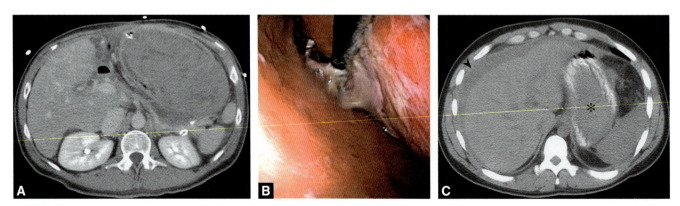

FIGURE 3.1.6 **Gastric hematoma.** CT (**A**) and EGD (**B**) images show a large intramural gastric hematoma that significantly compromises the gastric lumen. Note the displaced nasogastric tube. Noncontrast CT image (**C**) from a patient with hemophilia A shows a spontaneous intramural gastric hematoma (*asterisk*) that displaces the gastric folds. The high-attenuation peritoneal fluid represents hemoperitoneum (*arrowhead*).

3.2 Gastric Hernias

(Figures 3.2.1-3.2.8)

CLINICAL FEATURES

- Hiatal hernias can be classified as sliding, paraesophageal, or mixed; intrathoracic stomach represents an extreme form of hiatal hernia.
- Sliding hiatal hernias result from weakening of the phrenoesophageal membrane with elevation of the gastroesophageal junction into the thorax; although associated with reflux, either can exist without the other.
- Paraesophageal hernias maintain position of the gastroesophageal junction, with herniation of another portion of stomach or other viscus; risk for strangulation is much greater compared with the sliding type.
- Cameron lesions are found in about 5% of patients with hiatal hernias and represent a common cause of occult blood loss; they are most often seen in large hiatal hernias.
- Morgagni's hernias occur through an anteromedial diaphragmatic defect and more often contain omentum or colon.
- Traumatic diaphragmatic rupture often presents in delayed fashion if not repaired at the time of initial injury.

IMAGING FEATURES

- Hiatal hernias are best evaluated on real-time fluoroscopic GI studies; large persistent hernias are often apparent at other radiologic imaging studies and at EGD.
- Cameron lesions are characterized by mucosal erosions at the level of the diaphragmatic hiatus.
- Morgagni hernias present as right cardiophrenic angle masses on chest radiographs; CT is useful for confirmation and differentiation from other causes.
- Chest radiographs may demonstrate elevation of the "gastric bubble" in traumatic diaphragmatic injury, which can be confirmed with contrast evaluation; CT, however, is generally more accurate.

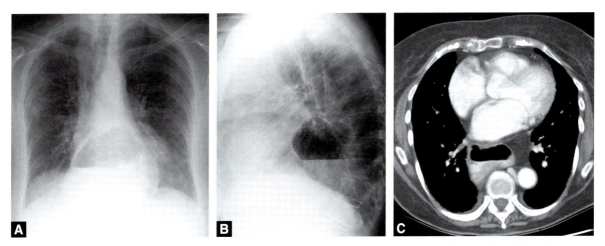

FIGURE 3.2.1 **Sliding hiatal hernia.** Frontal (**A**) and lateral (**B**) chest radiographs show a moderate to large hiatal hernia characterized as a middle mediastinal structure with an air-fluid level. CT image in the same patient (**C**) shows similar findings.

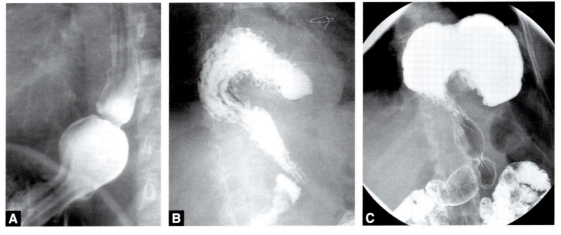

FIGURE 3.2.2 **Sliding hiatal hernia.** Barium UGI studies from three patients show small (**A**) and large (**B** and **C**) sliding hiatal hernias. The smaller hernia was associated with a Schatzki ring and gastroesophageal reflux.

Illustration continued on following page

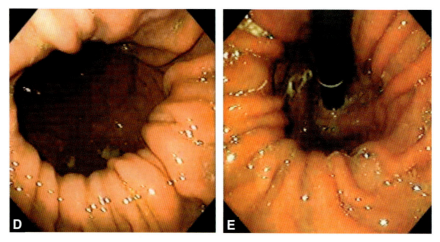

FIGURE 3.2.2 (Continued) **Sliding hiatal hernia.** EGD images from another patient show a sliding hiatal hernia from above (**D**) and below (**E**) the diaphragmatic hiatus.

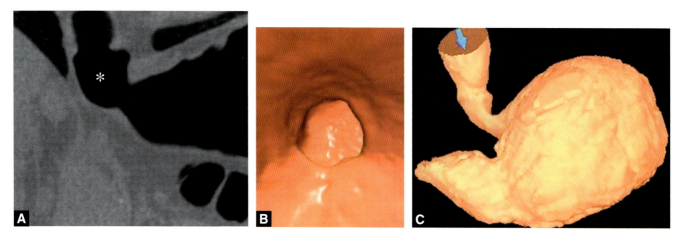

FIGURE 3.2.3 **Sliding hiatal hernia.** Coronal CT image (**A**) of a gas-filled stomach shows a small hiatal hernia (*asterisk*), separated from the esophagus by a slightly prominent B-ring. Endoluminal 3D view (**B**) from the vantage point demonstrated on the surface rendered map (**C**, *arrow*) shows the B-ring leading to the hiatal hernia.

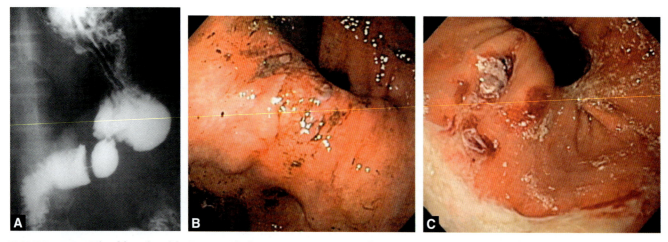

FIGURE 3.2.4 **Hiatal hernia with Cameron lesion.** Barium UGI (**A**) and EGD (**B** and **C**) images from three different patients show varying degrees of erosions, ulcerations, and old blood at the edge of the hernia sac at the level of the diaphragmatic hiatus.

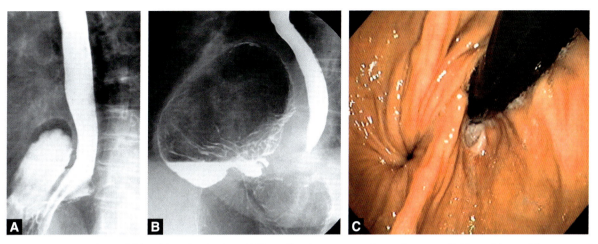

FIGURE 3.2.5 **Paraesophageal hiatal hernia.** Barium UGI studies from two patients show small (**A**) and large (**B**) paraesophageal hernias. Retroflexed view from EGD in a third patient (**C**) shows a narrowed orifice adjacent to the gastroesophageal junction that leads to a paraesophageal hernia. The narrow twisted appearance in **B** and **C** can suggest increased risk for torsion with vascular compromise.

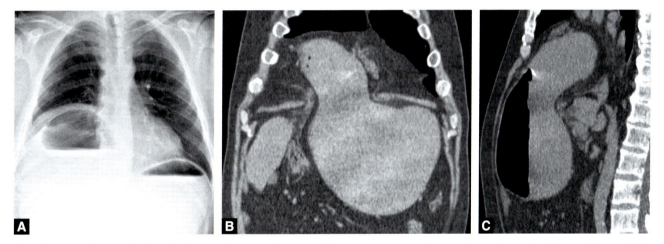

FIGURE 3.2.6 **Morgagni's hernia.** Upright frontal radiograph (**A**) shows an unusual large right-sided air-fluid level. Coronal (**B**) and sagittal (**C**) CT images show gastric herniation through a prominent anterior diaphragmatic defect, which gives rise to the radiographic appearance.

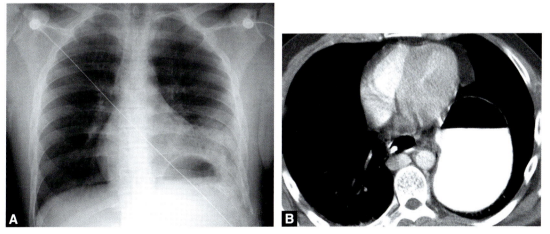

FIGURE 3.2.7 **Traumatic diaphragmatic herniation (acute).** Trauma chest radiograph (**A**) and CT image (**B**) from two different patients show acute diaphragmatic herniation of the stomach.

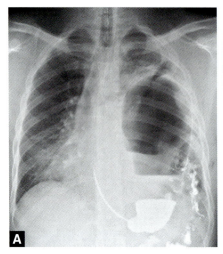
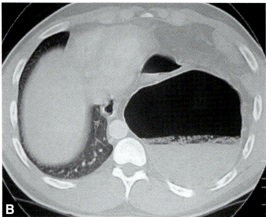

FIGURE 3.2.8 Traumatic diaphragmatic herniation (delayed). Upright chest radiograph **(A)** and CT image **(B)** show delayed diaphragmatic herniation of the stomach from prior trauma.

3.3 Gastric Fistulas

(Figures 3.3.1-3.3.3)

CLINICAL FEATURES

- Gastrocolic fistulas are among the most common acquired GI fistulas, often presenting as foul-smelling eructation or diarrhea.
- NSAID-induced gastric ulcers are the major cause of gastrocolic fistulas, followed by other causes such as Crohn's disease, malignancy, trauma, radiation, and percutaneous endoscopic gastrostomy (PEG) placement (see section 3.9).
- Gastroduodenal channels from prior PUD represent a localized fistula.
- In general, fistulas can conceivably occur between the stomach and nearly any adjacent structure; rare examples include gastropericardial, gastropleural, and gastrojejunal fistulas.

IMAGING FEATURES

- Fluoroscopic contrast studies are useful in evaluating for suspected fistulas; contrast enema is theoretically more effective than UGI evaluation for gastrocolic fistulas.
- CT and endoscopy both can play an important role in distinguishing benign from malignant causes.
- Gastroduodenal fistulas appear as a double-channel pylorus on imaging.

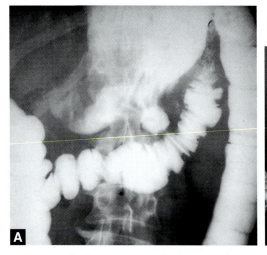
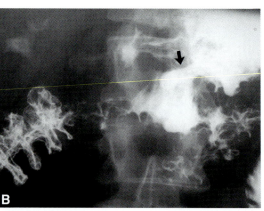

FIGURE 3.3.1 Gastrocolic fistulas. Image from BE **(A)** shows opacification of the stomach via a gastrocolic fistula due to a large penetrating greater curve ulcer from NSAID use. Note uniformly thickened folds leading to the ulcer crater. Barium UGI image **(B)** from another patient shows a gastrocolic fistula (*arrow*) due to Crohn's disease. (A, from Pickhardt PJ, Bhalla S, Balfe DM: Acquired gastrointestinal fistulas: Classification, etiologies, and imaging evaluation. Radiology 2002;224:9-23.)

Illustration continued on following page

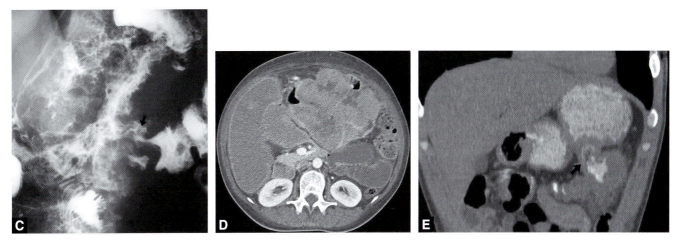

FIGURE 3.3.1 (Continued) **Gastrocolic fistulas.** Barium evaluation **(C)** and CT image **(D)** from two different patients with gastrocolic fistulas **(C,** *arrow*) from gastric adenocarcinoma. Invasion of the transverse colon in D has resulted in colonic obstruction. Coronal CT image **(E)** in a different patient shows a gastrocolic fistula (*arrow*) due to adenocarcinoma of the transverse colon.

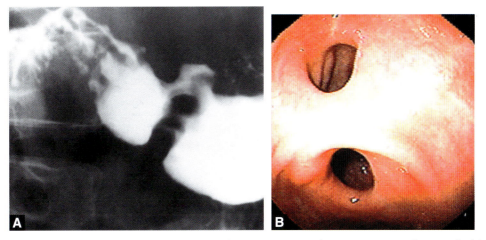

FIGURE 3.3.2 **Gastroduodenal channel.** Barium UGI **(A)** and EGD **(B)** images from two patients show a "double pylorus" appearance from gastroduodenal fistulas related to previous PUD.

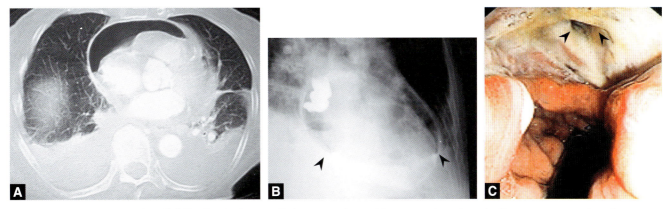

FIGURE 3.3.3 **Gastropericardial fistula.** CT image **(A)** from a patient with acute epigastric pain shows pneumopericardium. Subsequent fluoroscopic evaluation with water-soluble contrast **(B)** shows an air-contrast level within the pericardial space (*arrowheads*). At EGD **(C)**, a gastropericardial fistula due to a penetrating ulcer within a hiatal hernia was confirmed (*arrowheads*). *(From Pickhardt PJ, Bhalla S: Spontaneous pneumopericardium secondary to penetrating benign gastric ulcer. Clin Radiol 2000;55:798-800.)*

3.4 Heterotopic Pancreatic Rest

(Figures 3.4.1-3.4.2)

CLINICAL FEATURES

- This anatomic variant results from abnormal embryonic development; the majority of heterotopic rests involve the distal stomach and proximal small bowel.
- Most cases are asymptomatic, but some present as epigastric pain or GI bleeding due to inflammation.

IMAGING FEATURES

- Most often, this entity presents as a focal submucosal antral lesion located along the greater curvature.
- A central umbilication representing a rudimentary ductal system is highly suggestive of the diagnosis.
- CT may be useful for localizing the inflammatory process in symptomatic cases; intramural pseudocysts can be seen when pancreatitis involves the tissue rest.

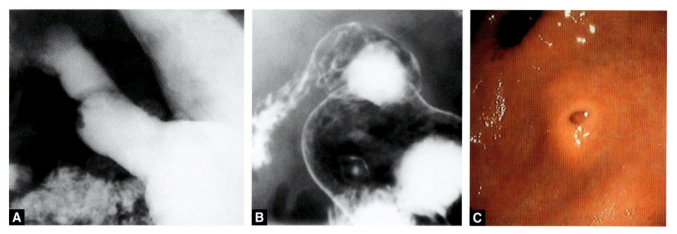

FIGURE 3.4.1 Heterotopic pancreatic rest. Barium UGI (**A** and **B**) and EGD (**C**) images from three different patients show smooth submucosal polypoid lesions with central umbilication along the greater curvature of the gastric antrum.

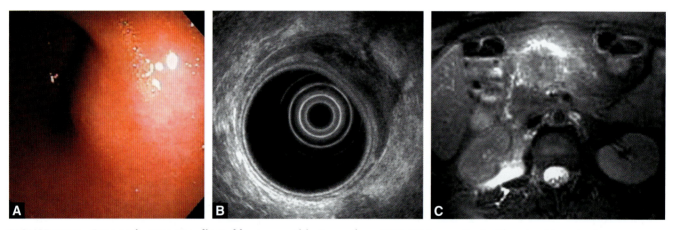

FIGURE 3.4.2 Pancreatic rests complicated by pancreatitis. Image from EGD (**A**) in a patient with epigastric pain shows a smooth, nonspecific gastric submucosal lesion, which appears hypoechoic at EUS (**B**). T2-weighted MR image (**C**) demonstrates the lesion, surrounded by high-signal inflammatory changes.

Illustration continued on following page

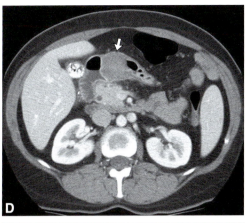
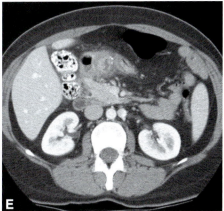
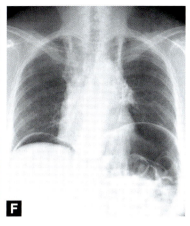
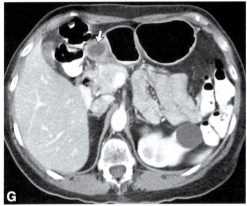

FIGURE 3.4.2 *(Continued)* **Pancreatic rests complicated by pancreatitis.** CT (**D** and **E**) confirms a submucosal mass in the distal antrum (**D**, *arrow*) with surrounding inflammatory changes. Pancreatitis within a heterotopic rest was confirmed by CT-guided biopsy. Upright chest radiograph (**F**) in another patient with acute onset of epigastric pain shows pneumoperitoneum with free air under the diaphragm. CT (**G**) shows an intramural gastric pseudocyst (*arrow*) related to pancreatitis of a heterotopic rest, which was also the cause of gastric perforation.

3.5 Duplication Cysts
(Figure 3.5.1)

CLINICAL FEATURES

- Congenital duplication cysts involving the stomach are uncommon and are usually detected as an incidental finding.
- Cysts containing functioning gastric mucosa are more often symptomatic and may present with bleeding or perforation.

IMAGING FEATURES

- Duplication cysts generally present as nonspecific broad-based intramural lesions on fluoroscopic or endoscopic evaluation.
- The overlying mucosa is usually intact; rarely, the cyst may communicate with the gastric lumen.
- Cross-sectional imaging such as CT or EUS provides more specific evaluation by demonstrating the fluid-filled cystic nature of these intramural lesions.

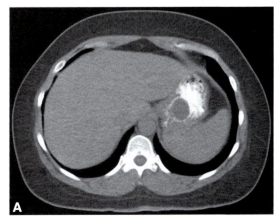
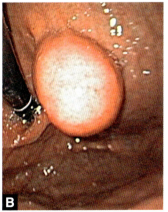

FIGURE 3.5.1 **Gastric duplication cyst.** Images from CT (**A**) and EGD (**B**) show a well-defined cystic, submucosal lesion at the gastric fundus.

Illustration continued on following page

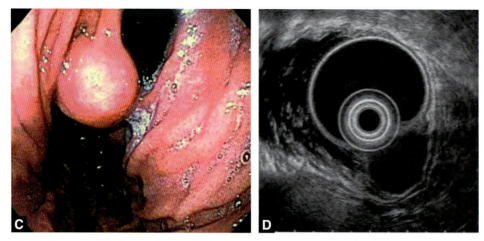

FIGURE 3.5.1 (Continued) **Gastric duplication cyst.** EGD **(C)** and EUS **(D)** images from a second patient show a similar simple-appearing cystic lesion involving the gastric cardia that originates from the submucosal layer. The anechoic appearance demonstrated by EUS distinguishes this cystic lesion from a solid submucosal mass.

3.6 Gastric Bezoars
(Figure 3.6.1)

CLINICAL FEATURES

- These are luminal concretions secondary to ingested material; phytobezoars are composed of plant material, and trichobezoars are undigested hair.
- Symptoms are related to the mechanical effects of the intragastric mass, including nausea, early satiety, and gastric outlet obstruction.

IMAGING FEATURES

- Conventional radiography may suggest an upper abdominal mass or fluid collection.
- Barium UGI evaluation will demonstrate a large intraluminal filling defect, often forming a cast of the dilated lumen; air and/or contrast may partially fill interstices of the lesion.
- Endoscopy can confirm the diagnosis and can sometimes offer therapeutic benefit.

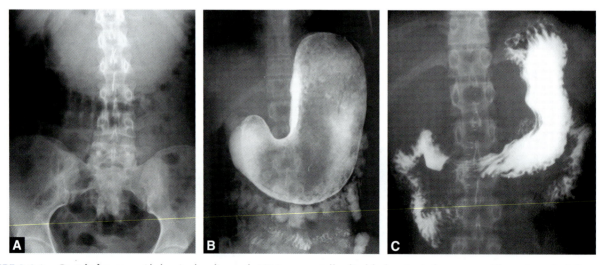

FIGURE 3.6.1 **Gastric bezoars.** Abdominal radiograph **(A)** in a mentally disabled patient shows mass-like epigastric fullness, with inferior displacement of the transverse colon. Image from subsequent barium UGI **(B)** shows a large gastric filling defect that forms a cast of the entire stomach. Note normal appearance to the stomach after open surgical removal of a large trichobezoar **(C)**.
Illustration continued on following page

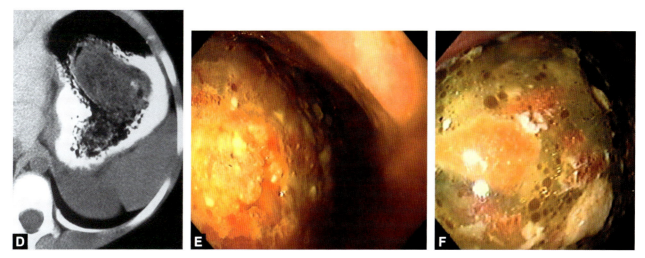

FIGURE 3.6.1 (Continued)   **Gastric bezoars.** Images from CT (**D**) and EGD (**E** and **F**) in three different patients show heterogeneous intraluminal masses representing gastric bezoars.

3.7 Gastric Volvulus
(Figures 3.7.1-3.7.2)

CLINICAL FEATURES

- Organoaxial volvulus involves rotation about the long axis of the stomach; it may present acutely or as an asymptomatic intrathoracic stomach.
- Mesoenteroaxial volvulus involves rotation about the short axis between the lesser and greater curvatures; it is less common and less often complete.
- Classic acute presentation of complete gastric volvulus consists of Borchardt's triad: abdominal pain, unproductive retching, and the inability to pass a nasogastric tube; this is a surgical emergency.
- Chronic gastric volvulus is likely under-recognized and manifests as nonspecific symptoms including epigastric discomfort, dysphagia, and bloating.

IMAGING FEATURES

- Fluoroscopic contrast evaluation and CT are perhaps the best means for diagnosis.
- In organoaxial rotation, the greater curvature assumes a more superior position relative to the lesser curvature; the stomach is usually at least partly intrathoracic.
- In mesenteroaxial rotation, the antrum rotates leftward and the fundus rotates to the right.

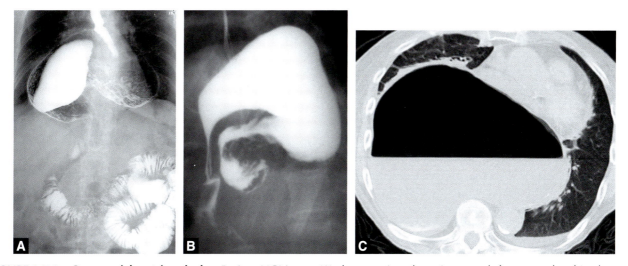

FIGURE 3.7.1   **Organoaxial gastric volvulus.** Barium UGI image (**A**) shows an intrathoracic stomach from complete hiatal herniation, which was asymptomatic. The orientation of the lesser and greater curvatures is reversed from normal. Barium UGI image (**B**) from a second patient shows organoaxial volvulus with the greater curvature located cephalad to the lesser curvature. CT image (**C**) from a patient with acute abdominal pain shows a massively dilated intrathoracic stomach with a large air-fluid level, related to volvulus with vascular compromise.

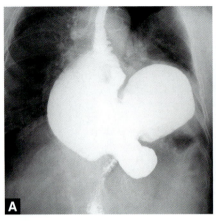
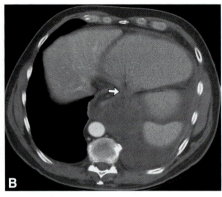
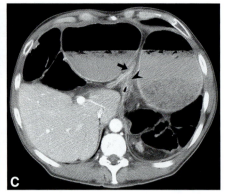

FIGURE 3.7.2 Mesenteroaxial gastric volvulus. Image from barium UGI **(A)** shows mesenteroaxial volvulus with reversal of the normal relationship between the gastric fundus and antrum. CT image **(B)** from a second patient shows an unusual gastric configuration, with a focal twist from gastric volvulus (*arrow*). Note the adjacent peritoneal fluid. CT image **(C)** in a patient with chronic intermittent symptoms shows close approximation of the gastric outlet (*arrow*) and esophagogastric junction (*arrowhead*). The appearance of the stomach was unchanged from prior CT studies.

3.8 Gastric Diverticula
(Figure 3.8.1)

CLINICAL FEATURES

- The vast majority of gastric diverticula occur as solitary outpouchings off the posterior fundus, near the gastric cardia.
- Gastric diverticula only rarely cause clinical symptoms but may present as hemorrhage or perforation.

IMAGING FEATURES

- The main importance of gastric diverticula is simply proper recognition, because they may simulate an exoenteric mesenchymal tumor or adrenal lesion on CT or MRI.
- Contrast or air within the diverticulum on radiologic studies avoids misdiagnosis.

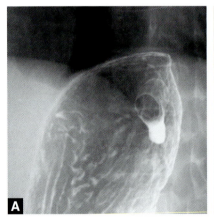
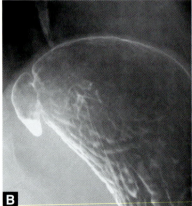
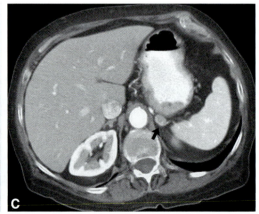

FIGURE 3.8.1 Gastric diverticula. Two images from barium UGI **(A** and **B)** show a typical gastric diverticulum extending off the posterior fundus. On CT **(C)**, gastric diverticula extend posteriorly to lie near the left adrenal gland and can simulate an adrenal lesion if not filled with air or oral contrast (*arrow*).

Illustration continued on following page

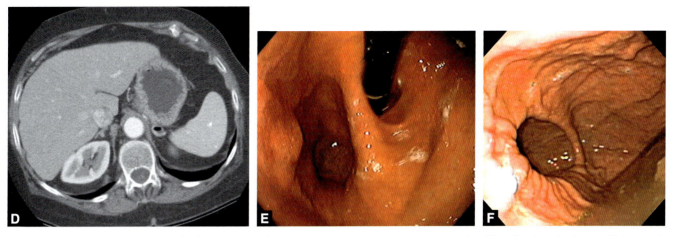

FIGURE 3.8.1 (Continued) **Gastric diverticula.** Subsequent CT in this patient (**D**) shows air within the diverticulum, which avoids the potential for misdiagnosis. EGD images (**E** and **F**) from two different patients show the endoscopic appearance of gastric diverticula.

3.9 Complications of Percutaneous Endoscopic Gastrostomy
(Figures 3.9.1-3.9.3)

CLINICAL FEATURES

- Complications of PEG can be divided into tube malpositioning and stomal complications.
- Tube malposition can be an early or late complication and includes extragastric location of the tip and fistula formation with the transverse colon.
- The "buried bumper syndrome" may present as GI bleeding, pneumoperitoneum, or peritonitis.
- Stomal complications include infection and metastatic tumor implantation due to scope-related seeding from a proximal malignancy (head/neck or GI tumor).

IMAGING FEATURES

- Contrast injection under fluoroscopy can easily confirm appropriate tip positioning.
- CT is valuable for precise localization of malpositioned tubes and detection of free peritoneal air and fluid.
- Absence or submucosal positioning of the PEG bumper at EGD is diagnostic of a buried bumper; radiologic evaluation is generally needed for localization of frankly extragastric PEG tubes.
- CT and EGD provide complementary evaluation of the tumor burden in cases of direct metastatic stomal seeding.

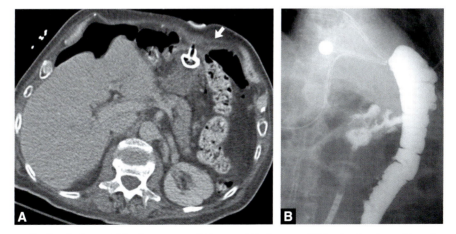

FIGURE 3.9.1 **Gastrocolic fistula from PEG placement.** CT image (**A**) shows a PEG tube in place. Note how the tube appears to traverse the transverse colon (*arrow*). Fluoroscopic image obtained after contrast injection through the PEG tube (**B**) shows communication with the colon.

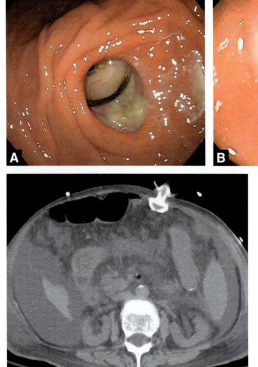

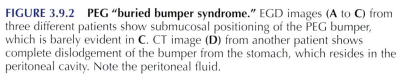

FIGURE 3.9.2 **PEG "buried bumper syndrome."** EGD images (**A** to **C**) from three different patients show submucosal positioning of the PEG bumper, which is barely evident in **C**. CT image (**D**) from another patient shows complete dislodgement of the bumper from the stomach, which resides in the peritoneal cavity. Note the peritoneal fluid.

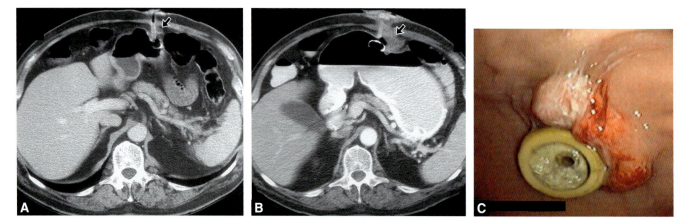

FIGURE 3.9.3 **Stomal metastasis from PEG placement.** Image from initial CT (**A**) from a patient with a PEG placed for squamous cell carcinoma of the tongue shows only minimal nonspecific soft tissue infiltration around the tube (*arrow*). Image from CT performed 3 months later (**B**) shows significant interval progression of soft tissue around the PEG (*arrow*). Stomal metastatic disease was confirmed at EGD (**C**). (From Pickhardt PJ, Rohrmann CA, Cossentino MJ: Stomal metastases complicating percutaneous endoscopic gastrostomy: CT findings and the case for radiologic tube placement. AJR 2002;179:735-739.)

CHAPTER 3

THE DUODENUM

Andrew D. Lee, MD • Perry J. Pickhardt, MD

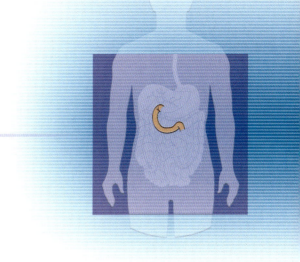

1. **DUODENAL TUMORS**
    1.1 Mucosal Neoplasms
    1.2 Submucosal Tumors
    1.3 Non-neoplastic Lesions
2. **INFLAMMATORY CONDITIONS**
    2.1 Peptic Ulcer Disease
    2.2 Duodenitis
3. **OTHER DUODENAL CONDITIONS**
    3.1 Vascular Lesions
    3.2 Aortoduodenal Fistula
    3.3 Duodenal Diverticula
    3.4 Duodenal Duplication Cyst
    3.5 Infiltrative Diseases

Despite continuing technical innovations in CT and MRI, endoscopic and fluoroscopic evaluations remain the mainstays for diagnosing pathologic conditions of the duodenum. Cross-sectional imaging, however, can be very valuable in certain clinical scenarios. Although many disease processes can affect the entire small bowel, a number of pathologic conditions are unique to the duodenum. In addition, the duodenum is much more accessible to standard endoscopic techniques compared with the mesenteric small bowel. Duodenal tumors, inflammatory conditions, and a variety of other duodenal conditions are covered in this chapter. The remainder of the small bowel and its associated pathology is covered in Chapter 4.

1. DUODENAL TUMORS

The majority of focal duodenal lesions are benign. Classification of duodenal tumors into mucosal neoplasms, submucosal tumors, and non-neoplastic lesions is useful for organizing these diverse entities.

1.1 Mucosal Neoplasms
(Figures 1.1.1-1.1.5)

CLINICAL FEATURES

- Duodenal mucosal neoplasms include adenomas and adenocarcinomas; non-neoplastic mucosal lesions are considered later.
- Unlike the stomach, most duodenal mucosal polyps are adenomatous.
- As with colonic neoplasms, an adenoma-carcinoma sequence generally applies and villous lesions have greater malignant potential.
- Malignancy risk is directly related to lesion size, particularly for tumors >4 cm.
- Unless periampullary in location, mucosal neoplasms are generally asymptomatic until large; they may ultimately present with occult blood loss, jaundice, or gastric outlet obstruction.
- Multiple adenomatous lesions are characteristic of familial adenomatous polyposis (FAP), with a periampullary predilection and increased risk of malignancy.
- Adenocarcinoma is rare but represents the most common duodenal malignancy; presentation may include nausea, epigastric pain, obstruction, weight loss, jaundice, or upper GI bleeding.
- Risk factors for developing duodenal adenocarcinoma include FAP, Peutz-Jeghers syndrome, hereditary nonpolyposis colorectal cancer, celiac disease, and neurofibromatosis.

IMAGING FEATURES

- At UGI evaluation and EGD, nonvillous duodenal adenomas usually appear as solitary sessile polyps in the first or second portion.
- Villous lesions usually appear as large, lobulated or sessile masses located near the ampulla of Vater; malignant

degeneration is suggested by an annular or shouldered appearance.
- Multiple lesions suggest a polyposis syndrome; multiple adenomas typify FAP syndrome.
- Duodenal adenocarcinoma typically arises at or distal to the ampulla; imaging appearances include an irregular annular or eccentric mass, with or without ulceration or lobulation (particularly if villous).
- Biliary and pancreatic ductal dilation are common with periampullary tumors.
- At CT, duodenal tumors may be difficult to differentiate from a pancreatic head neoplasm; the presence of metastatic disease confirms malignancy.

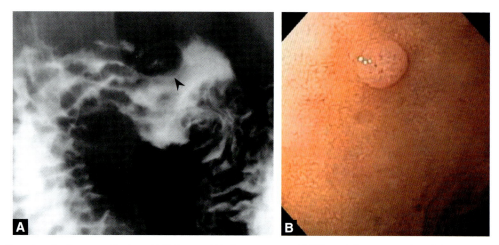

FIGURE 1.1.1 Duodenal adenoma. Barium UGI image (**A**) shows an ovoid filling defect (*arrowhead*) from an isolated adenoma. Smooth fold thickening is present from unrelated duodenitis. EGD image (**B**) from a different patient shows a small mucosal polyp that proved to be an adenoma.

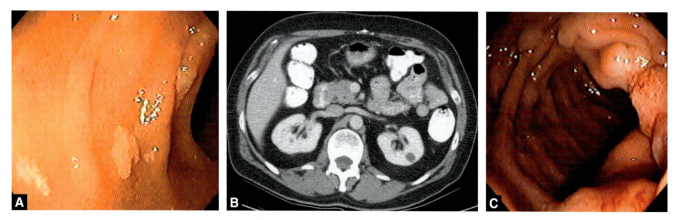

FIGURE 1.1.2 Multiple duodenal adenomas in FAP. EGD image (**A**) shows multiple, flat, white mucosal lesions typical of small duodenal adenomas. Contrast-enhanced CT (**B**) from another patient demonstrates focal irregular duodenal thickening involving the second portion, shown to be due to multiple large sessile adenomas at EGD (**C**).

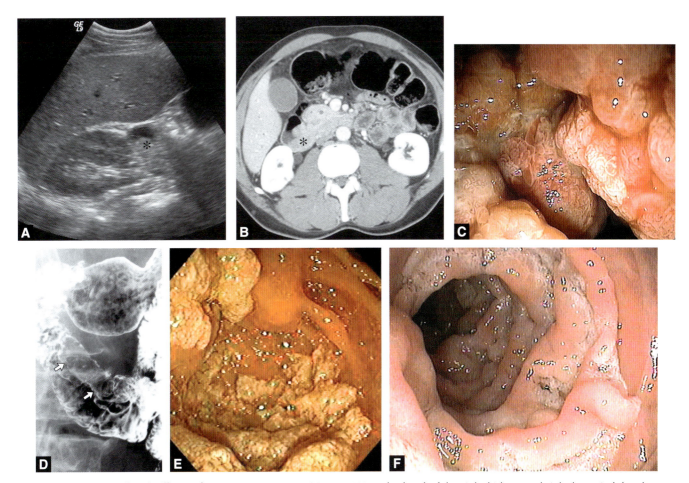

FIGURE 1.1.3 Duodenal villous adenoma. Transverse US image (**A**) at the level of the right kidney and right hepatic lobe shows a polypoid mass (*asterisk*) within the duodenum. Contrast-enhanced CT image (**B**) shows the lobulated mass (*asterisk*), which has a papillary frond-like appearance at EGD (**C**). Barium UGI image (**D**) from a second patient shows a long lobulated filling defect (*arrows*) in the periampullary duodenum. EGD images (**E** and **F**) from two different patients show villous lesions carpeting relatively long segments of duodenum.

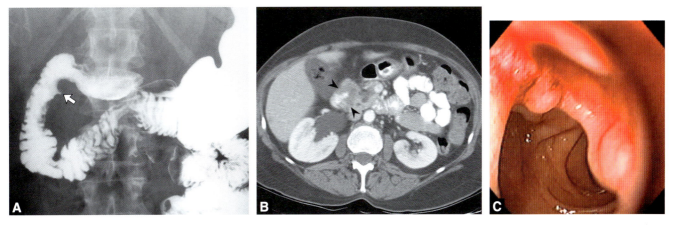

FIGURE 1.1.4 Duodenal adenocarcinoma. Barium UGI image (**A**) shows fixed irregular narrowing along the medial aspect of the second portion of the duodenum, with a focal barium collection (*arrow*) that suggests ulceration. Contrast-enhanced CT image (**B**) shows the same C-shaped ulcerated low-attenuation mass (*arrowheads*), which has a similar appearance at EGD (**C**).

Illustration continued on following page

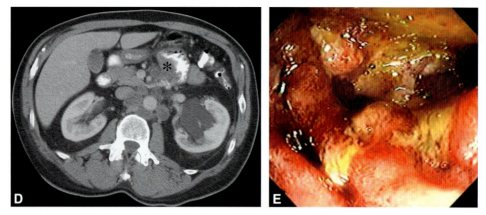

FIGURE 1.1.4 (Continued) **Duodenal adenocarcinoma.** Contrast-enhanced CT image (**D**) from a different patient shows an eccentric soft tissue mass (*asterisk*) involving the fourth portion of the duodenum, as well as para-aortic metastatic lymphadenopathy. EGD image (**E**) shows the mucosal irregularity and friability of the mass.

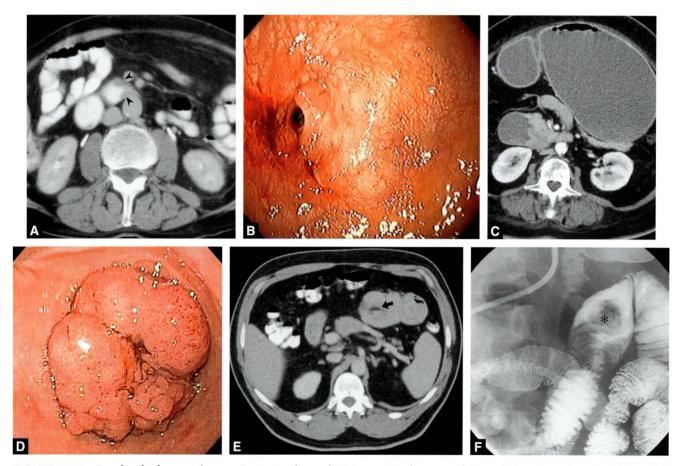

FIGURE 1.1.5 Duodenal adenocarcinoma. Contrast-enhanced CT image (**A**) shows a soft tissue lesion (*arrowheads*) with luminal narrowing involving the proximal third portion of the duodenum. Corresponding EGD image (**B**) shows the luminal appearance of the resulting malignant stricture. Contrast-enhanced CT image (**C**) from a second patient shows high-grade obstruction due to an irregular soft tissue mass involving the proximal third portion of the duodenum. Note the dilated fluid-filled stomach and proximal duodenum. EGD image (**D**) from a third patient shows a large duodenal villous tumor protruding through the pylorus, causing gastric outlet obstruction. Contrast-enhanced CT image (**E**) from a final patient shows a focally prominent bowel loop near the ligament of Trietz. Fat attenuation (*arrow*) projecting within this dilated loop is highly suggestive of mesenteric fat from intussusception, which was confirmed at enteroclysis (**F**). Note the "coiled spring" appearance of the intussusceptum and intussuscipiens. The polypoid lead mass (*asterisk*) proved to be duodenal adenocarcinoma.

1.2 Submucosal Tumors

(Figures 1.2.1-1.2.9)

CLINICAL FEATURES

- These varied entities include both benign and malignant neoplasms that arise deep to the mucosa.
- Mesenchymal tumors include lipomas, GI stromal tumors (GISTs), nerve sheath tumors, smooth muscle tumors, and hemangiomas.
- Lipomas are relatively common and usually an incidental finding; large lipomas can rarely cause obstruction.
- Previously, most GISTs were erroneously diagnosed as smooth muscle tumors, but they are now recognized as the most common intramural mesenchymal tumor of the GI tract.
- GISTs are believed to arise from the interstitial cells of Cajal and express the KIT receptor protein encoded by the *c-KIT* gene; presentation is often related to mass effect or GI bleeding from ulceration.
- B-cell non-Hodgkin's lymphoma and other lymphoproliferative disorders of the duodenum are more often the result of contiguous spread of disease rather than of primary duodenal origin.
- Hematogenous metastatic disease to the duodenum is rare and most often seen with breast cancer or melanoma; direct contiguous spread of tumor can be seen with pancreas, colon, and renal primary tumors.
- Other rare duodenal submucosal neoplasms include carcinoid tumor, Kaposi's sarcoma, gastrinoma, and other neurogenic tumors.

IMAGING FEATURES

- Submucosal duodenal lipomas may become pedunculated over time; although luminal studies may be highly suggestive of the diagnosis, CT is diagnostic for fat and obviates the need for tissue sampling.
- Intramural mesenchymal tumors typically manifest as smooth, broad-based impressions on barium UGI and EGD studies; when large, these may be difficult to distinguish from extrinsic lesions.
- Duodenal GISTs range from subcentimeter size to >10 cm; hepatic and peritoneal spread is common with malignant tumors.
- Duodenal lymphoma may appear as a nodular or ulcerated mass or with diffuse fold thickening.
- Hematogenous metastatic disease often manifests as discrete submucosal masses; central ulceration from necrosis can give a "bull's-eye" appearance from barium filling of the crater.
- Direct extension of extraduodenal malignancies may cause extrinsic compression or a focal mass, with or without ulcer or fistula formation.
- Duodenal carcinoid tumors typically manifest as polypoid lesions.
- Kaposi's sarcoma is almost always associated with AIDS, is often multifocal, and may ulcerate and bleed.
- Duodenal gastrinomas are hypervascular tumors; additional findings of Zollinger-Ellison syndrome may be present.

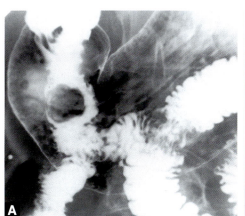 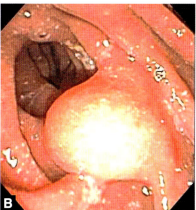 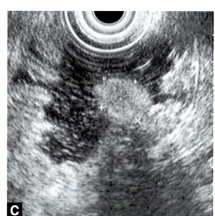

FIGURE 1.2.1 **Duodenal lipoma.** Barium UGI image (**A**) shows a relatively lucent polypoid filling defect in the second portion of the duodenum. EGD image (**B**) from a different patient shows a similar lesion, which was pliable at real-time examination. EUS image (**C**) shows that the lesion is echogenic with "dirty shadowing," compatible with a lipoma.

Illustration continued on following page

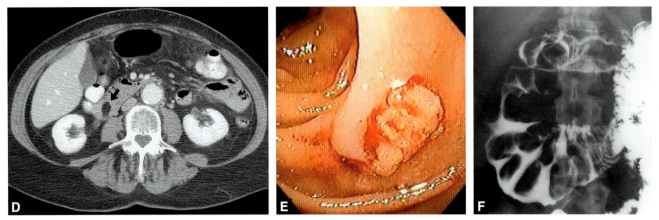

FIGURE 1.2.1 (Continued) **Duodenal lipoma.** Contrast-enhanced CT image **(D)** from a third patient shows a pedunculated fat-attenuation lesion (*arrow*) projecting into the duodenal lumen. EGD image **(E)** from a fourth patient shows extrusion of fatty tissue after multiple "bite on bite" biopsies of a pliable submucosal mass. Barium UGI image **(F)** from a final patient shows multiple polypoid filling defects throughout the duodenum representing "lipomatosis."

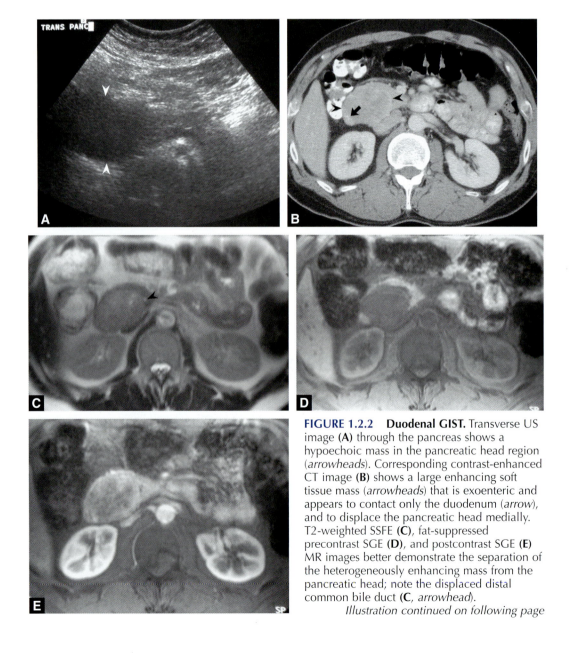

FIGURE 1.2.2 **Duodenal GIST.** Transverse US image **(A)** through the pancreas shows a hypoechoic mass in the pancreatic head region (*arrowheads*). Corresponding contrast-enhanced CT image **(B)** shows a large enhancing soft tissue mass (*arrowheads*) that is exoenteric and appears to contact only the duodenum (*arrow*), and to displace the pancreatic head medially. T2-weighted SSFE **(C)**, fat-suppressed precontrast SGE **(D)**, and postcontrast SGE **(E)** MR images better demonstrate the separation of the heterogeneously enhancing mass from the pancreatic head; note the displaced distal common bile duct (**C**, *arrowhead*).

Illustration continued on following page

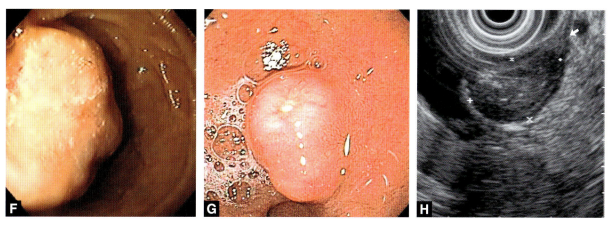

FIGURE 1.2.2 (Continued) **Duodenal GIST.** EGD image (**F**) from a different patient shows a large intramural GIST with a prominent submucosal impression. EGD (**G**) and EUS (**H**) images from a third patient show a smaller submucosal lesion in the duodenal bulb that originates from the muscularis propria layer (*arrow*) and demonstrates internal heterogeneity.

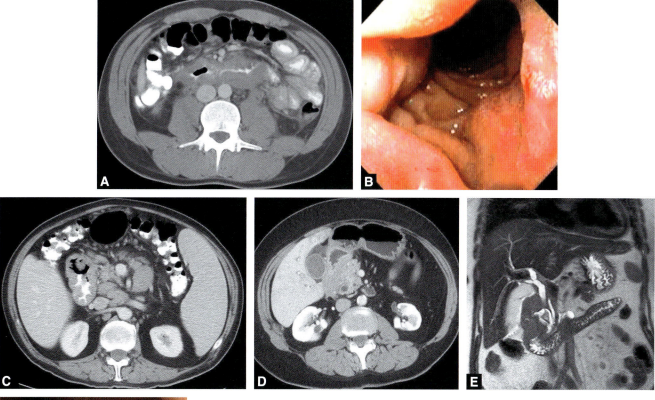

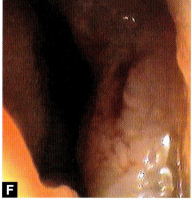

FIGURE 1.2.3 **Duodenal lymphoma.** Contrast-enhanced CT image (**A**) shows diffuse low-attenuation duodenal wall thickening without evidence of obstruction. Corresponding EGD image (**B**) shows diffuse fold thickening from submucosal lymphomatous infiltration. Contrast-enhanced CT image (**C**) from a second patient shows diffuse polypoid fold thickening of the duodenum, associated with luminal dilatation instead of compromise. Adjacent bulky lymphadenopathy is present at the mesenteric root. Contrast-enhanced CT image (**D**) from a third patient shows diffuse soft tissue thickening involving the proximal duodenum. Coronal T2-weighted SSFSE MR image (**E**) shows the bulky proximal duodenal mass with associated biliary obstruction. Subsequent EGD image (**F**) shows luminal narrowing and mucosal ulceration from the infiltrative submucosal tumor.

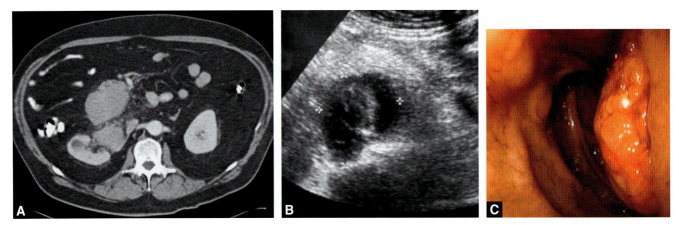

FIGURE 1.2.4 Duodenal plasmacytoma. Contrast-enhanced CT image **(A)** shows a bulky soft tissue mass centered on the second portion of the duodenum. The right renal pelvis is also involved. Transverse US image **(B)** shows hypoechoic duodenal wall thickening, which is the typical appearance of GI lymphoproliferative disorders. EGD image **(C)** from a different patient shows a lobulated submucosal mass from a duodenal plasmacytoma.

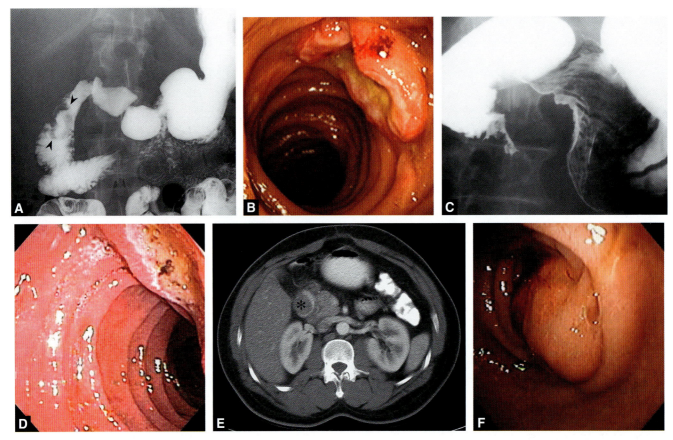

FIGURE 1.2.5 Duodenal metastases. Barium UGI **(A)** and EGD **(B)** images show an ulcerated submucosal mass **(A,** *arrowheads*) from metastatic melanoma, which demonstrates a "bull's-eye" fluoroscopic appearance due to barium filling of the central ulcer. Barium UGI image **(C)** from a second patient shows marked duodenal irregularity and obstruction due to direct invasion by pancreatic adenocarcinoma. EGD image **(D)** from a third patient shows another example of direct duodenal invasion by pancreatic adenocarcinoma. Contrast-enhanced CT **(E)** and EGD **(F)** images show a rounded duodenal submucosal mass (*asterisk*) from metastatic colonic adenocarcinoma, which causes significant luminal compromise.

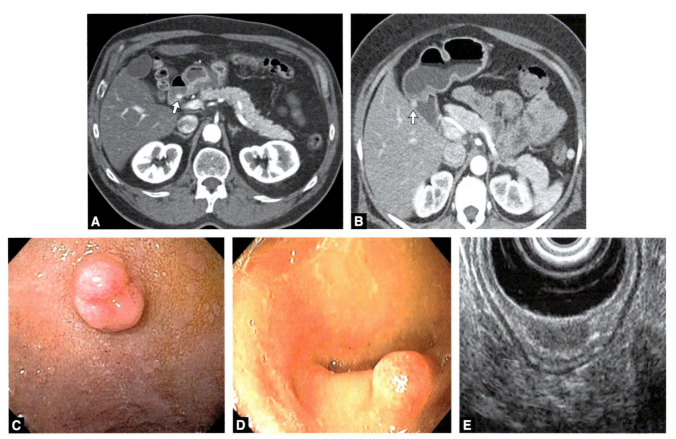

FIGURE 1.2.6 **Duodenal carcinoid tumor.** Contrast-enhanced CT images (**A** and **B**) from two different patients show subcentimeter hypervascular lesions (*arrows*) within the duodenal bulb. EGD images (**C** and **D**) from two additional patients show similar small submucosal carcinoid tumors. EUS image (**E**) from the last patient shows the well-circumscribed hypoechoic lesion originating from the submucosal layer.

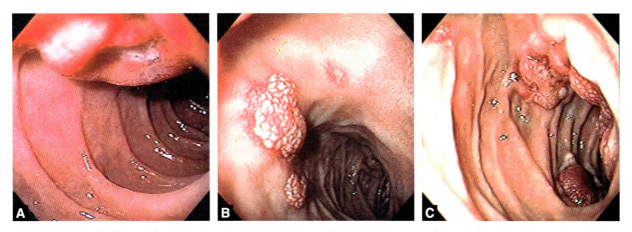

FIGURE 1.2.7 **Duodenal Kaposi's sarcoma.** EGD images (**A** to **C**) from two patients with AIDS show duodenal Kaposi's sarcoma manifesting as an ulcerated submucosal mass (**A**) and irregular multifocal submucosal lesions with a reddish purple appearance (**B** and **C**).

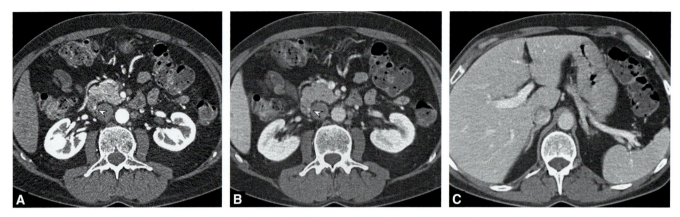

FIGURE 1.2.8 Duodenal gastrinoma. Arterial (**A**) and portal venous (**B**) phase CT images from a patient presenting with Zollinger-Ellison syndrome show a tiny hypervascular focus (*arrowheads*) within the medial wall of the second portion of the duodenum, which proved to be the causative gastrinoma. Diffuse gastric wall thickening related to the hypergastrinemic state was evident on more cephalad images (**C**).

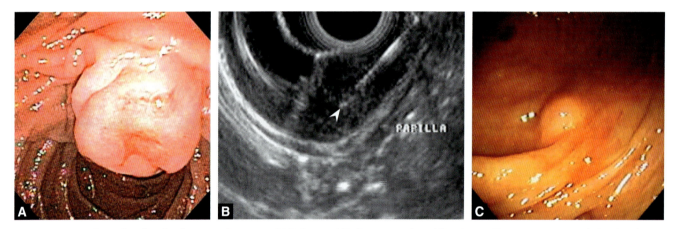

FIGURE 1.2.9 Rare duodenal submucosal tumors. EGD image (**A**) shows a polypoid periampullary mass, seen originating from the submucosa on endosonography (**B**). Note the aspiration needle (*arrowhead*) within the mass. Gangliocytic paraganglioma was confirmed after surgical resection. EGD image (**C**) from a different patient shows a small submucosal lesion, which proved to be a duodenal ganglioneuroma.

1.3 Non-neoplastic Lesions
(Figures 1.3.1-1.3.6)

CLINICAL FEATURES

- Brunner's glands are most numerous in the proximal duodenum and normally produce a protective alkaline secretion; hyperplasia of these glands is associated with gastric hypersecretion.
- Heterotopic gastric mucosa is typically seen in the proximal duodenal bulb and believed to be of no clinical significance.
- Heterotopic pancreatic rests are more common in the distal stomach than the duodenum; although usually asymptomatic, they may present as pain, bleeding, or even pancreatitis with pseudocysts.
- Hyperplastic and inflammatory fibroid polyps are uncommon lesions that do not have malignant potential.
- Multiple hamartomatous polyps may be seen in juvenile polyposis, Cowden's disease, Peutz-Jeghers syndrome, and Cronkhite-Canada syndrome.
- Duodenal lymphangiectasia is commonly found distal to the bulb; it is usually an incidental finding but has been associated with malabsorption and protein-losing enteropathy.

IMAGING FEATURES

- Brunner's gland hyperplasia usually appears as multiple polypoid lesions in the proximal duodenum; larger solitary lesions are sometimes referred to as "hamartomas" and often contain more fibrous tissue.
- Heterotopic gastric mucosa is typically found at the base of the duodenal bulb; the appearance on imaging may resemble normal gastric mucosa.
- Heterotopic pancreatic rests present as smooth, focal submucosal lesions; as with gastric antral lesions, cen-

tral umbilication is characteristic but may mimic other "bull's-eye" lesions on barium fluoroscopy.
- Hyperplastic and inflammatory fibroid lesions generally have a nonspecific sessile polypoid appearance on imaging; these lesions are typically solitary and rarely exceed 1 to 2 cm.
- Multiple polyps throughout the duodenum on imaging should suggest a polyposis syndrome.
- Lymphangiectasia may appear as small multifocal white spots on an otherwise normal duodenum or can be more focal and release white lymphatic fluid on biopsy.

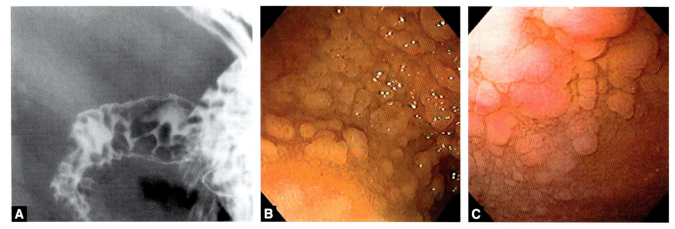

FIGURE 1.3.1 Brunner's gland hyperplasia. Barium UGI (**A**) and EGD (**B** and **C**) images from three different patients show multiple duodenal bulb lesions of various sizes representing Brunner's gland hyperplasia.

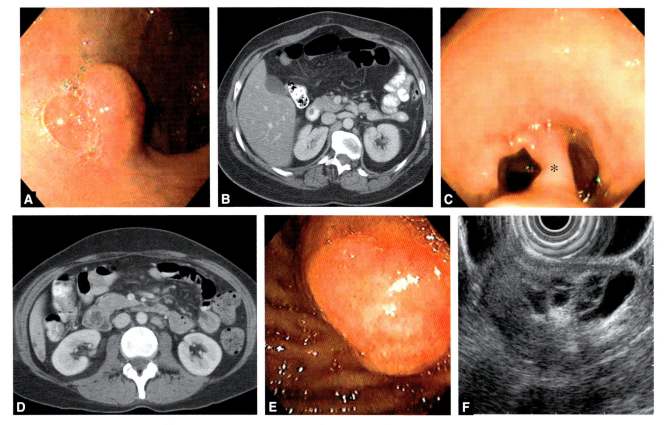

FIGURE 1.3.2 Brunner's gland hamartoma. EGD image (**A**) shows a small polypoid lesion with normal overlying mucosa. Contrast-enhanced CT image (**B**) from a second patient shows a soft tissue polyp projecting into the contrast-filled duodenal lumen. Corresponding EGD image (**C**) shows the stalk (*asterisk*) of this pedunculated hamartoma; the body of the polyp extends below the field of view. Contrast-enhanced CT image (**D**) from a third patient shows a complex cystic mass within the duodenum. Corresponding EGD image (**E**) shows the large submucosal polypoid mass. EUS image (**F**) demonstrates the complex cystic and solid nature of the lesion. The cysts represent dilated mucin-filled glands.

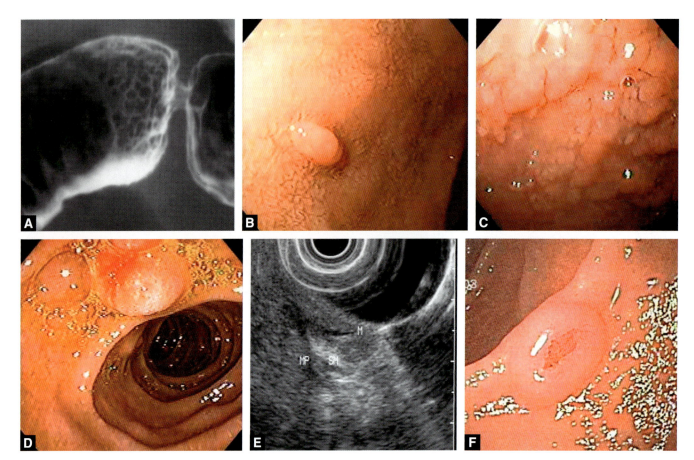

FIGURE 1.3.3 **Heterotopic gastric and pancreatic tissue.** Barium UGI image **(A)** demonstrates a mucosal pattern at the base of the duodenal bulb that has the appearance of prominent areae gastricae. EGD images **(B** and **C)** from two separate patients show heterotopic gastric epithelium in the bulb, manifesting as a small solitary polyp **(B)** and multiple sessile nodules **(C)**, that has an appearance similar to Brunner's gland hyperplasia. EGD **(D)** and EUS **(E)** images from a different patient show an enlarged minor papilla secondary to gastric heterotopia. Note the thickened mucosal layer (M) and the duct of Santorini coursing through it. EGD image **(F)** from a final patient shows a polypoid duodenal lesion with central umbilication representing a heterotopic pancreatic rest.

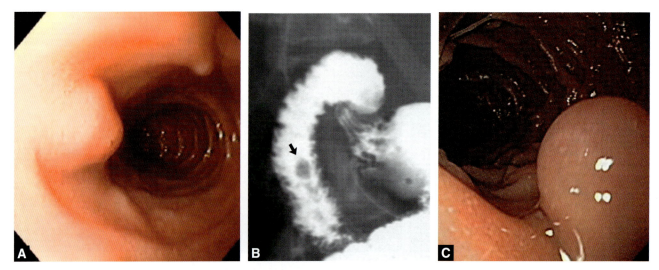

FIGURE 1.3.4 **Hyperplastic and inflammatory fibroid polyps.** EGD image **(A)** shows a duodenal polyp that proved to be hyperplastic at histologic evaluation. Note the minor papilla seen distally. Barium UGI **(B)** and EGD **(C)** images from a different patient show a smooth polypoid lesion (*arrow*) that proved to be an inflammatory fibroid polyp.

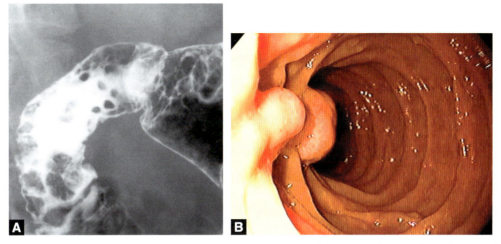

FIGURE 1.3.5 Duodenal hamartomatous polyposis. Barium UGI image **(A)** shows multiple irregular polyps involving the duodenum and stomach in a patient with Cronkhite-Canada syndrome. EGD image **(B)** from a second patient shows multiple hamartomatous polyps in a patient with Peutz-Jeghers syndrome.

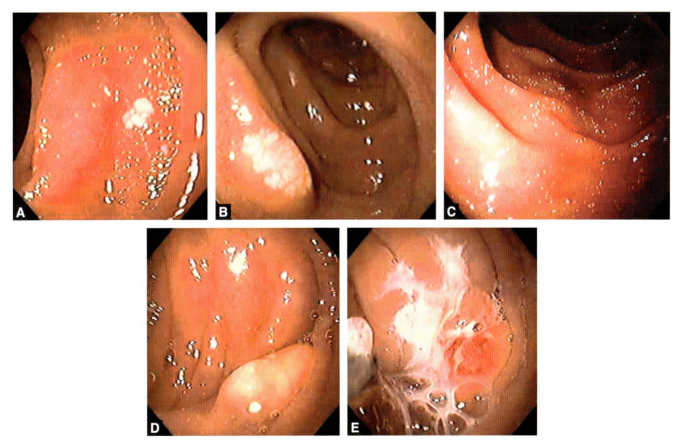

FIGURE 1.3.6 Focal duodenal lymphangiectasia. EGD images from four different patients demonstrate the varied endoscopic appearances: a focal flat white spot **(A)**, a small nodule with overlying punctate white foci **(B)**, innumerable miliary, white spots diffusely covering the duodenal mucosa **(C)**, and a yellowish nodule **(D)** that was soft on probing, similar to a lipoma. Biopsy of the nodule in the fourth case released milky lymphatic fluid **(E)**, confirming the diagnosis of focal lymphangiectasia.

2. INFLAMMATORY CONDITIONS

Duodenal peptic ulcer disease and duodenitis are two important inflammatory conditions discussed in this section. Although nearly all duodenal ulcers are benign, significant morbidity can result from peptic ulcer disease. Duodenitis is a nonspecific finding and may be due to a variety of underlying causes.

2.1 Peptic Ulcer Disease
(Figures 2.1.1-2.1.3)

CLINICAL FEATURES

- As with gastric ulcers, *Helicobacter pylori* and nonsteroidal anti-inflammatory drugs (NSAIDs) are the major risk factors for duodenal ulcer pathogenesis; if present, eradication of *H. pylori* is important to facilitate healing.
- The vast majority of duodenal ulcers are benign and located in the bulb.
- Duodenal ulcers tend to cause epigastric pain, which classically occurs several hours after a meal or awakens patients at night, but 25% to 50% of ulcers may be asymptomatic.
- Major complications include perforation, bleeding, and obstruction; giant duodenal ulcers (>2 cm) are at increased risk for complications.
- Perforated duodenal ulcers are the most common cause of pneumoperitoneum associated with peritonitis (see Chapter 4 for causes of small bowel perforation).
- Gastric outlet obstruction can result from edema, spasm, or post-inflammatory fibrosis.
- A postbulbar ulcer location is typical in Zollinger-Ellison syndrome.

IMAGING FEATURES

- Ninety-five percent of duodenal ulcers arise within the bulb, evenly split between anterior and posterior walls; multiple bulbar ulcers occur in 15% of cases.
- On barium UGI, the contrast-filled ulcer crater is typically surrounded by a smooth mound of edematous mucosa; persistence of the abnormal finding on multiple views increases diagnostic confidence.
- At EGD, these discrete excavated craters will typically have a white base, with adjacent mucosal inflammation; unlike gastric ulcers, follow-up EGD to document healing is not typically indicated.
- Endoscopic characteristics associated with higher rebleeding risk are the same for both gastric and duodenal ulcers (see Chapter 2, section 2.1 for a more detailed description).
- Duodenal ulcers can sometimes be detected on CT; CT is particularly useful for rapid diagnosis of a perforated ulcer, usually manifesting as extraluminal air.
- Associated imaging findings of *H. pylori* duodenitis are common in peptic ulcer disease.
- The presence of postbulbar duodenal ulcers should raise the possibility of Zollinger-Ellison syndrome or granulomatous disease, especially if the ulcers are multiple or associated with extensive duodenitis.

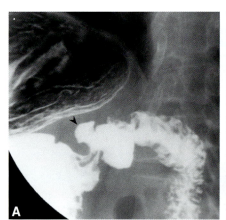 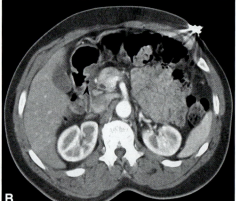 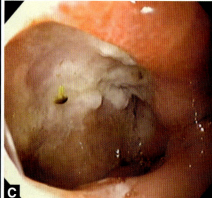

FIGURE 2.1.1 Duodenal ulcers. Imaging studies from nine different patients. Barium UGI image **(A)** shows a typical penetrating ulcer (*arrowhead*) of the duodenal bulb. Contrast-enhanced CT image **(B)** shows a small air-filled ulcer (*arrowhead*) with surrounding eccentric low-attenuation, intramural edema. EGD image **(C)** shows a giant duodenal ulcer that caused symptomatic gastric outlet obstruction from the surrounding edema.

Illustration continued on following page

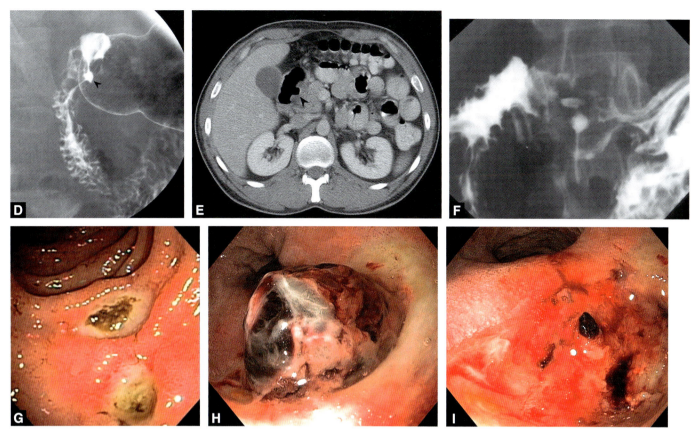

FIGURE 2.1.1 (Continued)   **Duodenal ulcers.** Barium UGI image (**D**) shows a barium-filled ulcer crater (*arrowhead*) with edematous folds extending to the base. Contrast-enhanced CT image (**E**) shows an ulcer (*arrowhead*) with a surrounding mound of low-attenuation edema. Barium UGI (**F**) and EGD (**G**) images each show two discrete duodenal ulcers—in the bulb and second portion, respectively. The location of the ulcers in **G** is atypical but they were secondary to NSAID use. EGD image (**H**) shows a large duodenal ulcer with an adherent clot. After clot removal (**I**), a large nonbleeding visible vessel is revealed.

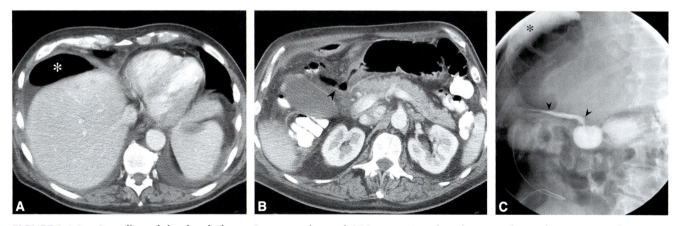

FIGURE 2.1.2   Complicated duodenal ulcers. Contrast-enhanced CT images (**A** and **B**) show extraluminal air (**A**, *asterisk*) tracking away from a perforated duodenal ulcer (**B**, *arrowhead*), associated with surrounding inflammatory changes. Barium UGI image (**C**) performed after surgery shows persistent extraluminal communication (*arrowheads*) with contrast streaming into the perihepatic air and fluid collection (*asterisk*).

Illustration continued on following page

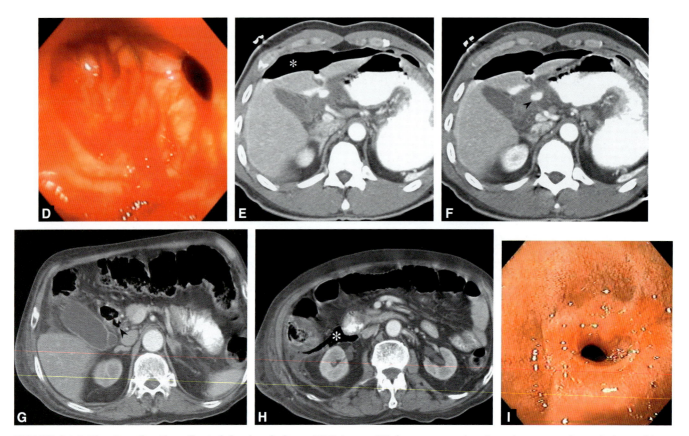

FIGURE 2.1.2 (Continued) **Complicated duodenal ulcers.** EGD image (**D**) from a second patient shows a perforated ulcer with associated bleeding and inflammation. Contrast-enhanced CT images (**E** and **F**) from a third patient show a contrast-filled perforated anterior duodenal ulcer (**F**, *arrowhead*) with pneumoperitoneum (**E**, *asterisk*) and extraluminal contrast. Note the marked low-attenuation intramural edema surrounding the ulcer. Contrast-enhanced CT images (**G** and **H**) from a fourth patient show a perforated posterior duodenal ulcer (**G**, *arrowhead*) with pneumoretroperitoneum (**H**, *asterisk*) and inflammation extending along the anterior pararenal space. EGD image (**I**) from a final patient shows a peptic stricture involving the duodenal bulb from healing and fibrosis of previous ulcer disease.

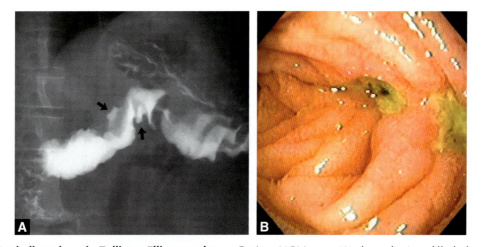

FIGURE 2.1.3 **Postbulbar ulcers in Zollinger-Ellison syndrome.** Barium UGI image (**A**) shows barium-filled ulcers (*arrows*), at least one of which is postbulbar, with surrounding lucent halos of edema. Gastric fold thickening is also present from the hypergastrinemic state. EGD image (**B**) from a different patient shows discrete ulcers in the second portion of the duodenum. A markedly elevated gastrin level (>1000 pg/mL) and positive octreotide scan confirmed the diagnosis of gastrinoma.

2.2 Duodenitis

(Figures 2.2.1-2.2.8)

CLINICAL FEATURES

- Duodenitis may be secondary to infection (primarily from *H. pylori*), Crohn's disease, vasculitis, pancreatitis, or other inflammatory causes; correlation with clinical history is often helpful.
- Typical symptoms from duodenitis include dyspepsia, epigastric pain, and nausea; erosive duodenitis is an uncommon cause of clinically significant gastrointestinal bleeding.
- Significance and treatment varies depending on the underlying cause; incidental detection of nonspecific inflammation is relatively common.

IMAGING FEATURES

- Radiologic features of duodenitis include nonspecific fold thickening at fluoroscopy and wall thickening at CT; more subtle barium findings include mucosal coarsening and tiny erosions.
- EGD is more accurate than radiologic imaging for diagnosis; endoscopic findings include erythema, fold thickening, raised patches, small white erosions, frank ulcers, and petechiae.
- Peptic erosions and ulcers are frequently superimposed on *H. pylori* duodenitis.
- Giardiasis, *Mycobacterium avium-intracellulare* (MAI), and Whipple's disease can all manifest as fold thickening and nodularity but may also appear normal in all of these infectious processes.
- Additional findings in MAI and Whipple's disease include low-attenuation adenopathy at CT and small white nodular lesions at EGD.
- Duodenal Crohn's disease is often associated with gastric antral involvement; imaging features include aphthoid or large ulcers, "cobblestone" mucosal pattern, and strictures.
- Duodenal findings that may be seen in celiac disease include irregularity on barium studies and fold scalloping and/or atrophy at EGD (see Chapter 4 for a more detailed description).
- Vasculitis, eosinophilic enteritis, and graft-versus-host disease are uncommon causes of duodenitis with a variable imaging appearance; clinical and histologic correlation is often required for diagnosis.
- Duodenal ischemia is uncommon, owing to its rich vascular supply, but it can be seen after arterial embolotherapy and other causes of vascular compromise.
- The endoscopic appearance of duodenal ischemia ranges from multiple ulcerations to dusky, necrotic mucosa.
- Pancreatitis is a common extrinsic cause of duodenitis from local surrounding inflammation.

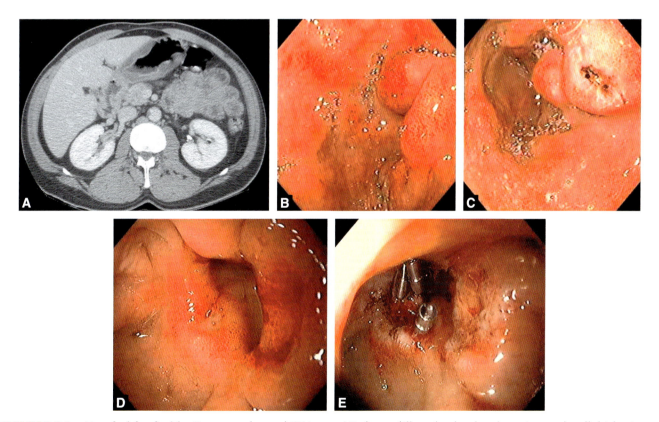

FIGURE 2.2.1 *H. pylori* **duodenitis.** Contrast-enhanced CT image **(A)** shows diffuse duodenal and gastric antral wall thickening. EGD image **(B)** shows the typical patchy erythema composed of multiple punctate spots classically seen in the duodenal bulb. EGD image **(C)** from a different patient demonstrates a similar but more diffuse mucosal pattern of erythema, associated with erosions and a shallow ulcer. EGD image **(D)** from a final patient shows bulbar duodenitis and two ulcers with recent bleeding, one of which has a visible vessel. Both ulcers were treated with bipolar electrocoagulation and hemoclips **(E)**.

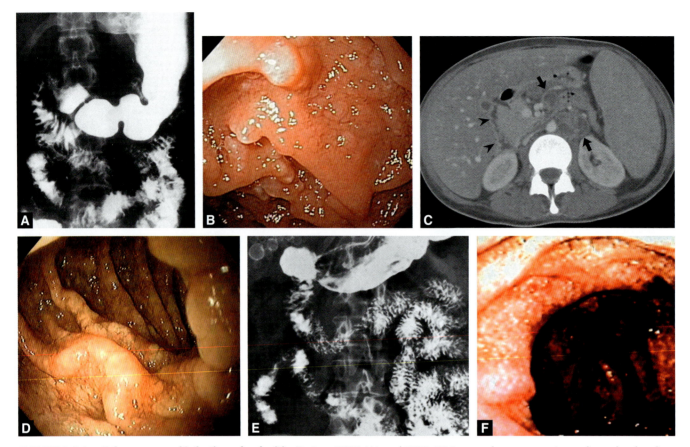

FIGURE 2.2.2 **Other causes of infectious duodenitis.** Barium SBFT (**A**) and EGD (**B**) images from two patients show duodenal fold thickening and nodularity from giardiasis. Jejunal fold thickening is also evident on the barium study. Contrast-enhanced CT image (**C**) from an AIDS patient with disseminated MAI shows splenomegaly, low-attenuation lymphadenopathy (*arrows*), and prominent duodenal folds (*arrowheads*). Corresponding EGD image (**D**) shows thickened duodenal folds with innumerable raised white mucosal nodules. Barium SBFT image (**E**) from a patient with Whipple's disease shows diffuse small-bowel fold thickening. EGD image (**F**) from another patient with Whipple's disease shows edematous and friable mucosa with punctate white spots.

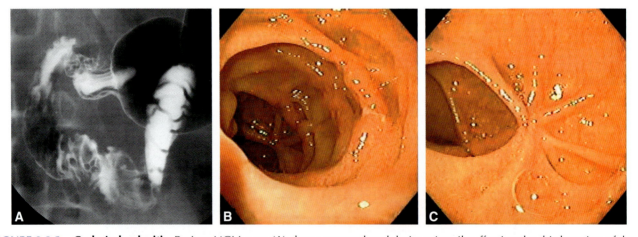

FIGURE 2.2.3 **Crohn's duodenitis.** Barium UGI image (**A**) shows mucosal nodularity primarily affecting the third portion of the duodenum. EGD images (**B** and **C**) from a second patient show shallow mucosal ulcers and fold thickening from active inflammation, as well as postinflammatory scarring and luminal narrowing.

Illustration continued on following page

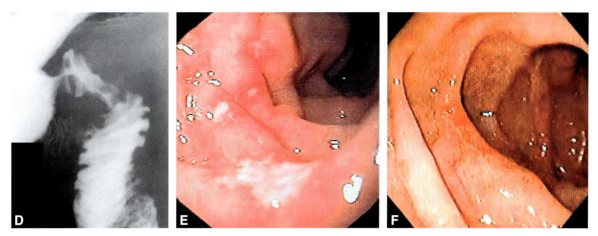

FIGURE 2.2.3 (Continued) **Crohn's duodenitis.** Barium UGI image (**D**) from a third patient shows irregular fold thickening of the proximal duodenum. Corresponding EGD image (**E**) shows multiple aphthoid ulcers and fold thickening. EGD image (**F**) from a final patient shows diffuse mucosal inflammation with aphthoid and linear erosions.

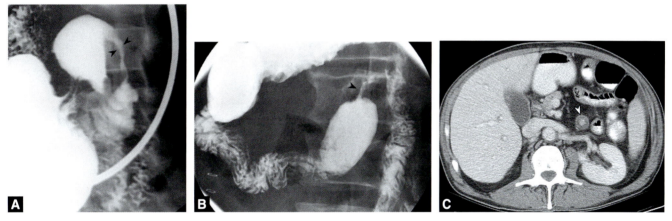

FIGURE 2.2.4 **Duodenal stricture from Crohn's disease.** Prone barium UGI image (**A**) shows a postbulbar stricture (*arrowheads*) from long-standing Crohn's disease. Barium UGI image (**B**) from a second patient shows high-grade narrowing of the fourth portion of the duodenum (*arrowhead*) with dilation of the segment proximal to the stricture. Contrast-enhanced CT image (**C**) shows circumferential duodenal wall thickening at the level of the stricture (*arrowhead*).

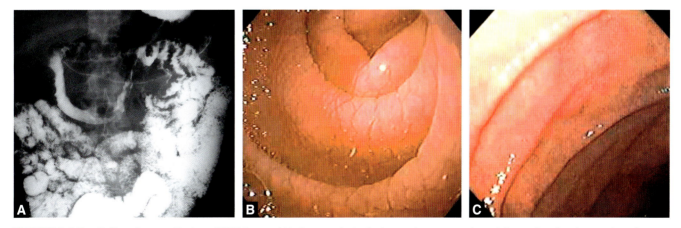

FIGURE 2.2.5 **Celiac disease.** Barium SBFT image (**A**) shows relatively featureless narrowing of the entire duodenum (moulage sign), as well as a decrease in the number of proximal jejunal folds, which also appear thickened. EGD image (**B**) from a second patient shows scalloping of the duodenal folds characteristic of celiac disease. EGD image (**C**) from a third patient shows marked atrophy of the duodenal folds.

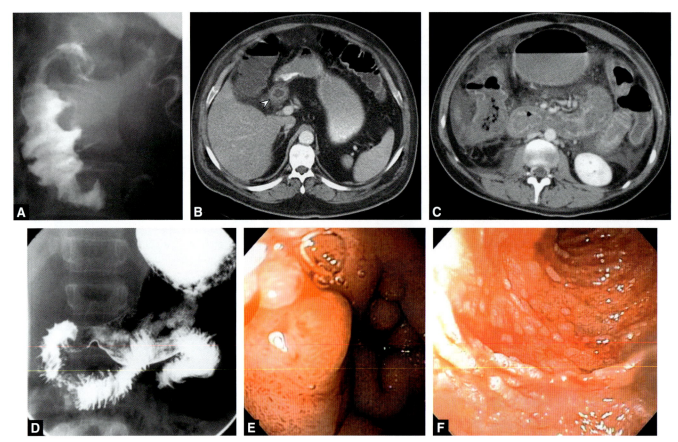

FIGURE 2.2.6 Other noninfectious causes of duodenitis. Barium UGI (**A**) and contrast-enhanced CT (**B**) images from two patients with Henoch-Schönlein purpura show prominent duodenal fold thickening and wall thickening (**B**, *arrowhead*), respectively, from submucosal hemorrhage and edema. Contrast-enhanced CT image (**C**) from a patient with new-onset Wegener's granulomatosis shows marked bowel wall thickening with mural striation due to severe vasculitis. Barium UGI image (**D**) from a patient with eosinophilic gastroenteritis shows diffuse duodenal fold thickening. EGD image (**E**) from a different patient with eosinophilic gastroenteritis shows thickened erythematous folds and an irregular ulcer. EGD image (**F**) from a patient with graft-versus-host disease shows extensive mucosal sloughing and exposed submucosa surrounding islands of remaining mucosa, creating a nodular appearance to the duodenum.

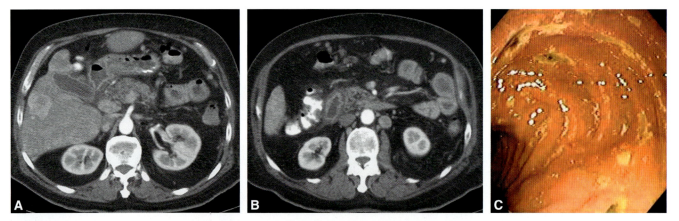

FIGURE 2.2.7 Duodenal ischemia after hepatic arterial chemoembolization. Contrast-enhanced CT images (**A** and **B**) from a patient status post hepatic artery chemoembolization for metastatic carcinoid tumor show diffuse duodenal wall thickening. Note the hypervascular hepatic metastatic disease. EGD image (**C**) shows edematous mucosa with superficial ulcerations involving the tops of folds in the second portion of the duodenum.

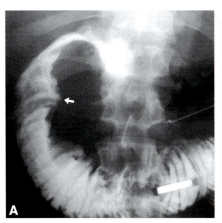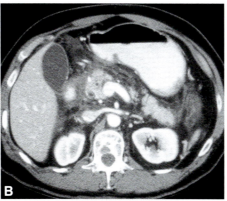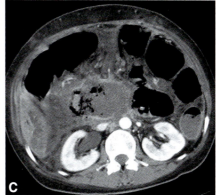

FIGURE 2.2.8 **Duodenal inflammation secondary to pancreatitis.** Image from contrast duodenography (**A**) shows luminal narrowing and fold thickening due to adjacent pancreatitis. Relative tethering at the level of the ampulla of Vater (*arrow*) gives rise to the "reverse 3 sign." Contrast-enhanced CT image (**B**) from a patient with edematous pancreatitis shows extensive peripancreatic inflammation, which includes the second portion of the duodenum. Contrast-enhanced CT image (**C**) from a patient with severe necrotizing pancreatitis shows duodenal pneumatosis from secondary ischemia.

3. OTHER DUODENAL CONDITIONS

3.1 Vascular Lesions
(Figures 3.1.1-3.1.4)

CLINICAL FEATURES

- Duodenal telangiectasias may be isolated or related to hereditary hemorrhagic telangiectasia or CREST variant of progressive systemic sclerosis; occult or clinically significant GI bleeding may be present.
- Duodenal varices are typically related to portal hypertension but are much less common than gastroesophageal varices; upper GI bleeding is the major complication.
- Superior mesenteric artery (SMA) syndrome results from compression of the third portion of the duodenum between the SMA and aorta; it is often associated with prior surgery or rapid weight loss.
- Intramural duodenal hematoma can result from blunt abdominal trauma (including nonaccidental trauma in children), endoscopic injury, and underlying coagulopathy.

IMAGING FEATURES

- Telangiectasias are readily identified at endoscopy as small cherry-red patches, sometimes surrounded by a halo of relatively white mucosa.
- Duodenal varices appear as smooth, often tortuous, submucosal lesions within the proximal duodenum.
- SMA syndrome is suggested by a dilated duodenum proximal to an abrupt cut-off from the crossing SMA; it is important to correlate for associated symptoms because the imaging findings alone are not diagnostic.
- At barium evaluation, duodenal hematoma appears as an intramural process that causes luminal narrowing; CT can readily confirm the diagnosis by directly demonstrating the hematoma.

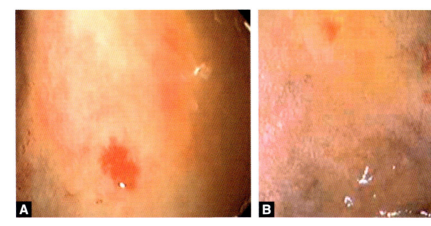

FIGURE 3.1.1 **Duodenal telangiectasias.** EGD images (**A** and **B**) from two patients show duodenal telangiectasias related to the CREST variant of scleroderma (**A**) and hereditary hemorrhagic telangiectasia (**B**).

134 THE DUODENUM

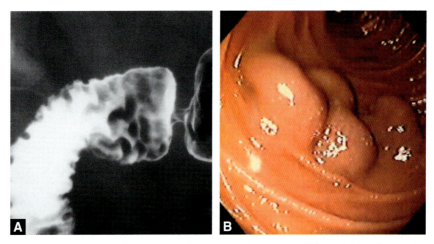

FIGURE 3.1.2 **Duodenal varices.** Barium UGI image **(A)** shows smooth, tortuous filling defects from submucosal varices. EGD image **(B)** shows varices in the second portion of the duodenum from a different patient with portal hypertension.

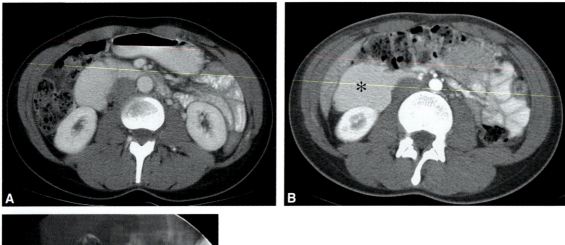

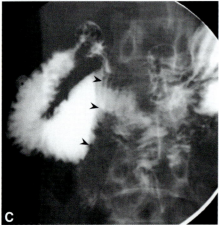

FIGURE 3.1.3 **SMA impression and syndrome.** CT image **(A)** from an asymptomatic patient shows a dilated contrast-filled duodenum that narrows at the third portion, where the SMA crosses over. In the absence of associated symptoms, such imaging findings should generally not be misinterpreted as pathologic. CT image **(B)** from a symptomatic patient shows prominent distention of the proximal duodenum (*asterisk*); cut-off related to SMA impression is well demonstrated at barium fluoroscopy **(C**, *arrowheads*).

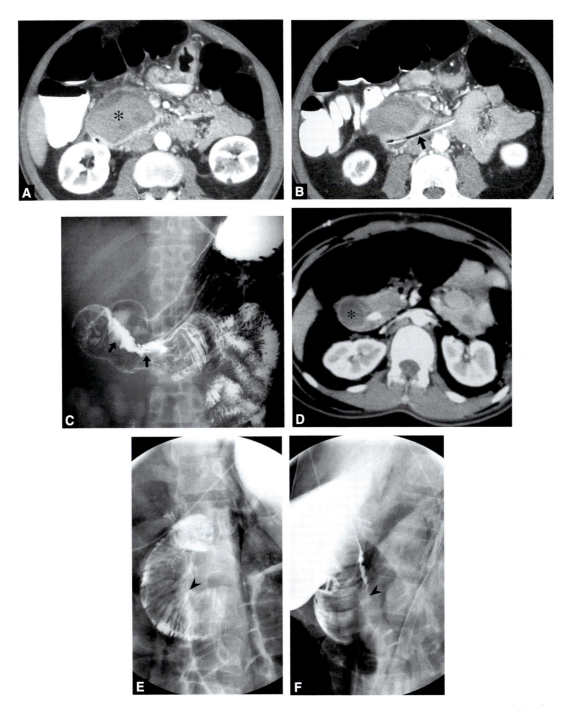

FIGURE 3.1.4 Duodenal hematoma. Contrast-enhanced CT images (**A** and **B**) demonstrate a large intramural duodenal hematoma (**A**, *asterisk*) due to endoscopic injury that causes significant luminal narrowing; note the enteric tube (**B**, *arrow*) within the compromised lumen. Barium UGI image (**C**) from a second patint shows eccentric narrowing of the duodenal lumen (*arrows*) from an intramural hematoma related to endoscopic trauma. Contrast-enhanced CT image (**D**) after ERCP from a third patient shows low-attenuation material (*asterisk*) within the duodenal wall, with medial compression of the crescent-shaped lumen where a biliary stent enters. The black areas represent extensive peritoneal, retroperitoneal, and subcutaneous gas. A large duodenal hematoma was confirmed on subsequent barium UGI, where frontal (**E**) and lateral (**F**) spot films demonstrate an extensive cast-like filling defect (*arrowheads*) that displaces the barium-filled lumen.

3.2 Aortoduodenal Fistula

(Figures 3.2.1-3.2.3)

CLINICAL FEATURES

- Aortoduodenal fistula represents a special subset of vascular lesions and can be a primary complication of an abdominal aortic aneurysm or, more commonly, secondary to prior aortoiliac surgery.
- It typically involves the third portion of the duodenum where it crosses and contacts the aorta.
- Aortic graft infection, typically from *Staphylococcus aureus* or *Escherichia coli*, is likely a major cause of the more common secondary fistula; this dreaded complication is seen in 2% or less of aortic repairs.
- Primary aortoduodenal fistula most often results from atherosclerotic disease; rare causes include aortitis, radiation therapy, and peptic ulcer disease.
- Presentations may include abdominal pain, GI bleeding, and a pulsatile abdominal mass; fatal exsanguinations are often preceded by a smaller "herald" hemorrhage days to weeks previously.

IMAGING FEATURES

- CT is usually abnormal; variable findings include periaortic hematoma, aortic pseudoaneurysm, contrast extravasation, extraluminal gas, focal duodenal wall thickening, and intraluminal duodenal blood.
- EGD can identify the site of herald bleed and occasionally even show aortic graft material at the fistula site; however, it is diagnostic in <25% of cases, often due to impaired visibility from pooling blood.
- Fluoroscopic findings are generally nonspecific, including extrinsic compression of the duodenum.
- Tagged red blood cell scintigraphy and angiography can demonstrate a herald hemorrhage but otherwise have limited roles in diagnosis.

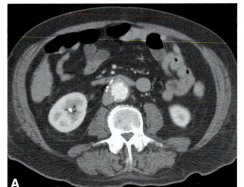
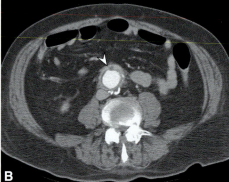
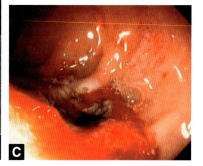

FIGURE 3.2.1 Aortoduodenal fistula. Contrast-enhanced CT images (**A** and **B**) from a patient with a UGI herald hemorrhage and history of previous aortic repair shows a subtle focus of low attenuation (**B**, *arrowhead*) that bridges the graft to involve the inferior aspect of the third portion of the duodenum. Subsequent EGD image (**C**) shows mucosal ulceration where the duodenum overlies the aortic graft, as well as evidence of recent bleeding. Unfortunately, this patient exsanguinated before surgical intervention could be performed.

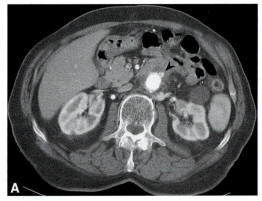
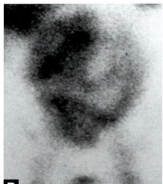
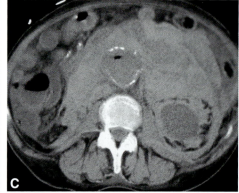

FIGURE 3.2.2 Aortoduodenal fistula. Contrast-enhanced CT image (**A**) shows a small focal aortic pseudoaneurysm (*arrowhead*) and surrounding low-attenuation hematoma between the aorta and overlying duodenum. Image from tagged red blood cell scintigraphy (**B**) from a second patient shows small bowel activity from a brisk herald hemorrhage; aortoduodenal fistula secondary to graft infection was confirmed and repaired at surgery. Noncontrast CT image (**C**) from a patient with an abdominal aortic aneurysm shows a massive high-attenuation para-aortic hematoma indicating aortic rupture. The patient presented with a massive gastrointestinal hemorrhage from a primary aortoduodenal fistula; note the intraluminal aortic gas indicative of this fistula.

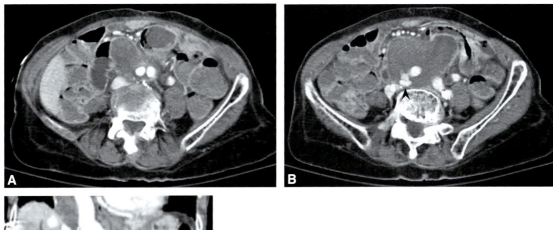
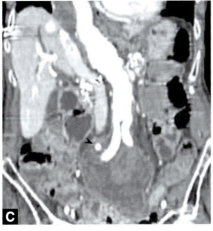

FIGURE 3.2.3 Aortoenteric fistula. Transverse (**A** and **B**) and coronal (**C**) contrast-enhanced CT images from a patient status post aortobifemoral bypass grafting show a large perigraft hematoma and enhancing graft leak (*arrowheads*) involving the right iliac limb. The patient presented with a GI herald hemorrhage related to an evolving fistula with the overlying mesenteric small bowel.

3.3 Duodenal Diverticula
(Figures 3.3.1-3.3.4)

CLINICAL FEATURES

- Duodenal diverticula are common acquired outpouchings; the vast majority are asymptomatic but rare complications include diverticulitis, bleeding, and various pancreaticobiliary complications.
- An intraluminal duodenal diverticulum is a rare congenital anomaly that develops from an incomplete membrane that elongates over time; it can present with nausea and vomiting related to partial obstruction.

IMAGING FEATURES

- Duodenal diverticula are commonly seen on barium UGI and EGD; diverticula most often project along the inner aspect of the duodenal sweep (postbulbar, often periampullary).
- On CT, diverticula contain varying combinations of gas, fluid, and debris; as such, incidental duodenal diverticula can sometimes be mistaken for abscess, cystic pancreatic lesions, or pneumobilia.
- Duodenal diverticulitis is rare, but CT can demonstrate peridiverticular inflammatory changes.
- Significant upper gastrointestinal bleeding from a duodenal diverticulum is also rare but can be localized at EGD.
- At fluoroscopy, an intraluminal diverticulum typically appears as a barium-filled "wind-sock" deformity originating in the second portion; it may simulate a polypoid lesion if it does not fill with contrast.

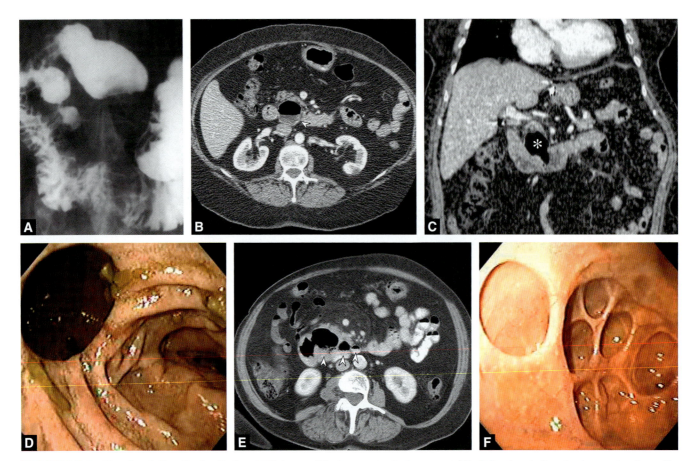

FIGURE 3.3.1 **Duodenal diverticula.** Barium UGI image **(A)** shows a typical contrast-filled duodenal diverticulum extending off the inner aspect of the duodenal sweep. Contrast-enhanced CT image **(B)** from a second patient shows a rounded focus (*arrowhead*) adjacent to the duodenum and pancreas that contains an air-fluid level. Curved reformatted coronal CT image **(C)** better demonstrates the duodenal origin of this uncomplicated diverticulum (*asterisk*) extending off the inner aspect of the sweep. EGD image **(D)** from a third patient shows the endoscopic appearance of a typical duodenal diverticulum. Contrast-enhanced CT image **(E)** from a fourth patient shows several duodenal diverticula (*arrowheads*) that vary in both size and luminal composition. EGD image **(F)** from a final patient shows multiple duodenal diverticula.

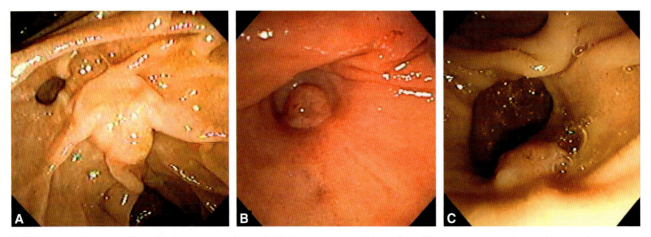

FIGURE 3.3.2 **Periampullary duodenal diverticula.** EGD images **(A to E)** from five different patients show periampullary diverticula of varying sizes and variable relationship to the ampulla. In some cases, cannulation for ERCP is made more challenging by the presence of these diverticula.

Illustration continued on following page

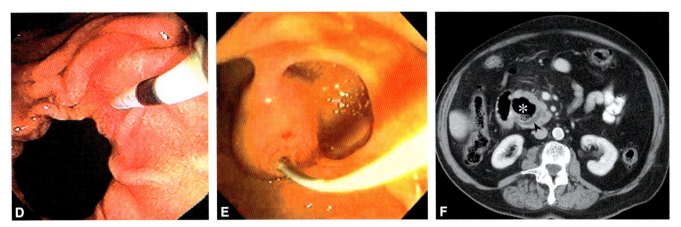

FIGURE 3.3.2 (Continued) **Periampullary duodenal diverticula.** Contrast-enhanced CT image **(F)** from a final patient shows a large periampullary diverticulum (*asterisk*) that deviates and compromises the main pancreatic duct (*arrowhead*), which is moderately dilated.

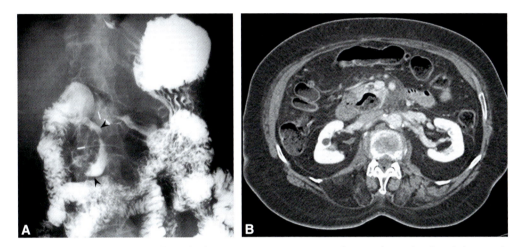

FIGURE 3.3.3 **Complications of duodenal diverticula.** Barium UGI image **(A)** shows a large duodenal diverticulum (*arrowheads*) that contains an irregular lobulated filling defect, which proved to be a villous adenoma. In the vast majority of cases, filling defects within diverticula simply represent intraluminal debris. Contrast-enhanced CT image **(B)** from a patient with acute abdominal pain shows a large debris-filled diverticulum with hazy soft tissue inflammatory changes in the surrounding fat. Although the CT findings suggest acute pancreatitis, this is an example of duodenal diverticulitis.

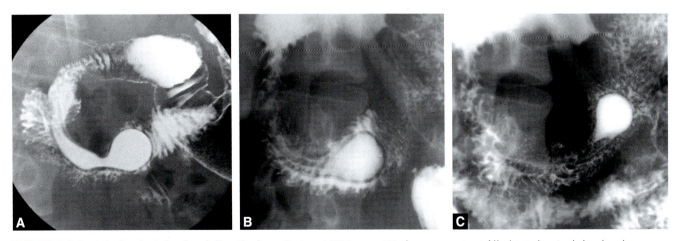

FIGURE 3.3.4 **Intraluminal duodenal diverticulum.** Barium UGI image **(A)** shows a contrast-filled intraluminal duodenal diverticulum, which demonstrates the "wind-sock" appearance. Note the radiolucent wall that separates the diverticular lumen from the rest of the duodenal lumen. Barium UGI images **(B** and **C)** from a different patient show a similar-appearing intraluminal diverticulum. Note how the diverticulum retains contrast longer than that passing through the remainder of the duodenum.

3.4 Duodenal Duplication Cyst
(Figure 3.4.1)

CLINICAL FEATURES

- Duplication cysts are uncommon congenital lesions of the alimentary tract that result in cystic masses generally involving the mesenteric aspect of the bowel wall.
- Duodenal duplication cysts comprise only about 5% of all intestinal duplications.
- Most duodenal duplication cysts involve the first or second portion; communication with the bowel lumen is very rare.
- The smooth muscle layer of the cyst is often contiguous with the adjacent duodenum; the mucosal lining may contain gastric, intestinal, pancreatic, or respiratory epithelium.
- Duplication cysts may present as incidental palpable masses or as pain, fever, bleeding, intussusception, or obstructive symptoms; cyst proximity to the ampulla of Vater can lead to pancreatitis or obstructive jaundice.

IMAGING FEATURES

- Contrast fluoroscopy will typically show a filling defect suggestive of an intramural or extrinsic mass; contrast opacification of the cyst itself is rare.
- Cross-sectional imaging studies, such as CT and US, elucidate the cystic nature of the mass and its relationship to the bowel wall.
- A striated appearance to the cyst wall at US represents the characteristic bowel layers and is highly suggestive of the diagnosis; echogenic internal material can be seen if the cyst is infected or hemorrhagic.
- Other cystic lesions can mimic a duodenal duplication cyst, including pancreatic pseudocysts, choledochal cysts, and mesenteric cysts.

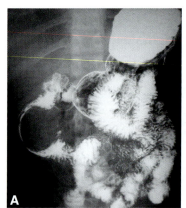
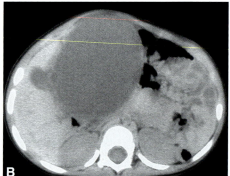
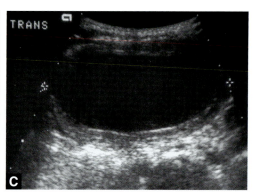

FIGURE 3.4.1 Duodenal duplication cyst. Barium UGI image (**A**) shows a large rounded filling defect that displaces the duodenal lumen laterally, suggestive of an intramural lesion or extrinsic pancreatic pseudocyst or mass. Noncontrast CT (**B**) and US (**C**) images from a different patient show a large right upper quadrant cystic mass. On US, a striated appearance to the cyst wall is characteristic of a duplication cyst. Hepatobiliary scintigraphy (not shown) demonstrated no evidence of communication with the biliary tree, which excluded choledochal cyst as a potential cause.

3.5 Infiltrative Diseases
(Figures 3.5.1-3.5.4)

CLINICAL FEATURES

- Non-neoplastic infiltrative diseases that can affect the duodenum include amyloidosis, mastocytosis, and lymphoid hyperplasia.
- Amyloidosis arises from abnormal protein deposition in the extracellular space; it can be a primary process or associated with multiple myeloma or various chronic inflammatory disorders.
- GI tract involvement by amyloidosis is common, especially in the small bowel and rectum; diagnosis is established with tissue biopsy.
- Abdominal manifestations of amyloidosis include dysmotility (e.g., diarrhea and pseudo-obstruction), malabsorption, pain, ascites, and hepatosplenomegaly.
- Mastocytosis results from mast cell infiltration of multiple organ systems; histamine and prostaglandin release cause the classic symptoms of flushing, headache, asthma, pruritus, and urticaria pigmentosa.
- GI manifestations of mastocytosis include abdominal pain, nausea, vomiting, and diarrhea; increased gastric acid secretion can lead to duodenal ulceration.
- Nodular lymphoid hyperplasia is typically seen in the setting of immunoglobulin deficiency, such as common variable immune deficiency; superimposed giardiasis is not uncommon, and some patients will develop frank lymphoma.
- Pseudomelanosis duodeni is a rare benign condition caused by the accumulation of hemosiderin pigment in the mucosa; it is associated with chronic renal failure, iron supplementation, and antihypertensive drugs.

IMAGING FEATURES

- Imaging findings in duodenal amyloidosis typically consist of nonspecific fold thickening and mucosal

nodularity; focal mass lesions (amyloidomas) are much less common.
- Duodenal mastocytosis also results in fold thickening and nodularity; endoscopy can show duodenal ulcers and urticaria-like lesions; associated sclerotic bone lesions and splenomegaly may suggest the diagnosis.
- Duodenal lymphoid hyperplasia manifests as prominent nodular fold thickening.
- Pseudomelanosis duodeni appears as varying degrees of peppery speckling of the mucosa.

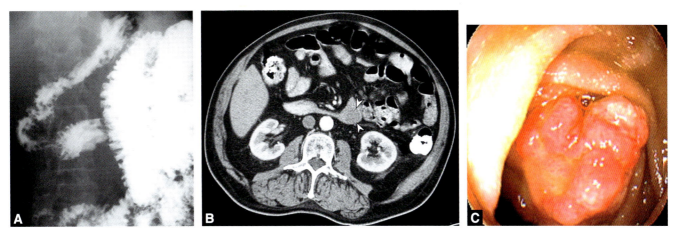

FIGURE 3.5.1 Amyloidosis. Barium SBFT image **(A)** shows diffuse nodular fold thickening that involves the stomach, duodenum, and mesenteric small bowel. Contrast-enhanced CT image **(B)** from a different patient shows focal dilatation of the fourth portion of the duodenum due to a subtle rounded mass lesion (*arrowheads*), which was confirmed at endoscopy **(C)** and proved to be an amyloidoma.

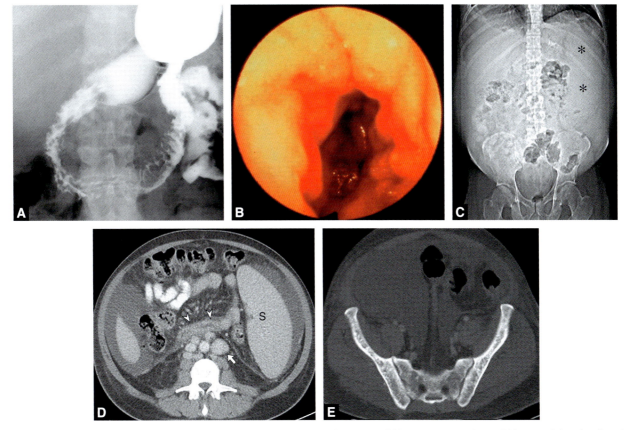

FIGURE 3.5.2 Mastocytosis. Barium UGI **(A)** and EGD **(B)** images from two different patients show diffuse nodular duodenal fold thickening. CT scout image **(C)** from a different patient shows massive splenomegaly (*asterisks*). Corresponding transverse CT image **(D)** shows duodenal fold thickening (*arrowheads*), retroperitoneal lymphadenopathy (*arrow*), and ascites, in addition to the splenomegaly (S) seen on the scout view. CT image **(E)** with bone windowing shows innumerable tiny sclerotic osseous foci throughout the bony pelvis.

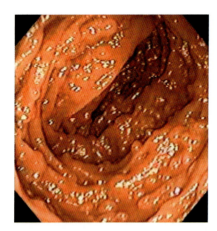 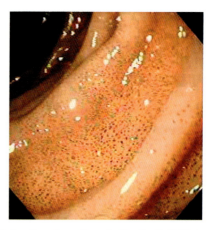

FIGURE 3.5.3 **Nodular lymphoid hyperplasia.** EGD image (A) from a patient with IgA deficiency shows innumerable mucosal nodules diffusely distributed throughout the duodenum. Both nodular lymphoid hyperplasia and giardiasis were present in this case.

FIGURE 3.5.4 **Pseudomelanosis duodeni.** EGD image from a patient with chronic renal failure and hypertension with the incidental finding of miliary black spots covering the duodenal mucosa.

CHAPTER 4

THE MESENTERIC SMALL BOWEL

David H. Kim, MD • Perry J. Pickhardt, MD

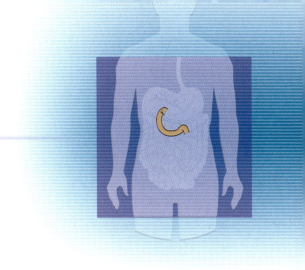

1. **SMALL BOWEL TUMORS**
   1.1 Adenocarcinoma
   1.2 Carcinoid Tumor
   1.3 Lymphoma
   1.4 Mesenchymal Tumors
   1.5 Metastatic Disease
2. **ENTERITIS**
   2.1 Crohn's Disease
   2.2 Infectious Enteritis
   2.3 Other Inflammatory Conditions
3. **OTHER SMALL BOWEL CONDITIONS**
   3.1 Small Bowel Obstruction
   3.2 Mesenteric Ischemia
   3.3 Small Bowel Herniation
   3.4 Celiac Disease
   3.5 Small Bowel Diverticula
   3.6 Malrotation
   3.7 Small Bowel Wall Thickening
   3.8 Small Bowel Perforation
   3.9 Vascular Ectasia

Often regarded as a "final frontier" owing to its relatively inaccessible location from a conventional endoscopic perspective, small bowel imaging distal to the ligament of Treitz has traditionally been the purview of the radiologist. However, the advent of capsule endoscopy and double-balloon enteroscopy has begun to shift this paradigm. Although barium evaluation remains an important component of small bowel imaging, newer modalities, most notably CT enterography and capsule endoscopy, continue to gain in importance. Perhaps the greatest strength of these studies lies in their complementary nature, because capsule endoscopy offers exquisite mucosal detail and the advanced radiologic techniques provide evaluation of the entire bowel wall and beyond. The broad topics of small bowel neoplasia, enteritis, small bowel obstruction, mesenteric ischemia, and a variety of other pathologic conditions are covered in this chapter.

1. SMALL BOWEL TUMORS

Overall, small bowel tumors are relatively uncommon, representing only 3% to 6% of GI neoplasms. The tumor types, however, are similar to those found in other portions of the GI tract. The specific entities range from benign mucosal polyps to intramural mesenchymal tumors to frankly malignant lesions. Traditionally, these tumors have generally presented late in their clinical course, but improvements in cross-sectional imaging and endoscopic technology now allow for an earlier diagnosis.

1.1 Adenocarcinoma
(Figures 1.1.1-1.1.2)

CLINICAL FEATURES

- Small bowel adenocarcinomas are relatively rare but still represent the most common malignancy of the small bowel.
- Most arise from the duodenum and proximal jejunum.
- Adenocarcinomas may present as unexplained abdominal pain, gastrointestinal bleeding (occult or overt), or obstructive symptoms.
- Routes of metastatic spread include regional lymph nodes, hematogenous to the liver, direct tumor extension, and peritoneal implantation.
- Risk factors include adult celiac disease, Crohn's disease, Peutz-Jeghers syndrome, and hereditary nonpolyposis colorectal cancer (Lynch syndrome).
- Small bowel carcinoma in the setting of long-standing Crohn's disease tends to involve the ileum.

IMAGING FEATURES

- Imaging findings include annular or eccentric focal bowel wall thickening and luminal narrowing; associated findings of ulceration and proximal dilatation may be seen.
- Classic "apple-core" appearance (irregular annular narrowing with shouldering) and proximal small bowel location are typical features that distinguish adenocarcinoma from carcinoid tumor, lymphoma, and GI stromal tumor (GIST).
- CT may demonstrate regional lymphadenopathy; widespread metastatic disease is relatively uncommon at initial presentation.

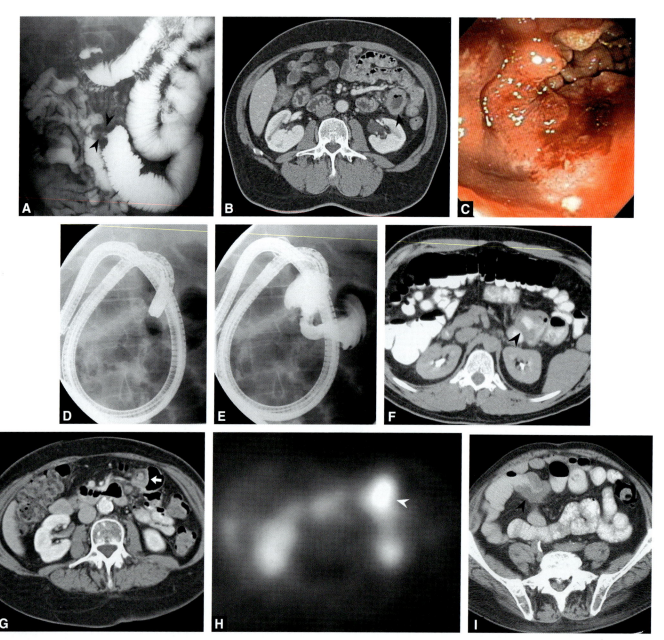

FIGURE 1.1.1. Small bowel adenocarcinoma. Image from barium UGI (**A**) shows partial obstruction from an annular, constricting jejunal mass (*arrowheads*) at the transition point to decompressed bowel. Contrast-enhanced CT image (**B**) from a different patient shows focal circumferential jejunal wall thickening (*arrowhead*). Corresponding image from push enteroscopy (**C**) shows an irregular ulcerated mucosal mass. Fluoroscopic spot films (**D** and **E**) taken during push enteroscopy in a patient with obscure GI bleeding show contrast opacification of an annular jejunal mass (**E**). The scope could not be advanced beyond this malignant stricture. Subsequent CT (**F**) confirms a focal jejunal mass (*arrowhead*) with luminal narrowing. Contrast-enhanced CT (**G**) and matched FDG PET (**H**) images from a different patient show focal jejunal wall thickening (*arrow*) that is hypermetabolic on PET (*arrowhead*). Contrast-enhanced CT image (**I**) from a patient with obscure GI bleeding shows an annular ileal soft tissue mass (*arrowhead*). (B and C, from Hara AK, Leighton JA, Sharma VK, et al: Imaging of small bowel disease: Comparison of capsule endoscopy, standard endoscopy, barium examination, and CT. Radiographics 2005;25:697-711.)

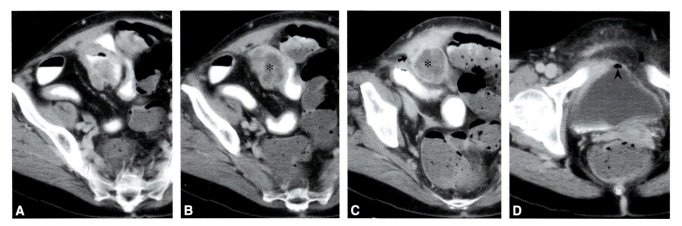

FIGURE 1.1.2. Ileal adenocarcinoma in Crohn's disease. Contrast-enhanced CT images (**A** to **D**) show a large heterogeneous soft tissue mass (**B** and **C**, *asterisks*) arising from an ileal loop with extraluminal extension. Surrounding enhancing soft tissue (**C**, *arrow*) denotes invasion of the anterior pelvic wall and urinary bladder. The gas bubble within the bladder (**D**, *arrowhead*) confirms an enterovesical fistula, which was responsible for the clinical presentation in this case. Note the underlying ileal wall thickening and fibrofatty mesenteric changes from long-standing Crohn's disease.

1.2 Carcinoid Tumor

(Figures 1.2.1-1.2.4)

CLINICAL FEATURES

- Carcinoid tumor is the second most common primary small bowel malignancy and is usually located in the ileum.
- It represents a submucosal lesion originating from neuroendocrine cells and produces vasoactive substances such as serotonin and bradykinin.
- It may be asymptomatic or manifest insidiously with nonspecific symptoms such as intermittent obstruction or vague abdominal pain; rarely, it presents as carcinoid syndrome or bleeding.
- Carcinoid syndrome due to systemic effects of serotonin includes episodic flushing, diarrhea, headache, nausea, and bronchospasm; 24-hour urine 5-HIAA level is usually elevated.
- Carcinoid syndrome typically occurs late in the disease course and generally requires hepatic metastatic disease to bypass metabolism of serotonin by the liver.
- Effects of serotonin may lead to subendothelial fibrosis in the right side of the heart with resultant tricuspid regurgitation; the left side of the heart is protected by the metabolizing effects of the pulmonary parenchyma.
- Benign versus malignant status is indistinguishable on histology; it is characterized instead by the presence or absence of metastatic spread.

IMAGING FEATURES

- Carcinoid tumor may appear as a submucosal mass at barium SBFT or on ileal intubation at colonoscopy.
- The overlying mucosa may ulcerate and result in occult or overt blood loss; rarely the lesion may serve as a lead point for intussusception.
- Detection of carcinoid tumors has improved with newer modalities such as capsule endoscopy and CT enterography.
- At CT, regional metastatic spread to the mesenteric root is more often identified than the primary tumor itself.
- The mesenteric nodal mass may calcify in up to 50% of cases; surrounding stellate desmoplasia is typical.
- Segmental ileal thickening at CT is often present and may be related to desmoplastic reaction or venous congestion from vascular compromise by a mesenteric root mass.
- Hepatic metastases are hypervascular at CT and MRI and often have a target appearance at US.
- Blastic osseous metastatic disease may be seen.
- Octreotide scintigraphy is useful for staging and evaluating for treatment response.
- Inferior vena cava and hepatic veins may rarely be enlarged secondary to tricuspid regurgitation from subendothelial fibrosis of the right side of the heart.

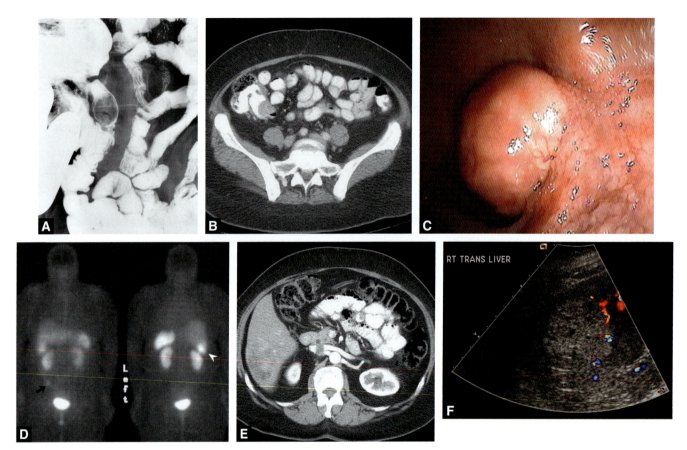

FIGURE 1.2.1 Ileal carcinoid tumor. Spot film from barium SBFT **(A)** shows a smooth, ovoid submucosal mass within the distal ileum. Contrast-enhanced CT image **(B)** shows that the soft tissue mass is located just proximal to the ileocecal valve. Image from ileal intubation at colonoscopy **(C)** confirms a submucosal lesion. Octreotide scintigraphy **(D)** shows subtle activity from the ileal primary (*arrow*), as well as focal hepatic activity (*arrowhead*) representing metastatic disease. Arterial phase CT **(E)** and color Doppler US **(F)** images show that the hepatic metastasis is hypervascular and hyperechoic, respectively, which are characteristic features.

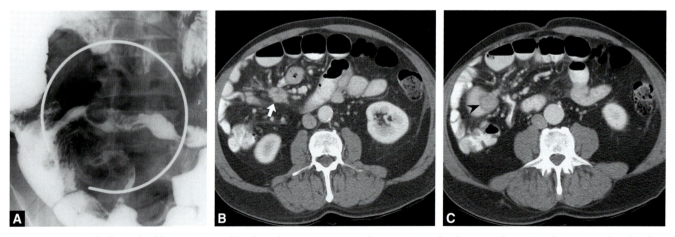

FIGURE 1.2.2 Ileal carcinoid tumor. Spot film from barium SBFT **(A)** shows a typical submucosal carcinoid tumor in the distal ileum. Contrast-enhanced CT images **(B** and **C)** from a different patient show local mesenteric spread **(B,** *arrow*) from the adjacent submucosal ileal mass **(C,** *arrowhead*).

Illustration continued on following page

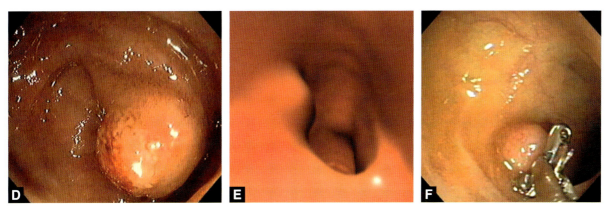

FIGURE 1.2.2 (Continued) **Ileal carcinoid tumor.** Image from ileoscopy (**D**) from a third patient shows a typical submucosal carcinoid tumor. 3D endoluminal image (**E**) of the distal ileum from CT colonography shows a small submucosal lesion in the distal ileum, which was proven to be a carcinoid tumor at optical colonoscopy with ileoscopy (**F**).

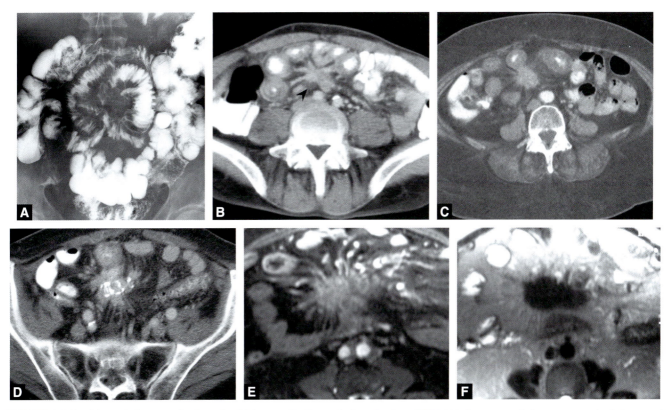

FIGURE 1.2.3 **Mesenteric spread of carcinoid tumor.** Radiograph from barium SBFT (**A**) shows a radial arrangement of abnormal small bowel loops with spiculated fold thickening due to desmoplastic tumor spread to the mesenteric root. Corresponding CT image (**B**) demonstrates the irregular mesenteric mass (*arrowhead*), with soft tissue tendrils radiating out to the thickened small bowel loops seen at SBFT. Contrast-enhanced CT images (**C** and **D**) from two different patients show typical spiculated central mesenteric masses, the second of which demonstrates calcification, and associated small bowel wall thickening. Fat-suppressed contrast-enhanced SGE MR (**E**) and T2-weighted MR (**F**) images show a large spiculated mesenteric mass, which demonstrates low T2 signal from the desmoplastic fibrosis.

Illustration continued on following page

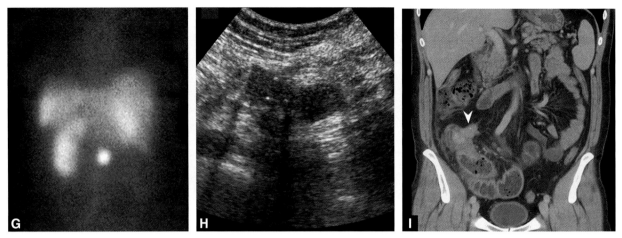

FIGURE 1.2.3 (Continued) **Mesenteric spread of carcinoid tumor.** Image from octreotide scintigraphy **(G)** in a different patient shows a central focus of increased activity from typical mesenteric spread. Right lower quadrant abdominal US **(H)** from a final patient shows a complex hypoechoic mass with punctate hyperechoic foci suggestive of calcifications. Coronal contrast-enhanced CT image **(I)** shows the mesenteric mass (*arrowhead*) and confirms the punctuate calcifications. Adjacent ileal soft tissue thickening represents the site of the primary tumor, which has resulted in partial small bowel obstruction.

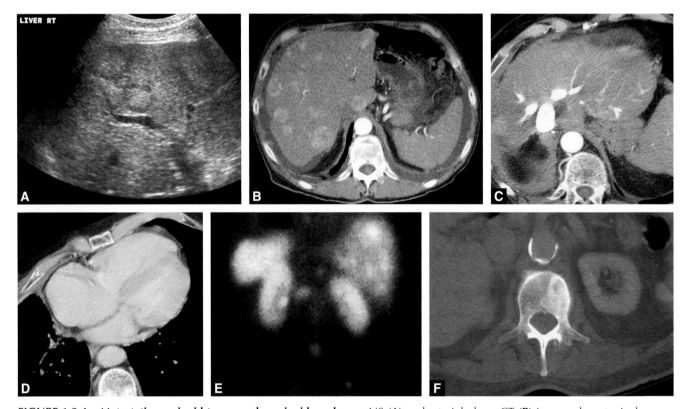

FIGURE 1.2.4 **Metastatic carcinoid tumor and carcinoid syndrome.** US **(A)** and arterial phase CT **(B)** images show typical carcinoid metastases with a target appearance, hypoechoic rim at US, and hypervascular enhancement at CT. Arterial phase CT image **(C)** from a patient with carcinoid syndrome shows evidence of tricuspid regurgitation with reflux of dense contrast into dilated hepatic veins. Partially treated hepatic metastatic disease is present. CT image through the thorax **(D)** shows a dilated right atrium from subendothelial fibrosis. Image from octreotide scintigraphy **(E)** in a final patient shows multiple metastatic foci, including osseous metastases that appear blastic on CT **(F)**.

1.3 Lymphoma
(Figures 1.3.1-1.3.6)

CLINICAL FEATURES

- Lymphomas may be primary or secondary but almost always of non-Hodgkin's histology (typically B cell).
- The small bowel is the second most common site for GI lymphoma after the stomach.
- The mid-distal small bowel is more often involved than the proximal small bowel.
- Lymphoma may present as abdominal pain, anemia, or weight loss; obstruction is uncommon.
- Acute presentation may be due to intussusception or massive GI hemorrhage.
- Risk for perforation is highest during treatment of cases with transmural bowel wall involvement.
- American Burkitt's lymphoma often presents as bulky ileocecal disease in children and young adults.
- Patients with autoimmune disease such as systemic lupus erythematosus are at an increased risk.
- Patients with celiac disease are prone to developing T-cell lymphoma (see section 3.4).

IMAGING FEATURES

- Massive segmental wall thickening with aneurysmal luminal dilatation is the classic appearance on imaging; multifocal submucosal nodules (lymphomatous polyposis) is typical of the mantle cell form.
- Mesenteric or peritoneal disease can be associated with or cause secondary bowel involvement.
- Obstruction is uncommon and may suggest an alternative diagnosis.
- CT is the imaging modality of choice for detecting typical bulky disease and can evaluate for associated lymphadenopathy.
- At US, lymphoma typically manifests as pronounced focal hypoechoic bowel wall thickening.
- Barium SBFT, enteroclysis, CT enterography, and capsule endoscopy can provide complementary imaging; luminal studies may be more sensitive for lymphomatous polyposis.
- Nodular lymphoid hyperplasia appears at barium evaluation as small, uniform filling defects most often involving the terminal ileum; these follicles should not be confused with lymphomatous polyposis.

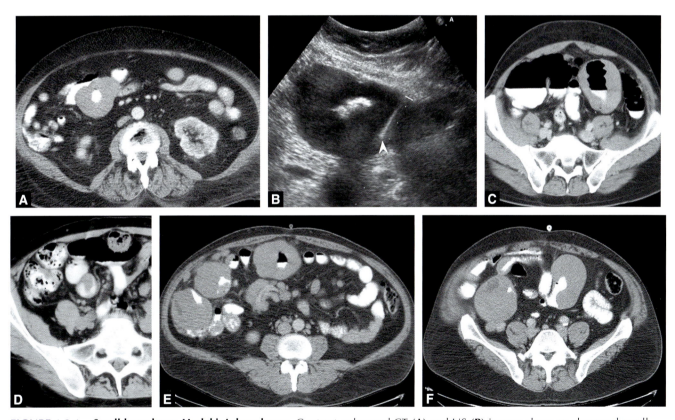

FIGURE 1.3.1 Small bowel non-Hodgkin's lymphoma. Contrast-enhanced CT (**A**) and US (**B**) images show an abnormal small bowel loop with marked circumferential wall thickening but relative preservation of the lumen. Diagnosis was made by percutaneous biopsy (*arrowhead*) of the hypoechoic wall under US. Contrast-enhanced CT image (**C**) from a second patient shows classic soft tissue thickening of a bowel loop with associated aneurysmal dilatation of the lumen. CT image (**D**) from a third patient shows an intraluminal polypoid mass; other lesions were present in this case of lymphomatous polyposis. Contrast-enhanced CT images (**E** and **F**) from a patient with mantle cell lymphoma show multiple areas of massive small bowel wall thickening without evidence of obstruction, which is typical of these tumors.

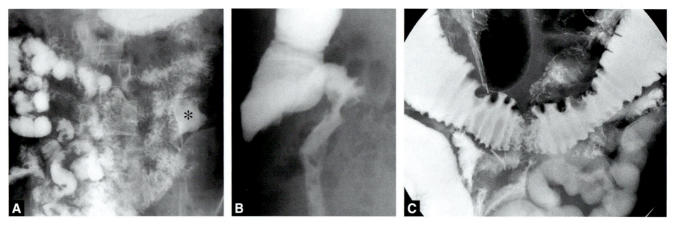

FIGURE 1.3.2 Barium findings in small bowel lymphoma. Radiograph from barium SBFT **(A)** shows a focal jejunal loop demonstrating featureless luminal dilation (*asterisk*). The degree of wall thickening can only be surmised on conventional barium studies. Spot film from barium evaluation **(B)** in a different patient shows mild narrowing and irregularity from ileocecal lymphoma. The lack of obstructive findings supports the diagnosis. Spot film from barium SBFT **(C)** in a third patient shows relatively diffuse and slightly nodular fold thickening involving a loop of small bowel.

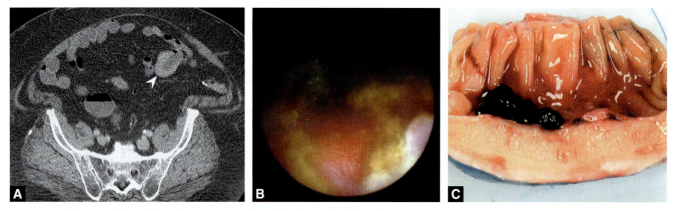

FIGURE 1.3.3 Small bowel lymphoma presenting with obscure GI bleeding. Contrast-enhanced CT image **(A)** shows focal eccentric wall thickening of a jejunal loop (*arrowhead*). Image from capsule endoscopy **(B)** demonstrates a corresponding ulcerated jejunal mass. Photograph of the resected gross specimen **(C)** again demonstrates the eccentric bowel wall thickening.

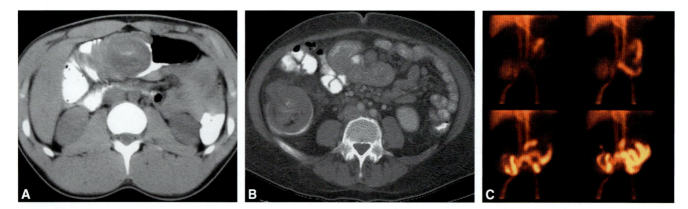

FIGURE 1.3.4 Acute presentation of small bowel lymphoma. CT image **(A)** from an adolescent with acute abdominal pain shows a prominent ileocolic intussusception extending into the transverse colon, which was later proven to represent Burkitt's lymphoma. CT image **(B)** from an adult shows ileocolic intussusception from ileal lymphoma, as well as extensive mesenteric lymphadenopathy. Collage of sequential images from tagged RBC scintigraphy **(C)** from a different patient shows progressive small bowel activity from an acute GI hemorrhage from lymphoma.

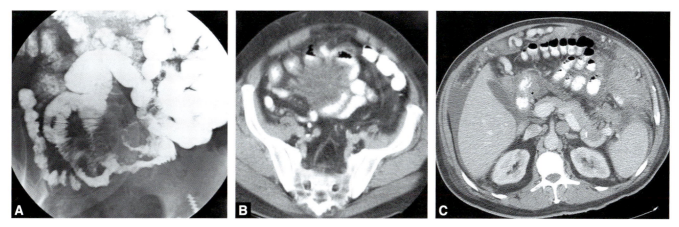

FIGURE 1.3.5 Mesenteric and peritoneal lymphoma with secondary bowel involvement. Spot film from barium SBFT (**A**) shows a cluster of ileal loops with luminal narrowing and fold thickening. Corresponding CT image (**B**) shows a large mesenteric soft tissue mass, which secondarily involves the small bowel and gives rise to the barium findings. Contrast-enhanced CT image (**C**) from a patient with peritoneal lymphomatosis shows diffuse omental and mesenteric soft tissue infiltration, as well as serosal bowel wall thickening and ascites.

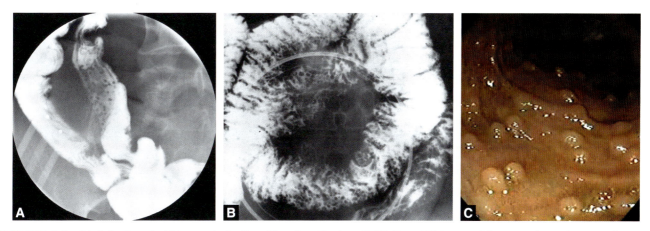

FIGURE 1.3.6 Nodular lymphoid hyperplasia. Spot films from barium SBFT (**A** and **B**) in two different patients show small uniform nodular filling defects from mild (**A**) and extensive (**B**) lymphoid hyperplasia. Image from ileoscopy during colonoscopy (**C**) in a third patient shows multiple well-circumscribed nodules. This benign finding is frequently encountered, particularly in young patients, and should not be mistaken for lymphoma.

1.4 Mesenchymal Tumors
(Figures 1.4.1-1.4.8)

CLINICAL FEATURES

- Mesenchymal tumors are a heterogeneous group of intramural lesions that arise deep to the mucosa.
- Gastrointestinal stromal tumor (GIST) accounts for the majority of solid mesenchymal neoplasms; these tumors arise from the interstitial cells of Cajal (GI pacemaker cells).
- Other mesenchymal tumors include smooth muscle tumors (e.g., leiomyoma), neurogenic tumors (e.g., schwannoma, neurofibroma), vascular tumors (e.g., hemangioma), and hamartomas.
- GISTs were previously misclassified as smooth muscle tumors.
- Mesenchymal tumors may present with acute or occult GI bleeding secondary to ulceration of the overlying mucosa.
- Malignant mesenchymal tumors typically spread via direct local extension, intraperitoneal seeding, or hematogenously (to liver).
- Small bowel lipomas are generally benign incidental findings but may lead to intussusception.
- Hamartomas consist of varying amounts of smooth muscle and epithelial tissue.
- Multiple small bowel hamartomas are a common finding in Peutz-Jeghers syndrome; these benign polyps may act as lead points for intussusception.
- Hemangiomas and lymphangiomas of the small bowel are usually asymptomatic incidental findings; see section 3.9 for discussion of vascular ectasia.
- Most nerve sheath tumors (i.e., schwannomas and neurofibromas) are benign.

IMAGING FEATURES

- Mesenchymal tumors are intramural masses that typically manifest as smooth, broad-based impressions on

barium studies; nonulcerated lesions may be difficult to distinguish from extrinsic impression.
- CT and MR are useful for demonstrating both the intramural and exoenteric tumor components, which are typically much more prominent than the endoluminal component.
- CT can evaluate for metastatic disease and monitor response to therapy (which is often striking in cases of GIST).
- A densely calcified lesion is suggestive of a leiomyoma.
- CT can provide an imaging-specific diagnosis for lipomas, obviating tissue sampling.
- Hemangiomas are typically small but can present as large polypoid lesions; the presence of phleboliths may allow for a specific diagnosis.
- Lymphangiomas may present as a polypoid or lobulated submucosal lesion and may be pliable at fluoroscopy and endoscopy; most will appear cystic on cross-sectional imaging.

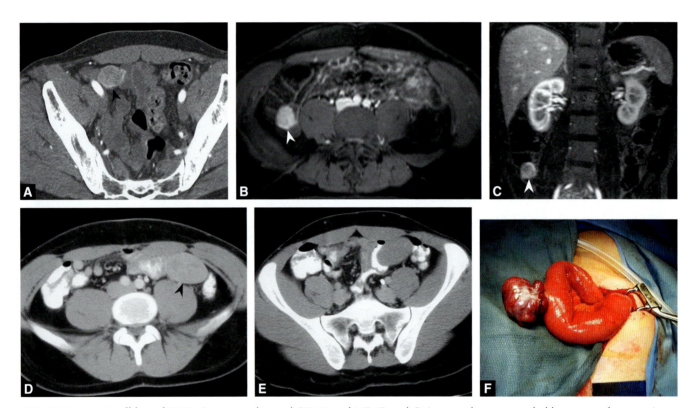

FIGURE 1.4.1 Small bowel GIST. Contrast-enhanced CT (**A**) and MR (**B** and **C**) images show a rounded hypervascular mass in the right lower quadrant (*arrowheads*), which proved to be an ileal GIST with predominately exoenteric growth. Dynamic (**D**) and delayed (**E**) contrast-enhanced CT images show an ovoid mass (*arrowhead*), which proved to be a jejunal GIST with exoenteric growth at laparotomy (**F**). Although gross ulceration is not identified at cross-sectional imaging, both cases presented as GI bleeding. Note also the relative mobility of these lesions, which appear to shift in location on different scans.

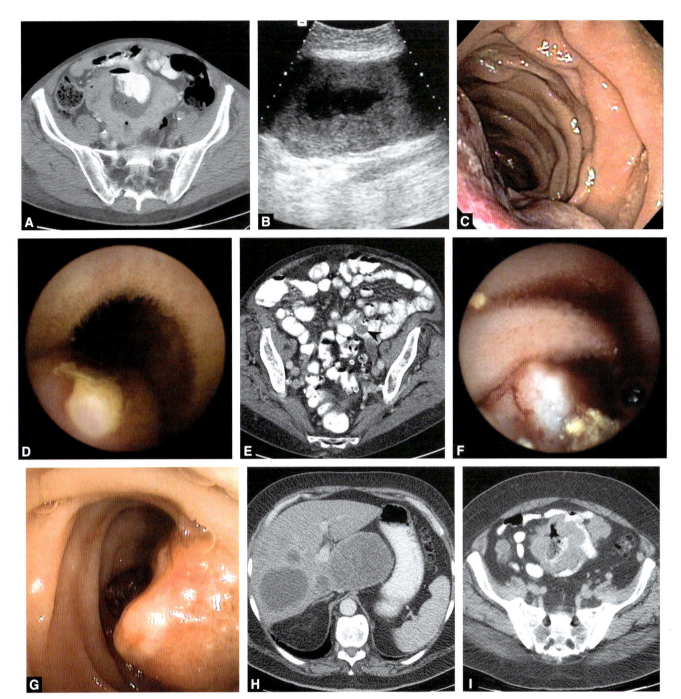

FIGURE 1.4.2 Ulcerated small bowel GIST. Contrast-enhanced CT image (**A**) shows a heterogeneous abdominal mass with a large central crater that contains air and oral contrast from ulceration. US image (**B**) from a different patient shows a large soft tissue mass with a central anechoic cavity from necrosis and ulceration. Image from push enteroscopy (**C**) from a third patient shows a large ulcerated mass. The exoenteric component cannot be assessed by luminal examination. Image from capsule endoscopy (**D**) from a fourth patient shows a polypoid GIST with central ulceration. CT image (**E**) from a patient with an acute GI hemorrhage shows a polypoid jejunal lesion (*arrowhead*). At capsule endoscopy (**F**), an ulcerated mass with evidence of active bleeding was seen, which was confirmed at subsequent push enteroscopy (**G**); note the ulcerated portion of the mass that appears dark red. Endoscopic biopsy was nondiagnostic, but a GIST was confirmed at surgery. Contrast-enhanced CT images (**H** and **I**) from a patient with obscure GI bleeding show a large ulcerated small bowel GIST with associated hepatic metastatic disease.

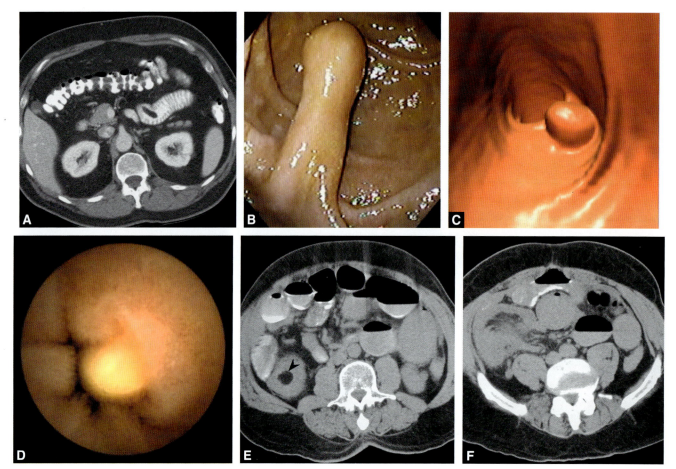

FIGURE 1.4.3 **Small bowel lipomas.** Contrast-enhanced CT (**A**) and EGD (**B**) images from two different patients show small bowel lipomas with a similar pedunculated appearance. 3D endoluminal small bowel image from CT colonography (**C**) and capsule endoscopy image (**D**) from two different patients show small bowel lipomas that were incidentally detected. CT images (**E** and **F**) from a symptomatic patient show small bowel obstruction from ileocecal intussusception. The rounded fat attenuation lead point (**E**, *arrowhead*) represents an ileal lipoma. Because of the presence of fat attenuation, CT is generally diagnostic for lipomas.

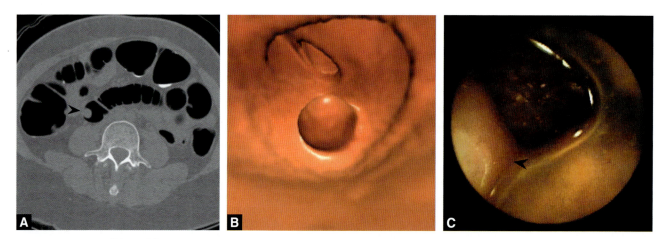

FIGURE 1.4.4 **Small bowel hamartomas.** Transverse 2D (**A**) and 3D endoluminal (**B**) images from a screening CT colonography study show an incidentally detected polypoid mass (*arrowhead*) located in the proximal ileum, which was confirmed at capsule endoscopy (**C**, *arrowhead*) and proven to be a hamartoma after surgery (**D**).

Illustration continued on following page

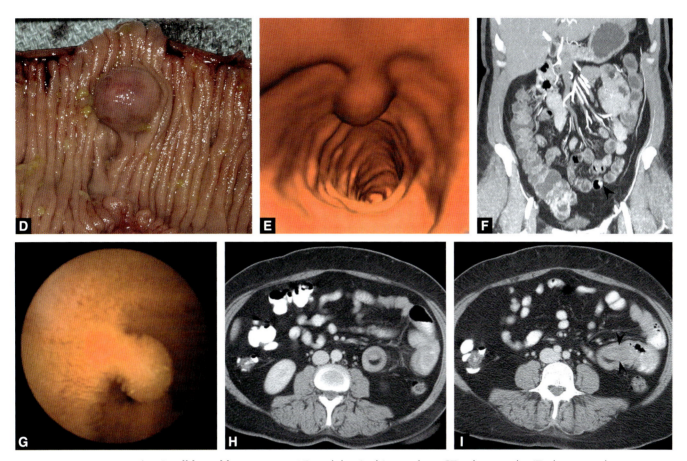

FIGURE 1.4.4 (Continued) **Small bowel hamartomas.** 3D endoluminal image from CT colonography (**E**) shows another incidentally detected small bowel lesion, which demonstrated enhancement at dedicated CT enterography (**F**, *arrowhead*) and was also confirmed at preoperative capsule endoscopy (**G**). Contrast-enhanced CT images (**H** and **I**) from a symptomatic patient show intussusception from an elongated jejunal soft tissue mass (**I**, *arrowheads*), which proved to be a large hamartoma after surgical resection.

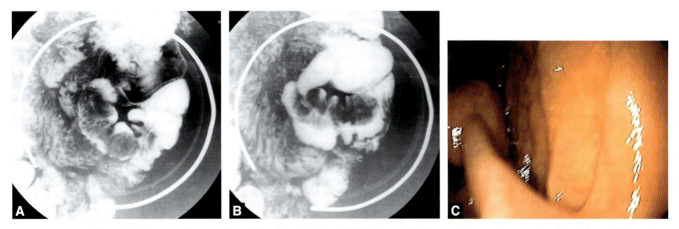

FIGURE 1.4.5 **Peutz-Jeghers syndrome.** Spot films from barium SBFT (**A** and **B**) show a large, elongated polypoid small bowel hamartoma. Endoscopic image (**C**) from a second patient with Peutz-Jeghers syndrome shows a large pedunculated small bowel hamartoma.

Illustration continued on following page

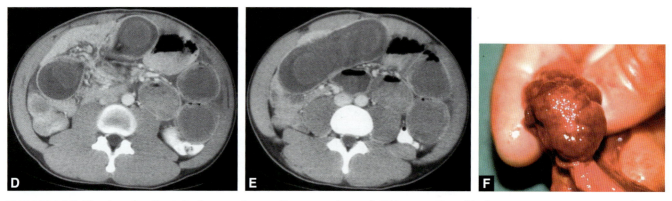

FIGURE 1.4.5 (Continued) **Peutz-Jeghers syndrome.** Contrast-enhanced CT images (**D** and **E**) from a symptomatic patient show a high-grade small bowel obstruction due to intussusception from a hamartomatous lead point (**F**).

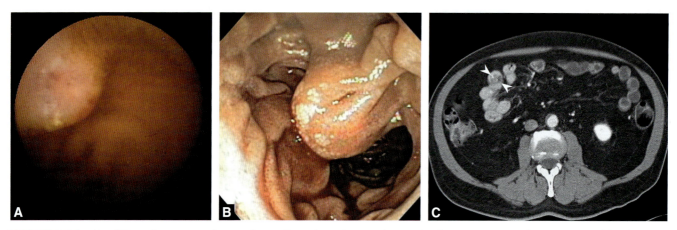

FIGURE 1.4.6 **Small bowel cavernous hemangioma.** Capsule endoscopy image (**A**) from a patient with recurrent GI bleeding shows an erythematous polypoid lesion. Subsequent push enteroscopy (**B**) shows a large polypoid submucosal lesion with active oozing. Surgical resection proved this to be a jejunal cavernous hemangioma. Contrast-enhanced CT image (**C**) from a patient with obscure GI bleeding shows a subtle small bowel lesion (*arrowheads*) containing punctate calcifications suggestive of phleboliths. A bleeding cavernous hemangioma was found at surgery.

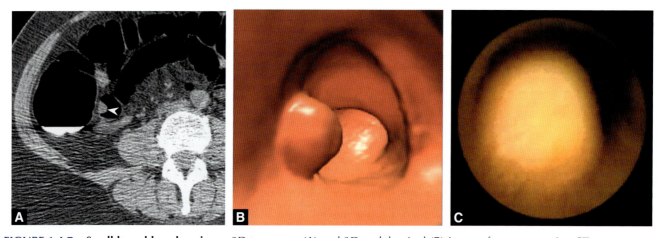

FIGURE 1.4.7 **Small bowel lymphangioma.** 2D transverse (**A**) and 3D endoluminal (**B**) images from a screening CT colonography study show a polypoid lesion (*arrowhead*) within the ileum, which was confirmed at capsule endoscopy (**C**) and found to be a lymphangioma after resection.

Illustration continued on following page

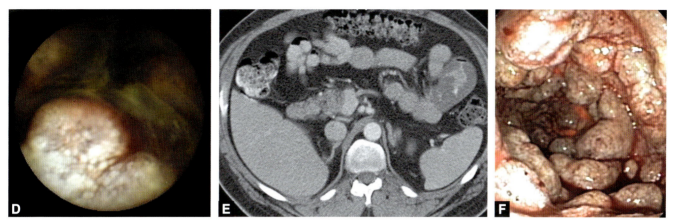

FIGURE 1.4.7 (Continued) **Small bowel lymphangioma.** Capsule endoscopy (**D**) from a different patient shows a jejunal lesion with overlying whitish mucosa and red specks. Contrast-enhanced CT image (**E**) shows prominent low-attenuation wall thickening involving a segment of jejunum. Intraoperative enteroscopy (**F**) confirms an extensive circumferential submucosal lesion. A large jejunal lymphangioma was confirmed after surgical resection. *(D to F, from Hara AK, Leighton JA, Sharma VK: Imaging of small bowel disease: Comparison of capsule endoscopy, standard endoscopy, barium examination, and CT. Radiographics 2005;25:697-711)*

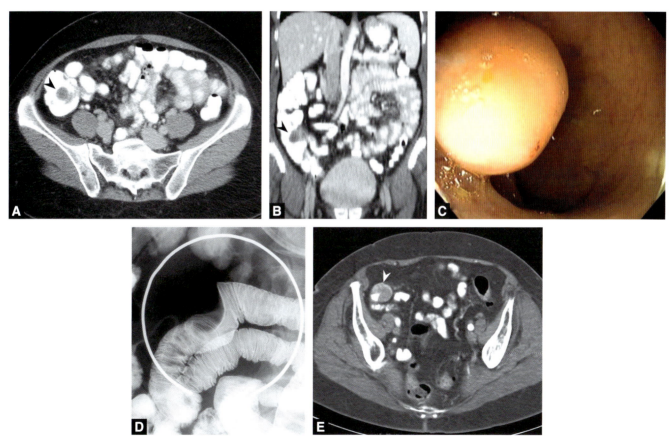

FIGURE 1.4.8 **Other mesenchymal tumors.** Transverse (**A**) and coronal (**B**) CT images show a rounded soft tissue lesion (*arrowheads*) in the ileocecal region, suggestive of a prominent ileocecal valve or a large polyp on the valve. Subsequent colonoscopy with ileoscopy (**C**) demonstrates a submucosal ileal polyp that proved to be a neurofibroma. Localized intussusception of the lesion had given the appearance of a primary colonic process at CT. Image from enteroclysis (**D**) in a second patient shows a classic submucosal lesion with smooth borders, which proved to be a rare leiomyoblastoma. Contrast-enhanced CT image (**E**) from a third patient shows a focal soft tissue mass involving the distal ileum (*arrowhead*), which proved to be a schwannoma at pathologic evaluation.

1.5 Metastatic Disease
(Figures 1.5.1-1.5.3)

CLINICAL FEATURES
- Intraperitoneal carcinomatosis with serosal small bowel involvement is more common than hematogenous spread; GI and ovarian primary tumors give rise to most serosal metastases.
- Serosal metastatic disease may cause symptoms from partial small bowel obstruction.
- Hematogenous implants involve the antimesenteric bowel wall where the vasa recta arborize into the submucosal plexus.
- Hematogenous metastatic spread to the small bowel submucosa is often multifocal and most often seen with melanoma and lung cancer; metastases may present with GI bleeding or intussusception.

IMAGING FEATURES
- Serosal implants may appear as multifocal soft tissue masses or as more diffuse bowel wall thickening.
- Hematogenous metastases appear as submucosal polypoid masses; central ulceration gives rise to a target appearance on barium studies.
- Intussusception related to hematogenous metastases may be the initial presentation of disease.

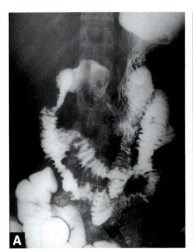 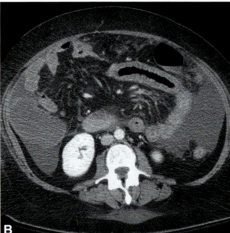 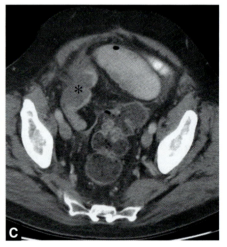

FIGURE 1.5.1 **Small bowel serosal metastatic disease.** Barium SBFT **(A)** from a woman with peritoneal carcinomatosis from breast cancer shows irregular fold thickening involving several loops of small bowel. Contrast-enhanced CT image **(B)** from a woman with metastatic ovarian cancer shows malignant ascites and segmental small bowel wall thickening that is analogous to the previous barium case. Contrast-enhanced CT image **(C)** from a patient with symptomatic peritoneal carcinomatosis shows marked eccentric luminal narrowing of a distal ileal segment by a low-attenuation serosal implant (*asterisk*), which results in small bowel obstruction.

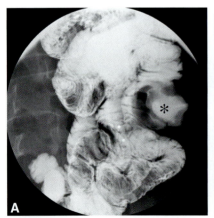 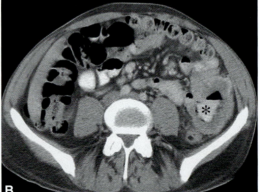 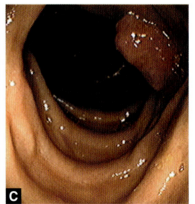

FIGURE 1.5.2 **Hematogenous small bowel metastatic disease from melanoma.** Images from barium SBFT **(A)** and contrast-enhanced CT **(B)** show a large jejunal mass with a central contrast-filled cavity (*asterisks*) from ulceration. EGD **(C)** shows additional smaller submucosal metastases involving the more proximal small bowel.

Illustration continued on following page

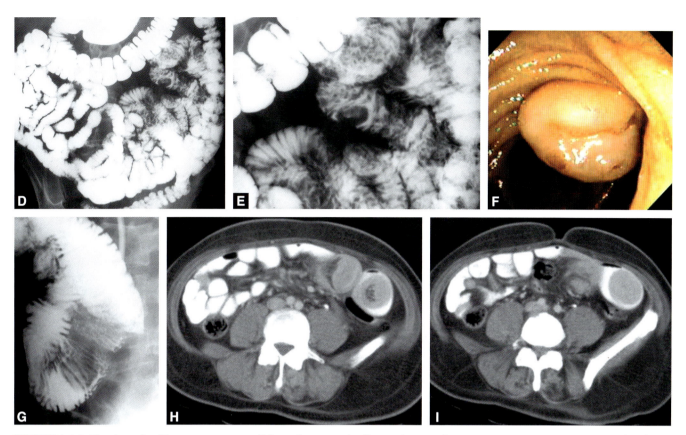

FIGURE 1.5.2 (Continued) Hematogenous small bowel metastatic disease from melanoma. Barium SBFT images (**D** and **E**) from a second patient show smaller submucosal hematogenous metastases from melanoma. Push enteroscopy (**F**) from a third patient shows a nonulcerated jejunal submucosal lesion. Barium SBFT (**G**) and contrast-enhanced CT (**H** and **I**) images from a final patient demonstrate jejunal intussusception from a submucosal melanoma metastasis.

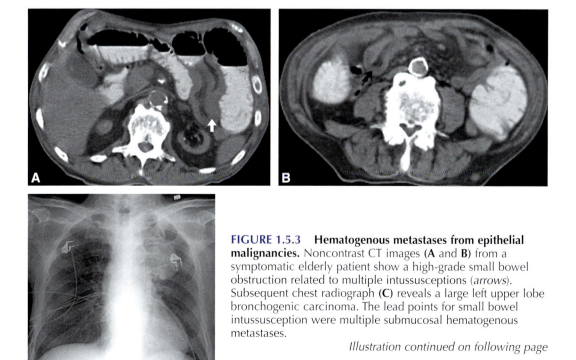

FIGURE 1.5.3 Hematogenous metastases from epithelial malignancies. Noncontrast CT images (**A** and **B**) from a symptomatic elderly patient show a high-grade small bowel obstruction related to multiple intussusceptions (*arrows*). Subsequent chest radiograph (**C**) reveals a large left upper lobe bronchogenic carcinoma. The lead points for small bowel intussusception were multiple submucosal hematogenous metastases.

Illustration continued on following page

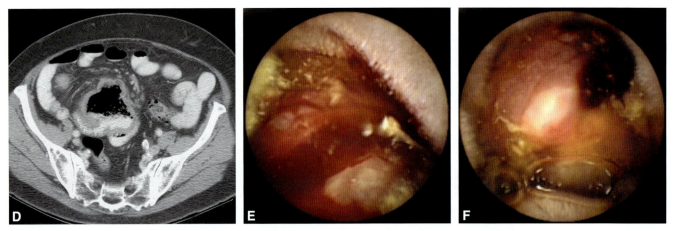

FIGURE 1.5.3 (Continued) **Hematogenous metastases from epithelial malignancies.** Contrast-enhanced CT image **(D)** from a patient with GI bleeding and a history of lung cancer shows a large ulcerated abdominal mass that communicates with the small bowel lumen. Although the appearance suggests a primary bowel tumor such as a GIST, unsuspected metastatic disease was subsequently proven as the cause. Capsule endoscopy images **(E** and **F)** from a patient with GI bleeding and a history of colon cancer show evidence of ongoing hemorrhage **(E)** related to an ulcerated submucosal mass **(F)**, which proved to be a metastasis.

2. ENTERITIS

Crohn's disease, infection, and other inflammatory conditions may all affect the small bowel. These processes typically begin with superficial involvement of the mucosa and submucosa, at which time endoscopy and possibly barium studies may be the most sensitive imaging tests. With disease progression, including involvement of deeper layers of the bowel wall and extension beyond the bowel, cross-sectional imaging studies such as CT become very useful for complementary evaluation.

2.1 Crohn's Disease
(Figures 2.1.1-2.1.9)

CLINICAL FEATURES

- This chronic, relapsing idiopathic inflammatory process can affect any part of the GI tract.
- Common features include a strong predilection for the distal ileum and "skip" lesions separated by uninvolved bowel.
- Age distribution is bimodal (typically 15 to 25 and 50 to 80 years); white and Jewish populations are more often affected.
- Typical presentation is abdominal pain, diarrhea, and weight loss.
- Diagnosis often requires synthesis of clinical, radiologic, endoscopic, and pathologic findings.
- Complications include stricture, fistula formation, and abscess formation.
- Distinguishing between an acute flare and fibrostenotic disease has important management implications with regard to medical versus surgical treatment.
- Common fistulas include enterocolic, enterocutaneous, and enterovesical types.
- Recurrence after prior ileocecal resection commonly affects the neo-terminal ileum.

IMAGING FEATURES

- Early Crohn's disease manifests as aphthoid ulcers (shallow 1- to 3-mm ulcers with mild surrounding edema) and fold thickening; endoscopy is most sensitive at this stage.
- The peroral pneumocolon, where air is insufflated per rectum at the conclusion of barium SBFT, increases accuracy for distal ileal evaluation.
- Progression of acute disease leads to deeper and coalescent ulceration, more severe wall thickening, and inflammatory polyp formation; advanced inflammation may have a "cobblestone" appearance.
- CT enterography can effectively delineate thick-walled segments of involved bowel, whether due to active inflammation or fibrostenotic disease.
- Other pertinent findings of disease activity at CT enterography include mucosal enhancement, mesenteric infiltration, increased vascularity, and free fluid.
- Fibrofatty mesenteric proliferation ("creeping fat") surrounding involved bowel loops is a characteristic and useful diagnostic finding at CT.
- CT can also evaluate for extraintestinal complications such as abscess and fistula formation.
- Contrast fluoroscopy studies are useful for fistula demonstration; CT fistulography can also provide for such evaluation.
- MR is sensitive for active disease; because ionizing radiation is not delivered, it may be preferred for evaluation of chronic relapsing disease.
- PET imaging may also be useful for assessing disease activity.
- Chronic ulcerative colitis can lead to a patulous ileocecal valve and granular terminal ileal fold pattern (termed *backwash ileitis*), which should not be confused with Crohn's disease.

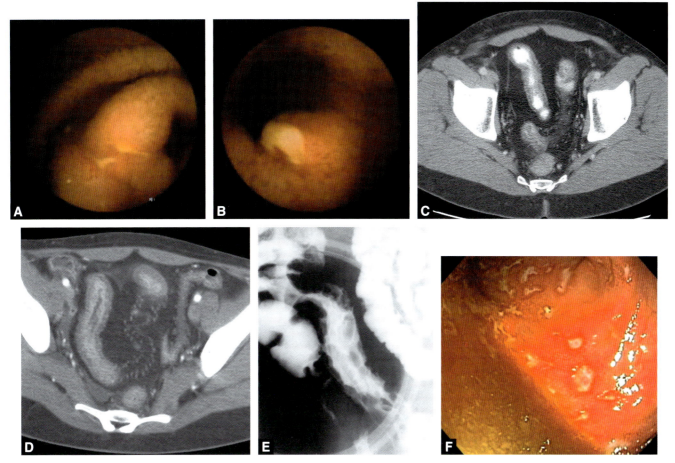

FIGURE 2.1.1 Ileal Crohn's disease. Images from capsule endoscopy (**A** and **B**) show ileal mucosal inflammation and ulceration typical of early Crohn's disease. Corresponding contrast-enhanced CT image (**C**) shows moderate diffuse wall thickening of the distal ileum and prominence of the surrounding mesenteric fat. Contrast-enhanced CT enterography image (**D**) from a second patient shows distal ileal wall thickening, as well as increased mucosal enhancement and prominence of the supplying vessels. Barium SBFT spot film (**E**) from a third patient shows mucosal irregularity of the terminal ileum, compatible with the ulceronodular form of Crohn's disease. Ileoscopy image (**F**) from a final patient shows diffuse mucosal inflammation with multifocal ulcerations.

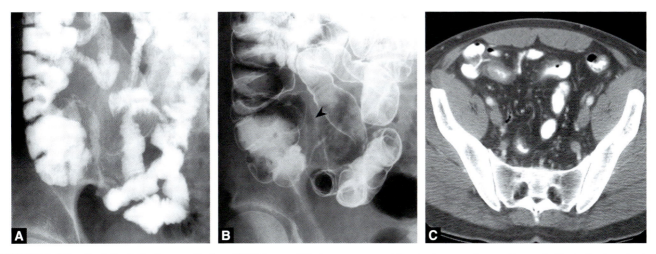

FIGURE 2.1.2 Ileal Crohn's disease. Barium SBFT image (**A**) shows apparent luminal narrowing and irregularity to the terminal ileum, but the segment is not well opacified or distended. Subsequent image (**B**) obtained after rectal air insufflation (peroral pneumocolon) demonstrates persistent terminal ileal irregularity and narrowing (*arrowhead*), despite good distention and double-contrast technique, indicative of true pathology. Contrast-enhanced CT (**C**) and endoscopic (**D**) images confirm terminal ileitis.

Illustration continued on following page

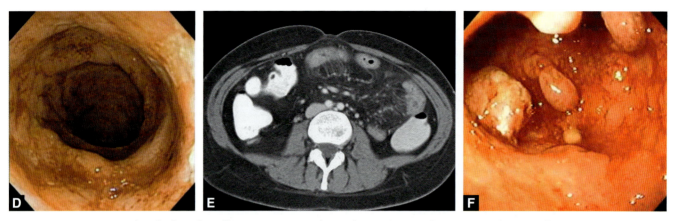

FIGURE 2.1.2 (Continued)   **Ileal Crohn's disease.** Contrast-enhanced CT image **(E)** from a second patient demonstrates an inflamed small bowel loop with associated prominence of the mesenteric vessels ("comb sign"). Endoscopic image **(F)** from a third patient shows acute ileitis with inflammatory pseudopolyps.

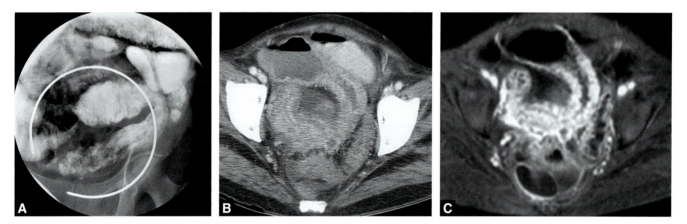

FIGURE 2.1.3   **Ileal Crohn's disease.** Barium SBFT image **(A)** shows a dilated ileal loop proximal to an area of narrowing. The patient was experiencing an acute flare of long-standing disease. Contrast-enhanced CT **(B)** and MR **(C)** images show segmental wall thickening with increased enhancement, as well as dilatation proximal to the involved loop. Note the conspicuity of mural enhancement from active disease on the fat-suppressed MR study.

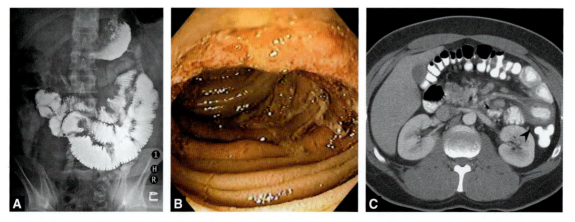

FIGURE 2.1.4   **Jejunal Crohn's disease.** Barium SBFT image **(A)** shows skip regions of irregular jejunal fold thickening and luminal narrowing. The ileum appeared normal on more delayed radiographs. Faint contrast within the colon was from a previous CT study, which showed similar findings. Push enteroscopy **(B)** confirms skip regions of circumferential jejunal fold thickening with ulceration and erythema. Contrast-enhanced CT image **(C)** from a previously healthy young man demonstrates segmental wall thickening involving the proximal jejunum (*arrowhead*), as well as localized mesenteric soft tissue infiltration and lymphadenopathy. Subsequent push enteroscopy (not shown) confirmed jejunal mucosal inflammation and ulceration.

Illustration continued on following page

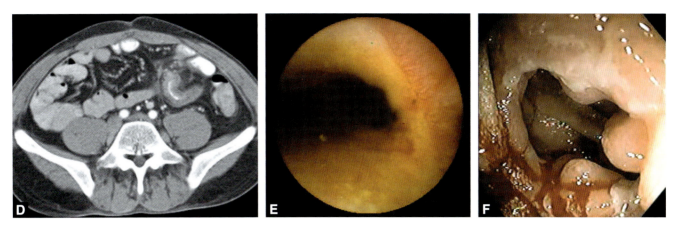

FIGURE 2.1.4 (Continued) **Jejunal Crohn's disease.** Contrast-enhanced CT image (**D**) from a third patient shows segmental jejunal wall thickening and surrounding inflammatory changes. Capsule endoscopy image (**E**) from a fourth patient shows extensive mucosal ulceration. Push enteroscopy image (**F**) from a final patient shows marked jejunal inflammation with nodular fold thickening and ulceration.

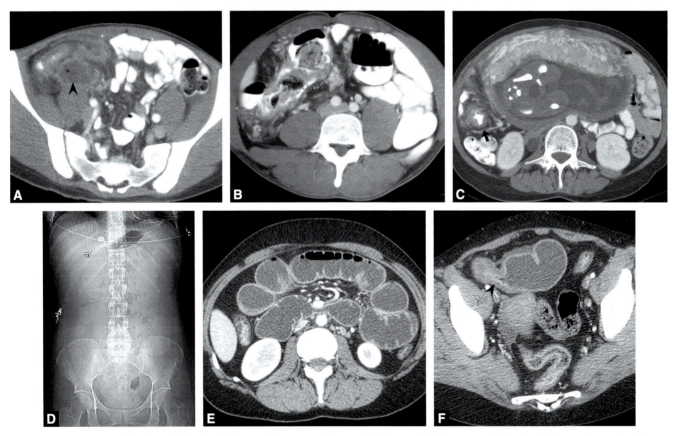

FIGURE 2.1.5 **Complications in Crohn's disease.** Contrast-enhanced CT image (**A**) shows an abdominal abscess (*arrowhead*) adjacent to the inflamed ileum, with extensive surrounding inflammatory changes. Contrast-enhanced CT image (**B**) from a second patient shows a more complex abscess associated with multiple interconnecting fistulas. Contrast-enhanced CT image (**C**) shows an acute flare of ileal Crohn's disease (*arrow*) complicating pregnancy. Note the fetus and enhancing placenta. CT scout image (**D**) from a patient with Crohn's disease and obstructive symptoms demonstrates a fairly unremarkable bowel gas pattern. The CT enterography images (**E** and **F**), however, demonstrate small bowel obstruction with abrupt transition at the point of fibrostenotic disease (**F**, *arrowhead*). Fluid-filled loops are a pitfall in conventional radiography.

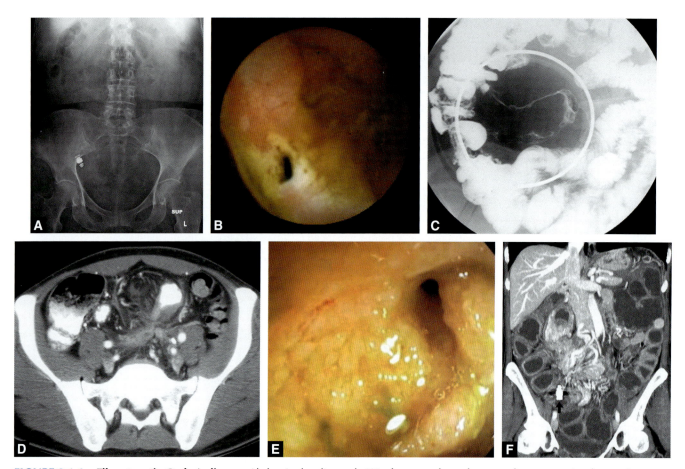

FIGURE 2.1.6   Fibrostenotic Crohn's disease. Abdominal radiograph **(A)** after capsule endoscopy shows a retained capsule located in the right lower quadrant due to a tight stricture **(B)** associated with mucosal ulceration. Segmental resection of the diseased small bowel was required for capsule removal. Barium SBFT spot film **(C)** from a second patient shows marked luminal narrowing of the distal ileum ("string sign"). The abnormal loop is separated from the other loops by fibrofatty proliferation of the mesentery. Contrast-enhanced CT image **(D)** from a third patient shows wall thickening and luminal narrowing of an ileal segment, associated with prominent surrounding inflammatory changes. Corresponding endoscopic image **(E)** shows a high-grade ileal stricture and mucosal irregularity. Coronal image from CT enterography **(F)** in a final patient shows diffuse bowel wall thickening and a retained video capsule (*arrow*) related to an ileal stricture.

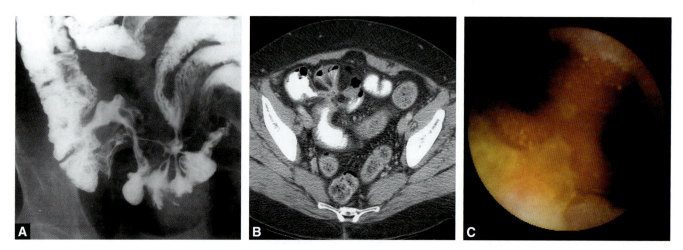

FIGURE 2.1.7   Fistulizing Crohn's disease. Barium SBFT spot film **(A)** shows a complex fistula located off the mesenteric aspect of the terminal ileum, with multiple communications involving small bowel and colon. Contrast-enhanced CT image **(B)** from a second patient shows a similar complex bowel-to-bowel fistula in the right lower quadrant. Capsule endoscopy image **(C)** from a third patient shows mucosal ulceration and fistula, which gives a double-barrelled appearance to the lumen. (*A, from Pickhardt PJ, Bhalla S, Balfe DM: Acquired gastrointestinal fistulas: Classification, etiologies, and imaging evaluation. Radiology 2002;224:9-23.*)

Illustration continued on following page

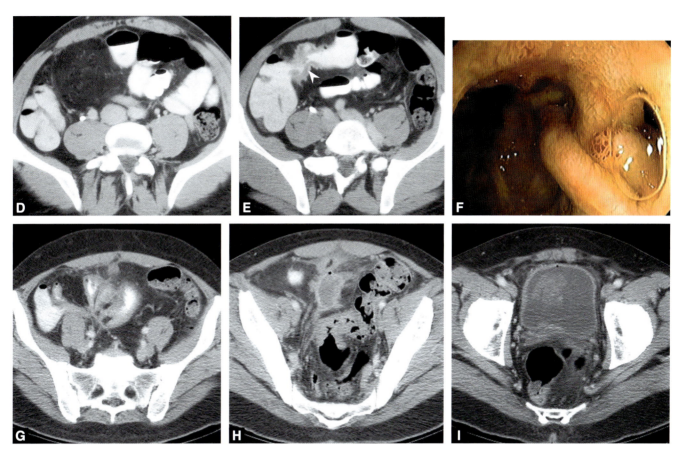

FIGURE 2.1.7 (Continued) **Fistulizing Crohn's disease.** Contrast-enhanced CT images (**D** and **E**) show an enterocolic fistula (**E**, *arrowhead*) with irregular soft tissue thickening and prominent fibrofatty proliferative changes of the adjacent mesentery. Colonoscopy image (**F**) shows the enterocolic fistula associated with chronic mucosal inflammatory changes. Contrast-enhanced CT images (**G** to **I**) from a final patient show complex bowel-to-bowel fistulas, as well as an enterovesical fistula. Note the inflammatory changes extending to the bladder and the tiny intraluminal gas bubble, suggestive of enterovesical fistula.

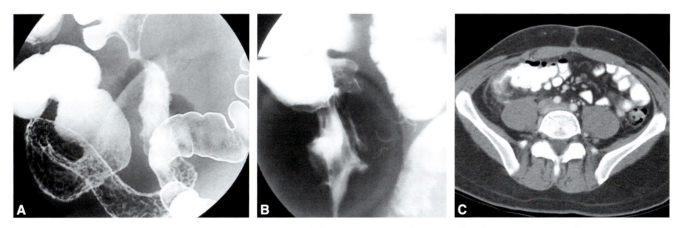

FIGURE 2.1.8 **Crohn's recrudescence at the neo-terminal ileum.** Barium studies (**A** and **B**) from two patients show acute mucosal inflammatory changes involving the neo-terminal ileum. In **A**, the ileal mucosa has a cobblestone appearance; also note the subtle aphthoid ulcers in the left colon. CT image (**C**) from a third patient shows wall thickening and mesenteric infiltration surrounding the neo-terminal ileum.

Illustration continued on following page

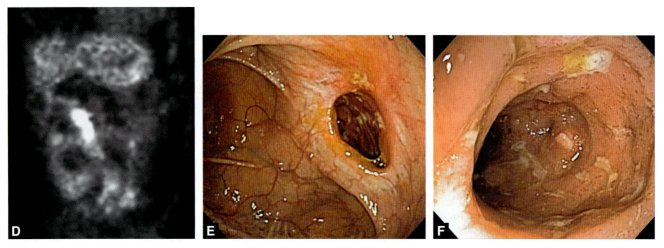

FIGURE 2.1.8 (Continued)   **Crohn's recrudescence at the neo-terminal ileum.** FDG PET image **(D)** from a fourth patient shows hypermetabolic activity centered on the neo-terminal ileum. The role of PET in Crohn's disease is currently evolving. Images from colonoscopy **(E)** and ileoscopy **(F)** in a final patient demonstrate marked acute mucosal inflammation and serpiginous ulceration involving the ileocolonic anastomosis **(E)** and neo-terminal ileum **(F)**.

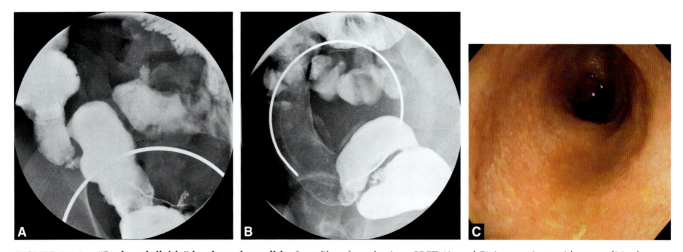

FIGURE 2.1.9   **"Backwash ileitis" in ulcerative colitis.** Spot films from barium SBFT **(A** and **B)** in a patient with pancolitis show a patulous ileocecal valve and a dilated terminal ileum. Peroral pneumocolon technique **(B)** shows subtle granularity to the ileal mucosa. Note also the distorted cone-shaped cecum **(A)**, which is typical of long-standing ulcerative colitis. Image from ileal intubation at colonoscopy **(C)** in a different patient shows a dilated terminal ileum and superficial mucosal inflammation, which extends only 5 cm proximal to the ileocecal valve. The more proximal ileal mucosa appeared endoscopically normal (not shown).

2.2 Infectious Enteritis
(Figures 2.2.1-2.2.10)

CLINICAL FEATURES

- Small bowel infection and infestation are still more prevalent in developing countries but are also being seen elsewhere due to increases in international travel and immunocompromise.
- Categories include bacterial, viral, parasitic, and fungal; medical and travel history may be important clues, because imaging findings are often nonspecific or absent.
- Mycobacterial infections affecting the small bowel include tuberculosis (TB) and *Mycobacterium avium-intracellulare* (MAI); most affected patients are immunocompromised.
- Small bowel mycobacterial disease may present as abdominal pain, weight loss, fever, and diarrhea.
- *Yersinia enterocolitica* is a gram-negative organism that can result in ileocecal inflammatory changes that clinically mimic appendicitis.
- Whipple's disease is a rare multisystem bacterial infection due to *Tropheryma whippelii* that has a predilection for the small bowel, joints, and central nervous system; it may present with symptoms of malabsorption.
- Cytomegalovirus (CMV) is an opportunistic DNA herpesvirus that most often affects the esophagus, stomach, or colon but can affect the small bowel; the virus induces a vasculitis that may result in focal ischemia and ulceration.
- Giardiasis is a relatively common protozoan infection that results in acute, self-limited diarrhea; there is an

association with dysgammaglobulinemia and IgA deficiency.
- Ascariasis infests one fourth of the world's population; the complex life cycle of this large nematode includes a small bowel location for the adult worm.
- Disseminated fungal infections may rarely involve the small bowel.

IMAGING FEATURES

- Gastrointestinal TB tends to involve the ileocecal region (cecum > ileum), often without associated pulmonary disease; nodular thickening may progress to ulceration, stricture, fistula, and abscess formation.
- TB peritonitis may predominate in some cases, with secondary bowel involvement.
- MAI may show diffuse nonspecific small bowel fold thickening; associated low-attenuation adenopathy and splenic microabscesses are helpful clues.
- *Yersinia* typically affects the ileocecal region (ileum > cecum); nodular wall thickening on imaging can closely mimic Crohn's disease.
- Whipple's disease manifests as micronodular duodenal and jejunal fold thickening; low-attenuation adenopathy (sometimes near fat density) may mimic MAI infection.
- CMV colitis may occasionally extend into the terminal ileum; rarely, the entire small bowel is affected.
- Giardiasis manifests on imaging with irregular fold thickening of the duodenum and jejunum (see also Chapter 3, section 2.2).
- Ascariasis typically manifests as elongated filling defects on barium studies, often with barium opacifying the nematode's GI tract.
- Multiple worms may have a whorled appearance and may cause obstruction at the level of the ileocecal valve.

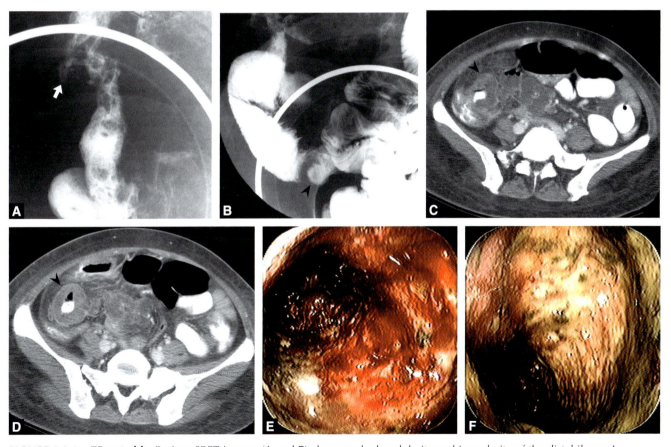

FIGURE 2.2.1 TB enteritis. Barium SBFT images (**A** and **B**) show marked nodularity and irregularity of the distal ileum. In addition, a deep ileal ulcer (**B**, *arrowhead*) is present and the cecum has a stenotic "coned" appearance (**A,** *arrow*). Contrast-enhanced CT images (**C** and **D**) show marked low-attenuation wall thickening of the terminal ileum (*arrowheads*), as well as extensive low-attenuation lymphadenopathy in the adjacent mesentery. The fixed stenotic appearance to the cecum is again demonstrated. Endoscopic images (**E** and **F**) show severely friable and inflamed ileal mucosa with circumferential ulceration and oozing.

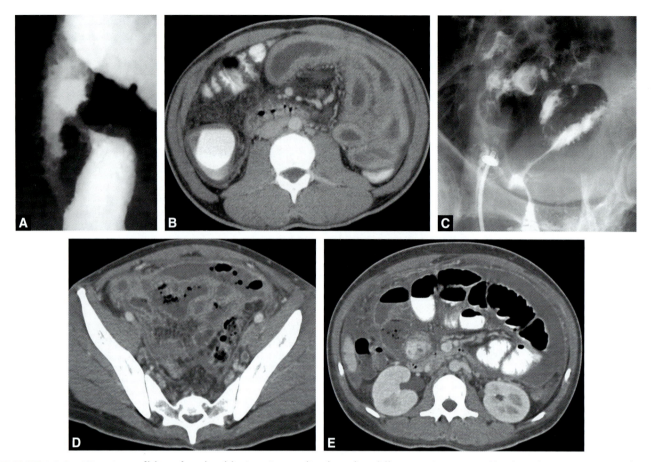

FIGURE 2.2.2 TB enterocolitis and peritonitis. Imaging studies from five different patients. Spot film from barium enema study (A) shows stenotic ileocecal disease with proximal ileal dilatation. The cecum has a coned appearance, and the colonic mucosa appears nodular. Contrast-enhanced CT image (B) shows diffuse small bowel wall thickening and lesser inflammatory changes to the right colon and mesentery. Contrast fistulogram study (C) shows complex enterocutaneous fistulas with external drainage to the pelvis. Contrast-enhanced CT images (D and E) from two different patients show extensive changes of TB peritonitis, with peritoneal thickening and enhancement surrounding loculated extraluminal air and fluid. Bowel wall thickening appears to be secondary to peritoneal disease in these cases.

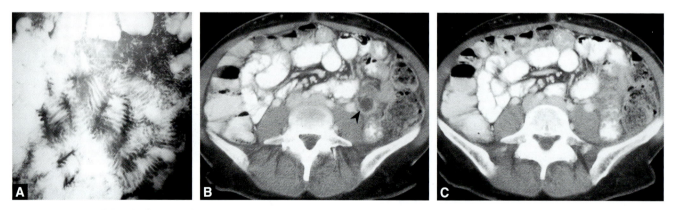

FIGURE 2.2.3 Abdominal MAI infection. Barium SBFT image (A) shows diffuse small bowel fold thickening. Contrast-enhanced CT images (B and C) from a patient with AIDS show a small abscess (B, *arrowhead*) adjacent to a segment of thick-walled jejunum.

Illustration continued on following page

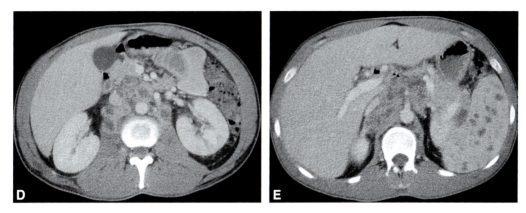

FIGURE 2.2.3 (Continued)   **Abdominal MAI infection.** Contrast-enhanced CT image **(D)** from a third patient shows extensive retroperitoneal and mesenteric lymphadenopathy with central low attenuation. Mild associated small bowel wall thickening is present. Contrast-enhanced CT image **(E)** from a final patient shows low-attenuation lymphadenopathy and splenic microabscesses.

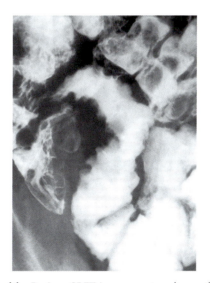

FIGURE 2.2.4   *Yersinia* **enteritis.** Barium SBFT image centered over the ileocecal region shows nodular fold thickening of the terminal ileum that mimics Crohn's' disease.

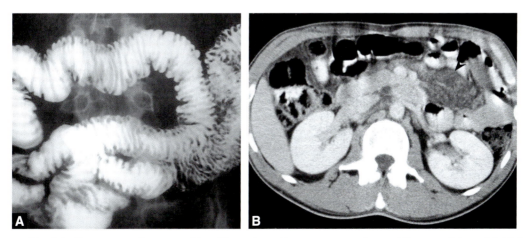

FIGURE 2.2.5   **Whipple's disease *(Tropheryma whippelii).*** Barium SBFT image **(A)** shows diffuse small bowel fold thickening of mild to moderate severity. Contrast-enhanced CT image **(B)** from a different patient shows mesenteric lymphadenopathy (*arrowhead*) that demonstrates an unusual mixed soft tissue and fatty appearance from lipid-laden macrophages.

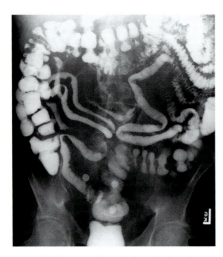

FIGURE 2.2.6 CMV enteritis. Abdominal radiograph from barium evaluation shows marked nonobstructive luminal narrowing involving the entire small bowel, which has a relatively featureless ribbon-like appearance due to loss of normal folds.

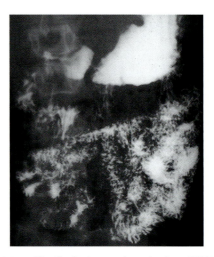

FIGURE 2.2.7 Giardiasis. Image from barium SBFT shows diffuse nodular fold thickening of the proximal small bowel, including both the duodenum and jejunum.

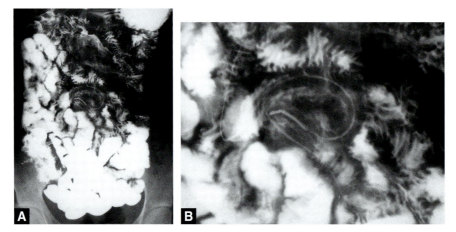

FIGURE 2.2.8 Ascariasis. Radiograph from barium SBFT **(A)** shows a thin linear density in the midabdomen, which is seen to correspond to a vermiform filling defect on a magnified view **(B)**. The central linear density represents luminal barium ingested by the roundworm itself.

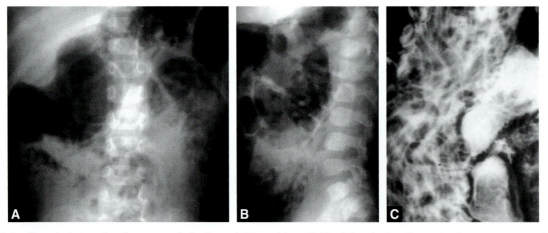

FIGURE 2.2.9 Bowel obstruction from ascariasis. Frontal **(A)** and lateral **(B)** abdominal radiographs from a young patient with obstructive symptoms show multiple dilated loops of bowel, as well as multiple linear and polypoid intraluminal soft tissue densities. Image from subsequent barium SBFT **(C)** shows innumerable vermiform filling defects within a markedly dilated small bowel loop that represents an obstructing bolus of roundworms.

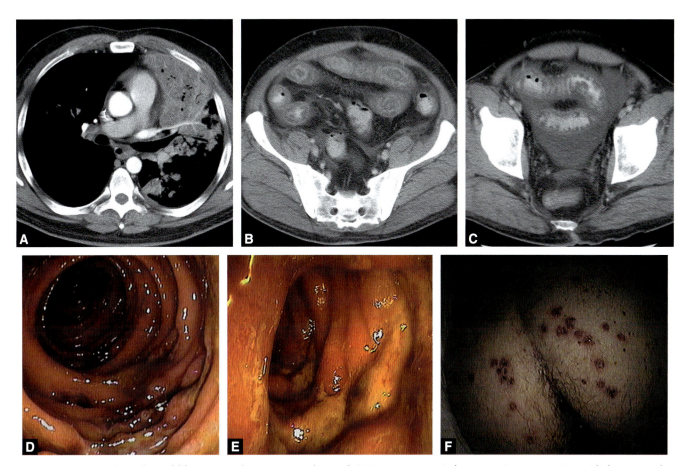

FIGURE 2.2.10 Disseminated blastomycosis. Contrast-enhanced CT images (**A** to **C**) from a patient presenting with fever, weight loss, dyspnea, joint pain, rash, and GI bleeding show extensive pulmonary consolidation from necrotizing pneumonia (**A**) and diffuse low-attenuation small bowel wall thickening (**B** and **C**). Peritoneal fluid and infiltration is also present. Image from push enteroscopy (**D**) shows mucosal inflammation of the jejunum with thickened, erythematous folds and focal ulceration. Ileoscopy during colonoscopy (**E**) reveals diffuse ileal mucosal ulceration. Cutaneous lesions over the buttocks were also noted at the time of colonoscopy (**F**). Pathologic specimens from multiple sites confirmed the diagnosis, and the patient's infection eventually responded to antifungal therapy.

2.3 Other Inflammatory Conditions
(Figures 2.3.1-2.3.6)

CLINICAL FEATURES

- Radiation enteritis is characterized by an obliterative endarteritis of the microvascular circulation; it may present subacutely or many years after exposure as pain, diarrhea, and malabsorption.
- Systemic vasculitides may affect the small bowel, particularly Henoch-Schönlein purpura (HSP).
- HSP is characterized by the clinical triad of palpable purpura, arthritis, and abdominal pain; small bowel involvement with submucosal hemorrhage is present in approximately 50% of cases.
- Systemic lupus erythematosus (SLE) is a multisystem autoimmune disorder that may affect the bowel via small vessel arteritis.
- NSAID enteropathy is characterized by intestinal ulcers, which may progress to short-segment strictures; it is a common cause of iron-deficiency anemia in patients with a normal EGD and colonoscopy.
- Eosinophilic gastroenteritis is associated with an atopic history; three overlapping forms exist: mucosal, intramural (predominantly involving the muscle layer), and serosal.
- Graft-versus-host disease (GVHD) is a complication of allogenic bone marrow transplant; the acute form often affects the gut, liver, and skin, whereas the chronic form typically affects the esophagus and skin.

IMAGING FEATURES

- Radiation enteritis is characterized by smooth fold thickening, associated with luminal narrowing; peristalsis is decreased at fluoroscopy and low-grade partial obstruction may be seen.
- Vasculitis from HSP presents as segmental uniform fold thickening of the proximal small bowel from submucosal edema and hemorrhage.
- Vasculitis from SLE presents as more diffuse uniform small bowel fold and wall thickening.
- NSAID ulcers of the small intestine are typically small but visible at capsule endoscopy; subsequent stricture

development often has a web-like or membrane appearance.
- Eosinophilic gastroenteritis has a variable endoscopic appearance, including erythematous folds, ulcers, and nodularity.
- Radiologic findings in eosinophilic gastroenteritis depend on the subtype: the mucosal form often shows fold thickening, the muscularis form can appear more mass-like, and the serosal form yields ascites.
- Acute GVHD is characterized by mucosal edema and sloughing, with wall thickening on radiologic imaging; some cases may progress to featureless ribbon-like narrowing of the bowel lumen.

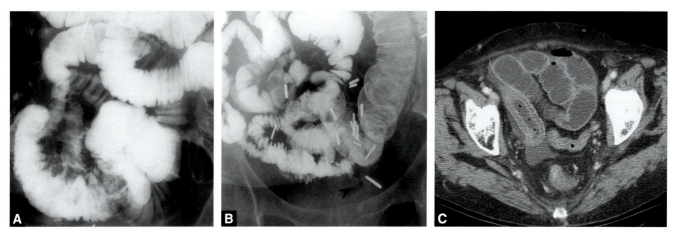

FIGURE 2.3.1 **Radiation enteritis.** Enteroclysis images (**A** and **B**) from two different patients show abnormal pelvic small bowel loops with luminal narrowing and fold thickening, which cause partial obstruction. A subtle enterovaginal fistula is present in the second case (**B**, *arrowhead*). CT enterography image (**C**) from a third patient shows analogous findings, including a narrowed, thick-walled segment associated with dilated proximal loops. Adjacent free peritoneal fluid is also present.

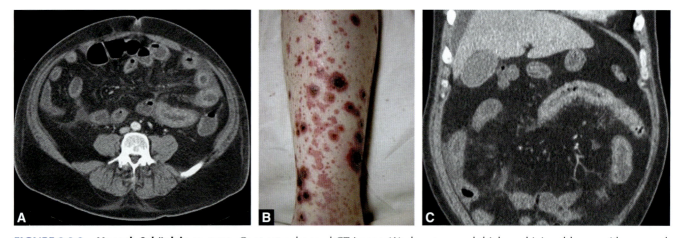

FIGURE 2.3.2 **Henoch-Schönlein purpura.** Contrast-enhanced CT image (**A**) shows several thickened jejunal loops with mucosal enhancement and low-attenuation intramural edema. Skin lesions consisting of nonblanching palpable purpura were present over the lower extremities (**B**). Coronal CT image (**C**) from a second patient shows proximal small bowel wall thickening and a small amount of free peritoneal fluid. The increased attenuation of the wall may be related to submucosal hemorrhage.

Illustration continued on following page

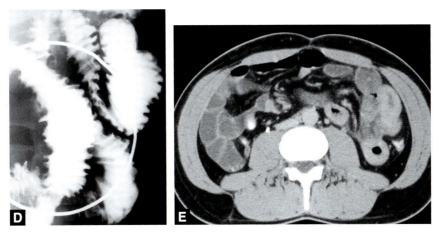

FIGURE 2.3.2 (Continued) **Henoch-Schönlein purpura.** Barium SBFT spot film (**D**) from a third patient shows uniform thickening of the jejunal folds, compatible with submucosal edema and/or hemorrhage. Corresponding CT image (**E**) shows relatively increased wall attenuation to the thickened loops, again suggestive of submucosal hemorrhage. Note the normal wall thickness of the right-sided small bowel loops.

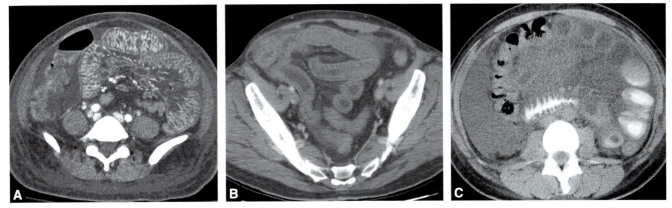

FIGURE 2.3.3 **Systemic lupus erythematosus.** Contrast-enhanced CT images (**A** to **C**) from three different patients with SLE show diffuse small bowel wall thickening from vasculitis, with variable amounts of mucosal enhancement and free peritoneal fluid.

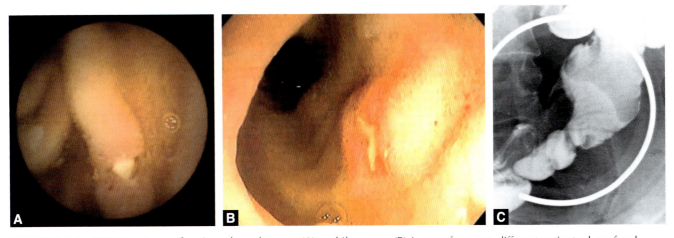

FIGURE 2.3.4 **NSAID enteropathy.** Capsule endoscopy (**A**) and ileoscopy (**B**) images from two different patients show focal mucosal ulceration and inflammation in the jejunum and ileum, respectively, related to NSAID use. Barium SBFT image (**C**) from a third patient shows a web-like NSAID stricture with proximal dilatation.

Illustration continued on following page

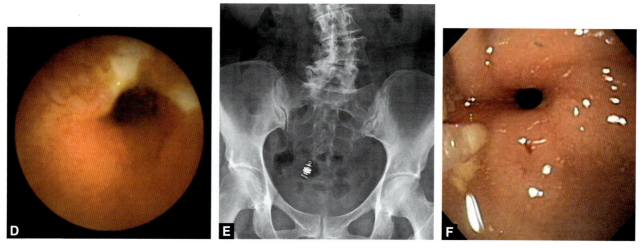

FIGURE 2.3.4 (Continued)   **NSAID enteropathy.** Capsule endoscopy image **(D)** from a fourth patient shows an ileal stricture and associated ulceration. The capsule was retained by the stricture and failed to pass **(E)**. Endoscopic image **(F)** from a final patient shows another web-like NSAID stricture.

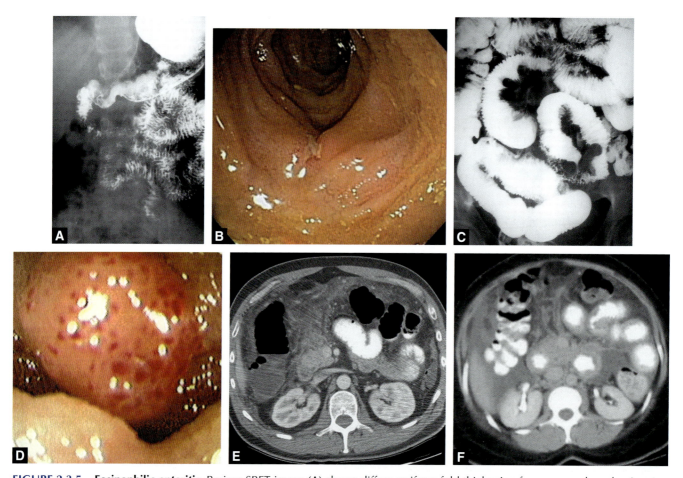

FIGURE 2.3.5   Eosinophilic enteritis. Barium SBFT image **(A)** shows diffuse uniform fold thickening from mucosal predominant disease. Ileoscopy **(B)** from a second patient shows fold thickening and ulceration from mucosal involvement. Barium SBFT image **(C)** from a third patient shows multifocal submucosal mass-like filling defects from muscularis-predominant disease. Ileoscopy **(D)** from a fourth patient shows a submucosal nodular mass with punctuate mucosal erythema. Contrast-enhanced CT image **(E)** from a fifth patient shows peritoneal soft tissue infiltration from serosal predominant disease (eosinophilic peritonitis). Ascites was present at other levels. Contrast-enhanced CT image **(F)** from a final patient with multilayer involvement shows irregular small bowel wall thickening, as well as peritoneal fluid and infiltration.

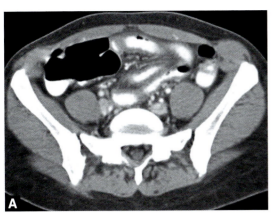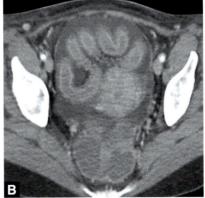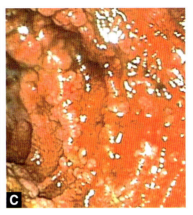

FIGURE 2.3.6 **Graft-versus-host disease.** Contrast-enhanced CT images (**A** and **B**) from two different patients show diffuse uniform small bowel wall thickening. Peritoneal thickening and ascites are present in the second case (**B**). EGD image (**C**) from a third patient shows markedly erythematous and eroded small bowel mucosa, giving it a diffusely nodular appearance.

3. OTHER SMALL BOWEL CONDITIONS

A number of important non-neoplastic, noninflammatory conditions can affect the small bowel. Once again, recent advances in bowel imaging, in addition to the more traditional modalities, have significantly improved the ability to diagnose and direct appropriate treatment for many of these entities.

3.1 Small Bowel Obstruction
(Figures 3.1.1-3.1.15)

CLINICAL FEATURES

- Small bowel obstruction (SBO) continues to be a common cause of the acute abdomen.
- Presentation is characterized by varying degrees of nausea, vomiting, abdominal pain, and distention.
- Adhesions and hernias account for the majority of cases (obstruction from hernia is covered in more detail in section 3.3).
- Other extrinsic causes include abdominal inflammatory processes, extrinsic masses, and endometriosis.
- Intrinsic causes of obstruction include tumor, inflammatory bowel conditions, stricture, hematoma, and intussusception.
- Intraluminal causes of obstruction include gallstones, ascariasis, bezoars, and foreign bodies.
- Closed loop obstruction (mechanical obstruction at two points) is at high risk for strangulation; causes include some combination of adhesive band, internal or external hernia, mesenteric mass, and volvulus.
- Afferent loop syndrome is a surgical complication representing at least partial obstruction of a jejunal pancreaticobiliary drainage limb; the symptoms are usually subacute or chronic in nature.
- The key clinical management issue in SBO is whether early laparotomy is required versus a trial of nonoperative management.

IMAGING FEATURES

- Because clinical evaluation is nonspecific and often unreliable, imaging plays a critical role in SBO.
- Conventional radiography is relatively sensitive for high-grade obstruction, typically showing dilated air-filled loops (>3 cm) and multiple air-fluid levels; radiography often is negative in patients with lower-grade obstruction.
- Because of the overlap of findings on conventional imaging, distinguishing mechanical obstruction from adynamic ileus can be difficult.
- Limitations of plain films include the general inability to locate a transition point, evaluate for the underlying cause, and assess for strangulation, which often necessitates additional imaging with CT.
- Contrast studies are of limited utility; enteroclysis can be useful in low-grade or intermittent obstruction.
- CT is ideal for evaluating acute small bowel obstruction because it is rapid, noninvasive, does not require oral contrast, and can provide comprehensive evaluation for degree, cause, and complications.
- CT can often demonstrate the transition point from dilated to decompressed bowel in cases of simple obstruction; multiplanar reformats may be useful in some cases.
- Abrupt transition without an identifiable cause suggests adhesion or benign stricture; in other cases, a specific cause is clearly identified (e.g., gallstone, mass, or hernia).
- Fecalization of luminal contents ("small bowel feces sign") usually indicates a significant subacute or chronic obstruction.
- CT findings of a closed-loop obstruction include a cluster of dilated fluid-filled loops with a fixed radial distribution that converge to a point; involved loops often have a grouped C-shaped configuration.
- CT signs of ischemia include bowel wall thickening, peritoneal fluid, delayed or decreased wall enhancement (or increased attenuation on noncontrast), pneumatosis, and portomesenteric venous gas.
- CT enterography can be useful for evaluating low-grade partial obstruction.
- US and MR can diagnose SBO but are not commonly employed for this indication.
- Beyond mechanical obstruction and adynamic ileus, much less common causes of small bowel dilation include scleroderma, idiopathic pseudo-obstruction, and celiac disease.

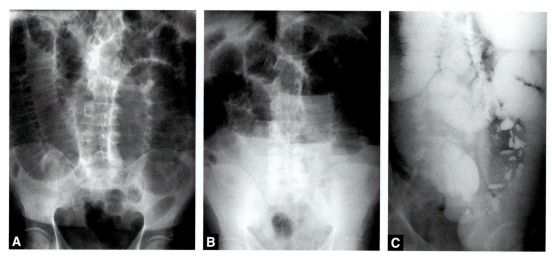

FIGURE 3.1.1 Small bowel obstruction on conventional imaging. Supine (**A**) and upright (**B**) frontal radiographs show prominently dilated small bowel loops with multiple air-fluid levels. Small bowel distention is clearly out of proportion to colonic gas, concerning for a high-grade mechanical obstruction. Radiograph from barium SBFT (**C**) shows dilated contrast-filled small bowel loops, as well as decompressed loops, which suggests a transition point. Conventional barium studies are often difficult to complete and interpret properly in the setting of mechanical obstruction owing to a variety of logistical factors. In general, CT is more informative and can be rapidly performed and interpreted.

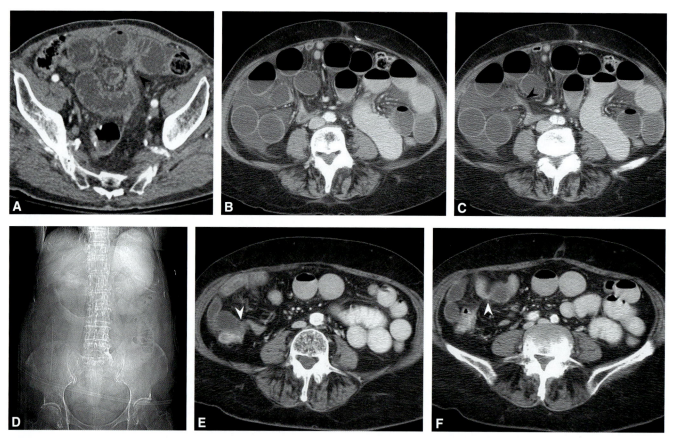

FIGURE 3.1.2 Small bowel obstruction from postoperative adhesions. Contrast-enhanced CT image (**A**) shows dilated fluid-filled small bowel loops with a relatively abrupt transition of two loops at the same point (*arrowhead*). Closed loop obstruction from postoperative adhesions was found at surgery. Contrast-enhanced CT images (**B** and **C**) from a second patient show multiple dilated small bowel loops that transition to decompressed loops at a point that appears tethered or kinked (**C**, *arrowhead*). The presence of peritoneal fluid is of concern and can suggest vascular compromise. Note how the addition of positive oral contrast added little diagnostic value yet likely worsened the patient's symptoms. CT scout radiograph from a third patient (**D**) shows a relatively unremarkable bowel gas pattern, but the contrast-enhanced CT images (**E** and **F**) show complex adhesive disease with two transition points (*arrowheads*). The use of positive oral contrast was again of little value in this case.

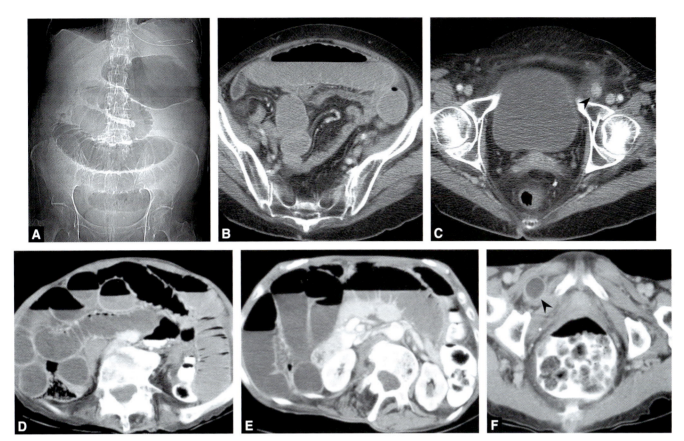

FIGURE 3.1.3 Small bowel obstruction from external hernias. CT scout radiograph (**A**) demonstrates stacked and dilated small bowel loops with a paucity of colonic gas, concerning for high-grade mechanical obstruction. Contrast-enhanced CT images (**B** and **C**) confirm a high-grade SBO with markedly dilated proximal loops and decompressed distal loops. A femoral hernia (**C**, *arrowhead*) was the underlying cause, which is not identifiable by conventional radiography. Contrast-enhanced CT images (**D** to **F**) from a different patient show a high-grade SBO due to an obturator hernia (**F**, *arrowhead*). Note how the administration of positive rectal contrast did not add any diagnostic value and could have been avoided.

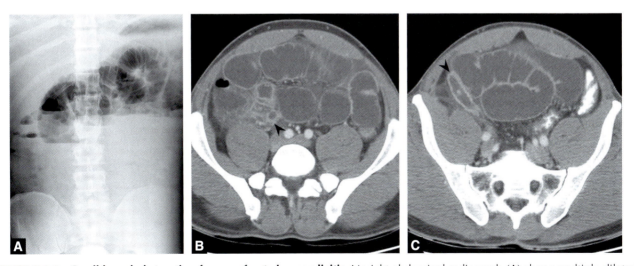

FIGURE 3.1.4 Small bowel obstruction from perforated appendicitis. Upright abdominal radiograph (**A**) shows multiple dilated small bowel loops with air-fluid levels. Contrast-enhanced CT images (**B** and **C**) show global small bowel dilatation likely related to both ileus and obstruction from inflammation related to a perforated appendicitis. Note the enhancing thick-walled appendix (*arrowheads*) with adjacent phlegmon. The administration of rectal contrast added no diagnostic information in this case.

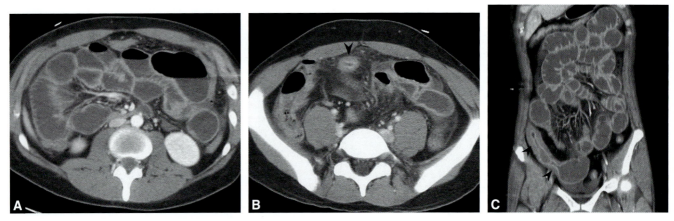

FIGURE 3.1.5 **Small bowel obstruction complicating Crohn's disease.** Transverse CT enterography images (**A** and **B**) show dilated small bowel loops with acute inflammatory changes surrounding the transition point (*arrowhead*). Coronal CT enterography image (**C**) from a second patient shows a distal SBO due to long-segment fibrostenotic disease (*arrowheads*).

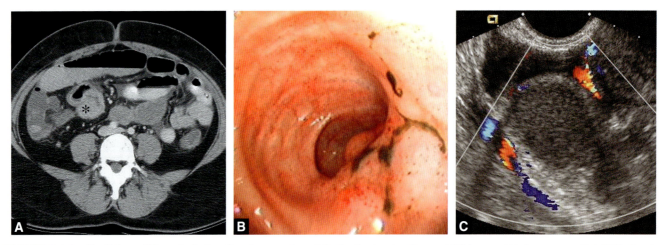

FIGURE 3.1.6 **Partial small bowel obstruction from endometriosis.** Contrast-enhanced CT image (**A**) shows a partial SBO due to a submucosal mass (*asterisk*) involving the distal ileum. Ileal intubation at colonoscopy (**B**) demonstrates luminal narrowing of the distal ileum by the submucosal process. Pelvic US image (**C**) with color Doppler shows a separate adnexal lesion with diffuse low-level internal echoes, which is typical for an endometrioma. At surgery, the ileal lesion proved to be serosal endometriosis with mural invasion.

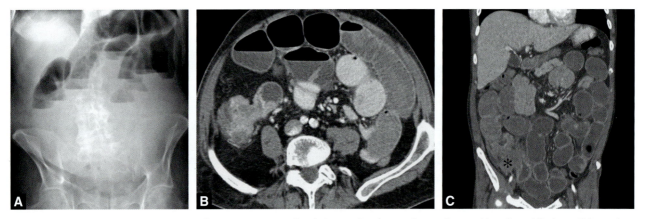

FIGURE 3.1.7 **Small bowel obstruction from tumor.** Upright abdominal radiograph (**A**) shows dilated air-filled small bowel loops with air-fluid levels and no discernible colonic dilatation. Subsequent contrast-enhanced CT (**B**) shows a cecal adenocarcinoma with direct invasion through the ileocecal valve as the obstructive cause. Coronal contrast-enhanced CT image (**C**) from a different patient shows a high-grade SBO related to an ileocecal soft tissue mass (*asterisk*), which proved to be a granulocytic sarcoma (chloroma).

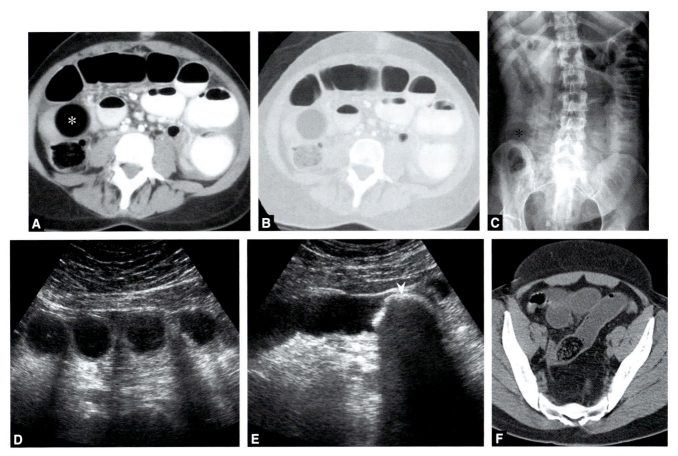

FIGURE 3.1.8 Small bowel obstruction from intraluminal foreign body. Contrast-enhanced CT image (**A**) from a mentally handicapped patient shows typical findings of a high-grade distal SBO. A spherical structure (*asterisk*) at the transition point mimics a dilated air-filled bowel loop on soft tissue windowing but is seen to be composed of lipid density on a wider lung window setting (**B**). This lucent structure is also evident in retrospect on the abdominal radiograph (**C**, *asterisk*). At surgery, an ingested "squeeze ball" was found. US images (**D** and **E**) from a second patient show dilated fluid-filled small bowel loops leading to a rounded echogenic shadowing focus (**E**, *arrowhead*), which appears as a low-attenuation structure with mottled internal gas on CT (**F**). This proved to be an obstructing small bowel bezoar related to a habit of eating persimmons.

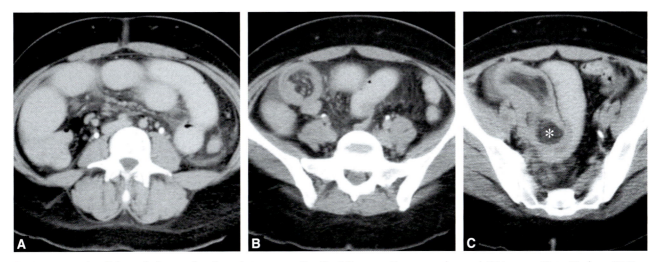

FIGURE 3.1.9 Small bowel obstruction from intussuscepting ileal lipoma. Contrast-enhanced CT images (**A** to **C**) show SBO caused by ileoileal intussusception, with telescoping mesenteric fat and vessels leading to a rounded lead point composed of fat attenuation (**C**, *asterisk*).

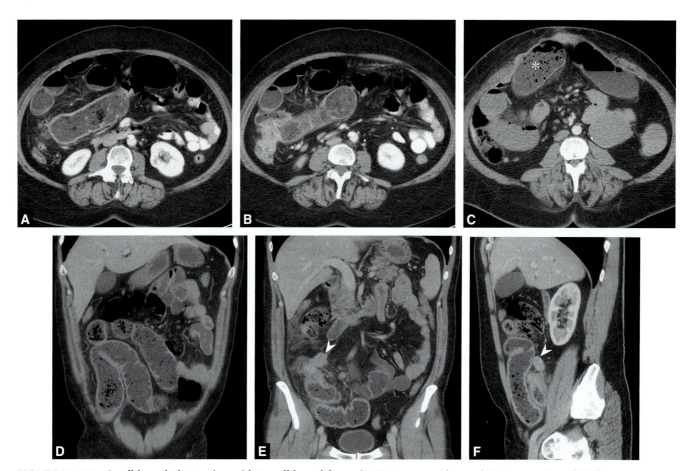

FIGURE 3.1.10 Small bowel obstruction with "small bowel feces sign". Contrast-enhanced CT images (**A** and **B**) from a patient with a subacute presentation show a markedly dilated terminal ileum filled with fecalized material, leading to a cecal soft tissue mass that proved to be an adenocarcinoma. Contrast-enhanced CT image (**C**) from a second patient shows a high-grade SBO, with a dilated small bowel loop near the transition point containing formed stool (*asterisk*). An adhesive band was the obstructive cause in this case. Coronal (**D** and **E**) and sagittal (**F**) contrast-enhanced CT images from a third patient show abundant fecalized contents within dilated ileal loops that lead to a segment of ileum that is thickened from carcinoid tumor. Note the adjacent mesenteric mass from metastatic spread of tumor (*arrowheads*).

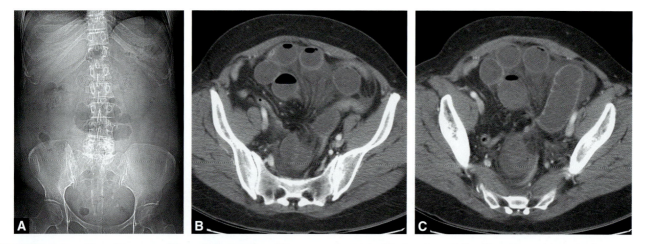

FIGURE 3.1.11 Closed loop small bowel obstruction. CT scout radiograph (**A**) shows a mildly dilated bowel loop in the midabdomen but is otherwise unremarkable. Corresponding contrast-enhanced CT images (**B** and **C**) show a classic closed loop obstruction, with dilated loops arranged in a radial configuration and mesenteric vessels that converge to a central point. The associated free fluid and mesenteric congestion implies vascular compromise. The bowel gas pattern on conventional radiography often underestimates the severity of disease in a closed loop obstruction because the involved segment is typically fluid filled.

Illustration continued on following page

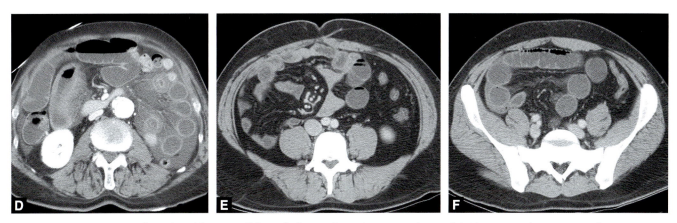

FIGURE 3.1.11 (Continued) **Closed loop small bowel obstruction.** Contrast-enhanced CT image (**D**) from a second patient shows an abnormal radial cluster of fluid-filled loops in the left hemiabdomen, associated with mesenteric fluid, congestion, and bowel wall thickening. Internal herniation of ischemic small bowel through an omental defect was found at surgery. Contrast-enhanced CT images (**E** and **F**) from a third patient show a radial cluster of fluid-filled small bowel loops, associated with high-attenuation free fluid concerning for hemorrhagic ascites. Note how the uninvolved bowel loops appear decompressed in this case.

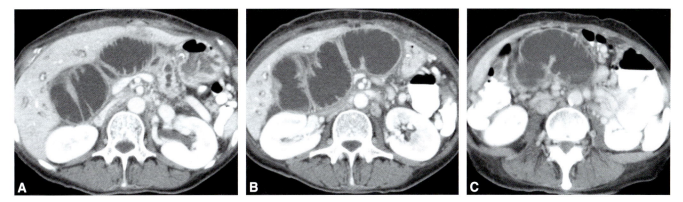

FIGURE 3.1.12 **Afferent loop (pancreaticobiliary limb) obstruction.** Contrast-enhanced CT images (**A** to **C**) from a patient who had previously undergone a Whipple procedure show marked dilatation of the jejunal pancreaticobiliary drainage limb, which is easily identified owing to lack of oral contrast opacification that is seen throughout the remainder of the gut. The increased back-pressure has also resulted in ductal dilatation of the pancreatic remnant and biliary tree. A benign stricture at the Roux-en-Y anastomosis was the obstructive cause in this case, which was suspected on CT based on the lack of a soft tissue mass.

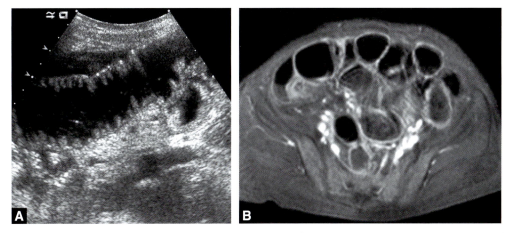

FIGURE 3.1.13 **Small bowel obstruction on US and MR.** US image (**A**) from a patient with SBO due to peritoneal carcinomatosis shows a dilated fluid-filled loop of jejunum. Fat-suppressed contrast-enhanced SGE MR image (**B**) from a patient with Crohn's disease demonstrates multiple dilated fluid-filled small bowel loops. Although these imaging modalities can depict SBO and can be useful in certain clinical scenarios, CT is generally employed in this clinical setting.

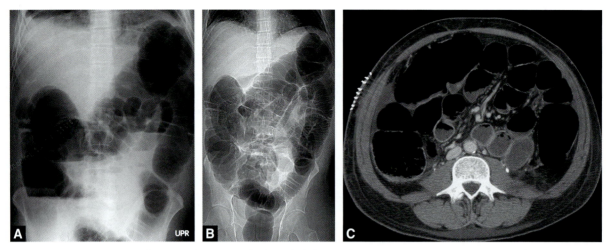

FIGURE 3.1.14 **Postoperative adynamic ileus.** Upright frontal abdominal radiograph (**A**) obtained 3 days after exploratory laparotomy shows dilated air-filled small and large bowel loops with air-fluid levels. The degree of colonic distention favors a nonobstructive adynamic ileus, but serial radiographic follow-up can be useful to exclude an evolving mechanical obstruction if clinical concern persists. Subsequent CT scout radiograph (**B**) performed 2 days later shows marked persistent dilatation of both small and large bowel. Contrast-enhanced CT image (**C**) also shows global bowel distention and excludes a mechanical obstruction.

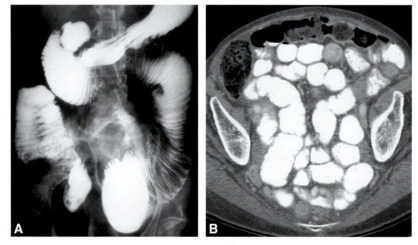

FIGURE 3.1.15 **Other causes of small bowel dilatation.** Delayed 3-hour radiograph from barium SBFT (**A**) in a patient with scleroderma shows extremely slow transit with markedly dilated loops of proximal small bowel, representing intestinal pseudo-obstruction. The close spacing of folds (valvular packing) despite the massive luminal dilatation has been called the "hide-bound" appearance and is characteristic of scleroderma. Contrast-enhanced CT image (**B**) from a patient with celiac disease shows mild to moderate dilatation of contrast-filled small bowel loops. Although nonspecific, nonobstructive small bowel dilatation is a common finding in celiac disease. *(A, from Pickhardt PJ: The "hide-bound" bowel sign. Radiology 1999;213:837-838.)*

3.2 Mesenteric Ischemia
(Figures 3.2.1-3.2.10)

CLINICAL FEATURES

- Categorized as acute or chronic; acute mesenteric ischemia is a life-threatening condition.
- Acute mesenteric ischemia may be occlusive, nonocclusive, or related to primary bowel pathology; the mucosa is most sensitive to decreased blood flow.
- Occlusive causes include superior mesenteric artery (SMA) thrombosis, SMA embolism, superior mesenteric vein (SMV) thrombosis, vasculitis, trauma, and dissection.
- Nonocclusive acute mesenteric ischemia typically involves a hypotensive episode (e.g., perioperative) in patients with underlying vascular compromise.
- "Shock bowel" seen in the setting of trauma is related to nonocclusive ischemia followed by reperfusion edema from vigorous volume resuscitation.
- Bowel conditions such as incarcerated hernia, intussusception, volvulus, or any closed-loop obstruction are at risk for localized mesenteric ischemia.
- In acute mesenteric ischemia, the pain is classically out of proportion to findings on physical examination.
- Chronic mesenteric ischemia may present as "intestinal angina" (pain after eating), sitophobia (fear of eating), or nonspecific complaints such as nausea and diarrhea.

IMAGING FEATURES

- Conventional radiography is nonspecific and insensitive for early signs of significant ischemia.
- CT can directly demonstrate occlusive causes of acute mesenteric ischemia involving the SMA or the SMV.
- SMA thrombosis typically involves the vessel origin associated with underlying atherosclerotic disease; SMA embolism tends to occlude beyond the vessel origin, often near branch points.
- CT findings of bowel ischemia include bowel wall thickening, delayed or decreased enhancement, pneumatosis, mesenteric and portal venous gas, and pneumoperitoneum.
- Acute mesenteric ischemia from arterial occlusion can manifest as small bowel wall thinning (instead of thickening) and luminal dilatation; bowel wall thickening is more common in SMV thrombosis.
- Small vessel vasculitis leading to acute mesenteric ischemia manifests with nonspecific signs of ischemia.
- CT is very effective for diagnosing primary bowel conditions, such as closed-loop obstruction, that result in mesenteric ischemia.
- Shock bowel typically demonstrates marked bowel wall thickening and prominent mucosal enhancement.
- Chronic mesenteric ischemia typically demonstrates advanced atherosclerosis of at least two of the three major splanchnic vessels (celiac, SMA, and inferior mesenteric artery); extensive collateral formation may be seen.

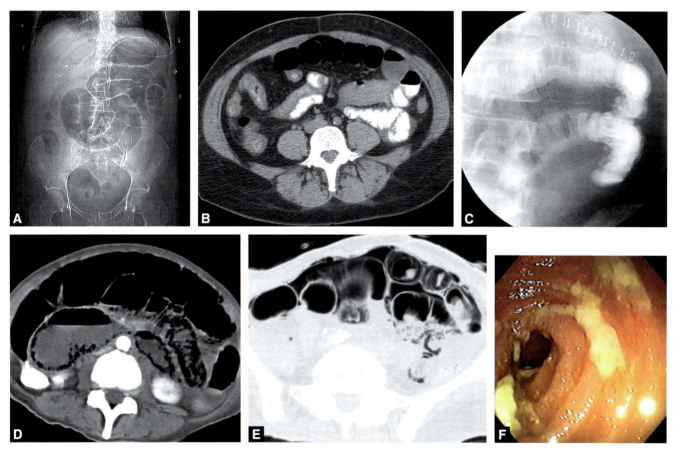

FIGURE 3.2.1 Small bowel findings in mesenteric ischemia. CT scout radiograph **(A)** and corresponding CT image **(B)** from a patient with acute mesenteric ischemia related to cocaine use show dilated small bowel loops with wall thinning, which can be seen with arterial occlusive processes. Contrast SBFT spot film **(C)** from a second patient shows diffuse jejunal wall thickening. Wall thickness can be assessed on this supine radiograph because massive pneumoperitoneum outlines the serosal bowel surface (Rigler's sign). Contrast-enhanced CT image **(D)** from a third patient shows diffuse bowel dilatation with extensive pneumatosis concerning for necrosis. CT image with lung window setting **(E)** from a fourth patient shows extensive pneumatosis, as well as free intraperitoneal air from perforation. Push enteroscopy image **(F)** from a final patient shows congested mucosa with multiple erosions and overlying exudate. In more severe cases, the mucosa may have a dusky appearance suggestive of impending infarction.

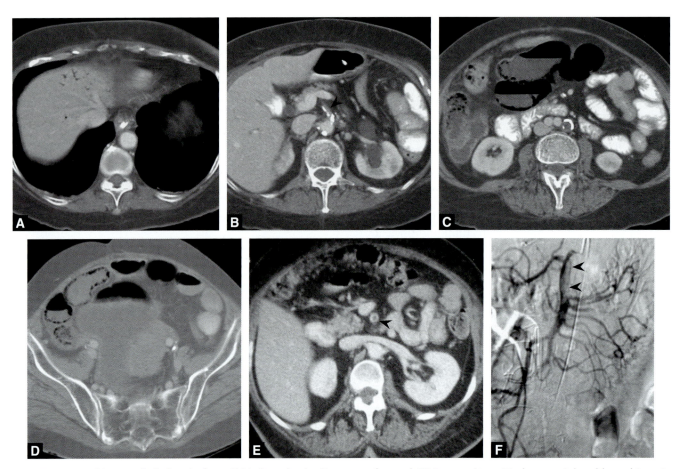

FIGURE 3.2.2 Mesenteric ischemia from SMA thrombosis. Contrast-enhanced CT images **(A to D)** show peripheral branching air within the liver **(A)** consistent with portal venous gas, SMA thrombosis **(B**, *arrowhead*) associated with advanced atherosclerotic disease, and small bowel pneumatosis **(C)**, which is better depicted on a wider window setting **(D)**. Contrast-enhanced CT image **(E)** and selective SMA angiogram **(F)** from a second patient show an extensive intraluminal filling defect (*arrowheads*), diagnostic of SMA thrombosis.

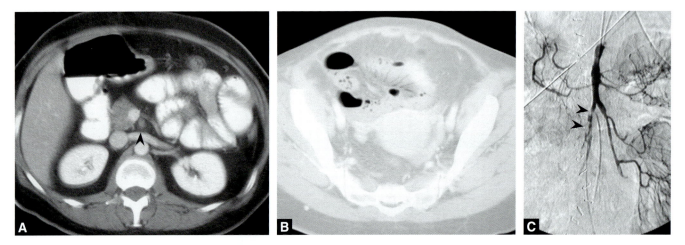

FIGURE 3.2.3 Mesenteric ischemia from SMA embolism. Contrast-enhanced CT image **(A)** shows a low-attenuation filling defect within the SMA (*arrowhead*). Lower CT image with lung window setting **(B)** shows subtle mesenteric venous gas extending from an ischemic small bowel loop. Selective SMA angiogram **(C)** shows multiple intraluminal filling defects (*arrowheads*), with absent visualization of several distal branches.

Illustration continued on following page

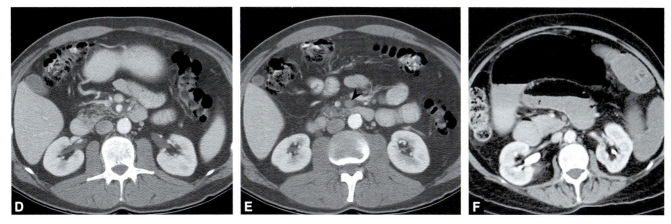

FIGURE 3.2.3 (Continued) **Mesenteric ischemia from SMA embolism.** Contrast-enhanced CT images (**D** and **E**) from a second patient show normal SMA enhancement proximally (**D**) with a low-attenuation embolus seen on the more inferior image (**E**, *arrowhead*). Contrast-enhanced CT image (**F**) from a third patient shows an SMA embolus associated with massive small bowel dilatation.

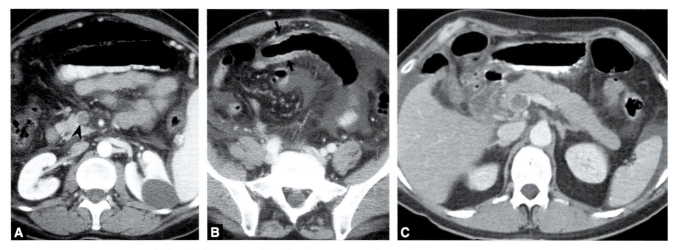

FIGURE 3.2.4 **Mesenteric ischemia from SMV thrombosis.** Contrast-enhanced CT images (**A** and **B**) show SMV thrombosis (**A**, *arrowhead*) associated with segmental small bowel wall thickening (**B**, *arrows*) and ascites. Contrast-enhanced CT image (**C**) from a different patient shows another example of SMV thrombosis.

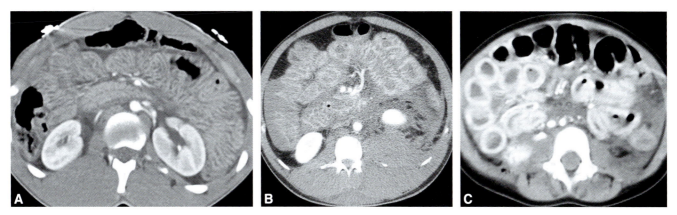

FIGURE 3.2.5 **Trauma-related "shock bowel."** Contrast-enhanced CT images (**A** to **C**) from three different trauma patients show diffuse small bowel wall thickening with prominent mucosal enhancement. Retroperitoneal hemorrhage is also seen in two cases (**B** and **C**).

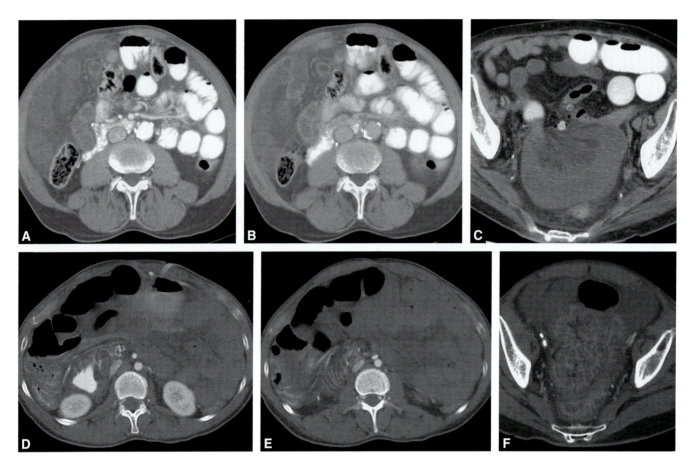

FIGURE 3.2.6 Ischemia from closed-loop bowel obstruction. Dynamic (**A**) and delayed (**B**) contrast-enhanced CT images show an internal hernia resulting from a small mesenteric defect that contains poorly enhancing small bowel loops and extensive mesenteric congestion. Subtle delayed enhancement of several thickened loops can be seen by comparing the two images. CT image (**C**) from a second patient shows a necrotic pelvic small bowel loop related to an internal hernia. Contrast-enhanced CT images (**D** to **F**) from a third patient show complete infarction of the midgut due to volvulus. Note the preserved mucosal enhancement seen with the duodenum and colon. The small bowel was diffusely necrotic at exploratory laparotomy and the patient died soon after.

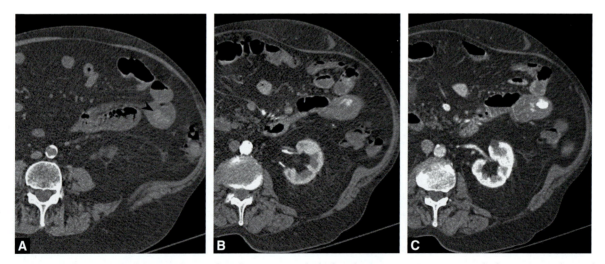

FIGURE 3.2.7 Gastrointestinal hemorrhage related to mesenteric ischemia. Precontrast (**A**), arterial phase (**B**), and portal venous phase (**C**) CT images show subtle high-attenuation material (**A,** *arrowhead*) within a jejunal loop on the precontrast image, followed by active extravasation after IV contrast administration, indicative of a brisk GI hemorrhage. Bowel ischemia was confirmed at surgery.

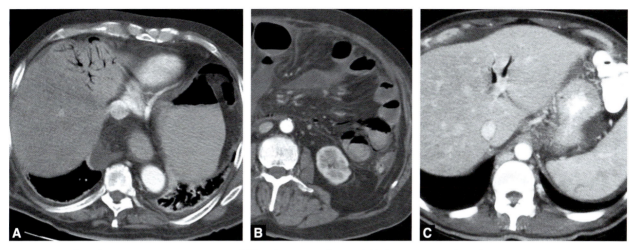

FIGURE 3.2.8 **Portal venous gas versus pneumobilia.** Contrast-enhanced CT images (**A** and **B**) show portomesenteric venous gas and small bowel pneumatosis related to mesenteric ischemia. The portal venous gas within the liver demonstrates a typical peripheral branching appearance. Compare this with pneumobilia (**C**) from a different patient, which typically appears more central with less extensive branching.

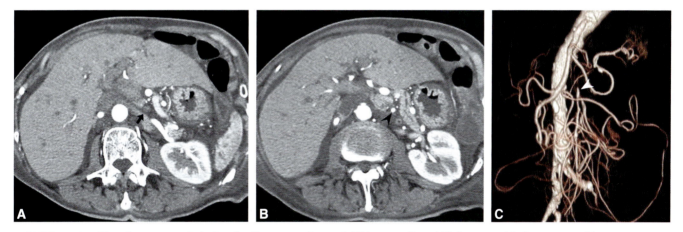

FIGURE 3.2.9 **Chronic mesenteric ischemia.** Contrast-enhanced CT images (**A** and **B**) from an elderly woman with symptoms suggestive of chronic mesenteric ischemia show thrombosis of the proximal SMA (**A**, *arrow*), with distal reconstitution (**B**, *arrowhead*). CT angiographic image (**C**) better depicts the findings of SMA reconstitution (**C**, *arrowhead*) and the extensive collateral formation.

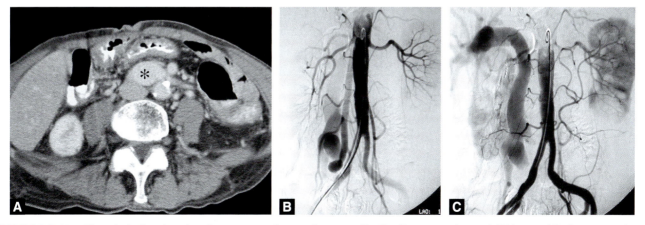

FIGURE 3.2.10 **Chronic ischemia related to mesenteric arteriovenous fistula.** Contrast-enhanced CT image (**A**) shows prominent dilatation of the SMV (*asterisk*), as well as small bowel wall thickening related to venous congestion. Early (**B**) and delayed (**C**) images from catheter angiography show an arteriovenous fistula connecting the SMA and SMV, which has led to massive dilatation of the SMV and portal vein. The fistula was believed to represent a complication from prior surgery.

3.3 Small Bowel Herniation
(Figures 3.3.1-3.3.10)

CLINICAL FEATURES

- Hernias are abnormal protrusions through fascial defects, which often contain loops of small bowel.
- Classified as external or internal; over 90% of diagnosed hernias are the external type.
- Inguinal hernias account for 75% of external cases; other types include ventral, umbilical, femoral, incisional, lumbar, parastomal, spigelian, obturator, and sciatic.
- Internal hernias are less common, occurring through various mesenteric and omental defects; named internal hernias include paraduodenal (left > right) and foramen of Winslow types.
- Incarceration of a bowel-containing hernia, leading to obstruction and strangulation, is a feared complication.
- Internal hernias and some external hernias are difficult to diagnose on physical examination; imaging can play an important role in these cases.

IMAGING FEATURES

- CT is the imaging study of choice for evaluating most hernias; US can be useful for some external hernias (particularly inguinal).
- CT not only identifies most hernias but can also assess for obstruction and vascular compromise.
- Multiplanar reformatted CT images may be useful for demonstrating the findings in selected cases.
- Internal hernias are more difficult to confidently diagnose; clustering of loops in certain locations is suggestive on CT; these hernias are at high risk for closed-loop obstruction.

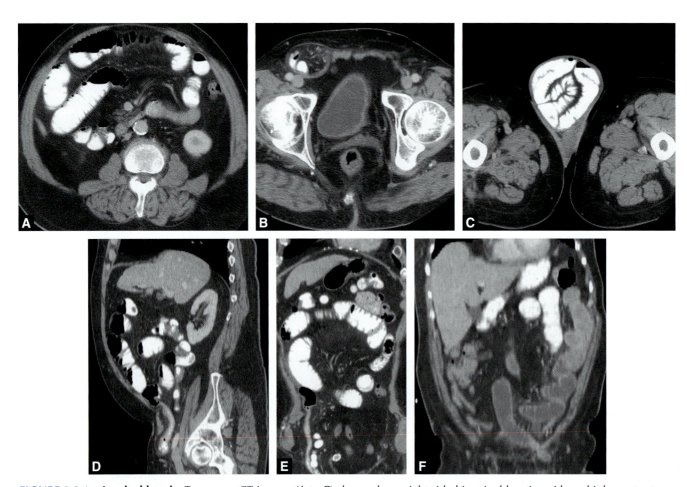

FIGURE 3.3.1 Inguinal hernia. Transverse CT images (**A** to **C**) show a large right-sided inguinal hernia, with multiple contrast-filled small bowel loops extending into the scrotum. Dilated proximal loops indicate partial obstruction. Curved reformatted sagittal (**D**) and coronal (**E**) CT images show the small bowel loops extending into the inguinal canal. Curved formatted coronal CT image (**F**) from a different patient shows a higher-grade SBO due to left-sided inguinal herniation. Note the decompressed loops within the right hemiabdomen.

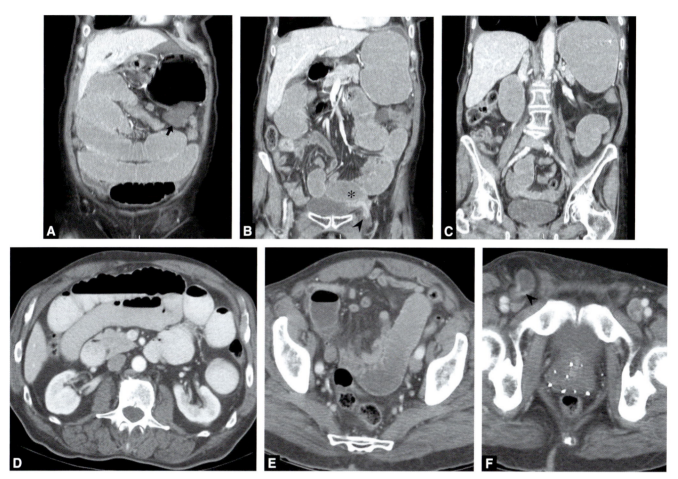

FIGURE 3.3.2 **Femoral hernia.** Coronal contrast-enhanced CT images (**A** to **C**) show a high-grade SBO caused by a left-sided femoral hernia, which was not evident clinically. The coronal plane nicely demonstrates the dilated afferent loop (**B**, *asterisk*), the herniated loop (**B**, *arrowhead*), and the decompressed efferent loop. The patient had other potential causes of SBO, including peritoneal implants from endometrial cancer (**A**, *arrow*) and prior abdominal surgeries. Transverse contrast-enhanced CT images (**D** to **F**) from a different patient show a high-grade SBO from a right-sided femoral hernia (**F**, *arrowhead*). Note the dilated pelvic loop and multiple distal decompressed loops.

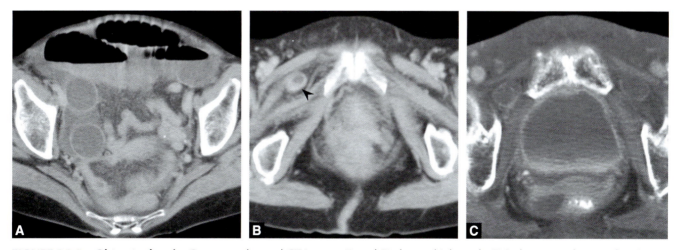

FIGURE 3.3.3 **Obturator hernia.** Contrast-enhanced CT images (**A** and **B**) show a high-grade SBO due to an obturator hernia, with a small bowel loop (**B**, *arrowhead*) located between fascicles of the obturator externus muscle. Extensive mesenteric congestion and free fluid are findings that suggest vascular compromise. Contrast-enhanced CT image (**C**) from a patient with increased intra-abdominal pressure shows bilateral obturator hernias, which did not result in SBO.

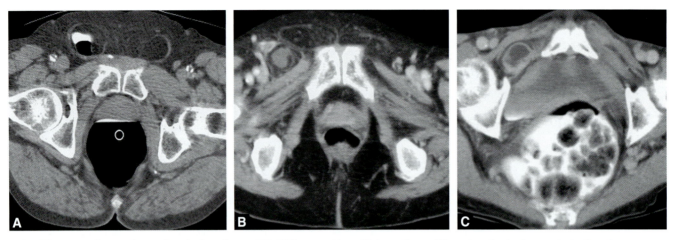

FIGURE 3.3.4 Comparison of groin hernias on CT. CT images (**A** to **C**) from three different patients demonstrate the close proximity of inguinal (**A**), femoral (**B**), and obturator (**C**) hernias. Care must be taken to correctly classify the hernia type, because the surgical approach may differ. The inguinal hernia in **A** is shown on a prone series from CT colonography.

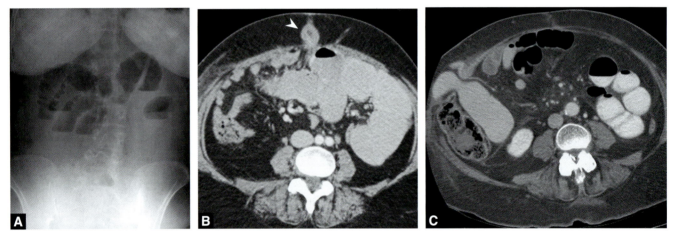

FIGURE 3.3.5 Incisional hernia. Upright abdominal radiograph (**A**) from a patient who had undergone recent laparoscopic surgery shows multiple dilated air-filled small bowel loops, differential air-fluid levels, and a paucity of colonic gas. Although the bowel gas pattern is suggestive of a mechanical SBO, an atypical-appearing postoperative ileus remains possible. Image from subsequent CT (**B**) demonstrates ventral herniation of small bowel through a laparoscopic port site (*arrowhead*), causing a high-grade SBO. CT can be very useful in cases of atypical radiographic bowel gas patterns in postoperative patients. Contrast-enhanced CT image (**C**) from a different patient shows a partial SBO due to an incisional hernia containing a small bowel loop.

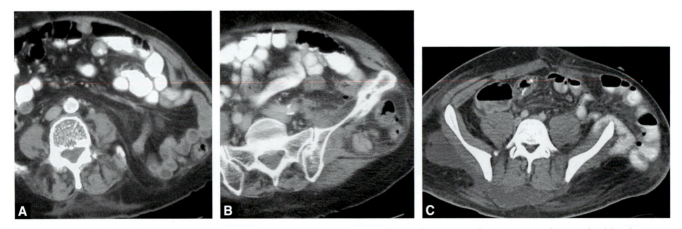

FIGURE 3.3.6 Lumbar hernia. Contrast-enhanced CT images (**A** and **B**) show a large, nonobstructive, wide-mouthed lumbar hernia containing multiple small bowel loops. Contrast-enhanced CT image (**C**) from a different patient shows an acute traumatic lumbar hernia resulting from a motor vehicle accident. Lumbar hernias rarely result in bowel obstruction.

SMALL BOWEL HERNIATION

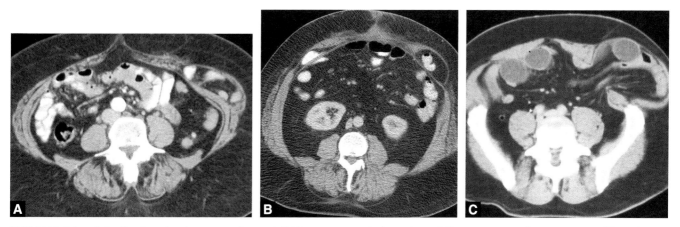

FIGURE 3.3.7 **Spigelian hernia.** Contrast-enhanced CT images (**A** to **C**) from three different patients show a variety of bowel-containing spigelian hernias, including a unilateral nonobstructive hernia (**A**), bilateral nonobstructive hernias (**B**), and a large unilateral hernia resulting in SBO (**C**).

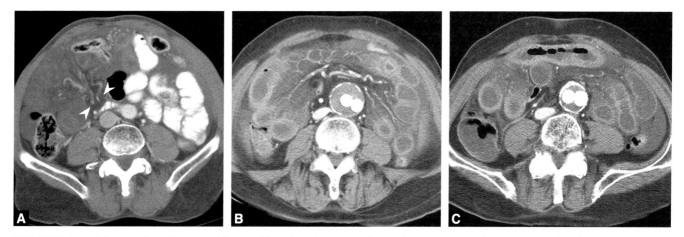

FIGURE 3.3.8 **Mesenteric and omental internal hernias.** Contrast-enhanced CT image (**A**) shows a strangulated internal hernia with a cluster of thick-walled, poorly enhancing small bowel loops in the right hemiabdomen. The supplying vessels appear to converge at the site of a small mesenteric defect (*arrowheads*). Contrast-enhanced CT images (**B** and **C**) from a different patient show multiple thick-walled small bowel loops with surrounding fluid and congestion. The supplying mesenteric vessels have an atypical appearance, which proved to be due to a strangulating internal herniation of nearly the entire midgut through an omental defect.

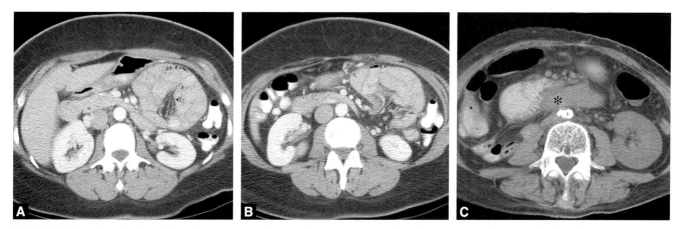

FIGURE 3.3.9 **Paraduodenal hernias.** Contrast-enhanced CT images (**A** and **B**) demonstrate a left paraduodenal hernia, consisting of an abnormal rounded cluster of small bowel loops extending into and expanding the fossa of Landzert. CT image (**C**) from a different patient shows a right paraduodenal hernia, with small bowel (*asterisk*) extending posterior to the SMA into the fossa of Waldeyer and causing a partial duodenal obstruction.

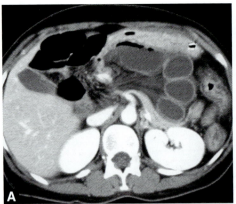 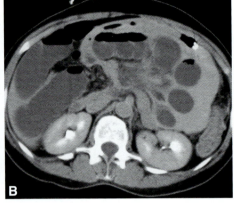 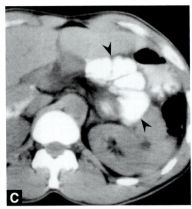

FIGURE 3.3.10 Foramen of Winslow hernia. Contrast-enhanced CT image **(A)** shows a radial cluster of dilated small bowel loops located posterior to the anteriorly displaced stomach, within the lesser sac. Note how the mesenteric fat and vessels converge between the portal vein and IVC at the foramen of Winslow. This closed-loop obstruction is at high risk for strangulation, which was demonstrated on a follow-up CT **(B)**, performed several hours later. Note the high-attenuation mesenteric fluid that outlines and expands the lesser sac. The involved bowel was necrotic at surgery. CT image **(C)** from a different patient shows a nonobstructive foramen of Winslow hernia containing contrast-filled small bowel loops (*arrowheads*).

3.4 Celiac Disease
(Figures 3.4.1-3.4.6)

CLINICAL FEATURES

- Celiac disease, also known as gluten-sensitive enteropathy and nontropical sprue, is caused by a complex immunologic response to gliadins in wheat, rye, and barley.
- Genetic predisposition and an immunologic component have been established; expression of HLA-DQ2 and HLA-DQ8 haplotypes is associated with the development of celiac disease.
- The highest incidence of disease is found in Western Europe, particularly in Celtic and Northern Ireland populations; the true prevalence of disease is not known because many afflicted individuals with the disease are relatively asymptomatic and undiagnosed.
- Presentation varies widely from vague abdominal complaints suggestive of irritable bowel syndrome to asymptomatic iron deficiency to classic disease (e.g., steatorrhea, diarrhea, weight loss).
- Serologic testing for endomysial and tissue transglutaminase antibodies is useful in cases where appropriate clinical suspicion exists.
- Approximately 5% of patients with celiac disease are IgA deficient, which can lead to a false-negative serology.
- Confirmation of disease requires small intestinal biopsy.
- The histologic spectrum of disease ranges from increased intraepithelial lymphocytes with normal villi to complete mucosal atrophy with loss of villi and crypt hyperplasia.
- Treatment with a gluten-free diet usually leads to resolution of symptoms and normalization of villous architecture; a minority of patients may require corticosteroids to achieve remission.
- Associated disorders include dermatitis herpetiformis, diabetes, selective IgA deficiency, and hyposplenism.
- Complications include ulcerative jejunoileitis, malignancy (particularly T-cell lymphoma), mesenteric lymph node cavitation, and stricture.

IMAGING FEATURES

- Endoscopic findings vary and include a normal-appearing mucosa, scalloping of the folds, an atrophic appearance, and a mosaic mucosal pattern; edematous folds may indicate malabsorption or jejunoileitis.
- Findings at barium evaluation include small bowel dilatation, reversal of the normal jejunoileal fold pattern, duodenal irregularity, and transient nonobstructive intussusceptions.
- The decrease in jejunal folds is a primary finding, with "jejunization" of the ileum representing an adaptive response; fold thickening may be seen if malabsorption findings predominate.
- Enteroclysis improves accuracy of radiologic diagnosis but is generally not necessary.
- Capsule endoscopy may be useful in evaluating the entire mesenteric small bowel in some cases, particularly those resistant to dietary therapy and to rule out the development of associated complications.
- CT findings include dilated small bowel, prominent lymph nodes, splenic atrophy, and transient intussusception.
- Extensive lymphadenopathy and bowel wall thickening suggests the possibility of enteropathy-associated T-cell lymphoma.
- Enlarged mesenteric nodes with fat-fluid levels indicate the rare cavitation syndrome.

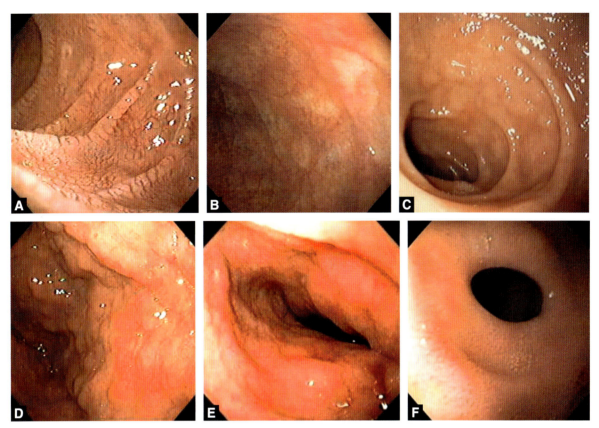

FIGURE 3.4.1 Endoscopic findings in celiac disease. Endoscopic images (**A** to **F**) from six different patients show the characteristic scalloping of folds (**A**), atrophy with loss of folds and visualization of submucosal vessels (**B**), atrophy with a subtle mucosal mosaic pattern (**C**), more extensive mucosal mosaic appearance with nodularity (**D**), loss of folds with diffusely edematous mucosa (**E**), and benign stricture (**F**). Strictures typically occur in patients with celiac disease complicated by ulcerative jejunoileitis. Absence of endoscopic findings does not rule out the diagnosis of celiac disease; and if clinical suspicion is present, biopsy specimens should be obtained for histologic evaluation.

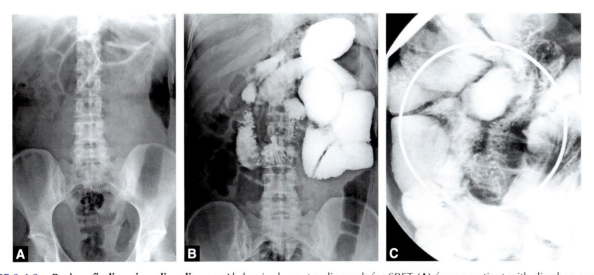

FIGURE 3.4.2 Barium findings in celiac disease. Abdominal scout radiograph for SBFT (**A**) from a patient with diarrhea and weight loss shows several abnormally dilated small bowel loops in the upper abdomen. Barium SBFT radiograph (**B**) shows dilated but nonobstructive jejunal loops with loss of folds giving a relatively featureless appearance. Mild duodenal irregularity is also present. Spot film (**C**) centered on the ileocecal region shows an increased ileal fold pattern, which may represent adaptive "jejunization."

Illustration continued on following page

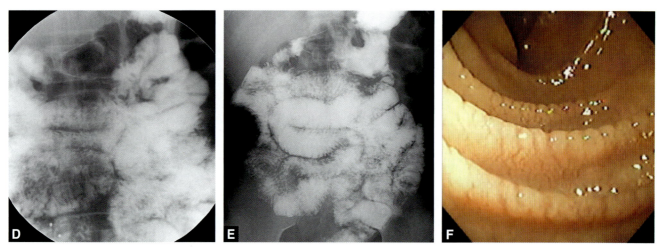

FIGURE 3.4.2 (Continued) **Barium findings in celiac disease.** Spot film (**D**) and overhead radiograph (**E**) from barium SBFT in a different patient show a fold reversal pattern with a decrease in jejunal folds and a relative increase in ileal folds. Mild to moderate dilatation of some loops is also present. Image from subsequent EGD (**F**) shows mucosal scalloping typical of celiac disease.

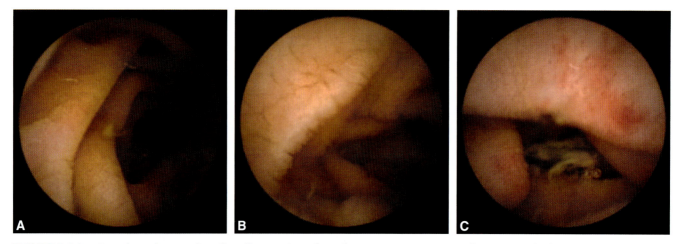

FIGURE 3.4.3 **Capsule endoscopy in celiac disease.** Capsule endoscopy images (**A** to **C**) demonstrate findings of marked villous atrophy (**A**), fold scalloping (**B**), and ulcerative jejunoileitis (**C**). Capsule endoscopy is a useful tool in patients who are refractory to a gluten-free diet to evaluate for the development of complications such as ulcerative jejunoileitis and lymphoma.

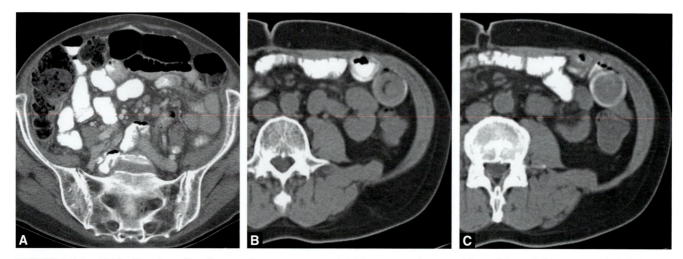

FIGURE 3.4.4 **CT findings in celiac disease.** Contrast-enhanced CT image (**A**) shows mild small bowel dilatation and slightly prominent mesenteric lymph nodes. CT images (**B** and **C**) from a second patient show jejunojejunal intussusception, which was nonobstructive and likely transient.

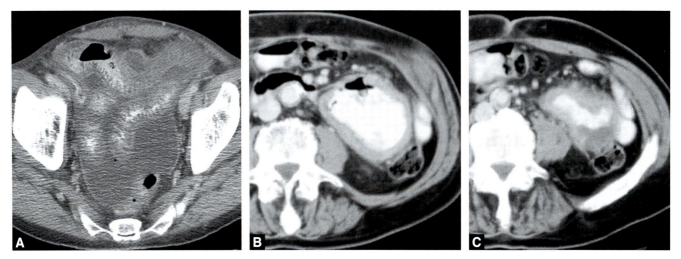

FIGURE 3.4.5 T-cell lymphoma in celiac disease. Contrast-enhanced CT image (**A**) shows small bowel wall thickening, peritoneal enhancement, and free fluid related to enteropathy-associated T-cell lymphoma. Contrast-enhanced CT images (**B** and **C**) from a different patient show prominent wall thickening and aneurysmal luminal dilatation of a jejunal loop from T-cell lymphoma complicating celiac disease.

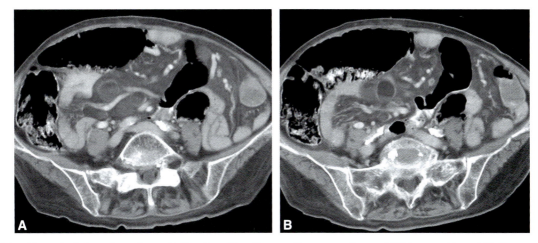

FIGURE 3.4.6 Mesenteric lymph node cavitation in celiac disease. Contrast-enhanced CT images (**A** and **B**) show multiple enlarged low-attenuation mesenteric lymph nodes, several of which demonstrate an unusual fat-fluid level from cavitation.

3.5 Small Bowel Diverticula
(Figures 3.5.1-3.5.10)

CLINICAL FEATURES

- Meckel's diverticulum represents incomplete involution of the vitelline (omphalomesenteric) duct, which connects the ileum to the umbilicus during development.
- Meckel's diverticulum is a true diverticulum that involves the antimesenteric aspect of the ileum, typically within 100 cm of the ileocecal valve.
- Meckel's diverticulum is usually asymptomatic; most symptomatic cases present early in childhood as bleeding (often due to heterotopic gastric mucosa).
- Other complications include inflammation (diverticulitis), inversion with intussusception, inguinal herniation (Littre's hernia), and ileal volvulus around a fibrous cord (vitelline remnant).
- Jejunal diverticulosis is characterized by multiple pseudodiverticula with mucosal and submucosal penetration through the muscularis at points where vessels penetrate along the mesenteric border.
- Jejunal diverticula are usually asymptomatic but may rarely present as bacterial overgrowth (blind loop syndrome), bowel dysmotility, bleeding, or diverticulitis.
- Ileal diverticula other than Meckel's diverticulum are uncommon; diverticulitis is a rare complication that can mimic other right lower quadrant inflammatory processes.

IMAGING FEATURES

- Meckel's diverticulum can be an incidental finding at contrast radiography or cross-sectional imaging.
- Technetium pertechnetate scintigraphy is sensitive for detecting gastric mucosa within Meckel's diverticulum and is typically performed in the setting of GI bleeding in an infant.
- CT can demonstrate complications such as Meckel's diverticulitis, intussusception, and volvulus.
- Jejunal diverticulosis can be identified at contrast radiography and CT; location along the mesenteric border can often be appreciated in advanced cases.
- Tagged red blood cell scintigraphy can localize bleeding from jejunal diverticula; the bleeding site may be confirmed with push enteroscopy or capsule endoscopy.
- The CT findings of small bowel diverticulitis are analogous to those of colonic diverticulitis.

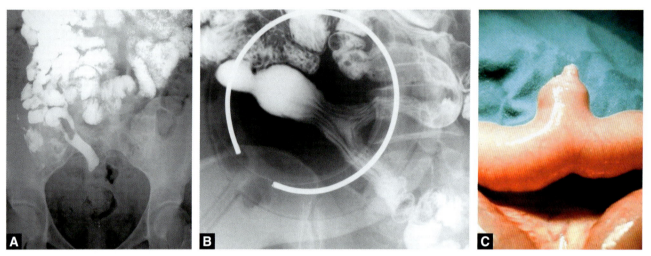

FIGURE 3.5.1   Meckel's diverticulum. Barium SBFT images **(A** and **B)** from two different patients show typical elongated Meckel's diverticula extending off the distal ileum. Both cases represent incidental detection because no complications were manifest. Intraoperative photograph **(C)** shows a Meckel's diverticulum that had presented with GI bleeding.

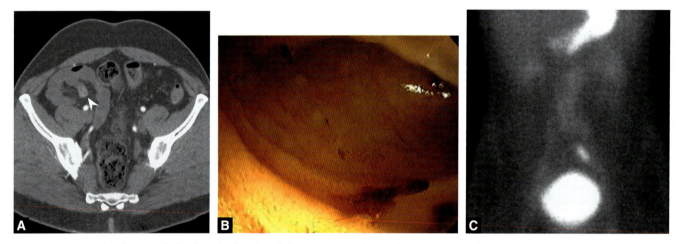

FIGURE 3.5.2   Bleeding Meckel's diverticulum in adults. Contrast-enhanced CT image **(A)** from a patient with obscure GI bleeding shows a Meckel's diverticulum (*arrowhead*) with a subtle increase in luminal attenuation relative to the remaining bowel loops due to ongoing hemorrhage. Ileoscopy during colonoscopy **(B)** from another patient with obscure GI bleeding shows luminal blood suggesting a small bowel source. Technetium pertechnetate scintigraphy **(C)** demonstrates a focus of lower abdominal activity above the bladder that corresponded to the temporal appearance of the gastric activity, consistent with a Meckel's diverticulum containing gastric mucosa.

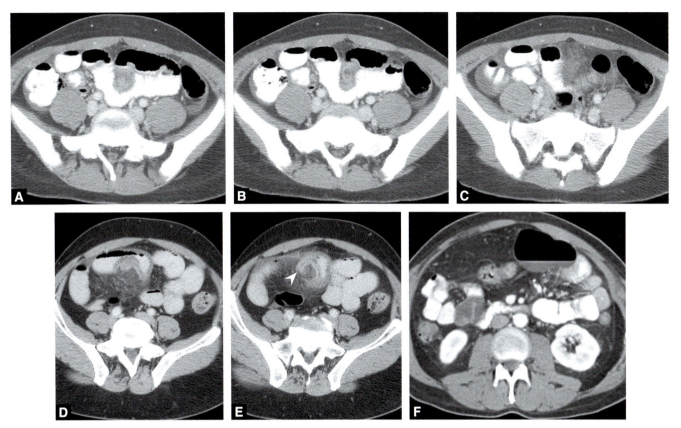

FIGURE 3.5.3 Meckel's diverticulitis. Contrast-enhanced CT images (**A** to **C**) show an inflamed Meckel's diverticulum extending anteriorly off a contrast-filled ileal loop. Soft tissue infiltration of the adjacent mesentery is evident. Contrast-enhanced CT images (**D** and **E**) from a second patient show a Meckel's diverticulum (**E**, *arrowhead*) with extensive mesenteric inflammation and secondary wall thickening of the adjacent ileum. Contrast-enhanced CT image (**F**) from a third patient shows a large, well-defined air- and fluid-filled cavity, which represents a dilated and inflamed Meckel's diverticulum. All three patients presented with acute symptoms and diverticulitis was surgically confirmed.

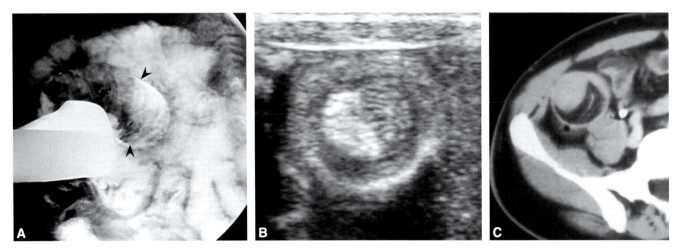

FIGURE 3.5.4 Intussusception of inverted Meckel's diverticulum. Spot film from barium SBFT (**A**) shows an ileoileal intussusception (*arrowheads*), which was confirmed at same-day US (**B**). The US image shows a cross section of the outer thick-walled intussuscipiens containing an echogenic region representing mesenteric fat and a hypoechoic region representing the inverted Meckel's diverticulum. Contrast-enhanced CT image (**C**) from a different patient shows the CT correlate of the US appearance, with the inverted Meckel's diverticulum and mesenteric fat projecting within an ileal loop.

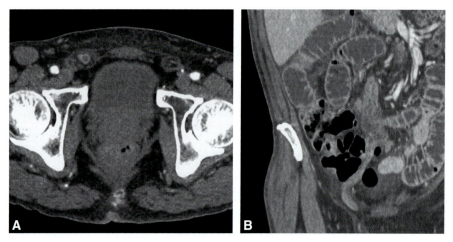

FIGURE 3.5.5 Inguinal herniation of Meckel's diverticulum (Littre's hernia). Transverse **(A)** and coronal **(B)** images from CT enterography demonstrate an indirect right inguinal hernia containing a slender Meckel's diverticulum.

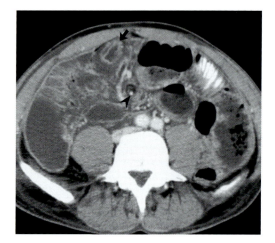

FIGURE 3.5.6 Ileal volvulus due to Meckel's diverticulum. Contrast-enhanced CT image from an acutely symptomatic patient shows an unusual configuration of abnormal bowel loops, as well as a whorled appearance around a mesenteric vessel (*arrowhead*), suggestive of volvulus. At surgery, a Meckel's diverticulum (*arrow*) was found be the cause of volvulus, owing to a persistent fibrous cord of attachment to the umbilicus.

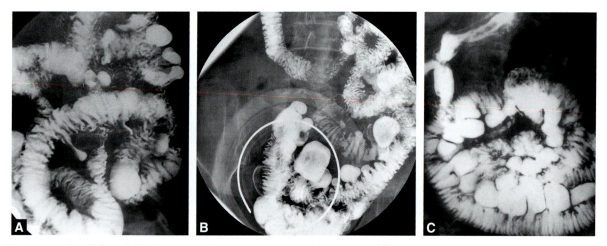

FIGURE 3.5.7 Jejunal diverticulosis. Barium SBFT images **(A to C)** from three different patients with varying degrees of bacterial overgrowth symptoms show multiple contrast-filled jejunal diverticula. The diverticula originate along the mesenteric aspect of the bowel, which is best appreciated in **C**.

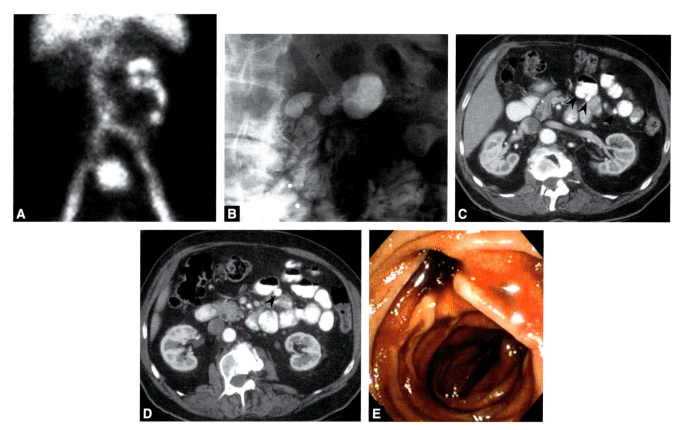

FIGURE 3.5.8 Bleeding jejunal diverticulum. Tagged red blood cell scintigraphy (**A**) from a patient on chronic anticoagulation with obscure but brisk GI bleeding demonstrates small bowel activity in the left upper quadrant, suggesting a jejunal source. Images from barium SBFT (**B**) and CT (**C** and **D**) reveal only multiple jejunal diverticula (*arrowheads*). Push enteroscopy (**E**) demonstrates ongoing bleeding from a jejunal diverticulum. Hemostasis was achieved by epinephrine injection into the base of the diverticulum and correction of the underlying coagulopathy. Segmental jejunal resection was not performed secondary to the patient's underlying comorbidities.

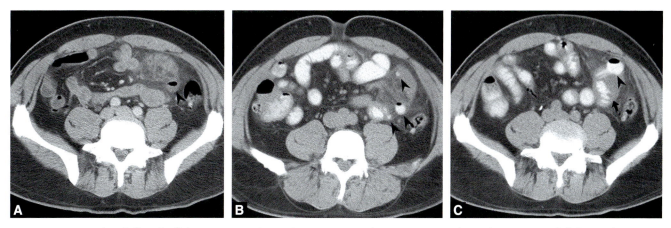

FIGURE 3.5.9 Jejunal diverticulitis. Contrast-enhanced CT image (**A**) from a patient with an abrupt onset of abdominal pain shows extensive left-sided mesenteric inflammatory changes and the suggestion of a jejunal diverticulum (*arrowhead*). The oral contrast had not yet emptied from the stomach. Delayed CT images (**B** and **C**) to allow for luminal opacification of the small bowel show multiple jejunal diverticula (**B, C,** *arrowheads*) and focal eccentric wall thickening (**C,** *arrow*), in addition to the mesenteric inflammation. Jejunal diverticulosis with perforated diverticulitis was confirmed at surgery.

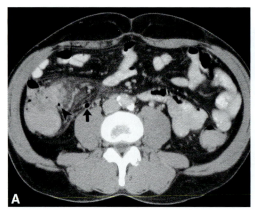 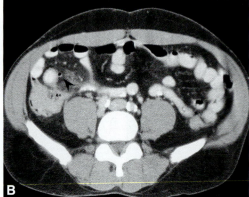

FIGURE 3.5.10 Ileal diverticulitis (non-Meckel's). Contrast-enhanced CT images (**A** and **B**) from a patient presenting with acute right lower quadrant pain show extensive soft tissue inflammatory changes in the ileocecal mesentery. Of note, the appendix was air filled and normal in appearance (**A**, *arrow*), and the terminal ileal wall was not thickened to suggest Crohn's disease. Terminal ileal diverticula, however, are present (*arrowheads*), one of which was the cause of the inflammatory process.

3.6 Malrotation
(Figures 3.6.1-3.6.6)

CLINICAL FEATURES

- Malrotation results from incomplete bowel rotation during development; nonrotation is most common, resulting in narrow mesenteric fixation that is prone to midgut volvulus.
- Most symptomatic cases present in the first month of life; other cases manifest in adolescence or adulthood or remain clinically silent.
- Acute presentation can manifest with hypotension and shock secondary to mesenteric ischemia or infarction requiring emergent surgical management.
- A history of unexplained abdominal complaints may be elicited in some adults with "incidental" malrotation detected on imaging.
- In addition to midgut volvulus, internal hernias can occur secondary to peritoneal bands (of Ladd).
- Malrotation is seen in the majority of patients with situs ambiguous (heterotaxy syndromes); in particular, polysplenia may go undiagnosed into adulthood.

IMAGING FEATURES

- On imaging, the small bowel is predominately right sided and the colon left sided; however, due to mobility, the cecum may appear in a normal position in 20% of cases.
- Reversal or vertical orientation of the SMA/SMV is a useful but inconstant finding at CT and US.
- Unsuspected malrotation in adults is an uncommon but not rare imaging finding.
- In infants with suspected malrotation, barium UGI remains a useful study; an incomplete duodenal sweep without normal positioning of the ligament of Treitz is diagnostic.
- A corkscrew or spiral appearance of the malpositioned bowel at barium UGI is evidence for midgut volvulus around the SMA axis; Ladd's bands typically result in a dilated proximal duodenum.
- Malrotation in symptomatic adults (whether causative or coincidental) is now most often seen at CT, because barium studies are seldom obtained in this setting.
- Midgut volvulus manifests with a whorled appearance around the SMA axis at CT and US.

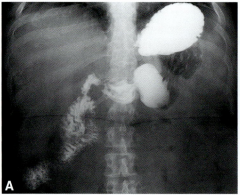 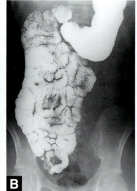 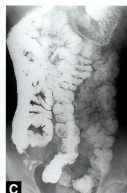

FIGURE 3.6.1 Unsuspected malrotation on barium examination. Barium UGI (**A**) performed after failed laparoscopic bariatric surgery reveals malrotation, which was the likely cause for the difficulty. Note the absence of the duodenal sweep and the right-sided positioning of the proximal small bowel. Barium SBFT study (**B** and **C**) from a different patient shows that the small bowel is located entirely on the right and the colon is entirely on the left.

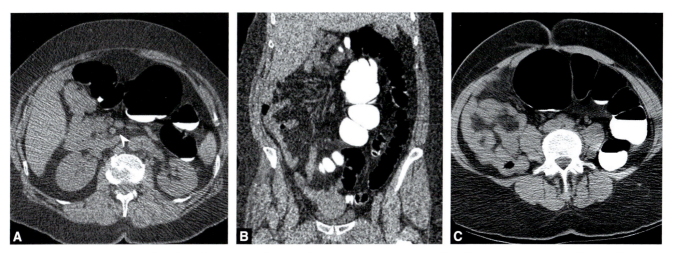

FIGURE 3.6.2 **Unsuspected malrotation at CT colonography screening.** Noncontrast low-dose transverse (**A**) and coronal (**B**) 2D CTC images demonstrate reversal of the normal SMA/SMV relationship (**A**, *arrowhead*), as well as malpositioning of the bowel. CTC image (**C**) from a different patient shows small bowel occupying the right hemiabdomen and the prepped and distended colon occupying the left.

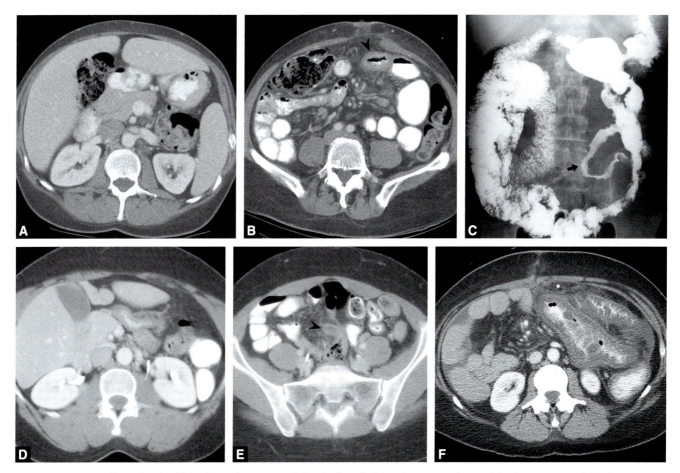

FIGURE 3.6.3 **Malrotation incidental to other acute abdominal pathology.** Contrast-enhanced CT images (**A** and **B**) show SMA/SMV reversal (**A**) and abnormal positioning of the bowel (**B**), including an inflamed segment of distal ileum (**B**, *arrowhead*) representing Crohn's disease. Barium SBFT (**C**) also demonstrates findings of malrotation and distal ileitis (*arrow*). Contrast-enhanced CT images (**D** and **E**) from a patient with acute left lower quadrant pain show SMA/SMV reversal (**D**) and bowel malpositioning (**E**), including an inflamed appendix extending off a left-sided cecum (**E**, *arrowhead*). Contrast-enhanced CT image (**F**) from a patient with fever and diarrhea demonstrates pancolitis with diffuse low-attenuation wall thickening and pericolonic stranding involving a left-sided colon, with small bowel occupying the right hemiabdomen. *Clostridium difficile* colitis was confirmed and treated. (D and E, from Pickhardt PJ, Bhalla S: Intestinal malrotation in adolescents and adults: Spectrum of clinical and imaging features. AJR 2002;179:1429-1435.)

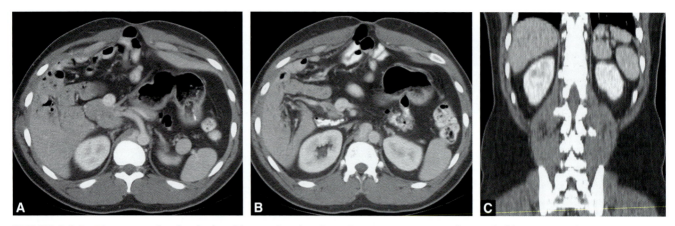

FIGURE 3.6.4 **Unsuspected polysplenia with associated malrotation.** Transverse (**A** and **B**) and oblique coronal (**C**) contrast-enhanced CT images show findings of polysplenia, including multiple spleens, azygous continuation of an interrupted inferior vena cava, preduodenal portal vein, and malrotation.

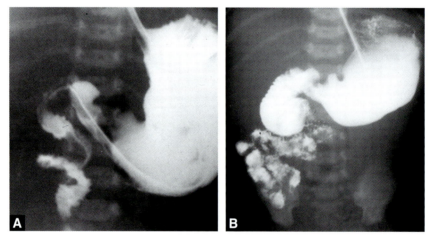

FIGURE 3.6.5 **Symptomatic malrotation in infants.** Barium UGI image (**A**) demonstrates a spiraled appearance to the malpositioned proximal small bowel, consistent with midgut volvulus complicating malrotation. Barium UGI image (**B**) from another infant with malrotation shows a dilated proximal duodenum representing partial obstruction from a Ladd's band.

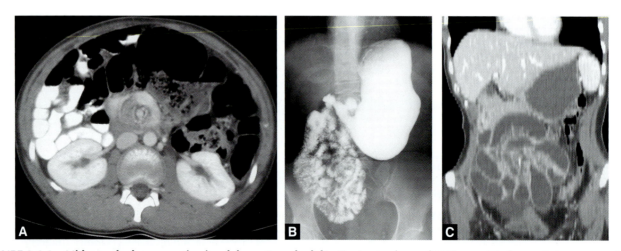

FIGURE 3.6.6 **Midgut volvulus presenting in adolescents and adults.** Contrast-enhanced CT image (**A**) demonstrates engorged mesenteric veins wrapping around the SMA axis. Note the malpositioned bowel. Midgut volvulus without bowel necrosis was confirmed at surgery. Barium SBFT image (**B**) from a woman with severe intermittent pain but asymptomatic at the time of this study shows findings of malrotation without significant complication. Coronal contrast-enhanced CT image (**C**) obtained during a symptomatic episode shows midgut volvulus with twisted and dilated fluid-filled small bowel loops.

Illustration continued on following page

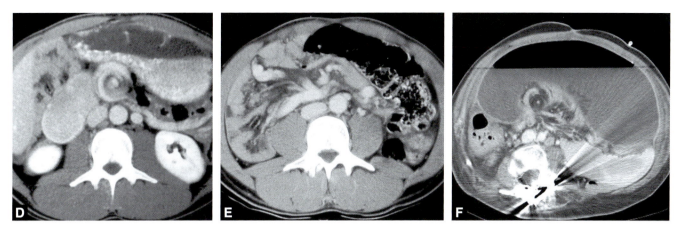

FIGURE 3.6.6 (Continued) **Midgut volvulus presenting in adolescents and adults.** Contrast-enhanced CT images (**D** and **E**) from a symptomatic patient with a previous history of severe episodic pain show malrotation with midgut volvulus. Note the whorl of congested vessels around the SMA axis. Contrast-enhanced CT image (**F**) from a chronically debilitated patient shows midgut volvulus with the "whorl sign" and massively dilated small bowel that was necrotic at surgery.

3.7 Small Bowel Wall Thickening
(Figures 3.7.1-3.7.5)

CLINICAL FEATURES

- Bowel wall thickening has numerous potential causes, which are mediated by common pathways such as edema, ischemia, hemorrhage, infection, inflammation, tumor, or an infiltrative process.
- The more common causes of bowel wall thickening have been discussed in preceding sections.
- Additional entities not previously discussed include hereditary angioedema, amyloidosis, lymphangiectasia, and immunodeficiency.
- Hereditary angioedema is an autosomal-dominant disorder manifested by recurrent swelling of skin, upper airway, GI tract, and other locations; the small bowel is often involved.
- Amyloidosis results from abnormal protein deposition in the extracellular space; nearly any organ system, including the GI tract, can be involved.
- Intestinal lymphangiectasia can be primary (congenital) or secondary (due to lymphatic blockage) and may be focal or diffuse; dilated lymphatics in the small bowel submucosa lead to fold thickening.
- Selective IgA deficiency is the most common primary immunodeficiency disorder, which manifests as nodular lymphoid hyperplasia and predisposes to certain diarrheal illnesses (e.g. giardiasis).

IMAGING FEATURES

- Luminal studies such as barium and endoscopic evaluation can demonstrate fold thickening but cannot truly assess bowel wall thickness.
- Cross-sectional imaging studies such as CT, US, and MR can directly assess the thickness of the bowel wall.
- Depending on the underlying cause, bowel wall thickening may be diffuse or focal, uniform or irregular, and smooth or nodular and range from mild to severe.
- Mural striation or a target-like appearance to the bowel wall at CT is suggestive of an inflammatory process and generally excludes tumor infiltration.
- Associated imaging findings such as lymphadenopathy and mesenteric disease may help narrow the differential diagnosis.
- Pseudothickening of the bowel wall at CT is most often seen in the proximal jejunum.

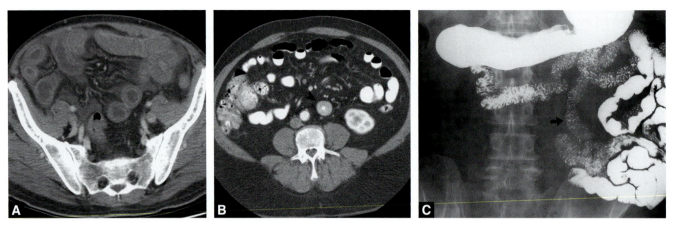

FIGURE 3.7.1 **True bowel wall thickening versus pseudothickening.** Contrast-enhanced CT image (**A**) from a patient with SLE shows true thickening of the bowel wall. The diffuse and uniform appearance with mural striation is compatible with an inflammatory process. Contrast-enhanced CT image (**B**) from a patient with breast cancer shows apparent focal thickening of a proximal jejunal loop (*arrowhead*), with a narrowed contrast-filled lumen. However, barium SBFT (**C**) performed the same day shows both a normal fold pattern and luminal caliber to the jejunal loop in question (*arrow*). Jejunal pseudothickening is a common pitfall at CT.

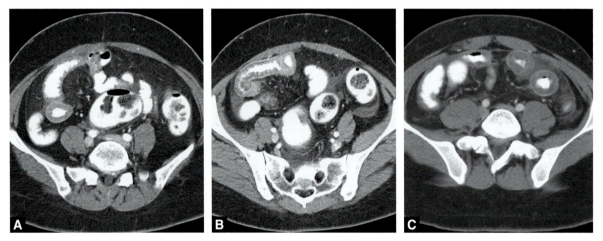

FIGURE 3.7.2 **Hereditary angioedema.** Contrast-enhanced CT images (**A** and **B**) show an ileal segment with uniform wall thickening and low-attenuation submucosal edema. Contrast-enhanced CT image (**C**) from another patient with hereditary angioedema shows bowel wall thickening with marked low-attenuation submucosal edema and surrounding mesenteric infiltration involving a jejunal loop.

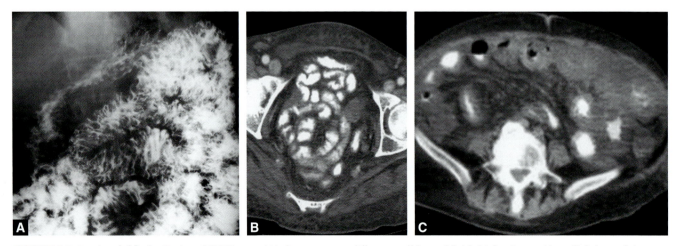

FIGURE 3.7.3 **Amyloidosis.** Barium SBFT image (**A**) demonstrates diffuse small bowel fold thickening, with a slightly nodular appearance. CT images (**B** and **C**) from two different patients with systemic amyloidosis show mild (**B**) and severe (**C**) bowel wall infiltration and thickening.

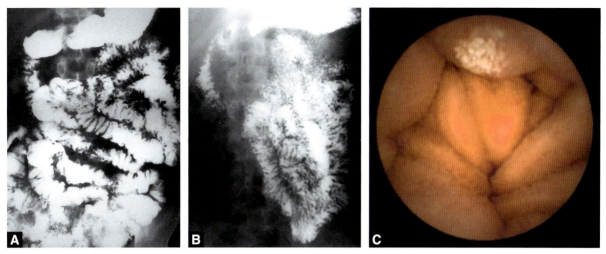

FIGURE 3.7.4 **Intestinal lymphangiectasia.** Barium SBFT radiographs (**A** and **B**) from two different patients with primary lymphangiectasia show diffuse small bowel fold thickening. Capsule endoscopy image (**C**) from a different patient shows an incidental finding of focal lymphangiectasia, consisting of multiple punctate white foci on a mucosal nodule.

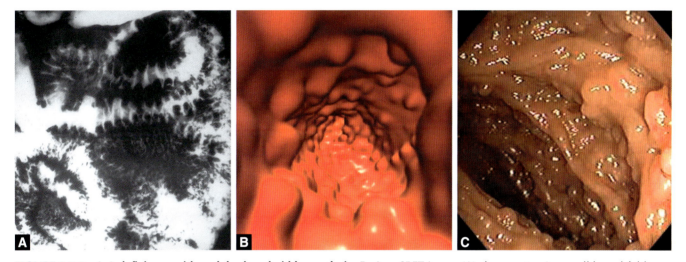

FIGURE 3.7.5 **IgA deficiency with nodular lymphoid hyperplasia.** Barium SBFT image (**A**) shows extensive small bowel fold thickening. 3D endoluminal CT image (**B**) from a second patient undergoing CTC evaluation shows innumerable polypoid nodules throughout the distal ileum. Endoscopic image (**C**) from a different patient shows diffuse nodular fold thickening.

3.8 Small Bowel Perforation
(Figures 3.8.1-3.8.6)

CLINICAL FEATURES

- Causes of mesenteric small bowel perforation include mesenteric ischemia, trauma, inflammation (both infectious and noninfectious), foreign bodies, iatrogenic injury, and complications of tumor.
- Peptic ulcer disease and procedure-related iatrogenic complications account for most duodenal perforations.
- Clinical presentation varies considerably, depending on the specific cause; surgical intervention is usually necessary.

IMAGING FEATURES

- Upright or lateral decubitus radiographs are sensitive for detecting pneumoperitoneum; however, this finding may be present in less than half of all proven cases.
- CT is the most useful imaging study for evaluation of suspected bowel injury; evaluation with lung windows improves sensitivity for detection of extraluminal gas.
- Beyond extraluminal gas, additional CT findings of bowel injury include extraluminal contrast, focal bowel wall thickening, peritoneal fluid, and peritoneal inflammation (peritonitis).
- Contrast fluoroscopy now plays a relatively minor diagnostic role for suspected bowel perforation.

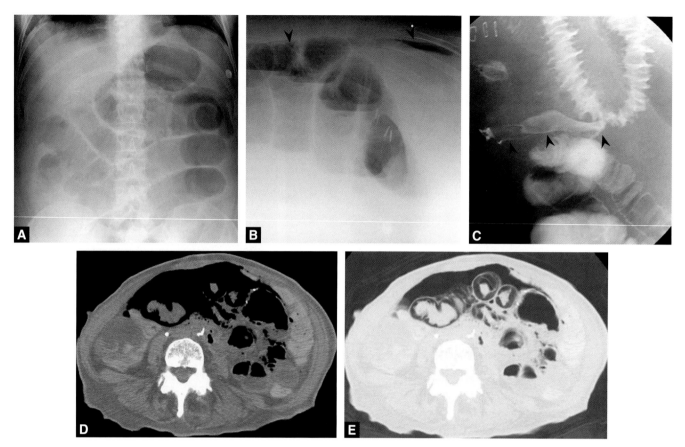

FIGURE 3.8.1 Small bowel perforation due to mesenteric ischemia. Supine abdominal radiograph (**A**) from a patient with mesenteric ischemia related to crack cocaine use shows nonspecific small bowel dilatation. Left lateral decubitus radiograph (**B**) shows free intraperitoneal air over the liver and between bowel loops (*arrowheads*), which was not identifiable on the supine view. Ileal perforation was confirmed at surgery. Water-soluble contrast SBFT (**C**) from a second patient shows marked fold thickening of an ischemic small bowel loop with focal leakage of contrast (*arrowheads*) indicative of necrosis with perforation. Pneumoperitoneum was also present, but the patient had recently undergone abdominal surgery. CT images with soft tissue (**D**) and lung (**E**) windows from a third patient show extensive pneumatosis and pneumoperitoneum from an ischemic-related perforation. Note how the lung windows better demonstrate the specific location of intra-abdominal gas collections.

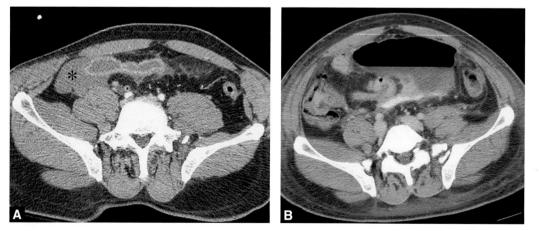

FIGURE 3.8.2 Mesenteric small bowel perforation from blunt trauma. Contrast-enhanced trauma CT image (**A**) from a patient who suffered a crush injury from a large concrete block shows a small bowel loop with abnormal enhancement and mild wall thickening adjacent to a mesenteric hematoma (*asterisk*). The abdominal injuries were initially managed conservatively in lieu of immediate exploratory laparotomy. Follow-up CT (**B** and **C**) performed 5 days later shows a large loculated peritoneal collection containing air, fluid, and oral contrast, diagnostic of perforated small bowel that was confirmed at subsequent surgery.

Illustration continued on following page

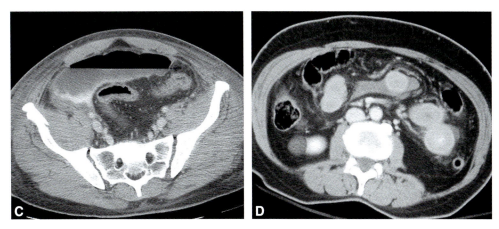

FIGURE 3.8.2 (Continued) **Mesenteric small bowel perforation from blunt trauma.** Contrast-enhanced CT image (**D**) from a patient involved in a motor vehicle accident shows several thickened small bowel loops surrounded by mesenteric fluid, which is of concern for significant injury. Jejunal perforation was confirmed at exploratory laparotomy.

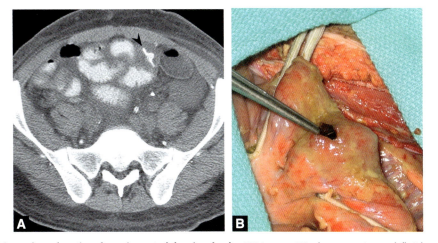

FIGURE 3.8.3 **Small bowel perforation from ingested foreign body.** CT image (**A**) shows peritoneal fluid and soft tissue infiltration related to peritonitis caused by perforation from an accidental ingestion of a pill still within its foil wrapper. The pill and its packaging are clearly identified as a dense structure (*arrowhead*). Photograph from subsequent exploratory laparotomy (**B**) shows the focal bowel perforation related to a corner of the foil wrapper.

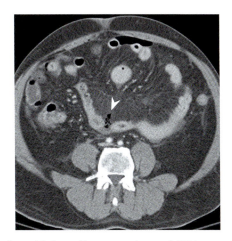

FIGURE 3.8.4 **Iatrogenic bowel injury.** Contrast-enhanced CT image shows a focal collection of extraluminal gas bubbles (*arrowhead*) adjacent to a small bowel loop, associated with hazy infiltration of its mesentery. Accidental enterotomy during a recent laparoscopic procedure was the cause of perforation in this case.

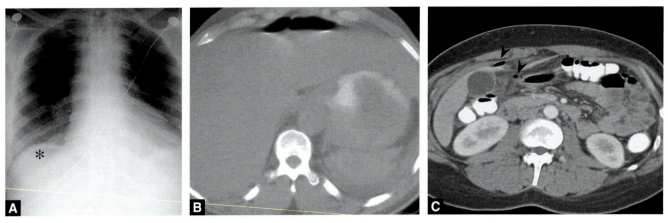

FIGURE 3.8.5 Perforated duodenal ulcers. Semi-upright frontal radiograph from a patient presenting to the emergency department with severe abdominal pain shows a subtle lucency (*asterisk*) over the right hemidiaphragm due to a perforated duodenal ulcer. CT image (**B**) with lung windows from a second patient with a perforated duodenal ulcer shows free intraperitoneal air outlining the falciform ligament. CT image (**C**) from a third patient shows small bubbles of extraluminal gas (*arrowheads*) with extensive peritoneal soft tissue inflammatory changes. CT detection of pneumoperitoneum is less dependent on technique as compared with conventional radiography and provides additional diagnostic information.

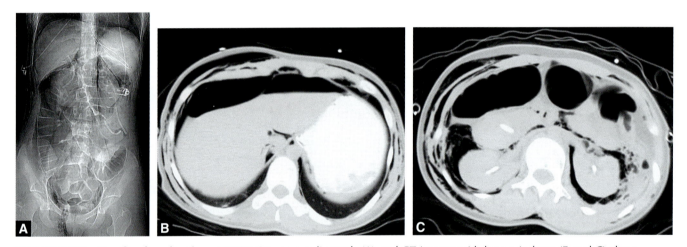

FIGURE 3.8.6 Duodenal perforation at ERCP. CT scout radiograph (**A**) and CT images with lung windows (**B** and **C**) show extensive extraluminal gas within the peritoneal, retroperitoneal, pleural, mediastinal, and subcutaneous spaces. This young woman had developed symptoms after an ERCP that was performed to evaluate suspected cystic duct stump leak following laparoscopic cholecystectomy. Sphincterotomy and biliary stenting was performed; additional stents have migrated to the jejunum (**A**).

3.9 Vascular Ectasia
(Figure 3.9.1)

CLINICAL FEATURES

- Vascular ectasia, also referred to as angiodysplasia or arteriovenous malformation, is the most common cause of occult or obscure GI bleeding involving the small intestine.
- It is predominantly seen in the elderly and in patients with renal insufficiency.
- It often presents as iron deficiency, but it can also manifest as overt bleeding (melena or hematochezia), hypotension, and a significant transfusion requirement.
- Typically sporadic, it can however be diffuse in the setting of hereditary hemorrhagic telangiectasia (Osler-Weber-Rendu syndrome).
- Actively bleeding lesions can be treated by either endoscopic or angiographic means.

IMAGING FEATURES

- Vascular ectasias typically appear as flat, red, spider-like lesions at endoscopy; primary venous ectasias (phlebectasias) often have a bluish appearance.
- Active hemorrhage may be detected on both scintigraphy and angiography; CT angiography may be useful for detection.
- Vascular ectasias are a common incidental finding at capsule endoscopy; treatment is generally not indicated in the absence of appropriate symptoms.

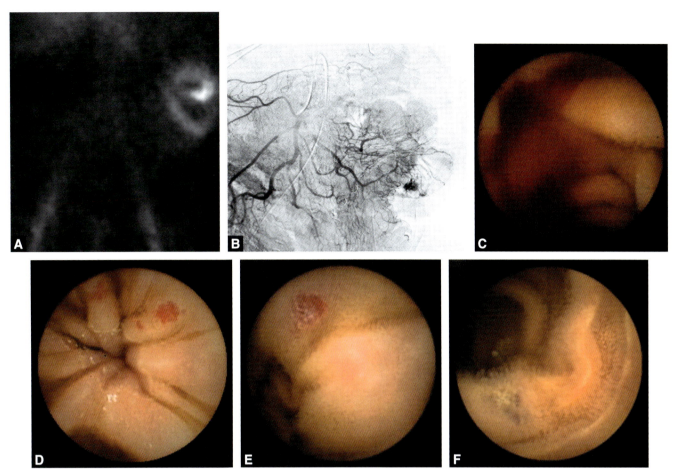

FIGURE 3.9.1 **Vascular ectasias.** Image from tagged red blood cell scintigraphy **(A)** shows active jejunal bleeding, which was shown to represent a focal telangiectasia at catheter angiography **(B)**. Capsule endoscopy **(C and D)** in a patient with obscure GI bleeding shows evidence of active hemorrhage **(C)**, as well as multiple telangiectasias **(D)**, which were believed to represent the source of bleeding. Capsule endoscopy image **(E)** from a patient with iron deficiency demonstrates a typical angioectasia. Capsule endoscopy image **(F)** from a final patient shows a venous ectasia (phlebectasia) with a bluish appearance.

CHAPTER 5

THE COLON AND RECTUM

Perry J. Pickhardt, MD

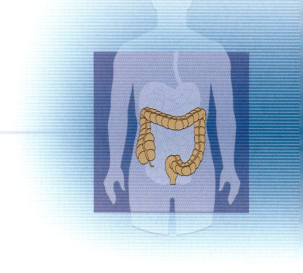

1. **COLORECTAL POLYPS AND MASSES**
   1.1 Benign Mucosal Neoplasms
   1.2 Non-neoplastic Mucosal Lesions
   1.3 Submucosal Lesions
   1.4 Colonic Adenocarcinoma
   1.5 Rectal Adenocarcinoma
   1.6 Other Colorectal Tumors
   1.7 CTC Diagnostic Tools
   1.8 CTC Pitfalls
2. **COLITIS**
   2.1 Ulcerative Colitis
   2.2 Crohn's Disease
   2.3 Infection
   2.4 Ischemia
   2.5 Other Colitides
3. **COLONIC DIVERTICULAR DISEASE**
   3.1 Diverticulosis
   3.2 Acute Diverticulitis
   3.3 Diverticular Fistulas and Strictures
   3.4 Diverticular Hemorrhage
   3.5 Giant Sigmoid Diverticulum
4. **THE APPENDIX**
   4.1 Appendicitis
   4.2 Appendiceal Tumors
5. **OTHER COLORECTAL CONDITIONS**
   5.1 Anorectal Disease
   5.2 Intussusception
   5.3 Vascular Lesions
   5.4 Colonic Volvulus
   5.5 Endometriosis
   5.6 Pneumatosis Coli
   5.7 Colonic Hernias
   5.8 Complications of Colonoscopy
   5.9 Epiploic Appendagitis
   5.10 Melanosis Coli

Imaging evaluation of the large intestine has undergone remarkable advances over the past decade, particularly with the advent of CT colonography (CTC, also referred to as virtual colonoscopy). Optical colonoscopy (also referred to as conventional or invasive colonoscopy) and CTC allow for complementary diagnostic evaluation of the colonic mucosa. Optical colonoscopy remains the therapeutic gold standard for nonsurgical interventions, whereas the role of CTC in colorectal cancer screening will likely continue to expand. Cross-sectional imaging modalities such as routine CT also provide for submucosal and extracolonic investigation, including evaluation of the vermiform appendix. Although the role of the barium enema (BE) for colorectal disease continues to wane as alternative modalities evolve, its demonstration of various disease entities remains instructive. The material presented in this chapter covers the broad topics of colorectal polyps, invasive carcinoma, colitis, diverticular disease, and the appendix, in addition to a variety of other colorectal conditions.

1. COLORECTAL POLYPS AND MASSES

A colorectal polyp represents any abnormal protrusion from the bowel wall into the lumen. Broad polyp categories include mucosal-based lesions (neoplastic and non-neoplastic) and submucosal lesions that originate deep to the mucosal surface. The most important colorectal mass is primary adenocarcinoma. Despite the fact that most colorectal adenocarcinomas are considered to be readily preventable through routine screening and that early detection markedly improves survival, it remains the second-leading cause of cancer-related mortality in the United States, primarily owing to poor screening compliance. Radiologic and endoscopic studies play a vital role in cancer detection, staging, and monitoring response to therapy. CTC is a rapidly evolving method for colorectal evaluation that complements the established technique of optical colonoscopy. A variety of CTC tools will be presented that are aimed at increasing accuracy and efficiency of interpretation. A number of diagnostic pitfalls at CTC are also discussed.

1.1 Benign Mucosal Neoplasms
(Figures 1.1.1-1.1.7)

CLINICAL FEATURES

- Over 95% of invasive colorectal cancers are believed to develop slowly from benign adenomatous precursors (adenoma-carcinoma sequence).
- Removal of adenomatous polyps, in particular advanced adenomas, interrupts the progression to carcinoma and is the rationale for screening.
- The clinical relevance of neoplastic polyps strongly correlates with lesion size and histology.
- Adenoma histology is as follows: tubular (80%-85%), tubulovillous (10%-15%), and villous (<5%).
- "Advanced adenomas" are defined as ≥10 mm or demonstrating a prominent villous component or high-grade dysplasia; these lesions are the primary target for screening.
- Malignant polyps are rare among the asymptomatic average-risk screening population; subcentimeter adenomas harbor cancer in <0.1% of cases.
- Tubular adenomas account for 30% to 40% of diminutive colonic polyps (≤5 mm); the vast majority do not progress to advanced neoplasia.
- Flat aggressive adenomas appear to be rare in the United States (particularly the "depressed" adenoma).
- Serrated adenomas represent an uncommon but distinct histopathologic subset that demonstrate features of both adenomas and hyperplastic polyps.
- Innumerable neoplastic polyps suggests familial adenomatous polyposis (FAP), especially in the setting of a positive family history or suggestive extracolonic findings.

IMAGING FEATURES

- In general, polyps can have a sessile, pedunculated, or flat morphology.
- Adenomas are composed of soft tissue at CTC and may appear erythematous or have a "cerebriform" pit pattern at colonoscopy; however, neither study can reliably distinguish adenomas from hyperplastic or other polyps.
- Tubulovillous and villous adenomas are typically larger than tubular adenomas and are often pedunculated; some villous tumors form "carpet lesions" that cover a relatively large surface area.
- The presence of high-grade dysplasia or malignancy cannot be reliably predicted from the radiologic or endoscopic appearance; thus, large lesions (≥1 cm) generally require histologic evaluation.
- Medium-sized polyps (6-9 mm) represent a relatively low-risk finding; current management of CTC-detected medium-sized lesions consists of CTC surveillance or optical colonoscopy referral for polypectomy.
- Diminutive polyps (≤5 mm) have questionable clinical significance and should not be reported at CTC, despite the fact that up to 30% to 40% may be adenomatous.

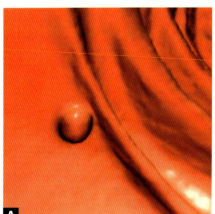 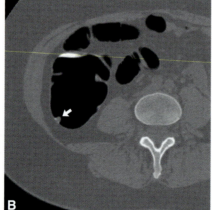 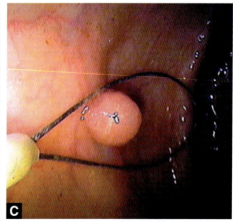

FIGURE 1.1.1 Sessile tubular adenomas. 3D endoluminal CTC image **(A)** shows a sessile 6-mm polyp in the ascending colon, which is confirmed on the transverse 2D CTC image **(B**, *arrow*) and was removed at same-day optical colonoscopy **(C)**.

Illustration continued on following page

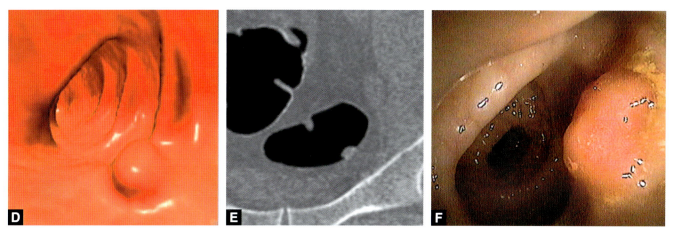

FIGURE 1.1.1 (Continued) **Sessile tubular adenomas.** 3D endoluminal CTC image (**D**), coronal 2D CTC image (**E**), and digital photograph from corresponding colonoscopy (**F**) from a different patient show another typical sessile polyp in the sigmoid colon (8-mm tubular adenoma).

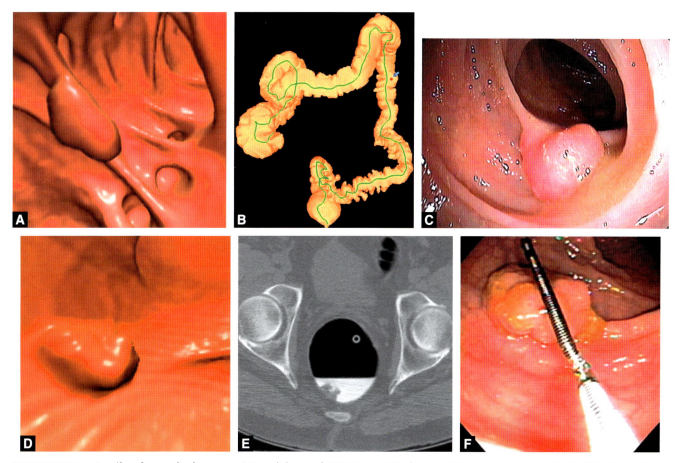

FIGURE 1.1.2 **Sessile advanced adenomas.** 3D endoluminal CTC image (**A**) shows a 1.5-cm polyp on a colonic fold. Note the adjacent diverticula. 3D colonic map (**B**) shows the location of the large polyp in the descending colon (*arrow*), in addition to multiple left-sided diverticula. Digital photograph from same-day colonoscopy (**C**) shows the same polyp on a fold, which proved to be a tubulovillous adenoma. Prone 3D endoluminal (**D**) and supine transverse 2D (**E**) images from a second patient show a 2-cm lobulated sessile polyp in the rectum, which is submerged on the supine view but visible due to contrast tagging of the fluid. Corresponding colonoscopy image (**F**) shows the same lesion, which proved to be a tubulovillous adenoma.

Illustration continued on following page

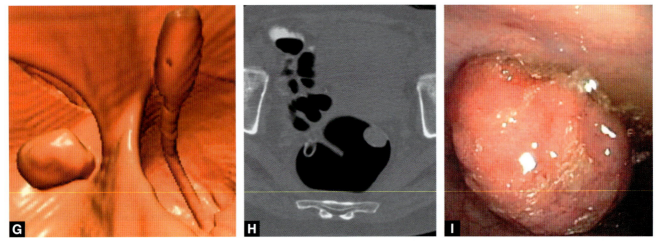

FIGURE 1.1.2 (Continued) **Sessile advanced adenomas.** 3D endoluminal CTC (**G**), 2D transverse CTC (**H**), and corresponding colonoscopy (**I**) images from a third patient show a large polypoid rectal mass, which is separated from the rectal catheter at CTC by a rectal fold. This 3-cm sessile mass proved to be a tubulovillous adenoma with high-grade dysplasia.

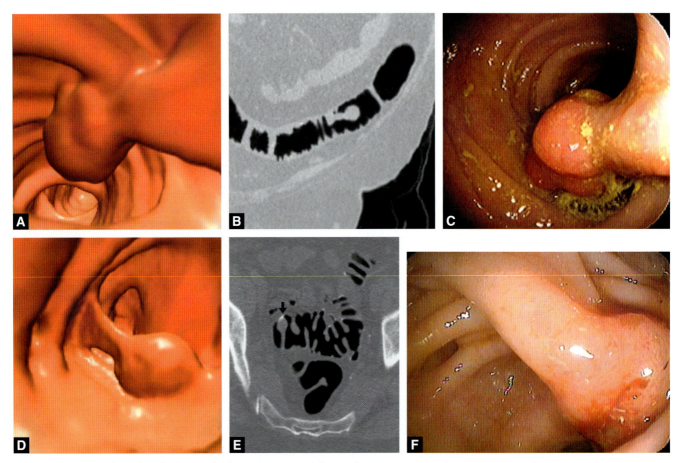

FIGURE 1.1.3 **Pedunculated advanced adenomas.** 3D endoluminal CTC (**A**), coronal 2D CTC (**B**), and corresponding colonoscopy (**C**) images show a large pedunculated tubulovillous adenoma in the sigmoid colon. 3D endoluminal CTC image (**D**) from a second patient shows a 1.7-cm pedunculated polyp in the sigmoid colon, which is less conspicuous on the 2D CTC images (**E**, *arrow*) due to the similar appearance of the sigmoid folds that are thickened by diverticular disease. The polyp was confirmed at same-day colonoscopy (**F**) and proved to be a tubulovillous adenoma.

Illustration continued on following page

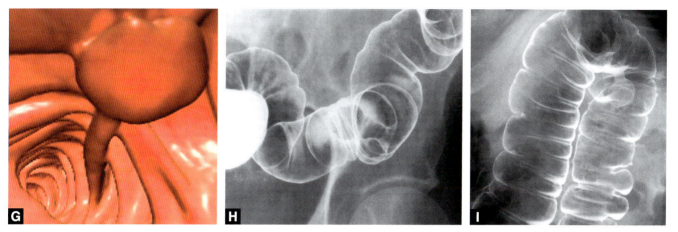

FIGURE 1.1.3 *(Continued)* **Pedunculated advanced adenomas.** 3D endoluminal CTC (**G**) and double-contrast BE (**H** and **I**) images from three different patients each show large pedunculated adenomas.

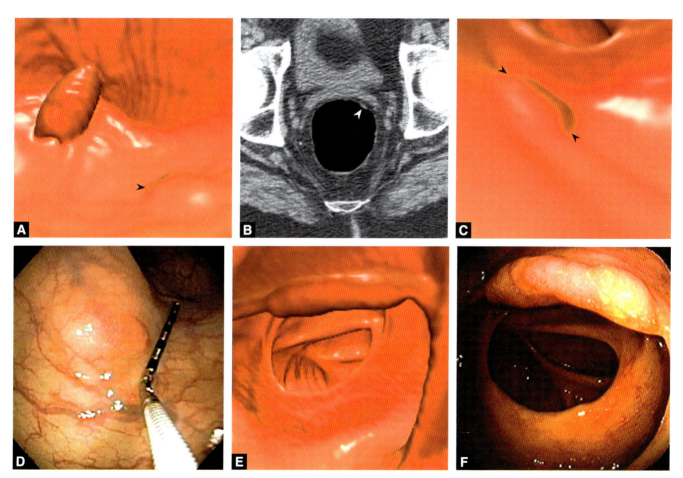

FIGURE 1.1.4 **Flat adenomas.** 3D endoluminal CTC image (**A**) and 2D CTC image with soft tissue windowing (**B**) show a slightly raised, flat 7-mm tubular adenoma (*arrowheads*) adjacent to the rectal catheter. 3D endoluminal CTC image (**C**) and corresponding colonoscopy image (**D**) from a second patient show a similar-appearing 6-mm, flat tubular adenoma (**C**, *arrowheads*) in the sigmoid colon. 3D endoluminal CTC (**E**) and corresponding colonoscopy (**F**) images from a third patient show a 3.5-cm tubulovillous adenoma with a broad elongated appearance. This lesion could be classified as flat or sessile, depending on the specific definition used. (A and B from Pickhardt PJ, Nugent PA, Mysliwiec PA, et al: Location of adenomas missed at optical colonoscopy. Ann Intern Med 2004; 141:352-359; C and D from Pickhardt PJ, Nugent PA, Choi JR, Schindler WR: Flat colorectal lesions in asymptomatic adults: Implications for screening with CT virtual colonoscopy. AJR 2004; 183:1343-1347.)

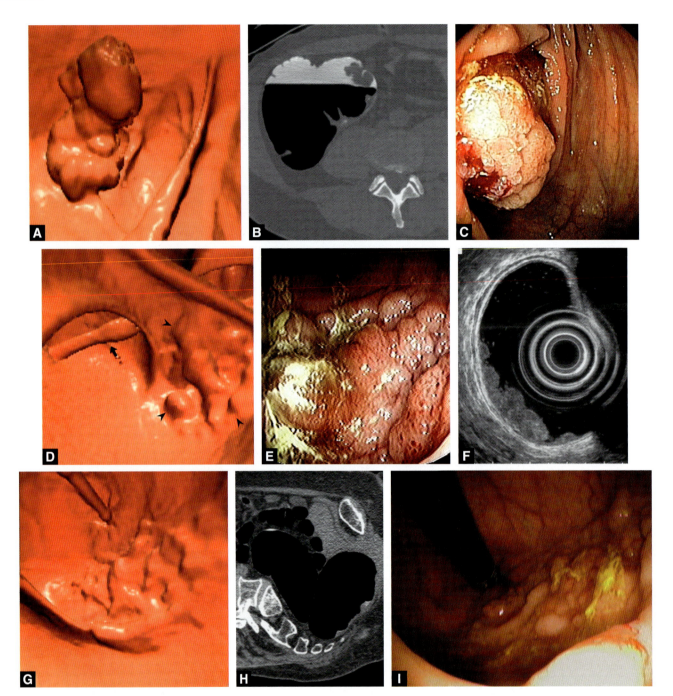

FIGURE 1.1.5 Villous adenomas. 3D endoluminal CTC (**A**) image shows a large, lobulated cecal mass. On prone 2D transverse CTC (**B**), the mass is submerged under the opacified fluid, which outlines its frond-like nature. The villous appearance is confirmed at colonoscopy (**C**). 3D endoluminal CTC image (**D**) from a second patient shows a relatively flat lobulated rectal mass (*arrowheads*), which carpets the mucosal surface. Note the rectal catheter (*arrow*). Images from subsequent colonoscopy (**E**) and EUS (**F**) show the same 5-cm mass. There is no evidence of submucosal extension at EUS, and this lesion proved to be a benign villous adenoma with high-grade dysplasia. 3D endoluminal CTC (**G**), 2D sagittal CTC (**H**), and colonoscopy (**I**) images from a third patient show another rectal villous adenoma manifesting as a flat carpet lesion, which involves a relatively large surface area and extends near the anorectal junction.

BENIGN MUCOSAL NEOPLASMS 217

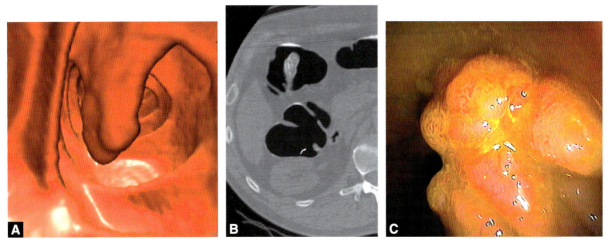

FIGURE 1.1.6 Serrated adenoma. 3D endoluminal CTC (**A**), 2D transverse CTC (**B**), and colonoscopy (**C**) images show a large, drooping pedunculated mass near the hepatic flexure that proved to be a serrated adenoma at histologic examination.

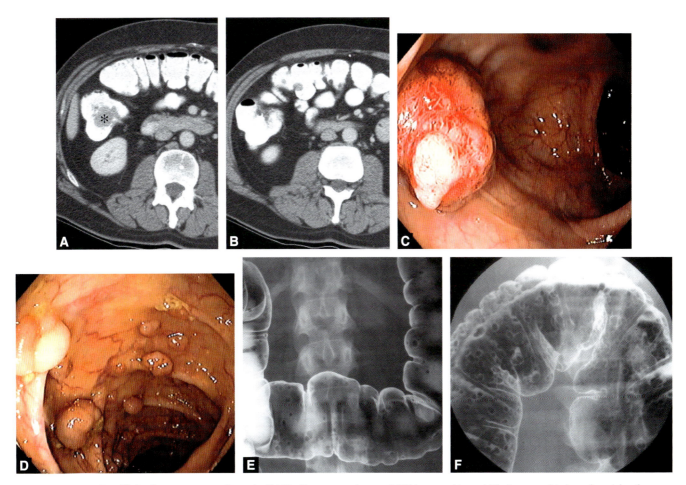

FIGURE 1.1.7 Familial adenomatous polyposis (FAP). Contrast-enhanced CT images (**A** and **B**) show multiple polypoid soft tissue lesions within the contrast-filled colon, including a dominant polypoid mass (*asterisk*) in the ascending colon. Images from subsequent colonoscopy (**C** and **D**) again demonstrate the multiple adenomatous polyps and the larger mass, which proved to be a tubulovillous adenoma with multiple foci of adenocarcinoma. Note the "cerebriform" appearance to the overlying mucosa often seen with adenomatous neoplasia. Double-contrast BE images (**E** and **F**) from two different patients with FAP show innumerable sessile filling defects representing adenomas. *(A to D from Pickhardt PJ: Differential diagnosis of polypoid lesions seen at CT colonography (virtual colonoscopy). Radiographics 2004; 24:1535-1559.)*

1.2 Non-neoplastic Mucosal Lesions

(Figures 1.2.1-1.2.7)

CLINICAL FEATURES

- Unlike the pathologic continuum seen with neoplastic lesions, nonadenomatous mucosal polyps are a heterogeneous group of unrelated entities.
- Nonadenomatous lesions predominate at smaller polyp sizes, whereas larger polyps are more often adenomatous.
- Hyperplastic (metaplastic) polyps account for the majority of resected nonadenomatous lesions.
- Although generally considered to be of no clinical significance, some have postulated that hyperplastic lesions may rarely have dysplastic potential.
- "Mucosal" polyps represent normal epithelial tags in a heaped-up or mammillated configuration; the vast majority are diminutive.
- Juvenile polyps are hamartomatous lesions that are typically seen in children, but solitary rectosigmoid lesions are occasionally identified in adults.
- Inflammatory polyps are thought to be extrusions related to peristaltic forces (not to be confused with inflammatory pseudopolyps and post-inflammatory polyps associated with inflammatory bowel disease [IBD]).
- Multiple hamartomas can be seen in juvenile polyposis, Cowden's disease, Peutz-Jeghers syndrome, and Cronkhite-Canada syndrome; some syndromes are associated with an increased risk for malignancy.
- Gastric heterotopia is rare and most often seen in the rectum; rectal bleeding is the most common presentation.

IMAGING FEATURES

- Non-neoplastic mucosal polyps are generally indistinguishable from adenomas; polyp size serves as the surrogate for histology and largely determines the need for polypectomy.
- CTC is less sensitive for non-neoplastic lesions compared with adenomas of a similar size, perhaps related to the irregular morphology of larger hyperplastic polyps and their tendency to flatten with luminal distention.
- Hyperplastic polyps are common in the rectosigmoid region and are typically small, sessile, and pale; right-sided lesions are less common but are more often large and irregular.
- Juvenile polyps are often pedunculated and may demonstrate a mottled appearance or cherry-red color at endoscopy.
- Inflammatory polyps may show a pale fibrinous cap at endoscopy.
- Multiplicity of polyps suggests a polyposis syndrome.
- Gastric heterotopia usually appears as a low rectal polypoid lesion, with or without associated ulceration.

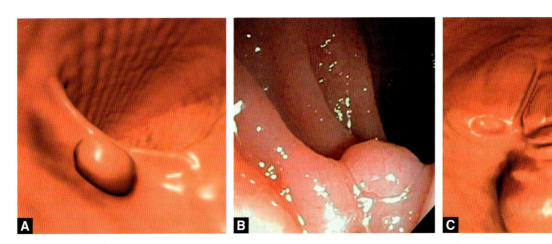

FIGURE 1.2.1 Hyperplastic (metaplastic) polyps. 3D endoluminal CTC (**A**) and corresponding optical colonoscopy (**B**) images show a sessile hyperplastic polyp, for which reliable distinction from an adenoma at imaging is not possible. 3D endoluminal CTC (**C**) from a second patient shows a flat 12-mm lesion adjacent to a normal-appearing ileocecal valve.

Illustration continued on following page

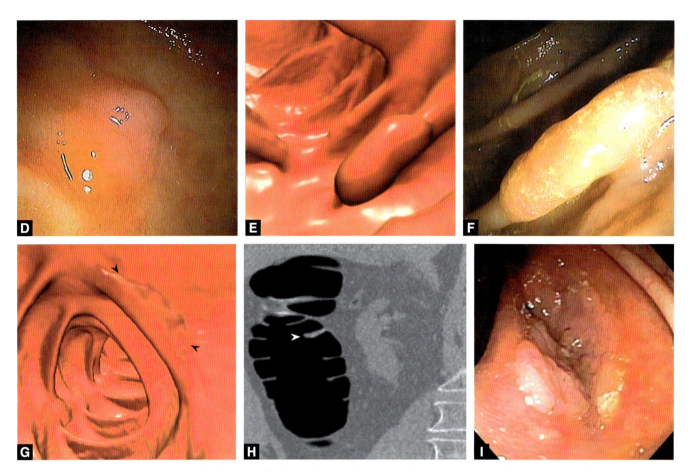

FIGURE 1.2.1 (Continued)   **Hyperplastic (metaplastic) polyps.** Subsequent colonoscopy (**D**) confirmed a subtle flat lesion, which proved to be hyperplastic. 3D endoluminal CTC (**E**) and colonoscopy (**F**) images from a third patient show an elongated hyperplastic polyp oriented along a fold. 3D endoluminal CTC (**G**), coronal 2D CTC (**H**), and colonoscopy (**I**) images show a 20-mm flat lesion that manifests with only subtle irregularity and fold thickening at CTC (**G, H,** *arrowheads*). Most large polyps missed at CTC are flattened hyperplastic lesions.

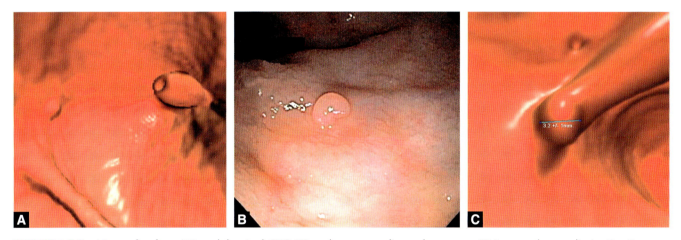

FIGURE 1.2.2   **Mucosal polyps.** 3D endoluminal CTC (**A**) and corresponding colonoscopy (**B**) images show a diminutive 3-mm polyp, which showed only normal mucosa at histologic evaluation. 3D endoluminal CTC image (**C**) from a different patient shows another diminutive mucosal polyp. *(A and B from Pickhardt PJ, Choi JR, Hwang I, Schindler WR: Nonadenomatous polyps at CT colonography: Prevalence, size distribution, and detection rates. Radiology 2004; 232:784-790.)*

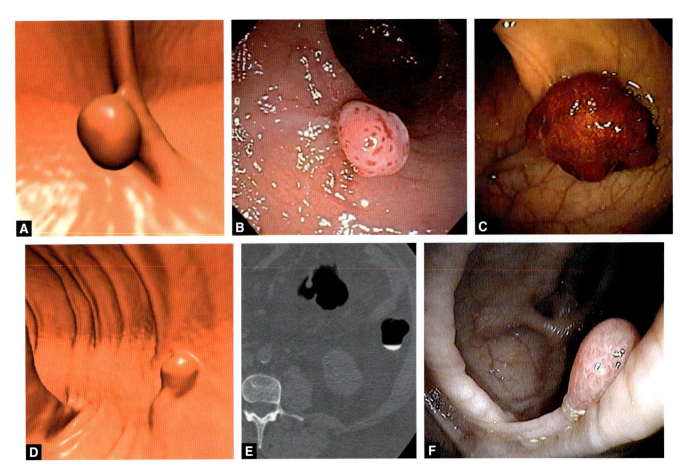

FIGURE 1.2.3 **Juvenile polyps.** 3D endoluminal CTC (**A**) and corresponding conventional colonoscopy (**B**) images show a solitary 1.5-cm pedunculated polyp located in the sigmoid colon in an asymptomatic adult undergoing primary screening. The erythematous and mottled appearance at colonoscopy is suggestive of a juvenile polyp. Colonoscopy image (**C**) from a child with rectal bleeding shows a typical large cherry-red juvenile polyp. 3D endoluminal CTC (**D**), transverse 2D CTC (**E**), and colonoscopy (**F**) images from an asymptomatic adult undergoing primary screening show a 1-cm pedunculated juvenile polyp in the sigmoid colon. *(A and B from Pickhardt PJ, Choi JR, Hwang I, Schindler WR: Nonadenomatous polyps at CT colonography: Prevalence, size distribution, and detection rates. Radiology 2004; 232:784-790.)*

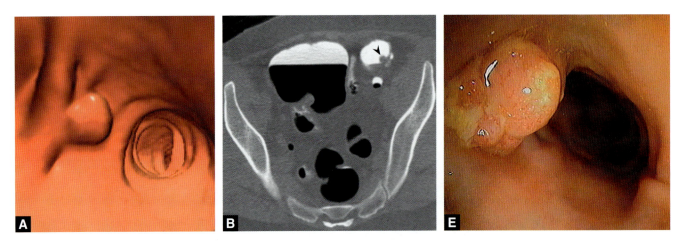

FIGURE 1.2.4 **Inflammatory polyps.** 3D endoluminal CTC (**A**), transverse 2D CTC (**B**), and colonoscopy (**C**) images from an asymptomatic screening patient show a 9-mm sessile polyp (*arrowhead*) in the sigmoid colon that showed only inflamed granulation tissue at histologic evaluation.

Illustration continued on following page

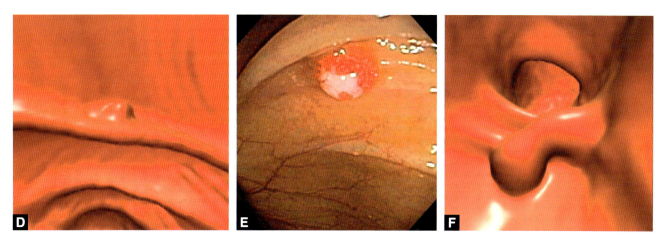

FIGURE 1.2.4 (Continued)   **Inflammatory polyps.** 3D endoluminal CTC (**D**) and colonoscopy (**E**) images from a different patient show a small sessile polyp adjacent to a fold that demonstrates a pale fibrinous cap at optical colonoscopy. 3D endoluminal CTC image (**F**) from a final patient shows a pedunculated 6-mm polyp that proved to be inflammatory at histologic evaluation.

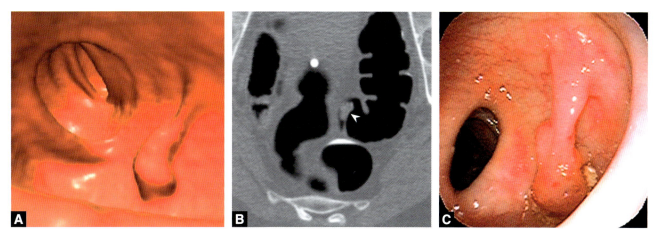

FIGURE 1.2.5   **Hamartomatous polyp.** 3D endoluminal CTC (**A**), transverse 2D CTC (**B**), and colonoscopy (**C**) images from an asymptomatic adult undergoing screening show a solitary 1.5-cm pedunculated polyp (*arrowhead*), which was found to be a hamartoma at histologic evaluation.

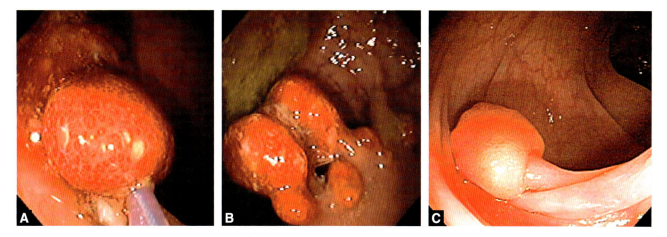

FIGURE 1.2.6   **Hamartomatous polyposis syndromes.** Optical colonoscopy images (**A** and **B**) from a child with hematochezia show multiple "cherry-red" polyps in the setting of juvenile polyposis. Colonoscopy image (**C**) from another patient with juvenile polyposis shows a large pedunculated juvenile polyp.

Illustration continued on following page

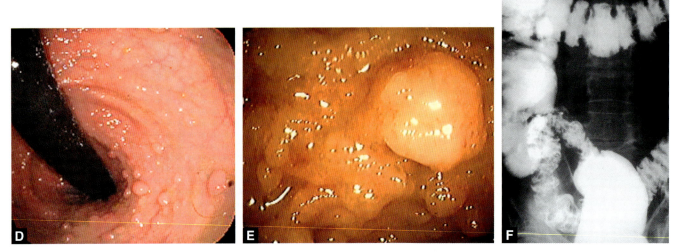

FIGURE 1.2.6 (Continued) **Hamartomatous polyposis syndromes.** Retroflexed rectal view from colonoscopy **(D)** in a patient with Cowden's disease shows innumerable small hamartomatous polyps. Similar lesions were present at EGD (not shown). Colonoscopy image **(E)** from a patient with Peutz-Jeghers syndrome shows multiple irregular polypoid lesions. Gastric and small bowel polyps were also seen at EGD (not shown). Image from single-contrast BE **(F)** in an elderly patient with Cronkhite-Canada syndrome shows irregular polypoid fold thickening throughout much of the colon. *(D from Pickhardt PJ: Differential diagnosis of polypoid lesions seen at CT colonography (virtual colonoscopy). Radiographics 2004; 24:1535-1559.)*

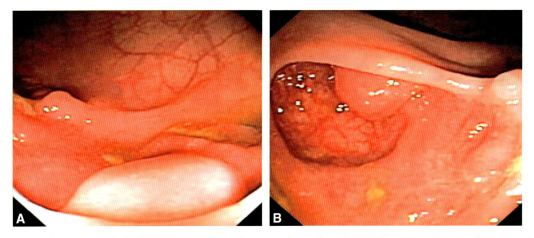

FIGURE 1.2.7 **Gastric heterotopia in the rectum.** Antegrade **(A)** and retroflexed **(B)** colonoscopy images from a patient with intermittent rectal bleeding show a large polypoid rectal mass with overlying erythematous mucosa. Heterotopic gastric mucosa was found at histologic evaluation.

1.3 Submucosal Lesions
(Figures 1.3.1-1.3.11)

CLINICAL FEATURES

- This varied group of entities range from incidental benign lesions to metastatic disease.
- Correlation with clinical history is useful in certain cases to refine the differential diagnosis.
- The colon is the most common GI site for lipomas; most lesions are right sided.
- Carcinoid tumors are more commonly encountered in the rectum, where they are typically an incidental finding; right-sided carcinoid tumors are rare but often bulkier and more aggressive (see section 1.6).
- Venous hemangiomas or vascular blebs of the colon may be seen in isolation or associated with blue rubber bleb nevus syndrome.
- Lymphoid polyps (nodular lymphoid hyperplasia) represent a benign condition; malignant lymphoma of the colon can rarely present as multiple polypoid lesions.
- Colorectal GI stromal tumor (GIST) is a rare but bulky lesion more often seen in the rectum; other mesenchymal tumors such as leiomyomas are likewise rare in the colon.
- Cystic lesions include lymphangiomas, duplication cysts, colitis cystica profunda, and retrorectal cystic hamartoma (tailgut cyst).

IMAGING FEATURES

- Submucosal lesions are typically smooth and broad based at endoluminal evaluation (e.g., BE, 3D CTC, and optical colonoscopy).
- 2D display at CTC allows for evaluation of the entire lesion, including internal composition, which is a distinct advantage over BE and traditional colonoscopy; transrectal US (TRUS) can provide similar diagnostic information for rectal lesions.
- Colonic lipomas can be confidently diagnosed at CT; at colonoscopy, lipomas are pale, have normal overlying mucosa, and are usually soft upon probing (pillow sign).
- Rectal carcinoid tumors are typically diminutive and often have a yellowish appearance.
- Venous hemangiomas can simulate soft tissue polyps at CTC; the bluish appearance at optical colonoscopy is diagnostic.
- A prominent exoenteric component suggests a mesenchymal tumor, such as a GIST or leiomyoma.
- Cross-sectional imaging demonstrates the cystic nature of lymphangioma and duplication cysts (colitis cystica profunda and retrorectal cystic hamartoma are covered in section 5.1).
- Central ulceration of a submucosal mass suggests hematogenous metastasis, Kaposi's sarcoma, carcinoid tumor, lymphoma, GIST, or other mesenchymal tumor.
- Extrinsic impressions may simulate submucosal lesions at BE and colonoscopy; 2D display at CTC avoids misdiagnosis in such cases.
- Pneumatosis can be diagnosed at both conventional radiography and CT (see section 5.6).

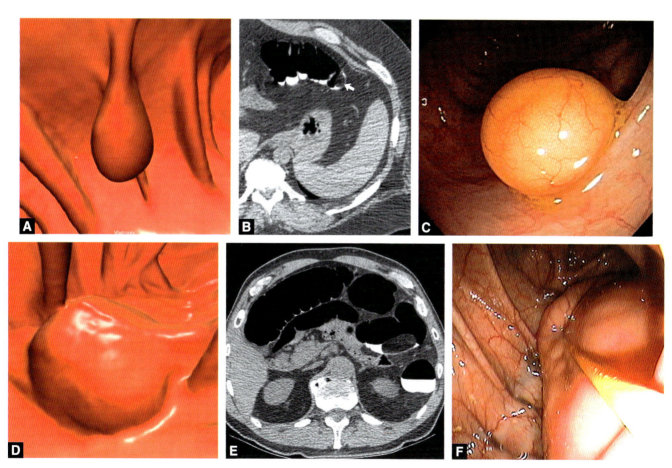

FIGURE 1.3.1   Colonic lipomas. 3D endoluminal CTC image (**A**) shows a smooth polypoid lesion that is composed of uniform fat attenuation on the transverse 2D CTC image (**B**, *arrow*), which is diagnostic of a lipoma. Optical colonoscopy image (**C**) from a different patient shows a similar ovoid lipoma with a typical yellowish endoscopic appearance. 3D endoluminal CTC image (**D**) from a third patient shows a large, broad-based mass that demonstrates uniform fat attenuation at 2D correlation (**E**). Image from colonoscopy (**F**) in this patient demonstrates the pliability of this soft mass, referred to as the "pillow sign."

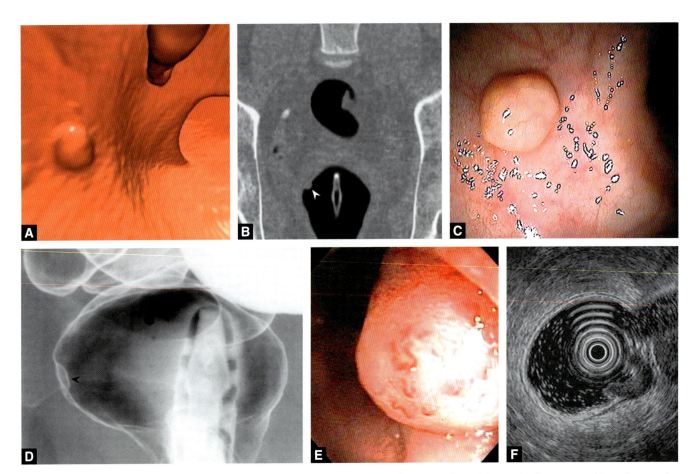

FIGURE 1.3.2 **Rectal carcinoid tumors.** 3D endoluminal CTC image **(A)** shows a polypoid lesion in the rectum. Note the rectal catheter at the 1 o'clock position. Coronal 2D CTC image **(B)** confirms a soft tissue polyp (*arrowhead*) involving the lateral rectal wall. Image from colonoscopy **(C)** shows the same polyp, which proved to be a rectal carcinoid. Image from double-contrast BE **(D)** from a second patient shows a small submucosal lesion involving the right lateral rectal wall (*arrowhead*). Colonoscopy image **(E)** from a third patient with a rectal carcinoid tumor shows a polypoid mass, which at TRUS **(F)** appears hypoechoic and originates from the submucosal layer of the rectal wall.

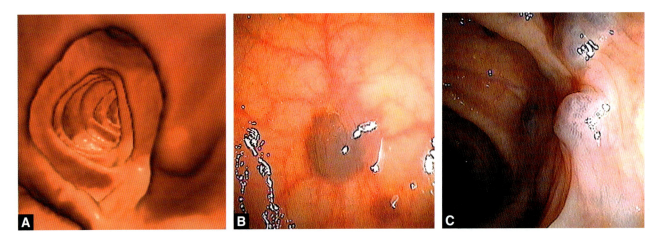

FIGURE 1.3.3 **Vascular blebs (venous hemangiomas).** 3D endoluminal CTC image **(A)** from an asymptomatic adult undergoing screening shows a polypoid lesion; multiple other similar subcentimeter lesions were identified at CTC (not shown). Corresponding colonoscopy image **(B)** shows a bluish hue to the polypoid lesion, diagnostic of a vascular bleb. Additional venous lesions were also identified at colonoscopy **(C)**.

Illustration continued on following page

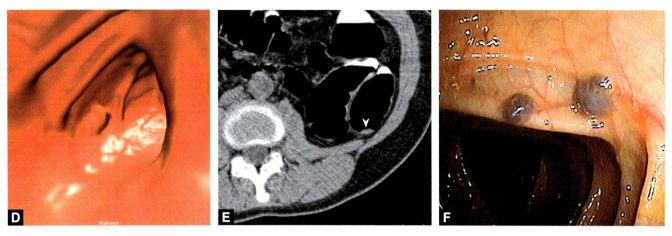

FIGURE 1.3.3 (Continued) **Vascular blebs (venous hemangiomas).** 3D endoluminal (**D**) and transverse 2D (**E**) CTC images from a second screening patient shows a relatively large polypoid soft tissue lesion; multiple subcentimeter lesions were also seen (not shown). At colonoscopy (**F**), all of the lesions corresponded to vascular blebs.

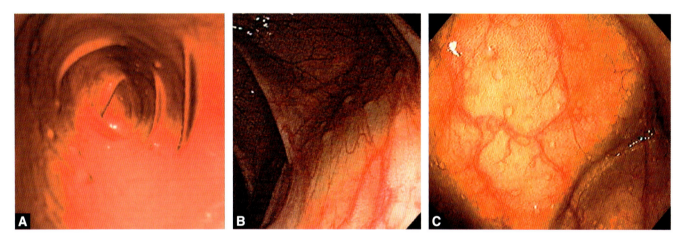

FIGURE 1.3.4 **Lymphoid polyps (nodular lymphoid hyperplasia).** 3D endoluminal CTC (**A**) and optical colonoscopy (**B** and **C**) images from three different patients show multiple diminutive polypoid lesions representing nodular lymphoid hyperplasia. The nodules are particularly well seen in the third case due to mild (pseudo)melanosis involving the background mucosa.

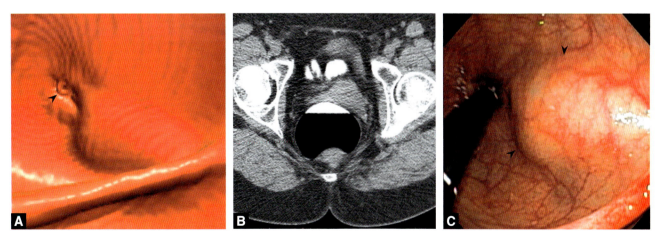

FIGURE 1.3.5 **Rectal gastrointestinal stromal tumor.** 3D endoluminal CTC image (**A**) shows a broad-based luminal impression in the low rectum. Note the tip of the adjacent rectal catheter (*arrowhead*). Transverse 2D CTC image (**B**) shows a lenticular mural soft tissue mass involving the posterior rectal wall. Image from corresponding colonoscopy (**C**) shows a broad but fairly subtle submucosal impression (*arrowheads*) in the low rectum that was initially missed at colonoscopy before correlation with CTC results. (*A to C from Pickhardt PJ: Differential diagnosis of polypoid lesions seen at CT colonography (virtual colonoscopy). Radiographics 2004; 24:1535-1559.*)

Illustration continued on following page

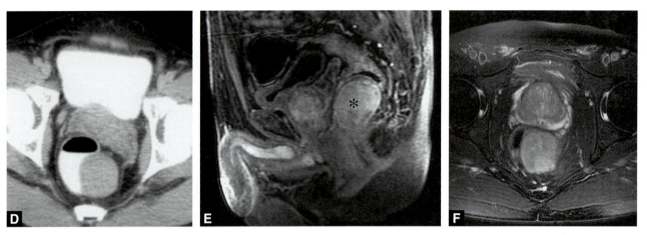

FIGURE 1.3.5 (Continued)   **Rectal gastrointestinal stromal tumor.** Transverse CT image (**D**) from a second patient shows a large rounded soft tissue mass associated with the rectal wall. Sagittal SGE post-contrast MR image (**E**) shows enhancement of the tumor (*asterisk*) and transverse T2-weighted MR image (**F**) shows increased signal throughout the lesion. A rectal GIST was confirmed after surgical resection. An enlarged prostate is also present.

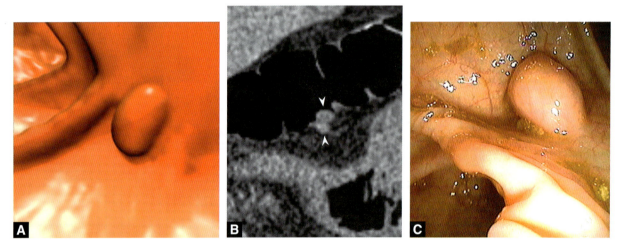

FIGURE 1.3.6   **Colonic leiomyoma.** 3D endoluminal CTC image (**A**) shows a well-defined polypoid lesion, which extends beyond the colonic wall and has a bilobed appearance on transverse 2D CTC (**B**, *arrowheads*). As with 3D CTC, only the endoluminal portion is apparent at conventional colonoscopy (**C**).

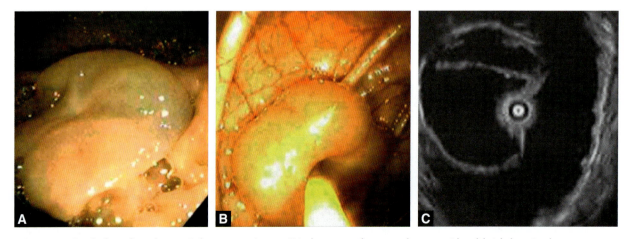

FIGURE 1.3.7   **Cystic lymphangioma.** Colonoscopy image (**A**) shows a submucosal mass with a bluish hue in the transverse colon. Probing with a closed forceps demonstrates pliability (**B**) similar to that seen with lipomas, but the lesion has a cystic appearance with internal septations at EUS (**C**). (**A** from Arluk GM, Drachenberg C, Darwin P: Colonic cystic lymphangioma. Gastrointest Endosc 2004; 60:98.)

Illustration continued on following page

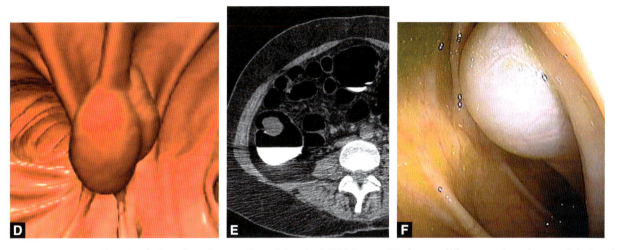

FIGURE 1.3.7 (Continued)   **Cystic lymphangioma.** 3D endoluminal CTC image **(D)** from a different patient shows a lobulated submucosal mass, which has a low-attenuation cystic composition at transverse 2D CTC **(E)**. Colonoscopy image **(F)** shows a tense-appearing submucosal lesion with a subtle bluish appearance.

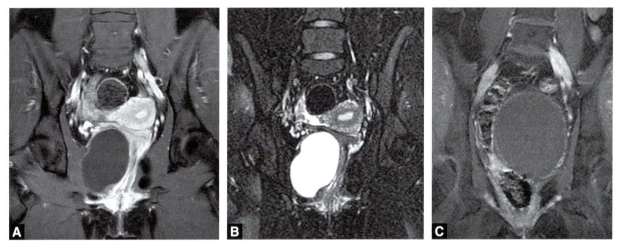

FIGURE 1.3.8   **Duplication cyst.** Coronal fat-suppressed contrast-enhanced SGE **(A)** and T2-weighted **(B)** MR images show a unilocular cystic lesion with broad rectal contact. Coronal fat-suppressed contrast-enhanced SGE MR image **(C)** from a different patient shows an even larger rectal duplication cyst, which displaces the rectum laterally.

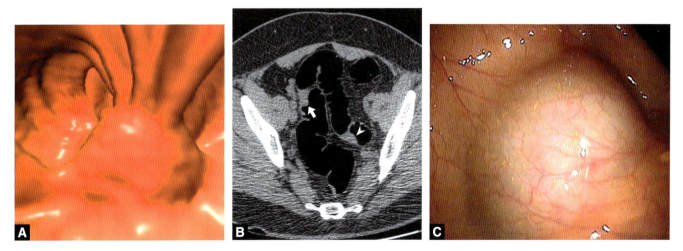

FIGURE 1.3.9   **Endometriosis.** 3D endoluminal image **(A)** from screening CTC shows a broad-based submucosal lesion involving the sigmoid colon. Transverse 2D CTC image **(B)** confirms a mural-based soft tissue mass (*arrowhead*), in addition to a second sigmoid lesion (*arrow*). Subsequent optical colonoscopy view **(C)** demonstrates a similar submucosal prominence.

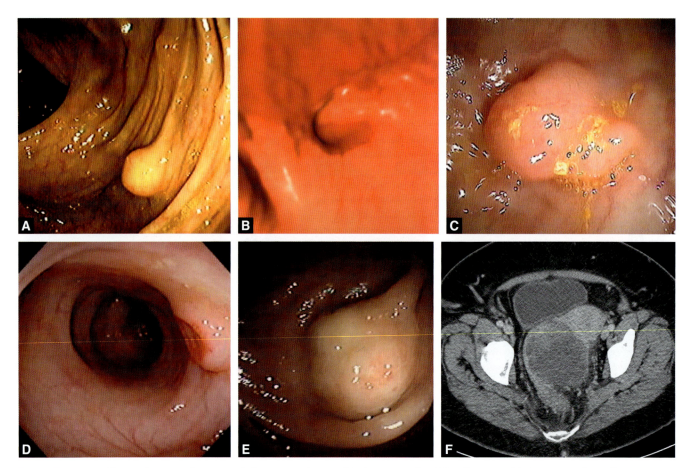

FIGURE 1.3.10 Rare submucosal tumors. Colonoscopy image **(A)** shows a yellowish submucosal lesion (granular cell tumor). 3D endoluminal CTC **(B)** and colonoscopy **(C)** images from a second patient show a lesion that simulates a mucosal polyp (ganglioneuroma). Colonoscopy image **(D)** from a third patient shows an ulcerated submucosal lesion (small cell lung carcinoma metastasis). Colonoscopy image **(E)** from a fourth patient shows a smooth submucosal mass (eosinophilic colitis). Contrast-enhanced CT image **(F)** from a patient with rectal bleeding shows a complex cystic lesion that was initially presumed to be ovarian in origin, but proved to represent a germ cell tumor originating from the sigmoid colon.

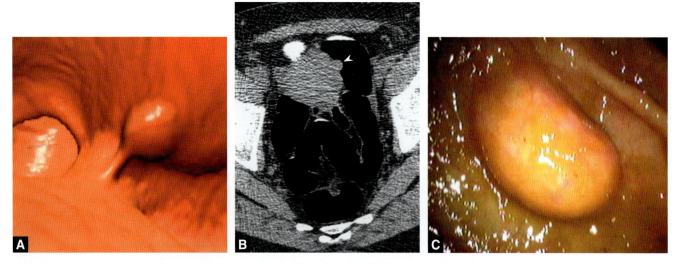

FIGURE 1.3.11 Impression from extrinsic structures. 3D endoluminal CTC image **(A)** shows a smooth polypoid lesion involving the sigmoid colon, which on 2D transverse CTC **(B)** is found to represent extrinsic impression from a small subserosal fibroid (*arrowhead*) extending off the adjacent uterus. Colonoscopy image **(C)** from a second patient shows a submucosal lesion that was also shown to be from an exophytic uterine fibroid at subsequent CTC (not shown).

Illustration continued on following page

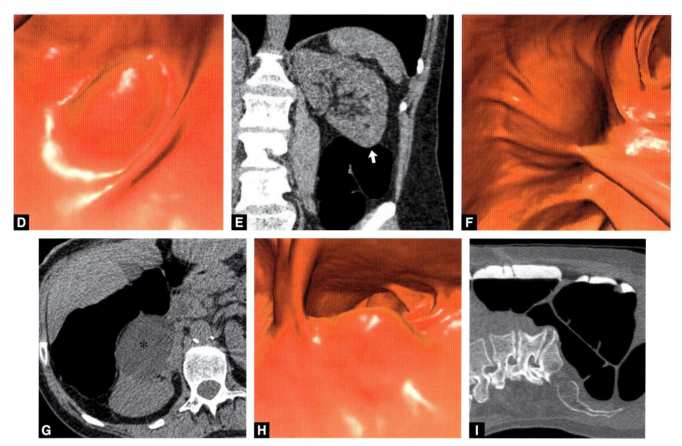

FIGURE 1.3.11 (Continued) **Impression from extrinsic structures.** 3D endoluminal CTC image (**D**) from a third patient shows an apparent submucosal mass, which is found to simply represent extrinsic impression of the left lower pole kidney on the coronal 2D CTC image (**E**, *arrow*). 3D endoluminal CTC image (**F**) from a fourth patient shows a prominent rounded submucosal bulge with inward displacement of the otherwise unaffected colonic folds. The cause is seen to be a large renal cyst (*asterisk*) at 2D CTC (**G**). 3D endoluminal (**H**) and sagittal 2D (**I**) CTC images from a final patient show extrinsic impression from a vertebral osteophyte related to degenerative disk disease. Extrinsic impressions are common and easily recognized as such on 2D correlation. Confident diagnosis may be more difficult at purely endoluminal studies such as conventional colonoscopy.

1.4 Colonic Adenocarcinoma
(Figures 1.4.1-1.4.8)

CLINICAL FEATURES

- The lifetime risk of developing colorectal cancer is approximately 6%, with a 2.5% chance of dying from it.
- Risk factors include age, diet, genetic predisposition (positive family history and various syndromes), and predisposing conditions (inflammatory bowel disease).
- Asymptomatic detection confers improved prognosis over presentation from symptoms (and is more cost effective).
- Subacute presentations include iron-deficiency anemia (usually right-sided lesions), change in bowel habits, and hematochezia; acute presentations include obstruction and perforation (usually left-sided lesions).
- Survival is highly dependent on stage of disease (5-year survival 95% for stage 1 but only 5% for stage 4).
- Pathologic prognostic factors include depth of wall penetration, nodal involvement, tumor histology, tumor morphology, and distant metastatic disease.
- Surgical resection remains the treatment of choice; the role of adjuvant chemoradiation therapy varies.
- Preoperative evaluation includes workup for synchronous lesions and metastatic disease (especially liver metastases).
- Unresectable obstructing tumors can be palliated by either diverting colostomy or placement of a self-expanding metallic stent.

IMAGING FEATURES

- Invasive adenocarcinomas are generally advanced in symptomatic patients, presenting as irregular annular constricting ("apple core") lesions; polypoid, plaque-like, or saddle lesions are more common in pre-symptomatic disease.
- A large frond-like or papillary appearance suggests villous histology.
- Prominent low attenuation within the tumor at CT suggests a mucinous lesion, especially if associated with stippled or punctuate calcifications.
- CT is valuable for detecting extracolonic spread (e.g., liver lesions, lymphadenopathy, mesenteric spread, and pulmonary nodules) but is not reliable for assessing depth of mural penetration.
- PET can be useful both for initial staging and for restaging of disease.
- Tumors are often initially detected at CT in patients with an acute presentation; preoperative diagnosis is typically confirmed at optical colonoscopy.

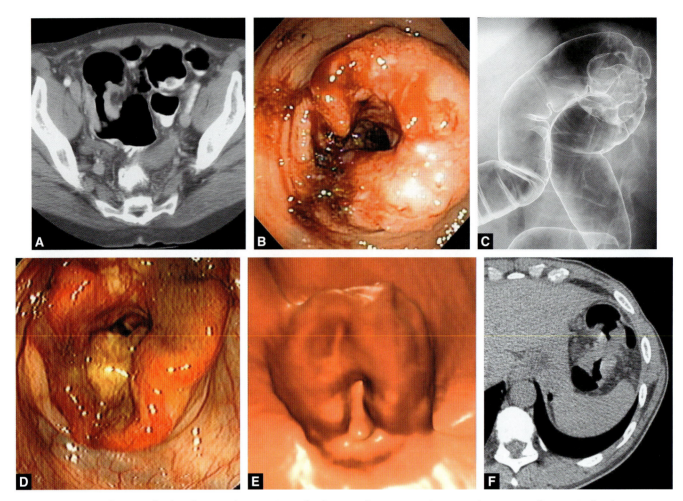

FIGURE 1.4.1 **Primary colonic adenocarcinoma.** Curved reformatted transverse CT **(A)** and corresponding optical colonoscopy **(B)** images show a typical annular constricting mass with shouldering. Double-contrast BE image **(C)** from a second patient shows an annular malignancy at the splenic flexure, which has an "apple core" appearance. Colonoscopy image **(D)** from a patient with an occlusive cancer at the splenic flexure, necessitating CTC for evaluation of the proximal colon. 3D endoluminal **(E)** and transverse 2D **(F)** images from subsequent CTC show the same annular constricting lesion. *(A and B from Pickhardt PJ: Differential diagnosis of polypoid lesions seen at CT colonography (virtual colonoscopy). Radiographics 2004; 24:1535-1559.)*

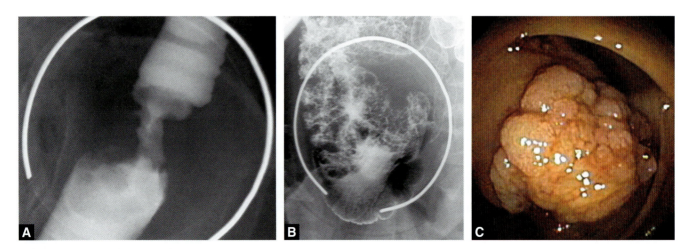

FIGURE 1.4.2 **Primary colonic adenocarcinoma.** Image from contrast enema **(A)** shows a typical annular cancer with an "apple core" appearance involving the descending-sigmoid junction. BE **(B)** and colonoscopy **(C)** images from two different patients with villous adenocarcinomas show large masses with a papillary or frond-like appearance. Extensive barium filling of the interstices of large villous tumors can sometimes simulate stool at BE examination.

Illustration continued on following page

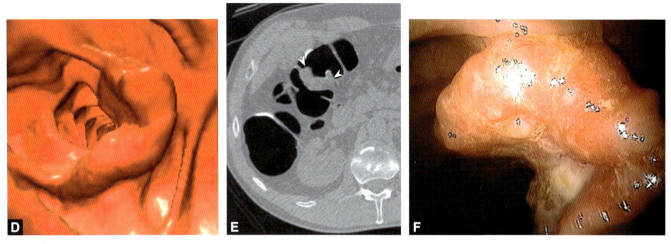

FIGURE 1.4.2 (Continued)   Primary colonic adenocarcinoma. 3D endoluminal (D) and transverse 2D (E) images from a screening CTC study in an asymptomatic adult show a hemi-circumferential mass (E, *arrowheads*) that has a saddle-like appearance. Image from subsequent colonoscopy (F) shows a similar endoscopic appearance.

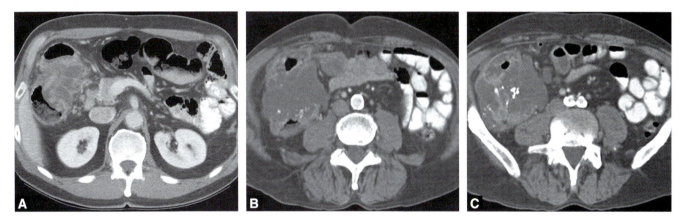

FIGURE 1.4.3   Mucinous adenocarcinoma of the colon. Contrast-enhanced CT image (A) shows a large colonic mass with prominent internal low-attenuation that is suggestive of a mucinous tumor. Contrast-enhanced CT images (B and C) from a second patient show an even larger low attenuation colonic mass, associated with calcifications that are even more suggestive of mucinous histology. Adjacent mesenteric lymphadenopathy is present in both cases.

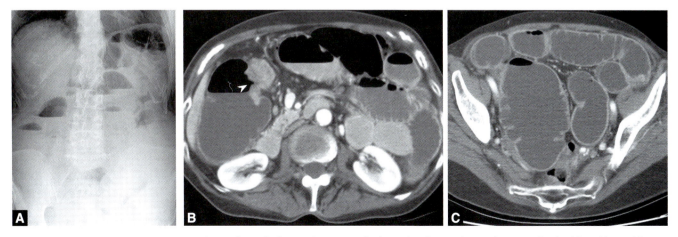

FIGURE 1.4.4   Colon cancer presenting as bowel obstruction. Upright frontal radiograph (A) shows multiple dilated bowel loops with air-fluid levels. Images from subsequent contrast-enhanced CT (B and C) confirm high-grade obstruction due to an enhancing soft tissue mass at the hepatic flexure (B, *arrowhead*).

Illustration continued on following page

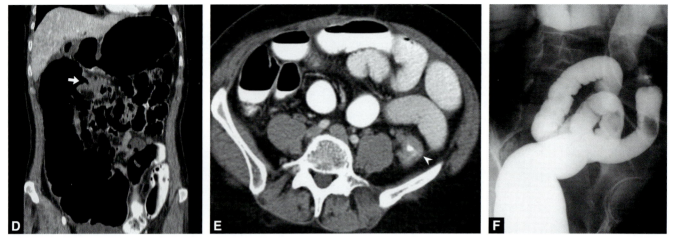

FIGURE 1.4.4 (Continued) **Colon cancer presenting as bowel obstruction.** Curved reformatted coronal CT image **(D)** from a second patient shows an obstructing tumor at the proximal transverse colon (*arrow*). Dilatation of the proximal colon relative to the small bowel likely relates to competence of the ileocecal valve. Contrast-enhanced CT image **(E)** from a third patient shows obstruction due to cancer involving the descending colon (*arrowhead*), which is confirmed on contrast enema **(F)**.

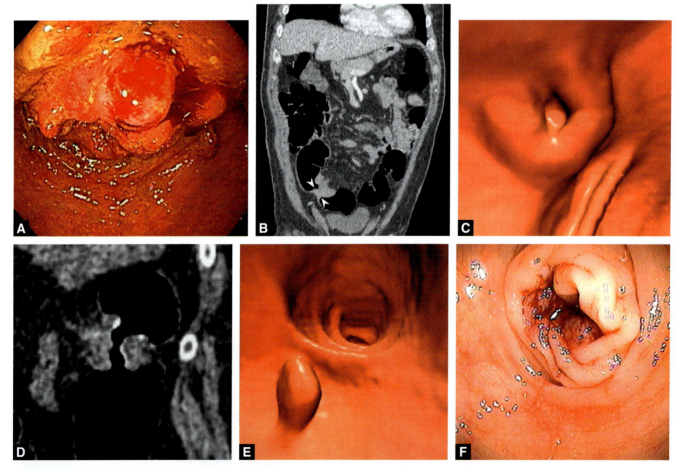

FIGURE 1.4.5 **Incomplete colonoscopy due to occlusive carcinoma.** Optical colonoscopy image **(A)** shows a friable, occlusive sigmoid cancer. Coronal image **(B)** from subsequent contrast-enhanced CTC shows the annular sigmoid lesion (*arrowheads*); a large synchronous polyp was also found in the proximal colon (not shown). 3D endoluminal **(C)** and coronal 2D **(D)** CTC images from an asymptomatic adult undergoing screening show an annular constricting carcinoma in the descending colon. A large synchronous polyp was also seen **(E)**. Malignancy was confirmed at same-day colonoscopy **(F)**.

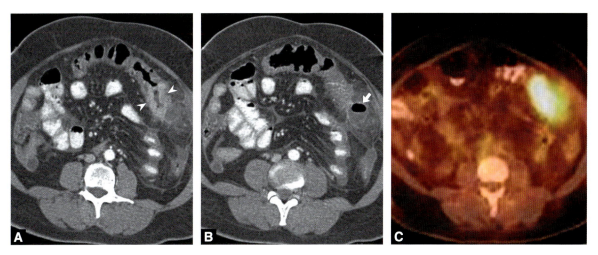

FIGURE 1.4.6 **Perforated colonic adenocarcinoma mimicking acute diverticulitis.** Contrast-enhanced CT images (**A** and **B**) from a patient presenting with fever and left lower quadrant pain show extensive inflammation of the pericolonic fat in the left abdomen, including a small extraluminal fluid collection consistent with a developing abscess (**B**, *arrow*). Segmental circumferential colonic wall thickening (**A**, *arrowheads*) is present, which could be inflammatory, ischemic, neoplastic, or some combination of these causes. Perforated colon cancer was subsequently diagnosed. Fused FDG PET/CT image (**C**) shows marked focal hypermetabolic activity representing the site of primary carcinoma.

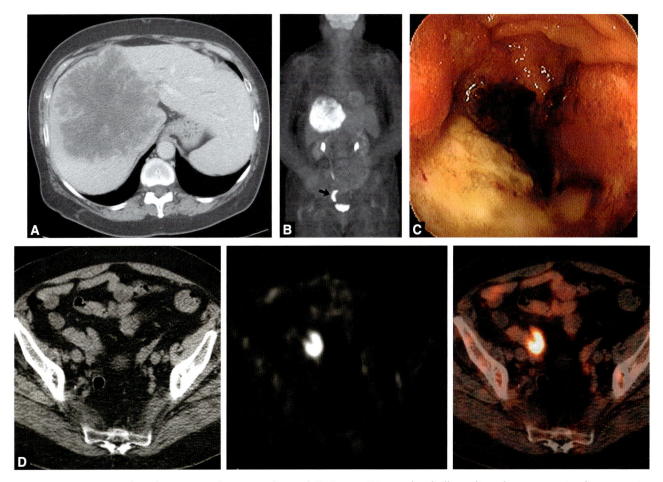

FIGURE 1.4.7 **Metastatic colon cancer.** Contrast-enhanced CT image (**A**) reveals a bulky, solitary low-attenuation liver mass in a patient without a prior history of cancer. Coronal FDG PET image (**B**) from subsequent PET/CT study demonstrates increased metabolic activity in the liver mass, as well as a crescentic focus of hypermetabolic activity in the right pelvis (*arrow*), which could be mistaken for ureteral activity. An ulcerated sigmoid cancer was found at subsequent colonoscopy (**C**). Additional transverse noncontrast CT, FDG PET, and fused CT/PET images (**D**) show that the abnormal activity appears to be located in the large bowel, although no obvious mass can be identified on CT. The liver mass proved to be a solitary metastasis.

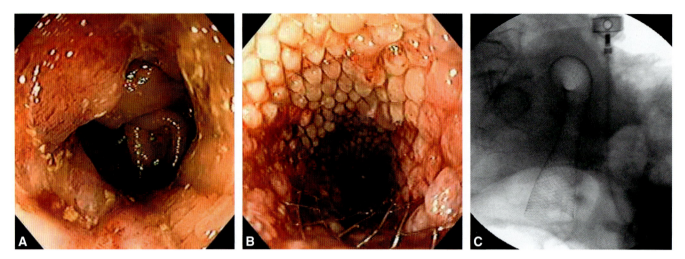

FIGURE 1.4.8 Endoscopic stenting of unresectable colon cancer. Colonoscopy images (A and B) from a patient with an unresectable primary sigmoid tumor show the appearance before (A) and after (B) endoscopic placement of a self-expanding metallic stent. Fluoroscopic image (C) also shows the deployed stent in place.

1.5 Rectal Adenocarcinoma
(Figures 1.5.1-1.5.7)

CLINICAL FEATURES

- Much of the previous discussion on colon cancer generally applies to rectal adenocarcinoma.
- Tumor location and degree of invasion largely determine the operative approach (e.g., low anterior resection vs. abdominoperineal resection); total mesorectal excision is now favored by some.
- Smaller tumors limited to the submucosa (T1) and without adenopathy often can be treated with transanal surgical excision.
- More advanced lesions generally receive preoperative chemoradiation therapy, which has been shown to decrease local recurrence rates.
- Nearly 80% of anal cancers are squamous cell carcinomas; anal adenocarcinomas are generally treated similarly to rectal adenocarcinomas.

IMAGING FEATURES

- The morphologic features described previously for colonic adenocarcinoma generally apply for rectal adenocarcinoma.
- TRUS and MRI are valuable for local tumor staging to guide preoperative therapy and for surgical planning.
- PET can be useful for distinguishing post-treatment fibrosis from local recurrence.

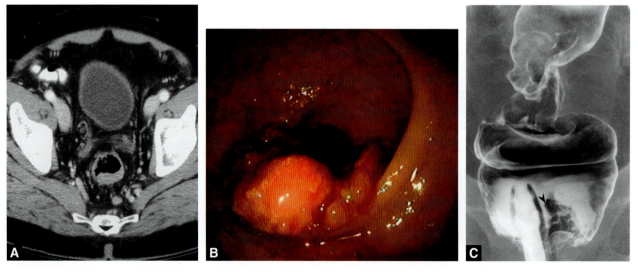

FIGURE 1.5.1 Primary rectal adenocarcinoma. Contrast-enhanced CT (A) and corresponding colonoscopy (B) images show an eccentric, lobulated hemi-circumferential mass involving the rectum. Note the perirectal lymphadenopathy (A, arrowhead). Double-contrast BE image (C) from a second patient shows a large annular, constricting rectal cancer. A second irregular filling defect (arrowhead) adjacent to the catheter tip in the distal rectum represents a synchronous malignancy.

Illustration continued on following page

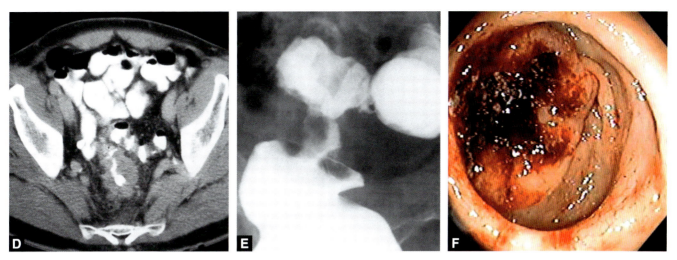

FIGURE 1.5.1 (Continued) **Primary rectal adenocarcinoma.** Contrast-enhanced CT (**D**), single-contrast BE (**E**), and colonoscopy (**F**) images from a third patient show an irregular annular constricting rectal ("apple core") lesion.

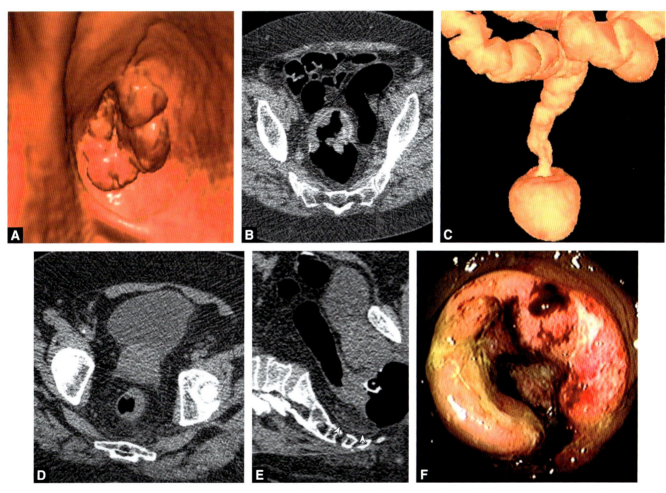

FIGURE 1.5.2 **Rectal adenocarcinoma at CTC.** 3D endoluminal (**A**) and transverse 2D (**B**) CTC images show a large irregular annular shouldered mass near the rectosigmoid junction. 3D colon map (**C**) from a second patient shows good distention of the distal rectum with abrupt luminal narrowing proximally due to cancer. Transverse (**D**) and sagittal (**E**) 2D CTC images, as well as an image from corresponding colonoscopy (**F**) show the nearly circumferential soft tissue mass responsible for the luminal narrowing. Note hazy soft tissue infiltration of the mesorectal fat (**E**, *arrowheads*).

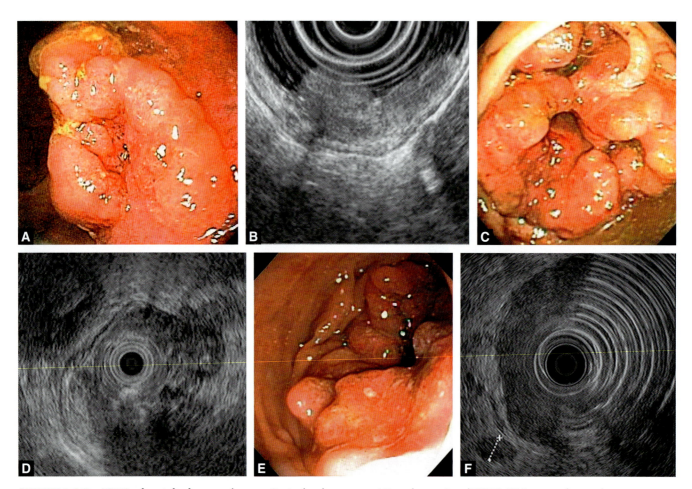

FIGURE 1.5.3 **TRUS of rectal adenocarcinoma.** Optical colonoscopy (**A**) and associated TRUS (**B**) images show a large lobulated rectal cancer limited to the mucosa and submucosa (T1 lesion). Note the intact hypoechoic muscularis propria layer. Colonoscopy (**C**) and associated TRUS (**D**) images from a second patient show a larger annular cancer that demonstrates extension of the tumor through the muscularis propria into the perirectal fat (T3 lesion). Colonoscopy (**E**) and associated TRUS (**F**) images from a third patient show a large lobulated mass that appears hypoechoic with an irregular outer border extending into the perirectal fat. No distinct wall layers are appreciated due to tumor infiltration. A round, hypoechoic perirectal lymph node with sharp borders is seen adjacent to the mass (T3N1 lesion).

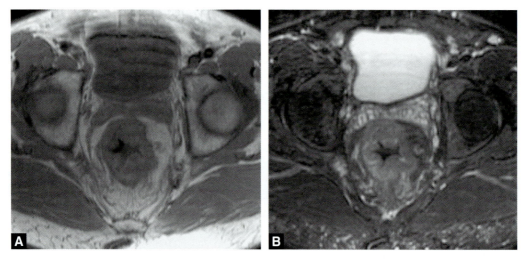

FIGURE 1.5.4 **MRI of rectal adenocarcinoma.** T1-weighted (**A**) and fat-suppressed T2-weighted (**B**) MR images show a circumferential rectal mass with soft tissue infiltration into the perirectal fat, which is of concern for transmural extension of tumor.

RECTAL ADENOCARCINOMA

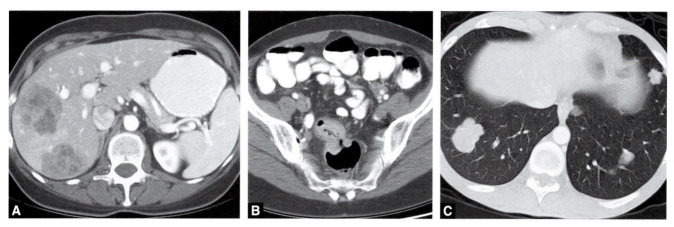

FIGURE 1.5.5 Metastatic rectal adenocarcinoma. Contrast-enhanced CT images **(A** and **B)** show heterogeneous low-attenuation liver metastases **(A)** from spread of an annular rectal adenocarcinoma **(B)**. CT image with lung windows **(C)** from a second patient shows multiple pulmonary metastases from rectal carcinoma.

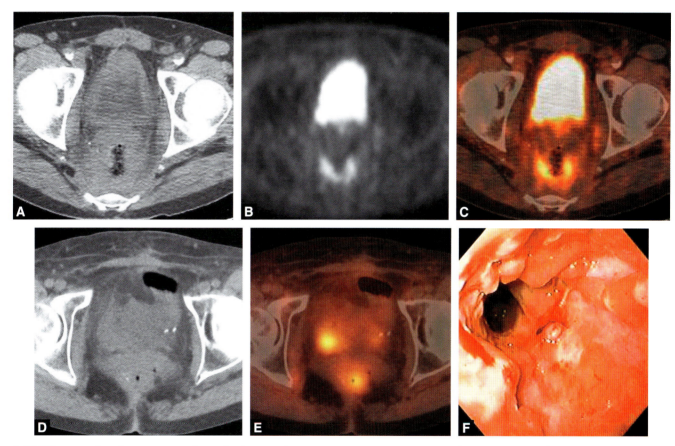

FIGURE 1.5.6 Local recurrence of rectal adenocarcinoma. Noncontrast CT image **(A)** from a patient with rising carcinoembryonic antigen (CEA) levels shows prominent perirectal and presacral soft tissue, which is a relatively common post-treatment imaging appearance and makes evaluation for recurrence difficult. Associated transverse FDG PET **(B)** and fused PET/CT **(C)** images show a curvilinear region of increased metabolic activity near the anastomosis posteriorly, which represented local recurrence. Noncontrast CT image **(D)** from a second patient with rising CEA levels shows nonspecific rectal and perirectal soft tissue thickening. Fused PET/CT image **(E)** at this level shows hypermetabolic activity centered on the rectal anastomosis, consistent with local recurrence. The focus more anteriorly is simply bladder activity. Colonoscopic image **(F)** of the anastomosis shows markedly irregular and nodular mucosa, which was confirmed on biopsy as recurrent adenocarcinoma.

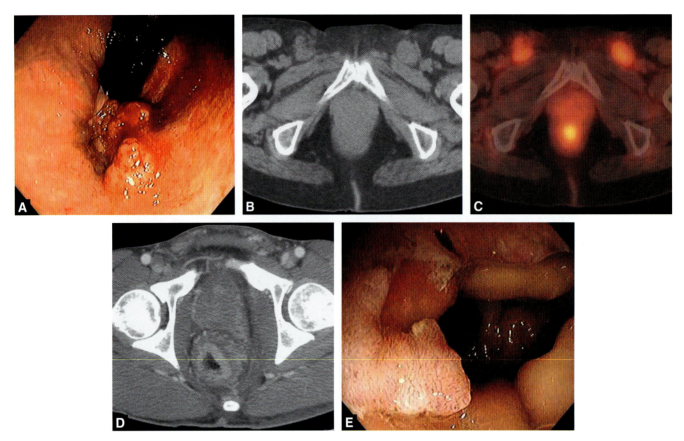

FIGURE 1.5.7 Anal cancer (squamous cell carcinoma). Colonoscopy image **(A)** with retroflexion from a patient with hematochezia shows an irregular mass arising at the dentate line that proved to be a squamous cell anal carcinoma. Noncontrast CT **(B)** and fused PET/CT **(C)** images demonstrate anorectal fullness and bilateral inguinal adenopathy, which demonstrate hypermetabolic activity consistent with the primary tumor and lymph node metastases, respectively. Contrast-enhanced CT **(D)** and colonoscopy **(E)** images from a patient with AIDS show extensive anorectal wall thickening and pericolonic infiltration.

1.6 Other Colorectal Tumors

(Figures 1.6.1-1.6.8)

CLINICAL FEATURES

- Metastatic involvement of the colon and rectum can occur via direct extension, ligamentous spread from adjacent organs, intraperitoneal seeding, or hematogenous dissemination.
- Ovarian and GI malignancies are the most common causes of peritoneal carcinomatosis with serosal colonic involvement.
- Primary colonic lymphoma most often involves the ileocecal region or the rectum; obstruction is rare.
- Carcinoid tumors involving the right colon are more often malignant and larger than those in the rectum (see also section 1.3).
- Malignant mesenchymal tumors of the colon are rare but typically large at presentation.

IMAGING FEATURES

- Location of metastatic involvement by direct invasion or ligamentous spread is predictable.
- Common sites for serosal metastatic disease from peritoneal spread include the rectosigmoid and ileocecal regions.
- Imaging manifestations of colonic lymphoma include smooth polypoid masses, annular lesions, ulcerating masses, and long-segment nodular wall thickening.
- Malignant carcinoid tumors tend to be large and involve the right colon.
- Malignant mesenchymal tumors are typically large masses with exoenteric growth, often with central necrosis and ulceration.
- Non-neoplastic causes such as diverticular disease, endometriosis, and atypical infections can mimic malignancy on imaging (see also Section 3.3).
- Benign strictures related to previous treatment may also simulate malignancy or at least limit colonoscopic evaluation of the proximal colon.

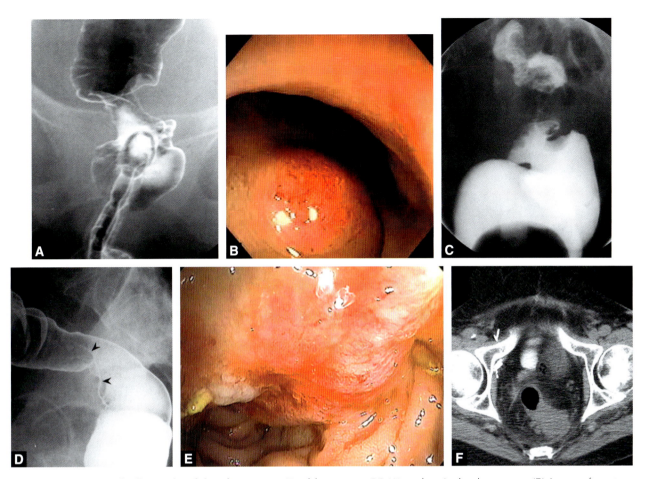

FIGURE 1.6.1 Metastatic disease involving the rectum. Double-contrast BE (**A**) and optical colonoscopy (**B**) images from two different patients demonstrate contiguous extension of cervical cancer to involve the rectum. BE image (**C**) from a third patient shows high-grade rectosigmoid narrowing from serosal metastatic involvement by ovarian cancer. Double-contrast BE image (**D**) from a fourth patient shows mass effect on the anterior rectal wall (*arrowheads*) from local extension of prostate cancer. Colonoscopy image (**E**) from a fifth patient shows a large ulcerating mass that was initially of concern for primary rectal cancer, but corresponding CT image (**F**) shows a predominately perirectal soft tissue mass, which proved to be local recurrence of prostate cancer.

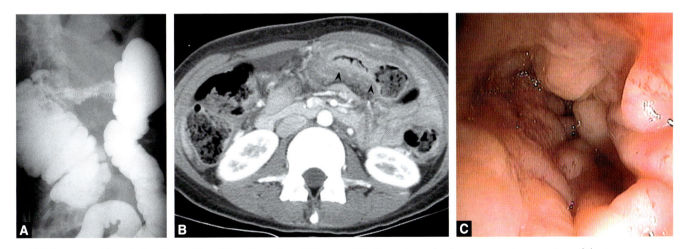

FIGURE 1.6.2 Metastatic disease involving the colon. BE image (**A**) shows irregular long-segment narrowing of the transverse colon due to contiguous spread of gastric adenocarcinoma via the gastrocolic ligament. Contrast-enhanced CT (**B**) and colonoscopy (**C**) images from a second patient show a similar case of diffuse transverse colonic wall thickening (*arrowheads*) from gastric cancer.

Illustration continued on following page

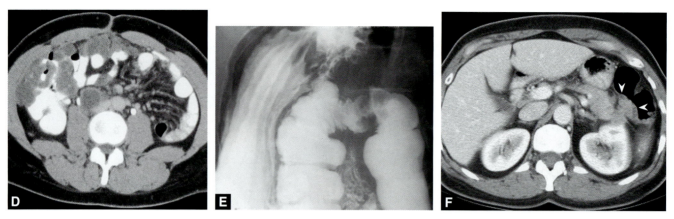

FIGURE 1.6.2 (Continued) **Metastatic disease involving the colon.** Contrast-enhanced CT image (**D**) from a third patient shows peritoneal carcinomatosis with multiple low-attenuation soft tissue masses involving the serosal surface of both small and large bowel. Images from barium study (**E**) and CT (**F**) from two different patients show direct extension of pancreatic adenocarcinoma to the splenic flexure (**F**, *arrowheads*). The barium findings simulate primary colon cancer.

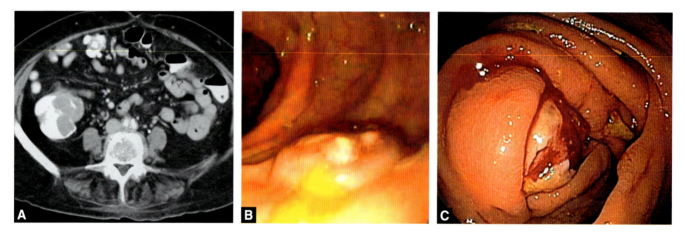

FIGURE 1.6.3 **Metastatic melanoma.** Contrast-enhanced CT image (**A**) from a patient with lower gastrointestinal bleeding shows a large lobulated soft tissue mass involving the right colon due to metastatic melanoma. Optical colonoscopy images (**B** and **C**) from two different patients show melanoma metastatic to the colon manifesting as an ulcerated submucosal lesion (**B**) and an obstructing mass (**C**), respectively.

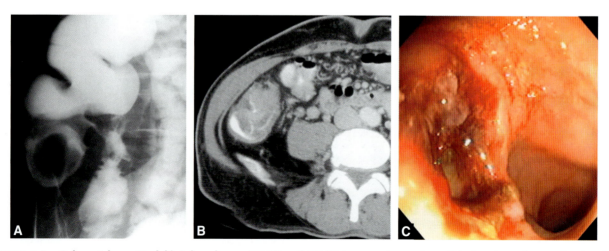

FIGURE 1.6.4 **Colorectal non-Hodgkin's lymphoma.** BE (**A**) and CT (**B**) images show a large lobulated cecal mass that involves the ileocecal region but does not result in obstruction. Regional lymphadenopathy is present on CT. Optical colonoscopy image (**C**) from a different patient shows an ulcerated submucosal mass within the right colon from lymphoma.

Illustration continued on following page

OTHER COLORECTAL TUMORS   241

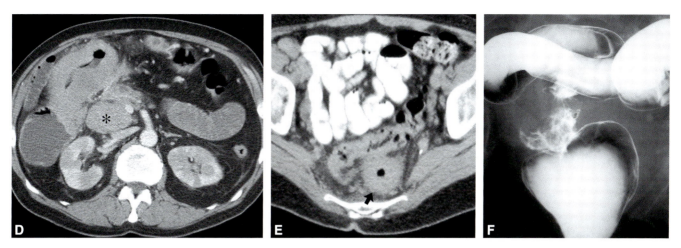

FIGURE 1.6.4 (Continued)   **Colorectal non-Hodgkin's lymphoma.** Contrast-enhanced CT image (**D**) from a third patient shows prominent enhancing circumferential soft tissue thickening at the hepatic flexure. Note also a large adjacent peripancreatic nodal mass (*asterisk*) and bilateral renal involvement. CT (**E**) and double-contrast BE (**F**) images from a patient with AIDS show an annular rectal soft tissue mass (**E**, *arrow*) without evidence of obstruction or lymphadenopathy.

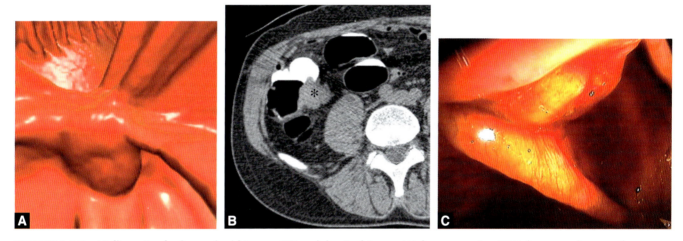

FIGURE 1.6.5   **Malignant colonic carcinoid tumor.** 3D endoluminal image (**A**) from screening CTC shows a submucosal mass within the ascending colon that simulates but was clearly separate from the ileocecal valve (not shown). A bulky soft tissue mass (*asterisk*) with adjacent mesenteric lymphadenopathy (not shown) was seen on the 2D CTC images (**B**). The submucosal mass was confirmed at subsequent optical colonoscopy (**C**), and malignant carcinoid tumor was proven after right hemicolectomy.

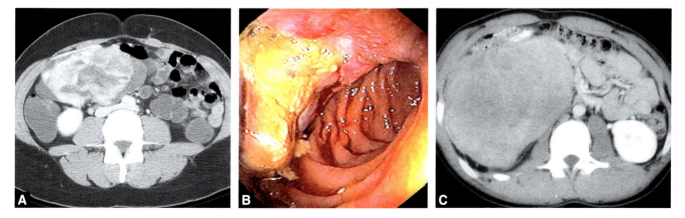

FIGURE 1.6.6   **Malignant colonic mesenchymal tumors.** Contrast-enhanced CT (**A**) and colonoscopy (**B**) images from two different patients show large heterogeneous masses, which are predominantly exoenteric at CT and ulcerated at endoscopy. Both masses proved to be colonic leiomyosarcomas. Contrast-enhanced CT image (**C**) from a third patient shows another large exoenteric soft tissue mass, which proved to be a colonic GIST.

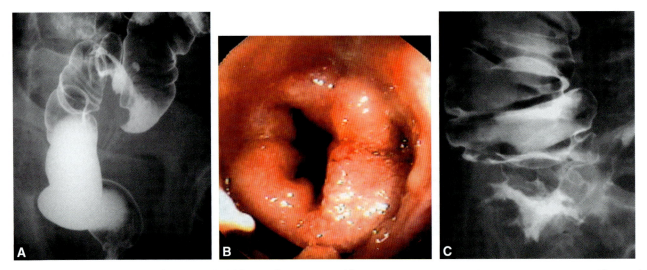

FIGURE 1.6.7 **Non-neoplastic diseases mimicking malignancy.** Double-contrast BE image **(A)** from a young woman with rectal bleeding shows an irregular fixed eccentric sigmoid mass from endometriosis that simulates primary cancer or serosal metastatic disease. Image from optical colonoscopy **(B)** from a second patient shows an irregular annular constricting mass that represents a histoplasmoma. Double-contrast BE image **(C)** from a third patient shows irregular circumferential cecal narrowing ("coned cecum") from amebiasis.

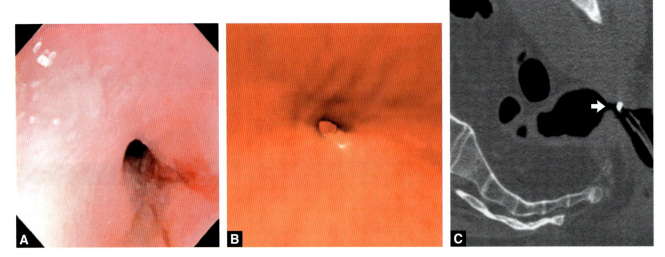

FIGURE 1.6.8 **Benign post-treatment rectal stricture.** Image from optical colonoscopy **(A)** shows a high-grade stricture in the low rectum related to prior treatment of rectal lymphoma. Biopsy specimens proved benign, but the colonoscope could not be advanced beyond this area of narrowing. 3D endoluminal **(B)** and sagittal 2D **(C)** images from subsequent CTC again demonstrate the stricture (**C**, *arrow*). The proximal colon was normal.

1.7 CTC Diagnostic Tools
(Figures 1.7.1-1.7.17)

IMAGING FEATURES

- Colonic segmentation allows for rapid endoluminal navigation at CTC.
- The 3D colonic map provides real-time orientation during CTC navigation and also provides precise polyp localization for subsequent follow-up or polypectomy.
- Translucency rendering is a 3D tool that combines an attenuation-dependent color scale with a transparency function; rapid interrogation of lesion composition can decrease overall interpretation time.
- Some CTC systems keep track of the visualized colonic surface during 3D endoluminal fly-through, ensuring comprehensive evaluation.
- Computer-aided detection (CAD) of significant polyps at CTC may allow for improved performance by less experienced or less skilled readers; achieving a low false-positive rate with acceptable sensitivity is critical.
- In addition to the standard endoluminal view that simulates conventional endoscopy, other 3D CTC projections include "virtual dissection" and "unfolded cube" displays.
- The 3D virtual dissection view "fillets" the colon to allow for more rapid visualization of the endoluminal

surface; current versions may be limited by spatial distortion introduced in the flattening process.
- Electronic cleansing or digital subtraction of opacified luminal fluid can increase 3D visualization of the endoluminal surface; current versions introduce artifacts that can simulate polypoid lesions.
- Gaseous distention of the colon can be achieved via manual room air insufflation or by automated carbon dioxide delivery; the latter provides overall improved distention with less post-procedural discomfort.
- CTC is useful for completing evaluation when optical colonoscopy fails to reach the cecum.
- Causes for incomplete colonoscopy include tortuosity, elongation, adhesions, strictures, masses, looping of the scope, and other complications.

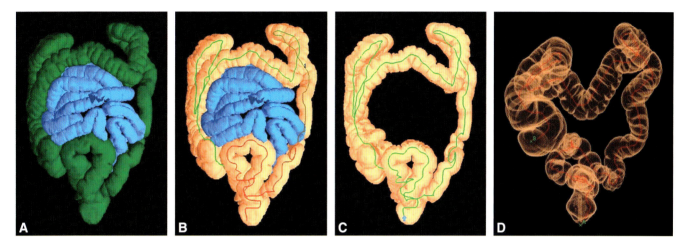

FIGURE 1.7.1 Colonic segmentation and 3D colon map at CTC. Sequential images of the 3D colon map from CTC (**A** to **C**) during the verification process before interpretation show automated extraction of a large portion of the small bowel (**A**, *blue*) in addition to colon (**A**, *green*). With this particular system, clicking on the colon (**B**) discards the unwanted small bowel portion, leaving only the colon with the automated centerline (**C**). 3D colon map (**D**) using a different CTC system shows a transparent display that simulates the appearance of double-contrast BE but is otherwise similar to the opaque map in C.

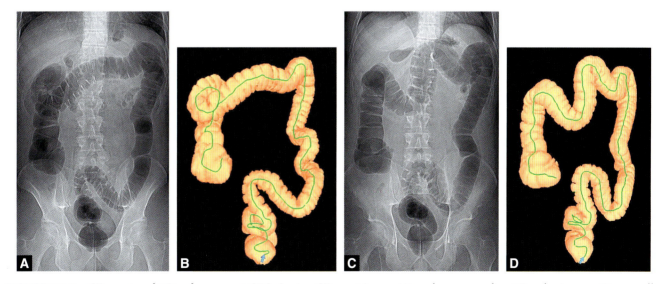

FIGURE 1.7.2 CT scout and 3D colon map at CTC. Supine CT scout image (**A**) and corresponding 3D colonic map (**B**), as well as prone CT scout (**C**) and corresponding map (**D**), show a normal, well-distended colon. Note the change in colonic contour from supine to prone. The green line represents the automated centerline for navigation, which greatly increases efficiency for interpretation. Of note, the CT scout can be inadequate for assessing distention of the sigmoid and descending colon, often necessitating online review of the 2D CTC images for this region.

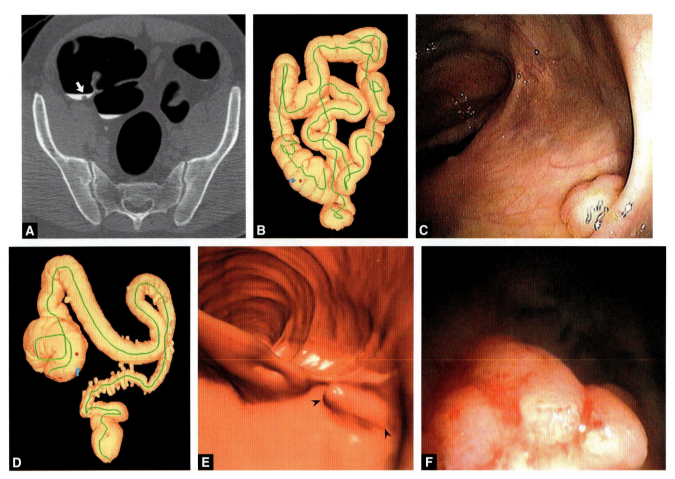

FIGURE 1.7.3 Colon map for polyp localization. Transverse 2D CTC image **(A)** from an asymptomatic adult undergoing screening shows an 8-mm polyp in the proximal ascending colon (*arrow*). The 3D colon map **(B)** marks the location of this polyp (*red dot*) and also demonstrates the extensive tortuosity and redundancy of the colon. The polyp was removed at colonoscopy **(C)** and proved to be a tubular adenoma. 3D colon map **(D)** from a different patient shows significant sigmoid diverticular disease, mild redundancy of the right colon, and a red dot indicating the location of a cecal polyp. The 3D endoluminal CTC image **(E)** shows a relatively subtle 1.5-cm lesion (*arrowheads*) located behind a fold and adjacent to the ileocecal valve. The lesion was found at optical colonoscopy, largely due to the specific CTC localization. Polypectomy was difficult due to the location behind the ileocecal valve and was performed in a piecemeal fashion. Histologic evaluation showed a tubulovillous adenoma with high-grade dysplasia. Follow-up colonoscopy **(F)** 3 months later revealed residual polyp tissue. Note the adjacent India ink tattoo left from the previous polypectomy.

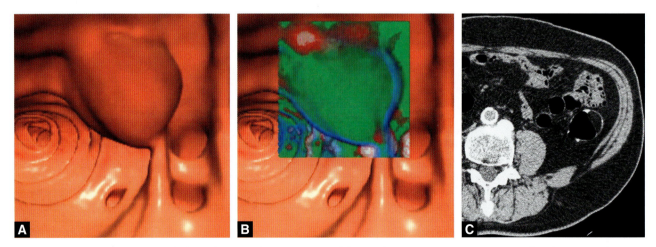

FIGURE 1.7.4 Translucency rendering of colonic lipomas. 3D endoluminal CTC images without **(A)** and with **(B)** translucency rendering show a large lobulated mass lesion with a green internal color signature characteristic of fat attenuation. Adjacent diverticula are incidentally noted. Transverse 2D CTC image with soft tissue windowing **(C)** confirms the fatty composition of the lesion.

Illustration continued on following page

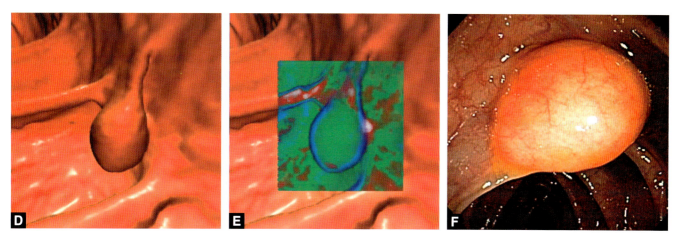

FIGURE 1.7.4 (Continued) **Translucency rendering of colonic lipomas.** 3D endoluminal CTC images without (**D**) and with (**E**) translucency rendering from a second patient show a pedunculated lipoma. Colonoscopy image (**F**) from a third patient shows the typical yellowish endoscopic appearance of a lipoma.

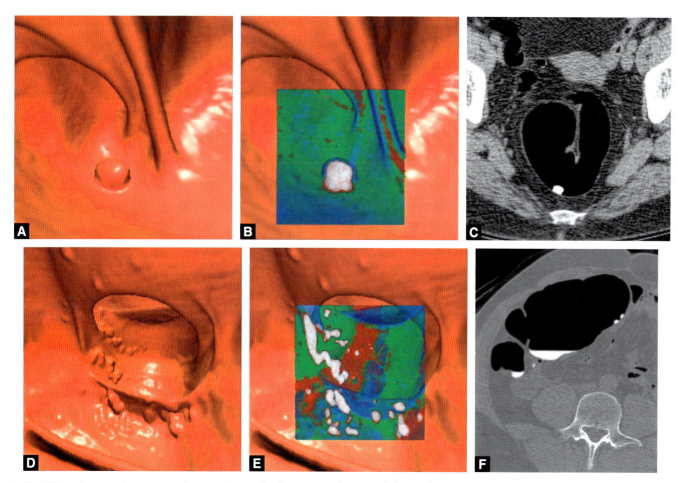

FIGURE 1.7.5 **Translucency rendering of tagged adherent stool.** 3D endoluminal CTC images without (**A**) and with (**B**) translucency rendering show a polypoid rectal lesion with a dense white color signature due to internal contrast tagging, which is also clearly demonstrated on 2D CTC (**C**). 3D endoluminal CTC images without (**D**) and with (**E**) translucency rendering from a second patient show multiple foci of well-tagged stool. In many cases, translucency rendering can reduce the number of 2D correlations (**F**) needed to exclude such false polyps. In general, contrast tagging of stool is necessary for confident distinction from true soft tissue polyps.

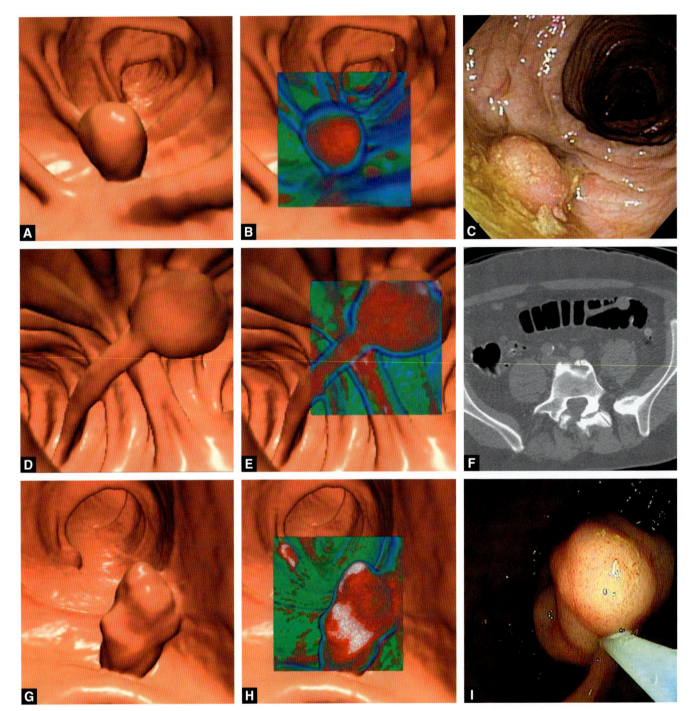

FIGURE 1.7.6 Translucency rendering of adenomatous polyps. 3D endoluminal CTC images without **(A)** and with **(B)** translucency rendering show the color signature of a soft tissue polyp (1.4-cm tubulovillous adenoma) with a central red core and concentric rings of color transition at the periphery. Colonoscopy image **(C)** shows the lesion before polypectomy. 3D endoluminal CTC images without **(D)** and with **(E)** translucency rendering from a second patient show a 2.2-cm pedunculated polyp on a long 5-cm stalk, which is also demonstrated on the curved reformatted 2D CTC image **(F)**. 3D endoluminal CTC images without **(G)** and with **(H)** translucency rendering from a third patient show a large lobulated mass (3.3-cm tubulovillous adenoma) with typical color signature. However, note another 1.3-cm tubulovillous adenoma in the background, which is more conspicuous on the translucency view. Colonoscopy image **(I)** obtained during polypectomy of the larger lesion also shows minimal bleeding from polypectomy of the smaller neoplasm.

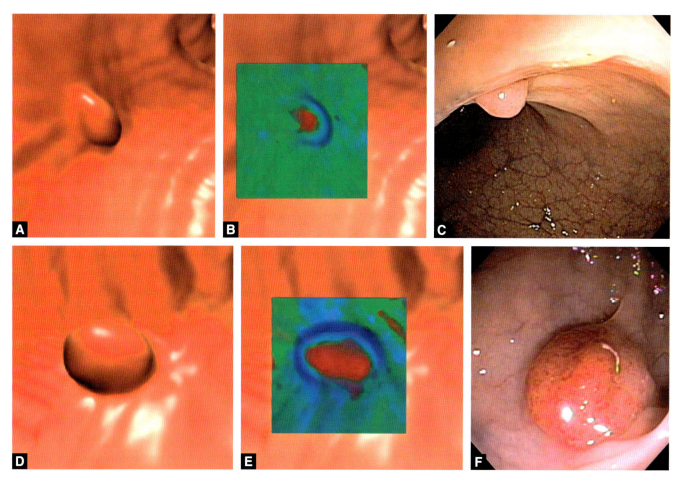

FIGURE 1.7.7 **Translucency rendering of hyperplastic polyps.** 3D endoluminal CTC images without (**A**) and with (**B**) translucency rendering show a sessile lesion with soft tissue characteristics at translucency rendering. Colonoscopy image (**C**) shows the endoscopic appearance of this hyperplastic polyp. Unfortunately, hyperplastic polyps cannot be reliably distinguished from adenomas at either CTC or conventional colonoscopy. 3D endoluminal CTC images without (**D**) and with (**E**) translucency rendering from a second patient show a large sessile soft tissue polyp, which also proved to be hyperplastic after polypectomy at colonoscopy (**F**). *(D to F from Pickhardt PJ: Translucency rendering in 3D endoluminal CT colonography: A useful tool for increasing polyp specificity and decreasing interpretation time. AJR 2004; 183:429-436.)*

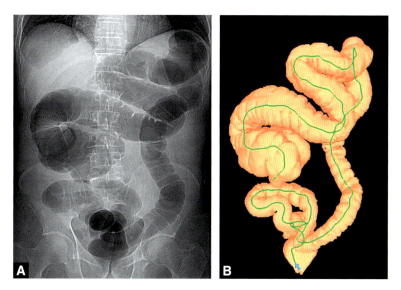

FIGURE 1.7.8 **Mucosal coverage at 3D CTC.** Supine CT scout (**A**) and corresponding 3D colon map (**B**) from CTC show a mildly tortuous and elongated colon with a rectal-cecal distance of 196 cm.

Illustration continued on following page

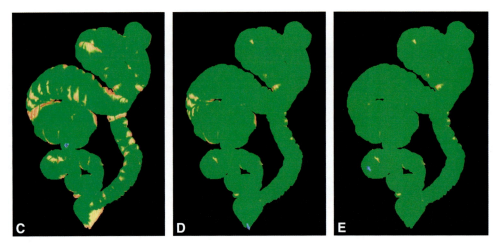

FIGURE 1.7.8 (Continued) **Mucosal coverage at 3D CTC.** 3D colon map after retrograde-only fly-through along the centerline from rectum to cecum (**C**) results in visualization of 70% of the mucosal surface in this case, indicated by the green color. 3D colon map after bidirectional fly-through (**D**) shows that surface coverage has increased to 95%. Coverage can easily be increased to 99% by viewing the larger remaining missed patches (**E**). The endoluminal field-of-view was set at 90 degrees in this case.

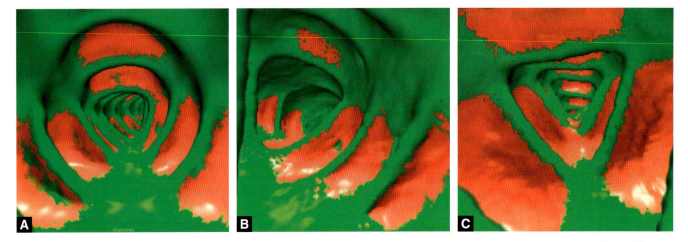

FIGURE 1.7.9 **Mucosal coverage at CTC after retrograde fly-through.** 3D endoluminal CTC images (**A** to **C**) from three different patients viewed toward the rectum show unpainted areas on the backside of folds that were not visualized during unidirectional fly-through toward the cecum, which approximates optical colonoscopy evaluation if efforts are not made to see behind the folds. This illustrates both why bidirectional flight is critical on the 3D endoluminal view and also why most polyps missed at colonoscopy are located behind folds.

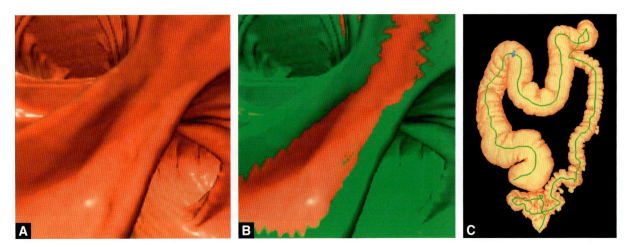

FIGURE 1.7.10 **Missed region tool after bidirectional fly-through.** 3D endoluminal CTC images after bidirectional fly-through both without (**A**) and with (**B**) visualized areas colored green show a typical missed region, which is located at the inner turn of a flexure as seen by the 3D colon map (**C**, *blue arrow*).

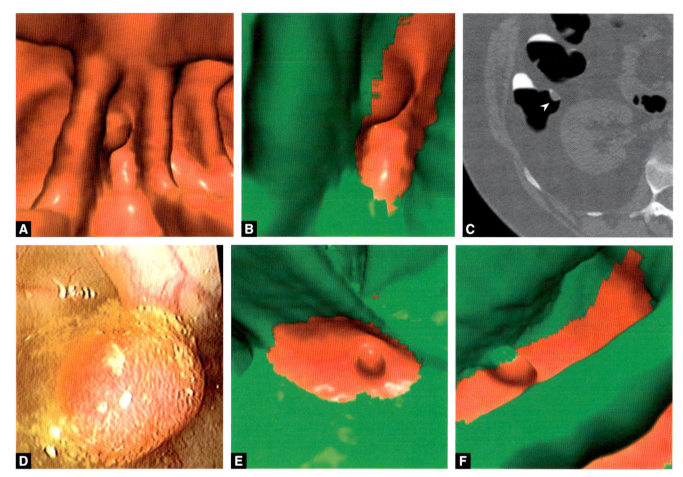

FIGURE 1.7.11 **Polyps identified by missed region tool.** 3D endoluminal CTC image (**A**) shows a 10-mm polyp located between folds within a segment with suboptimal distention, which was not seen after bidirectional fly-through along the automated centerline but was detected on review of missed patches (**B**). The lesion was confirmed on 2D CTC (**C**, *arrowhead*) and at subsequent colonoscopy (**D**). 3D endoluminal CTC images (**E** and **F**) from two additional patients show 6-mm (**E**) and 10-mm (**F**) polyps identified during review of missed patches. In the majority of such cases, the lesion can be more readily identified on the alternate 3D view and also at 2D evaluation, which demonstrates the redundancy built into CTC polyp detection.

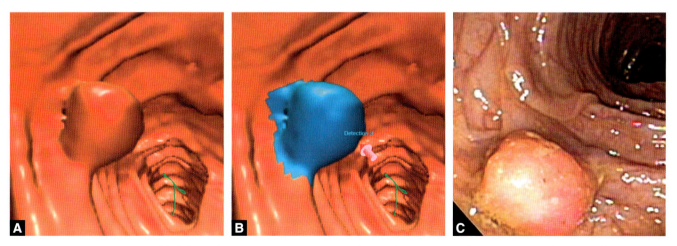

FIGURE 1.7.12 **Computer-aided detection (CAD) at CTC.** 3D endoluminal CTC images show a 1.4-cm polyp (**A**), which was also identified by the CAD system (**B**) and confirmed at subsequent colonoscopy (**C**).

Illustration continued on following page

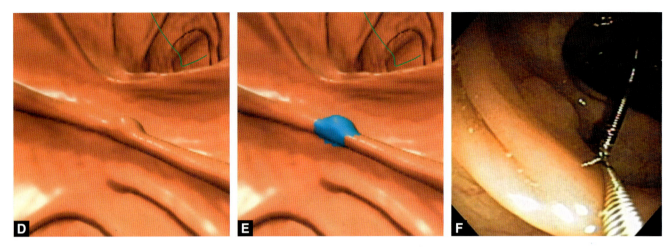

FIGURE 1.7.12 (Continued) **CAD at CTC.** 3D endoluminal CTC images from a second patient show a more subtle flat 6-mm lesion **(D)** also identified by the CAD system **(E)** and confirmed at colonoscopy **(F)**. *(From Summers RM, Yao J, Pickhardt PJ, et al: Computed tomographic virtual colonoscopy computer-aided polyp detection in a screening population. Gastroenterology 2005; 129:1832-1844.)*

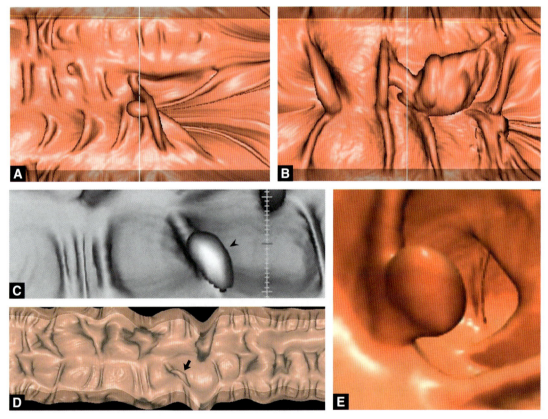

FIGURE 1.7.13 **3D virtual dissection display at CTC.** A 3D virtual dissection or "perspective filet" view **(A)** obtained by flattening the tubular colonic surface shows a polyp on a fold at the level of the white line, as well as a diverticulum on the left. The image display encompasses over 360 degrees by including a 20-degree overlap. Distortion is present but does not affect polyp detection in this case. 3D virtual dissection CTC image **(B)** from a second patient shows the white line crossing the stalk of a large pedunculated polyp, which is significantly distorted by the unfolding algorithm. 3D virtual dissection images **(C** and **D)** from a third patient using a different CTC software system shows the increased distortion by increasing the degree of coverage from 120 degrees **(C)** to 360 degrees **(D)**. A 12-mm pedunculated tubulovillous adenoma is readily identified on the narrow strip **(C,** *arrowhead*) but is seen only in retrospect on the wider strip **(D,** *arrow*). Compare the appearance of this polyp on the 3D endoluminal view **(E)**.

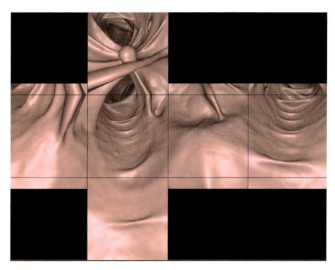

FIGURE 1.7.14 **3D unfolded cube display at CTC.** 3D CTC view obtained by simultaneously displaying six projections at 90-degree viewing angles (an unfolded cube display) shows a relatively undistorted polyp in the upper pane.

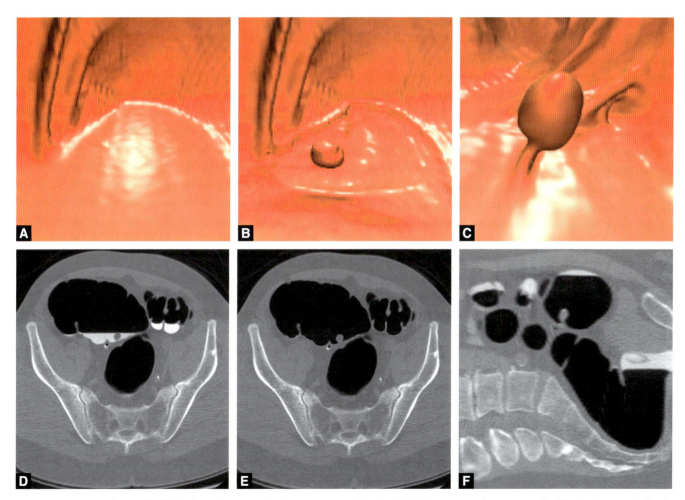

FIGURE 1.7.15 **Electronic fluid cleansing at CTC.** Supine 3D endoluminal CTC images without (**A**) and with (**B**) electronic fluid cleansing show a submerged 1.6-cm tubulovillous adenoma in the cecum that is "uncovered" by the digital subtraction of the opacified fluid. The artifact seen at the interface of the air, fluid, and colonic wall is common. Note, however, that the polyp is readily identified on the prone 3D view (**C**) without the need for fluid subtraction. Supine transverse 2D CTC images without (**D**) and with (**E**) electronic cleansing show the same polyp. Note that fluid subtraction is unnecessary on 2D because the fluid is opacified by contrast and therefore submerged polyps can be seen. Such cleansing can only introduce artifacts. The lesion is also confirmed on prone 2D (**F**).

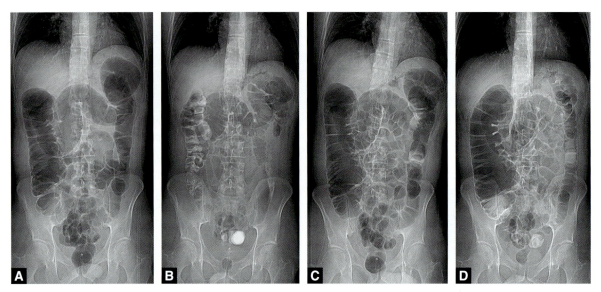

FIGURE 1.7.16 **Colonic distention with room air versus carbon dioxide.** Supine CT scout views from screening CTC examination show the colonic gas pattern before scanning (**A**) and 15 minutes after scanning (**B**) using carbon dioxide, compared with similar CT scouts before (**C**) and after (**D**) scanning using room air. Note the striking difference in gas resorption, which is significant with carbon dioxide but only minimal with room air. The patient noted no discomfort with carbon dioxide after cessation of gas delivery but prolonged discomfort with the room air technique. *(From Shinners TJ, Pickhardt PJ, Taylor AJ, et al: Patient-controlled room air insufflation versus automated carbon dioxide delivery for CT colonography. AJR 2006; 186:1491-1496.)*

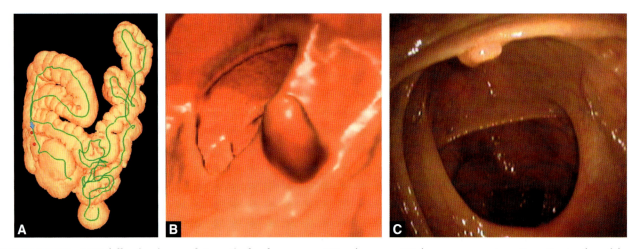

FIGURE 1.7.17 **CTC following incomplete optical colonoscopy.** 3D colon map (**A**) from an asymptomatic patient referred for CTC after incomplete colonoscopy shows a markedly tortuous and elongated colon, which measured over 260 cm in total length along the centerline. The red dots mark the location of large polyps found in the ascending colon at CTC. 3D endoluminal CTC image (**B**) shows one of the lesions, which was located on the back side of a fold. Subsequent colonoscopy (**C**) by a very experienced and skilled endoscopist confirmed the polyps, both of which were advanced adenomas.

Illustration continued on following page

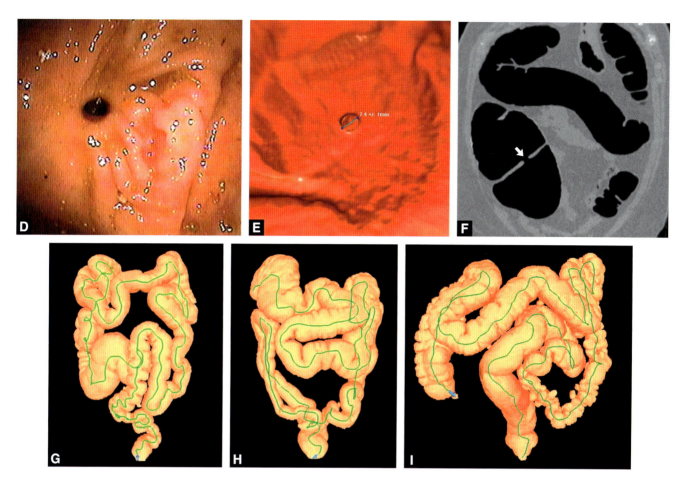

FIGURE 1.7.17 (Continued)   **CTC following incomplete optical colonoscopy.** Colonoscopy image (**D**) from a second patient shows a high-grade stricture in the ascending colon without an obvious mass that resulted in failure to reach the cecum. Biopsies revealed only normal colonic mucosa. 3D endoluminal (**E**) and coronal 2D (**F**) images from subsequent CTC show a web-like diaphragm (**F**, *arrow*) with a central aperture measuring 7 to 8 mm in diameter. The colon proximal to the abnormality can be well evaluated at CTC. 3D colon maps (**G** to **I**) from three different patients referred to CTC for incomplete colonoscopy show tortuous and redundant colonic anatomy.

1.8 CTC Pitfalls
(Figures 1.8.1–1.8.14)

IMAGING FEATURES

- Adherent residual colonic feces represents the major source of false-positive results; stool tagging with oral contrast increases specificity of CTC by significantly reducing this pitfall.
- A thin coating of contrast often adheres to true polyps, particularly larger adenomas with a villous component, and should not be mistaken for the internal tagging seen with residual stool.
- Prominent or thickened folds may simulate pathology at CTC; in general, the 3D endoluminal view provides for better evaluation than 2D displays by demonstrating the elongated nature of the fold.
- Inadequate colonic distention can severely limit CTC evaluation; online monitoring by the CT technologist, with addition of a decubitus view if needed, can limit nondiagnostic studies to < 1% of screening cases.
- Impacted diverticula often appear polypoid on 3D, but the 2D images clearly demonstrate the larger extraluminal component.
- The ileocecal valve is easily recognized at CTC by its location and appearance, including a frequent lipomatous composition; however, both true and false polyps may be seen on or near the valve.
- Foreign bodies such as undigested capsules are easily recognized by their shifting position and varied internal density.
- Pedunculated polyps can mimic stool by shifting to dependent locations on supine and prone positioning; however, the polyp stalk is readily apparent on 3D imaging and the lesion is composed of soft tissue on 2D imaging.
- Extrinsic impression from a variety of normal and abnormal structures can create smooth, broad-based pseudolesions on 3D; correlative 2D imaging easily confirms the extraluminal nature.

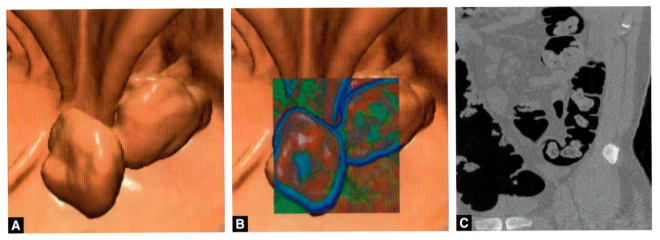

FIGURE 1.8.1 **Untagged residual stool at CTC.** 3D endoluminal CTC image (**A**) shows prominent retained formed stool in a patient who failed to follow the colonic preparation instructions. 3D translucency rendering (**B**) and coronal 2D (**C**) images show the internal heterogeneity of the fecal material. Because of the lack of both catharsis and contrast tagging, the study is largely nondiagnostic.

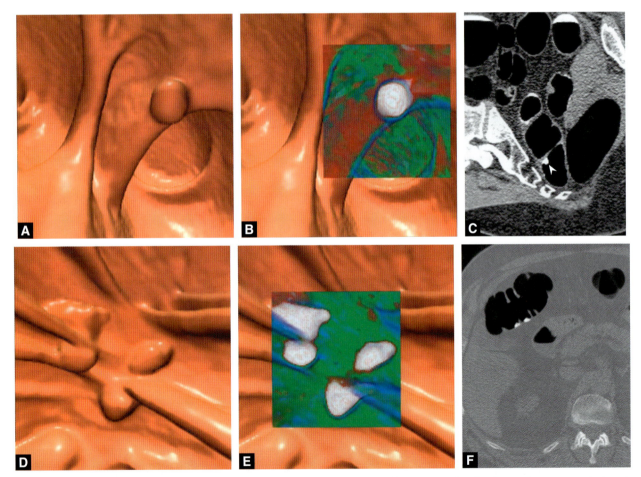

FIGURE 1.8.2 **Tagged residual stool at CTC.** 3D endoluminal CTC images without (**A**) and with (**B**) translucency rendering show a polypoid lesion that represents tagged adherent stool. This is also apparent on the 2D display (**C**, *arrowhead*). 3D endoluminal CTC images without (**D**) and with (**E**) translucency rendering show a cluster of small polypoid lesions, which are shown to represent tagged stool on both translucency rendering and on 2D correlation (**F**). Contrast tagging of solid stool greatly increases specificity for polyp detection.

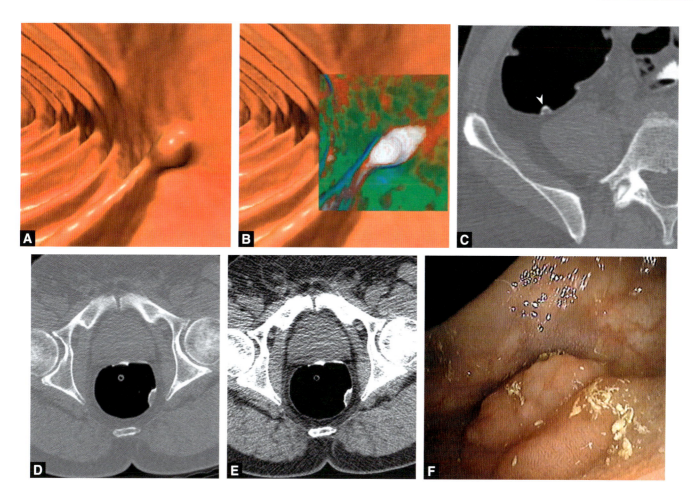

FIGURE 1.8.3 **Contrast coating of polyp surfaces at CTC.** 3D endoluminal CTC images without (**A**) and with (**B**) translucency rendering show a polypoid lesion that would appear to represent tagged adherent stool. However, 2D correlation (**C**) reveals a small polyp coated with a thin rim of contrast (*arrowhead*). Transverse 2D CTC images with polyp (**D**) and soft tissue (**E**) windows from a second patient show a sessile 1.5-cm rectal lesion, which demonstrates a thin coating of contrast. The lesion proved to be a large tubulovillous adenoma after colonoscopic polypectomy (**F**). The key to avoiding this pitfall is recognition of the central core of homogeneous soft tissue density under the thin layer of contrast, which essentially acts as a beacon for pathology.

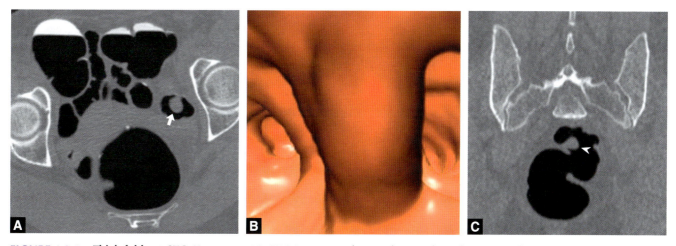

FIGURE 1.8.4 **Thick folds at CTC.** Transverse 2D CTC image (**A**) shows a large polypoid-appearing lesion (*arrow*) that is seen to represent a prominent fold on the 3D endoluminal view (**B**). Coronal 2D CTC image (**C**) from a second patient shows a pedunculated-appearing lesion (*arrowhead*) that represents another thick fold as seen on 3D (**D**).

Illustration continued on following page

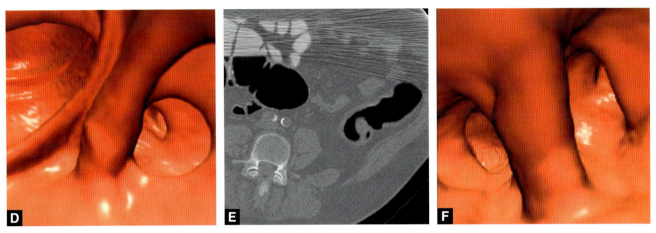

FIGURE 1.8.4 (Continued) **Thick folds at CTC.** Transverse 2D **(E)** and 3D endoluminal **(F)** CTC images from a third patient show another thick fold simulating pathology on 2D.

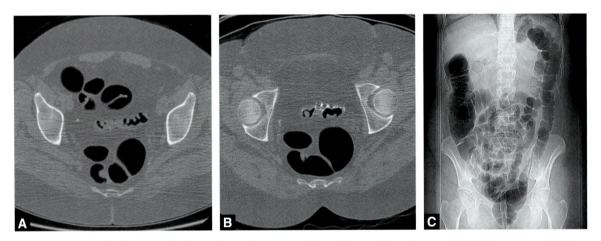

FIGURE 1.8.5 **Segmental collapse on both supine and prone positions.** Supine **(A)** and prone **(B)** 2D transverse CTC images show near-total collapse of the same portion of sigmoid colon on both views, which precludes adequate evaluation for polyps. Note how the prone CT scout **(C)** overestimates sigmoid distention in this case. An additional decubitus view would be indicated to further evaluate this area. If the segmental evaluation remains nondiagnostic, a flexible sigmoidoscopy could be performed the same day without sedation to complete screening. Fortunately, persistent segmental collapse is uncommon (<1%) with automated carbon dioxide delivery.

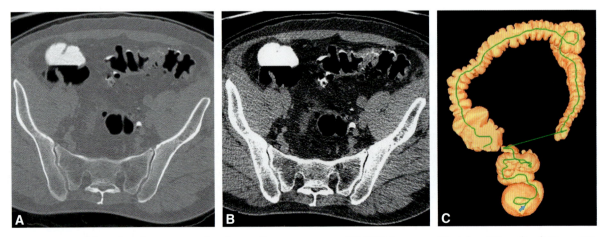

FIGURE 1.8.6 **Decubitus view for segmental collapse.** Prone transverse 2D CTC images with polyp **(A)** and soft tissue **(B)** windows show advanced sigmoid diverticular disease with fold thickening and focal collapse. The prone 3D colon map **(C)** shows the segmental collapse of the sigmoid colon, which was also the case for the supine view (not shown).

Illustration continued on following page

CTC PITFALLS 257

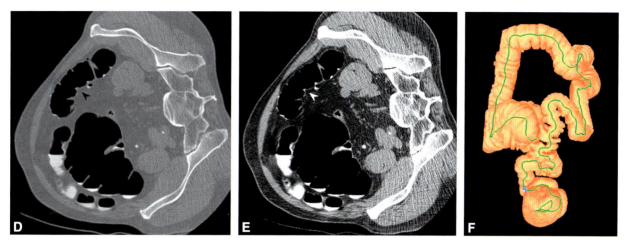

FIGURE 1.8.6 (Continued)   **Decubitus view for segmental collapse.** Fortunately, right lateral decubitus positioning (**D** to **F**) yielded optimal sigmoid distention (**D**, **E**, *arrowheads*), which avoided nondiagnostic examination and the need for flexible sigmoidoscopy.

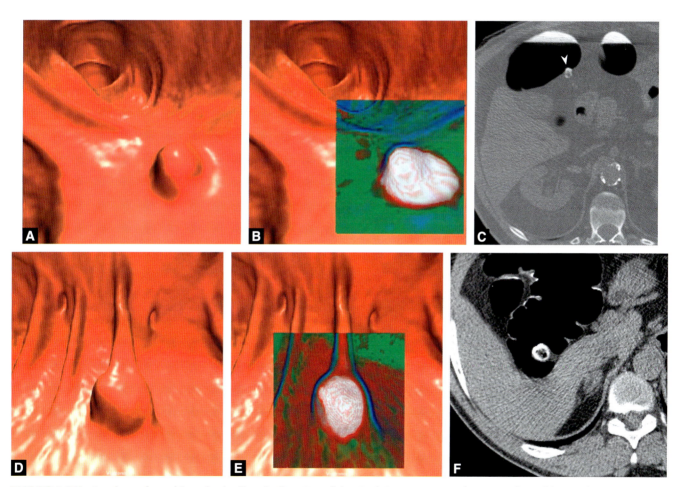

FIGURE 1.8.7   **Inspissated stool in colonic diverticula.** 3D endoluminal CTC image (**A**) shows a polypoid lesion that appears densely white and appears to "bloom" at translucency rendering (**B**). The increase in size on translucency rendering results from depiction of the extraluminal component of this impacted diverticulum, which is also apparent on 2D (**C**, *arrowhead*). 3D endoluminal CTC image (**D**) from a different patient shows a pedunculated lesion or a lesion on a fold that also demonstrates a white internal appearance at translucency rendering (**E**). An impacted diverticulum is confirmed on 2D correlation (**F**).

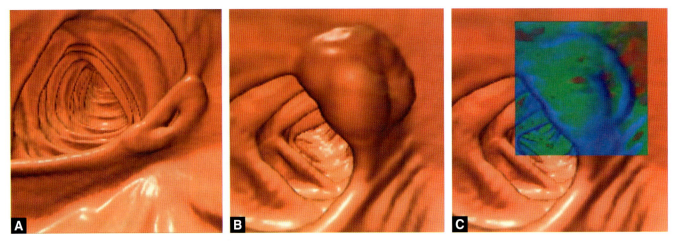

FIGURE 1.8.8 **The ileocecal valve at CTC.** The normal ileocecal valve usually has a labial **(A)** or polypoid **(B)** appearance at 3D endoluminal CTC. Its anatomic location and frequent lipomatous composition **(C)** allow for confident diagnosis.

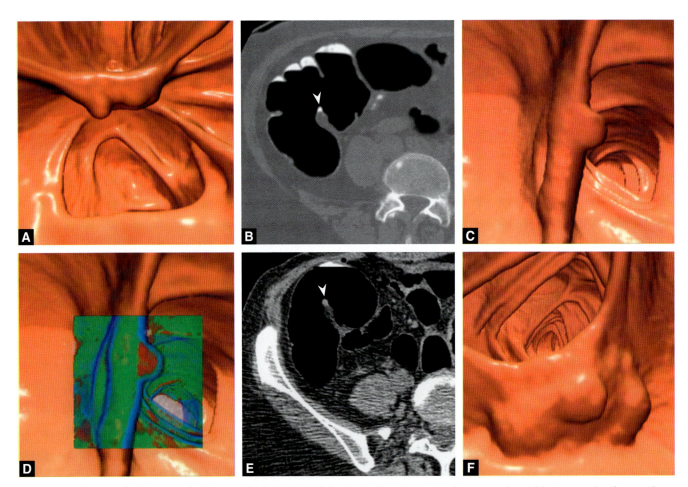

FIGURE 1.8.9 **Focal lesions on the ileocecal valve.** 3D endoluminal CTC image **(A)** shows a polypoid lesion on the ileocecal valve, which is shown on 2D **(B)** to represent a drop of opacified fluid (*arrowhead*). 3D endoluminal CTC image **(C)** from a second patient shows a similar appearance to the ileocecal valve, but in this case the lesion is composed of soft tissue on translucency rendering **(D)** and 2D **(E,** *arrowhead*), consistent with a true polyp. 3D endoluminal CTC image **(F)** from a third patient shows another polyp on the valve, which proved to be a small tubular adenoma.

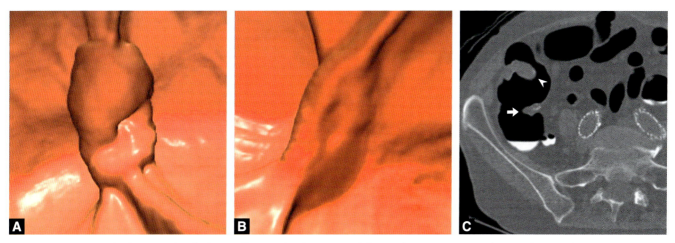

FIGURE 1.8.10   **Colonic mass simulating an ileocecal valve.** 3D endoluminal CTC image (**A**) shows a large polypoid mass within the right colon that resembles the ileocecal valve. However, a normal valve is separately identified nearby on 3D fly-through (**B**). 2D correlation (**C**) demonstrates both the lobulated mass (*arrowhead*) and the ileocecal valve (*arrow*). The mass proved to be invasive adenocarcinoma.

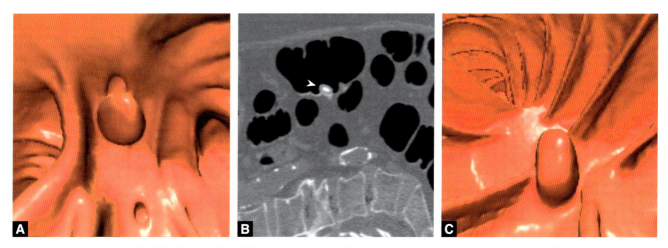

FIGURE 1.8.11   **Endoluminal foreign bodies (pills).** 3D endoluminal CTC image (**A**) shows a rounded polypoid lesion and adjacent diverticula. Correlation with a sagittal 2D image (**B**) shows internal high density within the lesion (*arrowhead*). 3D endoluminal CTC image (**C**) from a different patient shows another ingested pill (multi-vitamin) that simulates a polyp. In addition to having an internal density incompatible with a soft tissue polyp, both pills shifted to dependent positions between supine and prone views.

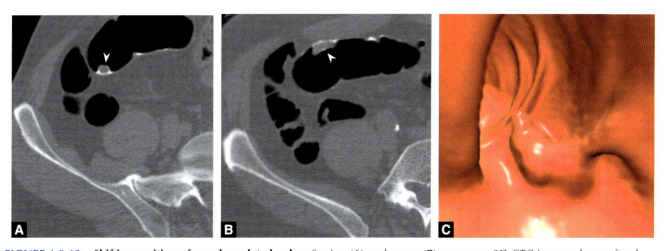

FIGURE 1.8.12   **Shifting position of a pedunculated polyp.** Supine (**A**) and prone (**B**) transverse 2D CTC images show a focal lesion (*arrowheads*) that lies dependently on both views, simulating mobile untagged stool. The homogeneous soft tissue composition of the lesion, however, is an important clue. Supine (**C**) and prone (**D**) 3D endoluminal CTC images clearly demonstrate a large pedunculated polyp (tubulovillous adenoma) with a prominent stalk. Careful inspection of the 2D images will often demonstrate the constant position of the stalk attachment to the colonic wall.

Illustration continued on following page

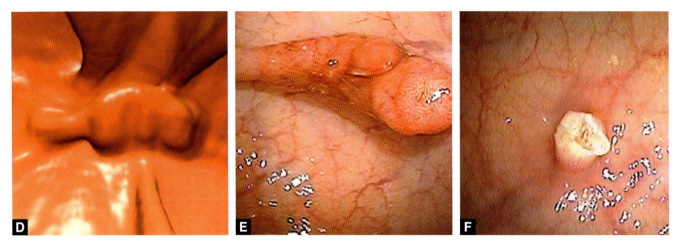

FIGURE 1.8.12 *(Continued)* **Shifting position of a pedunculated polyp.** Images from optical colonoscopy (**E** and **F**) show the pedunculated polyp (**E**) and subsequent polypectomy site (**F**).

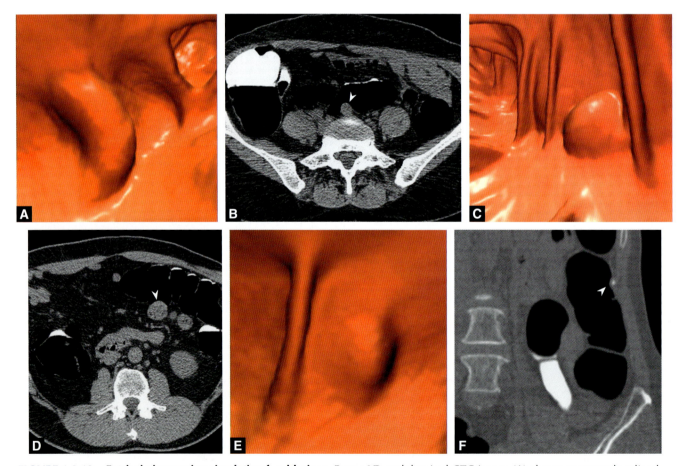

FIGURE 1.8.13 Extrinsic impression simulating focal lesions. Prone 3D endoluminal CTC image (**A**) shows apparent localized fold thickening. The finding, however, is shown to represent extrinsic impression from the left common iliac artery (*arrowhead*) on the transverse 2D CTC image (**B**). The finding was much less apparent on the supine view (not shown). 3D endoluminal CTC image (**C**) from a second patient shows a broad-based mass suggestive of a submucosal lesion, but 2D correlation (**D**) shows that it is simply due to an adjacent small bowel loop (*arrowhead*). 3D endoluminal CTC image (**E**) from a third patient shows a small focal lesion resulting from extrinsic impression from the chondral portion of a rib (**F**, *arrowhead*).

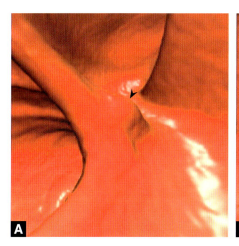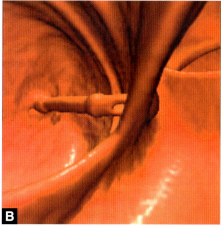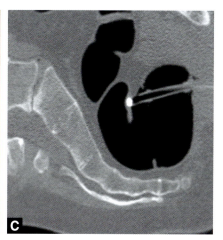

FIGURE 1.8.14 Catheter tip simulating a rectal polyp. 3D endoluminal CTC image (**A**) shows a subtle focal bulge (*arrowhead*) involving a rectal fold that is simply due to the rectal catheter pushing up from underneath (**B** and **C**).

2. COLITIS

The main differential diagnosis for acute colitis includes idiopathic inflammatory bowel disease (ulcerative colitis [UC] and Crohn's disease), infection, and ischemia. Although there is great overlap in presenting symptoms and imaging features, the treatment will greatly differ depending on the specific cause. CT is often useful in the setting of acute colitis, when direct endoluminal examination with conventional colonoscopy or BE is generally best avoided. Specific diagnosis often combines histologic findings with the available clinical data. Some colitides, such as lymphocytic and collagenous colitis, have no notable imaging features.

2.1 Ulcerative Colitis
(Figures 2.1.1-2.1.7)

CLINICAL FEATURES

- UC is an idiopathic inflammatory disorder that characteristically involves the rectum, with variable but contiguous proximal involvement of the colon (pancolitis in 20%).
- It most often presents in young adults, particularly among white and Jewish populations; a markedly higher incidence is seen in westernized areas of the world.
- Crampy abdominal pain, bloody diarrhea, and rectal urgency are common presenting features.
- UC typically behaves as a chronic illness with intermittent exacerbations, but it may be fulminant in 15% of cases.
- Unlike Crohn's disease, inflammation is more superficial in UC and often limited to the mucosa.
- Diagnosis is usually based on combined clinical, imaging, and histologic data.
- Long-standing UC carries a significantly increased risk for the development of colon cancer.
- Total proctocolectomy (preferably with rectal mucosal stripping and ileoanal pouch formation) is curative.

IMAGING FEATURES

- Contiguous mucosal involvement extending proximally from the rectum is characteristic; focal periappendiceal inflammation discontinuous from distal colitis represents an exceptional variant.
- Loss of the normal vascular pattern and hyperemia are the earliest findings at colonoscopy.
- A granular appearance to the mucosa from mild to moderate inflammation can be seen at BE and colonoscopy.
- Ulceration signifies progressive inflammation; friability and bleeding may be present at colonoscopy.
- CT manifestations of UC include mild to moderate uniform wall thickening with pericolonic inflammatory changes, a "target" or "halo" appearance to the bowel wall, and increased perirectal fat.
- Inflammatory pseudopolyps represent edematous mucosal islands surrounded by denuded mucosa.
- In fulminant UC, conventional radiographs and CT may show evidence of toxic colitis.
- Chronic UC is characterized by a narrowed, foreshortened, ahaustral appearance ("lead pipe").
- Postinflammatory polyps represent areas of regenerative granulation and often appear filiform at BE.
- A patulous ileocecal valve with an altered terminal ileal fold pattern has been termed "backwash ileitis."
- Dysplastic mucosa may be visible on colonoscopy as a "dysplasia-associated lesion or mass" (DALM).
- Not all strictures in UC are malignant, but they are generally treated with surgical resection.
- Chronic UC can rarely be complicated by rectal fistulas, but these are much more characteristic of Crohn's disease.

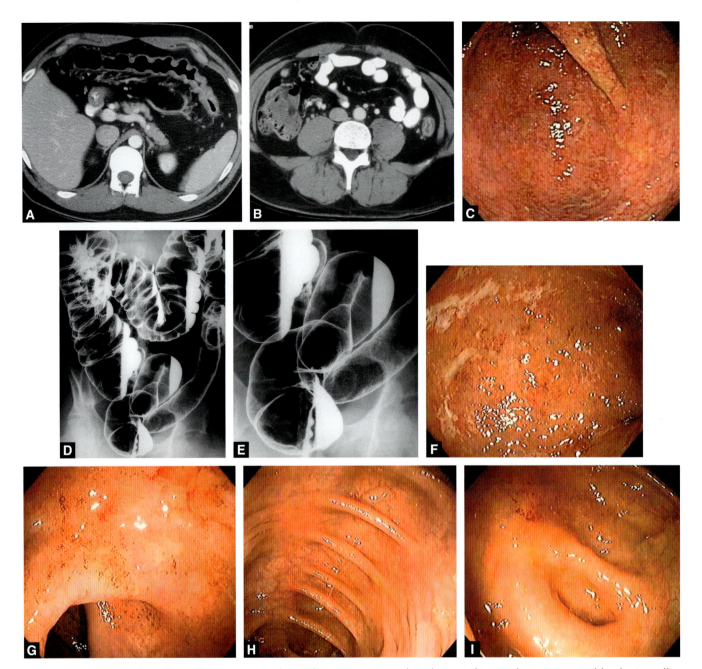

FIGURE 2.1.1 Mild ulcerative colitis. Contrast-enhanced CT images (**A** and **B**) show uniform and contiguous mild colonic wall thickening of the left colon and rectum that returns to normal near the hepatic flexure. Note prominent pericolonic vasculature supplying the involved areas. Optical colonoscopy image (**C**) from a second patient shows a granular mucosal pattern with patchy erythema. Double-contrast BE image (**D**) and magnified view (**E**) from a third patient show diffuse granularity of the distal colonic and rectal mucosa. Note the contiguous extension with abrupt transition to normal proximally. Colonoscopy image (**F**) from a fourth patient shows mucosal granularity, patchy erythema, and mucopus. Colonoscopy images (**G** to **I**) from a final patient show mild rectal inflammation (**G**). The remainder of the colonic mucosa was normal (**H**), except for a focal area of periappendiceal inflammation (**I**). This discontinuous mucosal inflammation is a variant seen in distal UC and should not be confused with Crohn's disease.

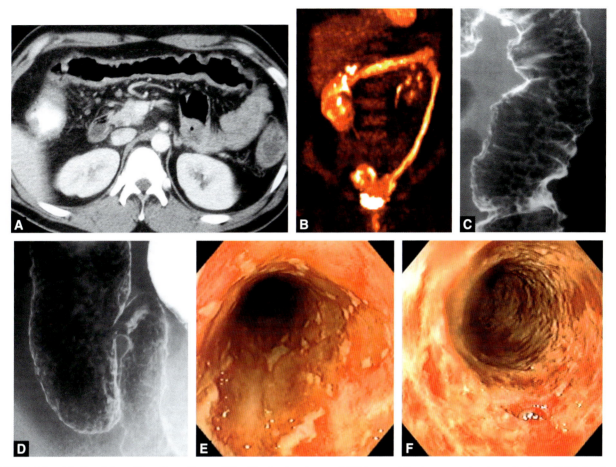

FIGURE 2.1.2 Moderately active ulcerative colitis. Contrast-enhanced CT image **(A)** shows moderate colonic wall thickening and pericolonic inflammation. FDG PET image **(B)** from a second patient shows diffusely increased metabolic activity throughout the large intestine from pancolitis. Double-contrast BE images **(C** and **D)** from two different patients show multifocal ulceration and nodularity. The patulous ileocecal valve and mild inflammatory changes of the terminal ileum in **D** are features of "backwash ileitis." Colonoscopy images **(E** and **F)** from two different patients show more advanced mucosal inflammation, with focal ulcerations and purulent exudates.

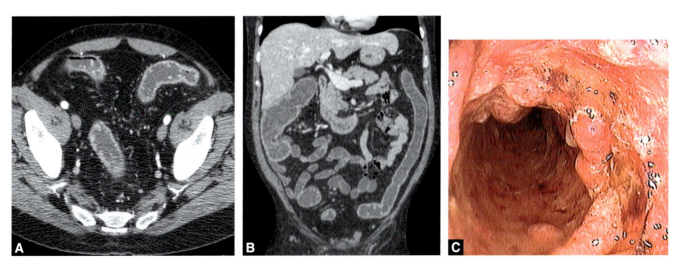

FIGURE 2.1.3 Severe ulcerative colitis. Transverse **(A)** and coronal **(B)** contrast-enhanced CT images show multiple enhancing polypoid lesions in the sigmoid colon, representing inflammatory pseudopolyps. Note the changes of long-standing UC, consisting of ahaustral foreshortening of the entire colon and mild uniform wall thickening. At colonoscopy **(C)**, the pseudopolyps are evident and the mucosa appears friable and ulcerated.

Illustration continued on following page

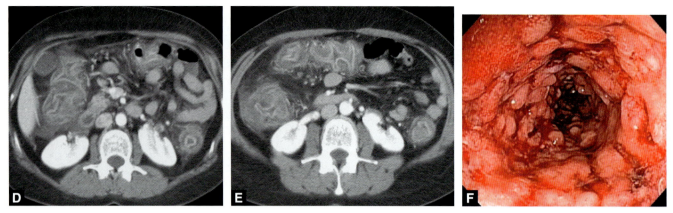

FIGURE 2.1.3 (Continued) **Severe ulcerative colitis.** Contrast-enhanced CT images **(D** and **E)** from a second patient show marked low-attenuation wall thickening of the entire colon, with mucosal and serosal enhancement. Pancolitis in this case is more prominent than usual for UC, and the CT appearance may suggest *Clostridium difficile* or granulomatous colitis. Colonoscopy image **(F)** from a third patient shows extensive pseudopolyp formation with advanced hemorrhagic inflammation and mucosal friability.

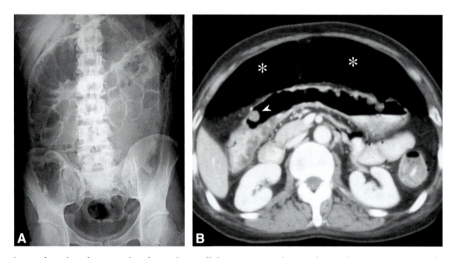

FIGURE 2.1.4 **Colonic perforation from toxic ulcerative colitis.** Supine radiograph **(A)** from a patient with severe abdominal pain and leukocytosis shows colonic fold thickening ("thumbprinting") and massive pneumoperitoneum (Rigler's sign) related to perforation from toxic colitis. This was the initial presentation of UC in this patient. Contrast-enhanced CT image **(B)** from another patient with colonic perforation from UC shows massive intraperitoneal air (*asterisks*) anterior to an inflamed transverse colon. Note the prominent inflammatory pseudopolyp (*arrowhead*).

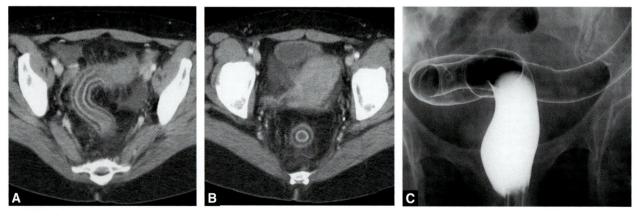

FIGURE 2.1.5 **Long-standing ulcerative colitis.** Contrast-enhanced CT images **(A** and **B)** show a striated appearance to the rectosigmoid, with high-attenuation mucosal enhancement and low-attenuation submucosal fat deposition. Prominence of the perirectal fat is also typical. An acute flare of chronic UC is present in this case with superimposed inflammatory stranding. Double-contrast BE images **(C** and **D)** from a second patient show uniform luminal narrowing, prominent foreshortening, and loss of the normal haustral appearance, giving the "lead pipe" appearance typical of long-standing UC.

Illustration continued on following page

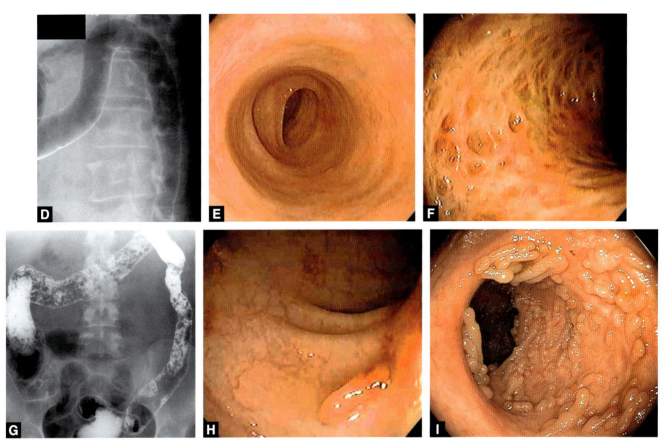

FIGURE 2.1.5 (Continued)   **Long-standing ulcerative colitis.** Colonoscopy images (**E** and **F**) from two separate patients with long-standing disease show loss of the normal mucosal vascular pattern (**E**) and irregular mucosal scarring from prior inflammation (**F**). Double-contrast BE image (**G**) from a different patient shows a foreshortened ahaustral colon with innumerable postinflammatory "filiform" polyps. Colonoscopy images (**H** and **I**) from two patients with UC show endoscopic examples of filiform postinflammatory polyps.

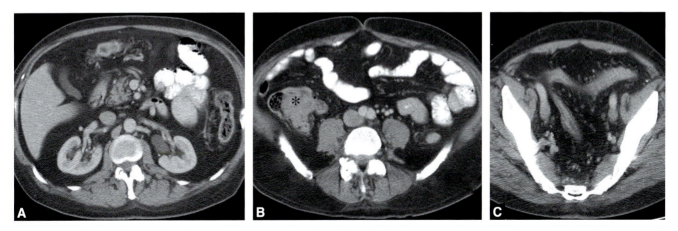

FIGURE 2.1.6   **Dysplasia and carcinoma in long-standing ulcerative colitis.** Contrast-enhanced CT images (**A** to **C**) show a cecal carcinoma (**B**, *asterisk*) superimposed on features of long-standing UC, including a foreshortened, ahaustral appearance with prominence of the pericolonic vessels.

Illustration continued on following page

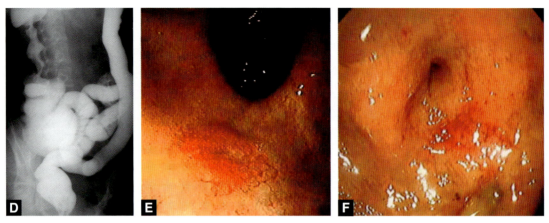

FIGURE 2.1.6 *(Continued)*   **Dysplasia and carcinoma in long-standing ulcerative colitis.** BE image **(D)** from a second patient with long-standing UC shows irregular long-segment narrowing of the ascending colon from adenocarcinoma. Note again the foreshortened, ahaustral colon and findings suggestive of "backwash ileitis." Colonoscopy image **(E)** from a third UC patient shows a flat reddish lesion that demonstrated low-grade dysplasia on biopsy. Unfortunately, the patient was lost to follow-up and returned 2 years later with a malignant stricture in this region **(F)**.

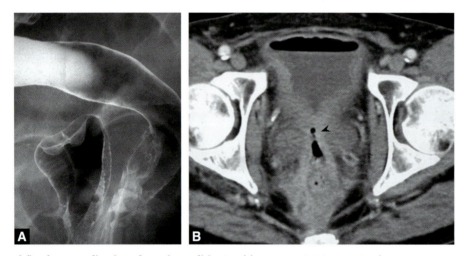

FIGURE 2.1.7   **Rectal fistulas complicating ulcerative colitis.** Double-contrast BE image **(A)** shows contrast communication with the vagina due to a rectovaginal fistula. The fistula itself involved the low rectum and is not well demonstrated on this image. Note the typical rectosigmoid features of chronic UC, including widening of the presacral space. Contrast-enhanced CT image **(B)** from a second patient with UC shows fistulous communication (*arrowhead*) between the rectum and bladder (rectovesical fistula). Note air within the bladder and the prominent bladder wall thickening from inflammation. In general, fistulas are much more common in the setting of Crohn's disease. *(B from Pickhardt PJ, Bhalla S, Balfe DM: Acquired gastrointestinal fistulas: Classification, etiologies, and imaging evaluation. Radiology 2002; 224:9-23.)*

2.2 Crohn's Disease
(Figures 2.2.1-2.2.6)

CLINICAL FEATURES

- Crohn's disease is a chronic idiopathic inflammatory condition that can affect any portion of the alimentary tract but has a strong predilection for the ileocecal region.
- Age distribution is bimodal (roughly at 15-25 and 50-70 years); white and Jewish populations are more often affected.
- Clinical manifestations are protean: common features include diarrhea, abdominal pain, and hematochezia; less common presentations include malabsorption, fistula, and intra-abdominal abscess.
- In distinction to UC, inflammation is typically transmural and can be discontinuous ("skip lesions"); granulomas may be present histologically but are not a constant feature.
- The disease is initially confined to the colon in up to 25% of cases.
- Diagnosis requires synthesis of clinical, radiologic, endoscopic, and pathologic findings.

IMAGING FEATURES

- Ileocecal distribution is classic, but any portion of the colon and rectum can be involved.
- Aphthoid ulcers seen at BE and colonoscopy are an early manifestation of active disease.
- The endoscopic appearance of mild confluent disease can mimic UC, sometimes leading to an incorrect diagnosis.

- More advanced endoluminal findings of early disease include deep ulcers and cobblestoning (inflammatory pseudopolyps); asymmetrical involvement and skip lesions are common.
- Changes in more severe disease include fistulas, stricture formation, and postinflammatory polyps (perianal fistulas are covered in section 5.1).
- Wall thickening and pericolonic inflammation is generally more pronounced with Crohn's disease than UC.
- CT is useful in evaluating for intra-abdominal abscess and other extraintestinal complications.
- The risk for colon cancer is increased, albeit less so than long-standing UC.

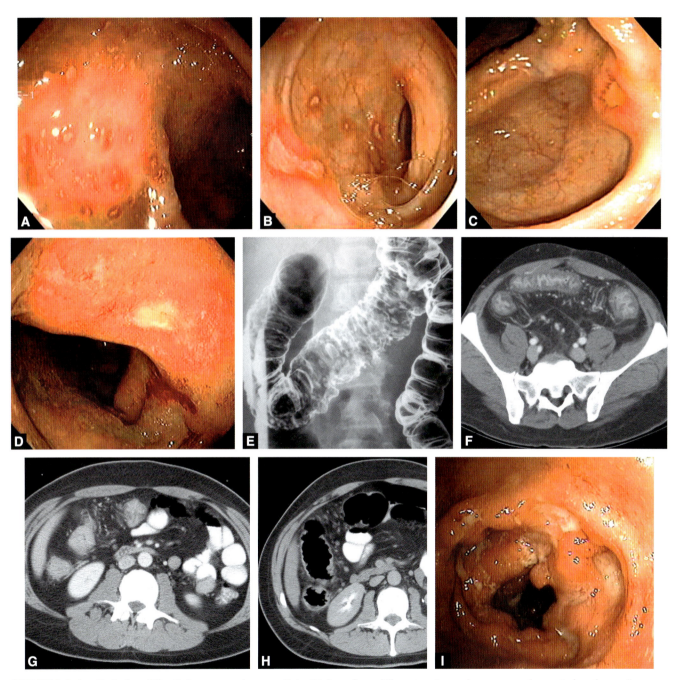

FIGURE 2.2.1 Crohn's colitis. Colonoscopy images (**A** to **D**) from four different patients demonstrate the varied endoscopic appearance of Crohn's colitis, including diffuse, shallow aphthoid ulcers (**A**), linear ulcers (**B**), deep ulceration (**C**), and diffuse mucosal inflammation (**D**), which mimics ulcerative colitis. Double-contrast BE image (**E**) from a different patient shows severe inflammatory changes with deep ulcerations involving the transverse colon. Compare this appearance with the chronic changes seen 8 years later in this patient (see Figure 2.2.5F). Contrast-enhanced CT image (**F**) from another patient shows pancolitis with extensive colonic wall thickening, mucosal enhancement, and engorgement of the pericolonic vasculature (comb sign). Contrast-enhanced CT image (**G**) from a final patient shows findings of active colitis involving the hepatic flexure region, but the degree of pathologic wall thickening is difficult to assess due to nondistention. Delayed CT image (**H**) after low-pressure carbon dioxide delivery (CTC technique) shows persistent segmental colonic wall thickening despite good luminal distention. Colonoscopy image (**I**) shows circumferential inflammation with cratered mucosal ulcerations.

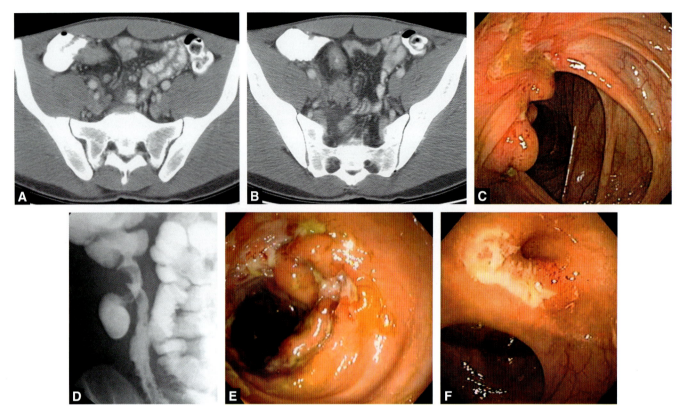

FIGURE 2.2.2 **Ileocecal Crohn's disease.** Contrast-enhanced CT images (**A** and **B**) in a patient with right lower quadrant abdominal pain demonstrate circumferential terminal ileal wall thickening extending to the ileocecal valve. Colonoscopy image (**C**) shows marked inflammation of the ileocecal valve and surrounding cecal mucosa. SBFT image (**D**) from a second Crohn's patient shows irregular cecal narrowing and terminal ileitis. Ileocecal inflammation with deep ulceration was seen at colonoscopy (**E**). Colonoscopy image (**F**) in a final patient with obstructive symptoms shows severe stenosis of the ileocecal valve.

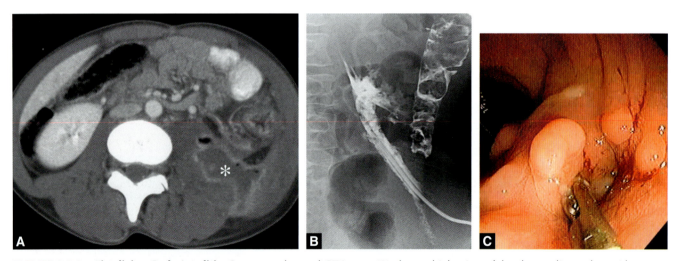

FIGURE 2.2.3 **Fistulizing Crohn's colitis.** Contrast-enhanced CT image (**A**) shows thickening of the descending colon with pericolonic inflammation extending to a retroperitoneal abscess (*asterisk*). Subsequent placement of an abscess drainage catheter (**B**) shows communication of the collection with the descending colon after contrast injection. Colonoscopy image (**C**) from a second patient shows a colovesical fistula with surrounding polypoid inflammatory reaction and pus extruding from the orifice.

Illustration continued on following page

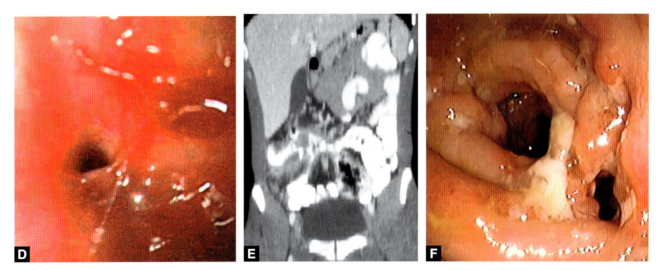

FIGURE 2.2.3 (Continued) **Fistulizing Crohn's colitis.** Colonoscopy image (**D**) from a patient with a rectovaginal fistula shows the site of communication. Coronal CT (**E**) and colonoscopy (**F**) images from a patient with a complex enterocolic fistula show abnormal communication of the ileum, ascending colon, and sigmoid colon. Soft tissue inflammatory changes surround the fistulas on CT.

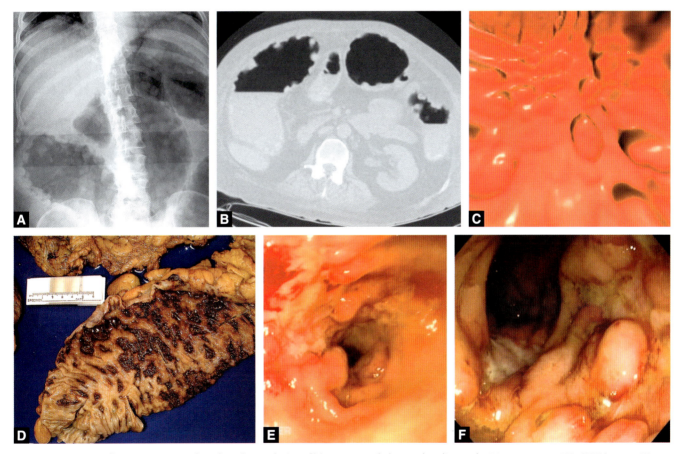

FIGURE 2.2.4 **Inflammatory pseudopolyps in Crohn's colitis.** Supine abdominal radiograph (**A**), transverse 2D CTC image (**B**), and 3D endoluminal CTC image (**C**) show innumerable colonic polypoid lesions in a patient with fulminant Crohn's colitis. The appearance simulates a polyposis syndrome. Photograph of colectomy specimen (**D**) shows hemorrhagic areas of denuded mucosa between areas of edematous mucosa that represent the inflammatory pseudopolyps. Colonoscopy images (**E** and **F**) from two different patients show severe inflammation with heaped up adjacent mucosa forming inflammatory pseudopolyps.

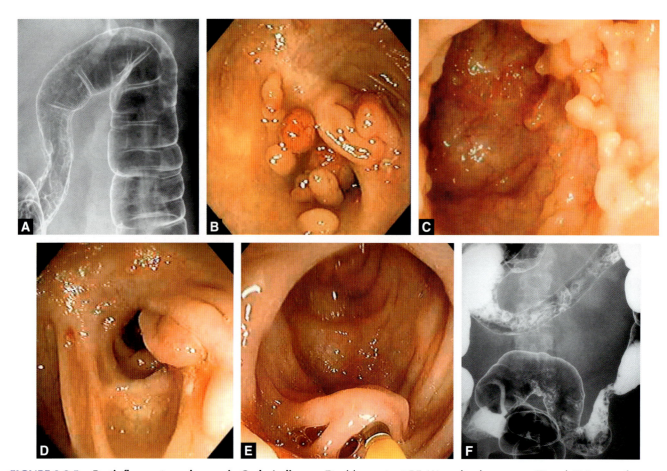

FIGURE 2.2.5 Postinflammatory changes in Crohn's disease. Double-contrast BE **(A)** and colonoscopy **(B** and **C)** images from three different patients show nodular mucosal lesions representing a reparative response. Healing of the mucosa occasionally leads to the development of benign strictures **(D)** and mucosal bridges **(E)**. Double-contrast BE **(F)** shows postinflammatory filiform polyps within the transverse and sigmoid colon, associated with luminal narrowing. The appearance of the involved segments resembles long-standing UC, but skip lesions without contiguous involvement excludes UC. Compare this chronic appearance to the acute inflammation seen in Figure 2.2.1E (same patient 8 years earlier).

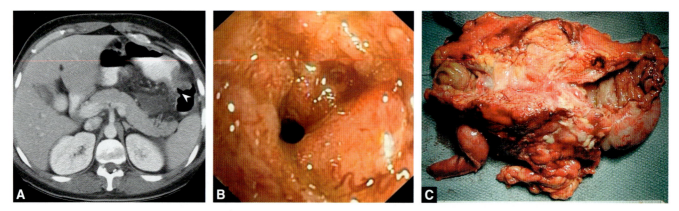

FIGURE 2.2.6 Colonic adenocarcinoma complicating Crohn's disease. Contrast-enhanced CT **(A)**, colonoscopy **(B)**, and gross resected specimen **(C)** images show an annular carcinoma resulting in a malignant stricture at the splenic flexure **(A,** *arrowhead*). Note the infiltration of the pericolonic fat on CT.

2.3 Infection
(Figures 2.3.1-2.3.6)

CLINICAL FEATURES

- *Clostridium difficile* accounts for the vast majority of cases of pseudomembranous colitis, typically associated with recent antibiotic therapy (antibiotic-associated colitis); stool testing for the toxin is straightforward.
- Although GI tuberculosis is usually secondary to pulmonary disease, thoracic involvement is not apparent in many patients.
- Viral infections such as cytomegalovirus (CMV) and herpes simplex virus (HSV) are often associated with immunocompromise (e.g., HIV/AIDS), but HSV proctitis can also be seen in immunocompetent patients.
- Lymphogranuloma venereum (LGV) is a sexually transmitted chlamydial disease that primarily affects pelvic lymphatics; proctitis with deep ulceration, perirectal abscess, rectal fistula, and rectal stricture may develop.
- Acute bacillary dysentery is caused by *Shigella*, but infectious colitis may be caused by a variety of bacterial organisms (e.g., *Salmonella*, *Campylobacter*, *Yersinia*, and *Escherichia coli*); stool culture is necessary for diagnosis.
- Notable parasitic infections include amebiasis, schistosomiasis, and various worms (e.g., pinworms, whipworms, and tapeworms).

IMAGING FEATURES

- *C. difficile* colitis manifests on CT with prominent low-attenuation colonic wall thickening, often associated with ascites; at colonoscopy, discrete pseudomembranes may be seen overlying intensely inflamed mucosa.
- Ileocecal tuberculosis can closely mimic inflammatory bowel disease, with ulceration, nodularity, and fibrostenotic changes; low-attenuation lymphadenopathy may suggest the diagnosis.
- CMV is usually a right-sided process with variable distal extension; radiographic studies show ulceration (BE) and marked low-attenuation wall thickening (CT); erythematous patches and ulcerations are typical colonoscopy findings.
- BE can demonstrate ulceration, fistula, or stricture in LGV; CT can also show perirectal and pelvic disease.
- Acute bacterial infections generally manifest as nonspecific inflammatory findings on radiographic and colonoscopic evaluation and can be indistinguishable from noninfectious inflammatory bowel disease.

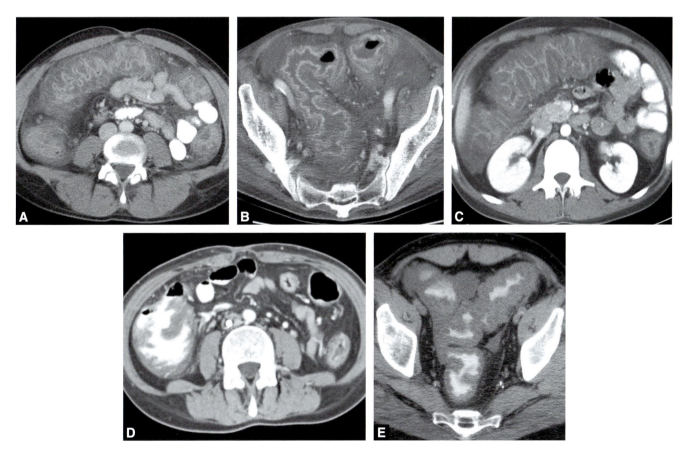

FIGURE 2.3.1 *Clostridium difficile* colitis (pseudomembranous colitis). CT images (**A** to **E**) from five different patients show prominent diffuse low-attenuation colonic wall thickening and mucosal enhancement, associated with pericolonic inflammation. Ascites is seen best in **B**.

Illustration continued on following page

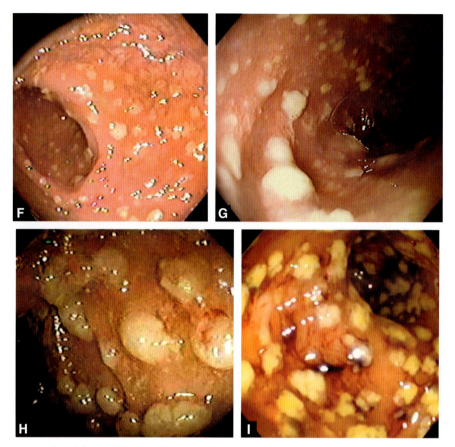

FIGURE 2.3.1 (Continued) ***Clostridium difficile* colitis (pseudomembranous colitis).** Optical colonoscopy images (**F** to **I**) from four different patients show varying severity of disease consisting of pseudomembranes that overlie areas of inflamed mucosa. Because endoscopic absence of pseudomembranes does not rule out *C. difficile* infection, stool evaluation for toxin should be performed whenever clinical suspicion exists.

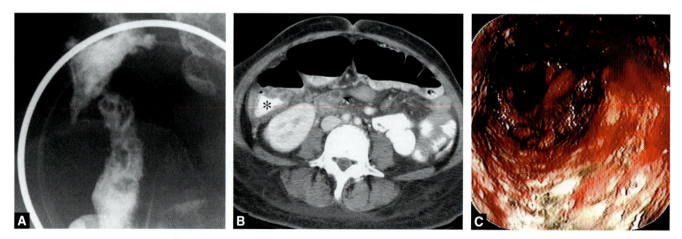

FIGURE 2.3.2 **Tuberculosis of the colon.** SBFT image (**A**) shows ileocecal inflammatory changes with mucosal nodularity and a coned appearance to the cecum. Associated contrast-enhanced CT image (**B**) shows concentric cecal wall thickening (*asterisk*) and low-attenuation lymphadenopathy (*arrowhead*). Colonoscopy (**C**) shows a diffusely friable mucosa with circumferential ulceration.

Illustration continued on following page

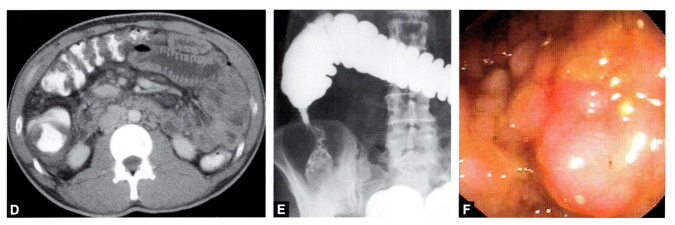

FIGURE 2.3.2 (Continued) **Tuberculosis of the colon.** Contrast-enhanced CT image **(D)** from a second patient shows diffuse wall thickening of the small intestine and right colon, associated with mesenteric inflammation and lymphadenopathy. BE image **(E)** from a third patient shows focal ileocecal narrowing with loss of the normal anatomic landmarks (Stierlin sign). Nodularity of the terminal ileal mucosa is present. Colonoscopy image **(F)** from a final patient shows mucosal nodularity of the right colon.

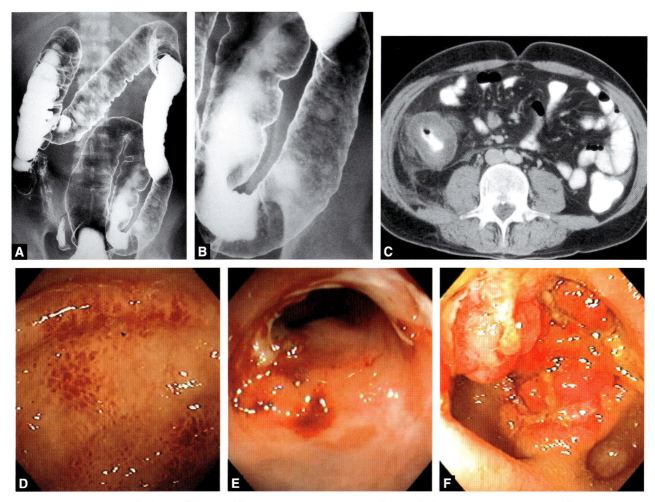

FIGURE 2.3.3 **Cytomegalovirus colitis.** Double-contrast BE image **(A)** and magnified view **(B)** show innumerable colonic aphthoid ulcers similar to those seen in early Crohn's disease. Contrast-enhanced CT image **(C)** from a second patient shows marked low-attenuation wall thickening of the right colon with extensive pericolonic infiltration. The left colon is spared. Colonoscopy images **(D** to **F)** from three patients with CMV show erythematous mucosal patches **(D)**, focal ulceration **(E)**, and nodular mass-like fold thickening **(F)**.

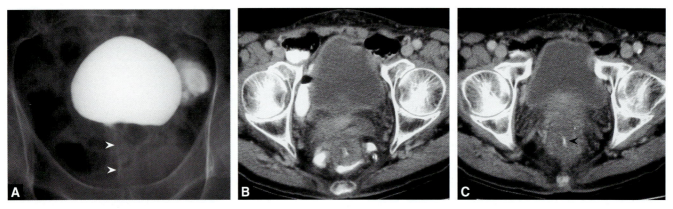

FIGURE 2.3.4 Lymphogranuloma venereum. BE image **(A)** shows a high-grade rectal stricture (*arrowheads*). Contrast-enhanced CT images **(B** and **C)** show extensive rectal/perirectal soft tissue infiltration resulting in a stricture (**C**, *arrowhead*).

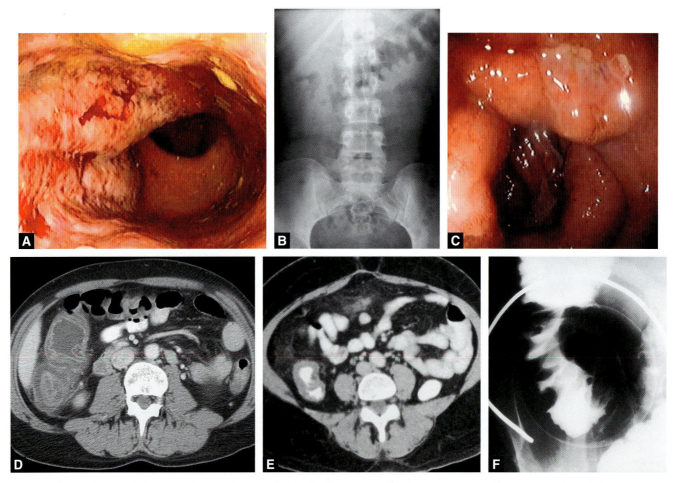

FIGURE 2.3.5 Other viral and bacterial infections. Optical colonoscopy **(A)** from an immunocompetent patient with HSV proctitis shows hemorrhagic and ulcerated rectal mucosa. The asymmetrical involvement would be atypical for idiopathic ulcerative proctitis. Conventional radiograph **(B)** and colonoscopy **(C)** from two patients with colitis from *Salmonella* show thickened, edematous colonic folds (thumbprinting). Contrast-enhanced CT image **(D)** from a patient with bloody diarrhea from enterohemorrhagic *E. coli* (O157:H7) shows prominent right-sided colonic wall thickening. Contrast-enhanced CT image **(E)** from a patient with *Yersinia* colitis also shows right-side colonic wall thickening. BE image **(F)** from a patient with *Campylobacter* colitis shows marked fold thickening of the cecum and ascending colon.

Illustration continued on following page

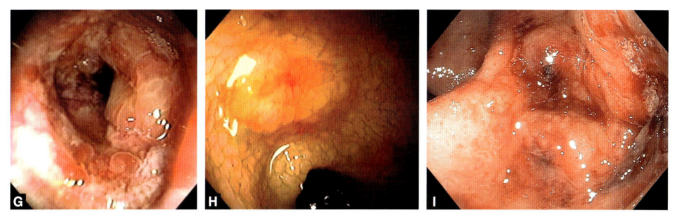

FIGURE 2.3.5 (Continued) **Other viral and bacterial infections.** Colonoscopy image **(G)** from a patient with *Aeromonas sobria* colitis shows extensive mucosal inflammation and submucosal hemorrhage involving only the splenic flexure and descending colon. This was originally misdiagnosed as ischemic colitis. Colonoscopy image **(H)** from a patient with disseminated *Mycobacterium avium intracellulare* infection shows a nodule with a central depression surrounded by diffusely edematous mucosa. Colonoscopy image **(I)** from an HIV-positive patient with a positive RPR and proctalgia shows severe ulcerative and hemorrhagic inflammation of the distal rectum. Histologic evidence of spirochetes confirmed the diagnosis of syphilitic proctitis.

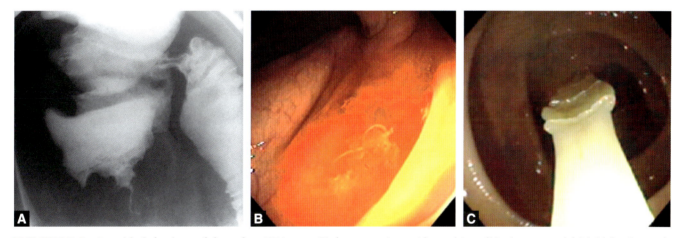

FIGURE 2.3.6 **Parasitic infections of the colon.** BE image **(A)** from a patient with amebic colitis shows cecal fold thickening and luminal narrowing, with sparing of the terminal ileum. Pinworms **(B)** may be found incidentally in the rectum and are typically thin, small worms no longer than 1 cm in length. Tapeworms **(C)** are broad and flat and can grow to be meters long. Note the scolex of the worm seen here.

2.4 Ischemia
(Figures 2.4.1-2.4.6)

CLINICAL FEATURES

- A common cause of colitis in the elderly, ischemia often presents as pain and bloody diarrhea.
- No precipitating vascular event or condition is identified in most cases.
- There is a wide spectrum of clinical disease; most cases are self-limited, but gangrene or fulminant colitis can rarely occur.
- The healing phase of transmural disease can result in stricture formation.
- Any portion of the colon can be involved, but the transverse colon, splenic flexure, and descending colon are most often affected (classic "watershed" distribution) and the rectum is typically spared.
- Segmental ischemia can be seen either proximal or distal to a colonic adenocarcinoma.
- Bowel necrosis can rarely be seen in uremic patients taking Kayexalate (sodium polystyrene sulfonate).

IMAGING FEATURES

- CT is often the initial imaging study; BE and colonoscopy should generally be avoided if extensive ischemia is suspected.
- The degree of wall thickening and pericolonic stranding at CT correlate with severity of disease.
- Sharp demarcation between involved and uninvolved segments is often apparent on radiologic and endoscopic imaging.
- Mucosal pallor and petechial hemorrhages are early findings at endoscopy.
- Progressive ulceration, mucosal sloughing, and pneumatosis are findings of more extensive disease.
- Strictures resulting from healing of severe ischemia appear smooth at imaging.

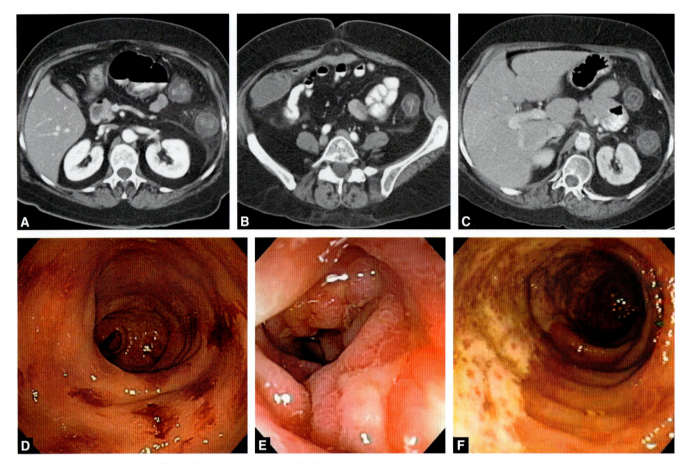

FIGURE 2.4.1 Ischemic colitis with classic "watershed" distribution. Contrast-enhanced CT images (**A** and **B**) from an older patient with crampy pain and bloody diarrhea show segmental low-attenuation wall thickening involving only the splenic flexure region and descending colon. Contrast-enhanced CT image (**C**) from a second patient shows moderate wall thickening but only mild pericolonic infiltration centered at the splenic flexure. Colonoscopy images (**D** to **F**) from three different patients show endoscopic findings of ischemia, with patchy mucosal erythema (**D**), diffusely edematous folds with shallow ulcerations (**E**), and confluent ulceration in a single stripe pattern (**F**).

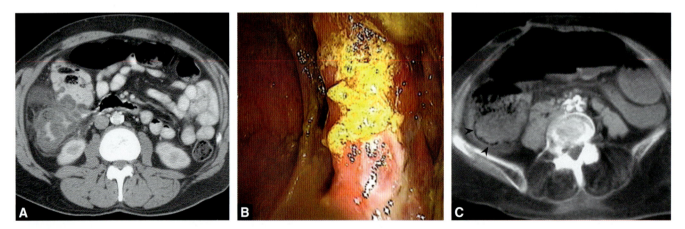

FIGURE 2.4.2 Ischemic colitis with less typical distribution. Contrast-enhanced CT (**A**) and corresponding colonoscopy (**B**) images show prominent segmental colonic fold thickening near the hepatic flexure with abrupt transition to normal colon. CT image (**C**) from a second patient shows wall thickening with pneumatosis (*arrowheads*) involving the right colon.

Illustration continued on following page

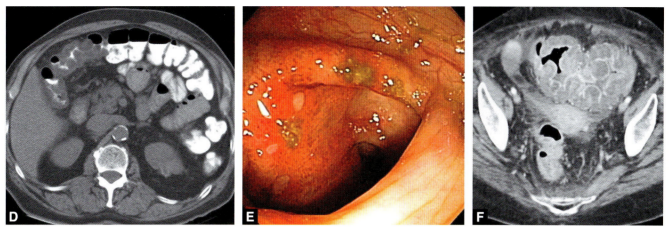

FIGURE 2.4.2 (Continued)   **Ischemic colitis with less typical distribution.** CT **(D)** and colonoscopy **(E)** images from a third patient show localized ischemia involving the hepatic flexure and proximal transverse colon, with an abrupt transition to normal. Contrast-enhanced CT image **(F)** from a final patient shows marked segmental wall thickening isolated to the sigmoid colon. Colonic ischemia is confined to such atypical regions in a minority of cases.

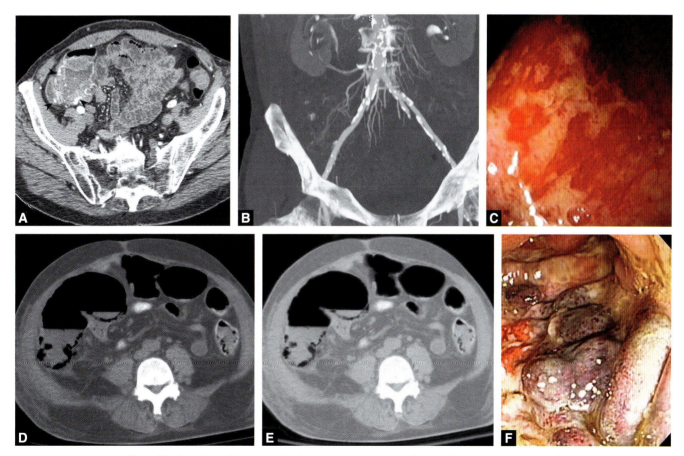

FIGURE 2.4.3   **Complicated ischemic colitis.** Arterial phase transverse **(A)** and coronal MIP **(B)** CT images from an elderly patient with GI bleeding show cecal wall thickening with multiple punctate foci of contrast (*arrowheads*) related to ischemic ulceration and bleeding. Cecal ischemia with hemorrhagic ulceration was confirmed at optical colonoscopy **(C)**. CT images with soft tissue **(D)** and lung **(E)** window settings from a second patient show colonic pneumatosis from gangrenous necrosis of the right colon. Colonoscopy image **(F)** from a third patient with extensive colonic necrosis shows patchy areas of purplish dusky mucosa, as well as submucosal bullae due to pneumatosis.

Illustration continued on following page

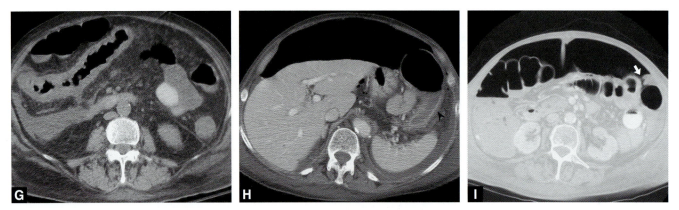

FIGURE 2.4.3 (Continued) **Complicated ischemic colitis.** CT image (**G**) from a patient with fulminant ischemic colitis shows diffuse colonic wall thickening, mesenteric infiltration, and peritoneal fluid. Contrast-enhanced CT images with soft tissue (**H**) and lung (**I**) windows from a final patient show pneumoperitoneum related to perforation from ischemic colitis. Note the colonic wall thickening (**H**, *arrowhead*) and apparent site of perforation (**I**, *arrow*) at the splenic flexure.

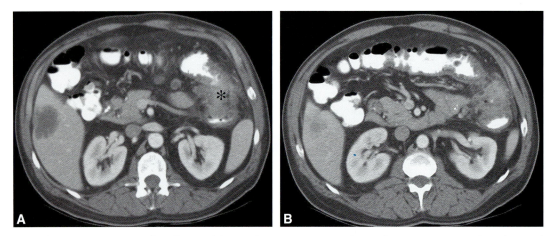

FIGURE 2.4.4 **Ischemia associated with colonic adenocarcinoma.** Contrast-enhanced CT images (**A** and **B**) show a focal soft tissue mass at the splenic flexure (*asterisk*) representing primary adenocarcinoma. Milder and more uniform segmental wall thickening involving the transverse colon is related to ischemia. A liver metastasis is also demonstrated.

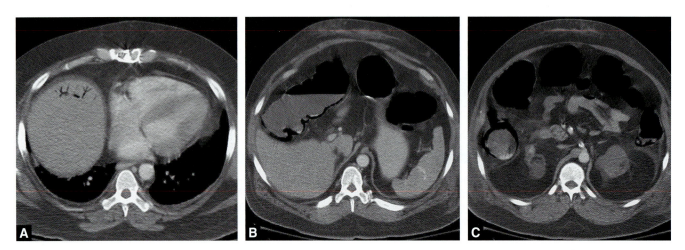

FIGURE 2.4.5 **Colonic necrosis from Kayexalate.** Contrast-enhanced CT images (**A** to **C**) from a renal transplant patient show extensive colonic pneumatosis, portal venous gas in the liver, and mesenteric venous gas due to colonic necrosis as a complication of sodium polystyrene sulfonate administration. Note the atrophic native kidneys.

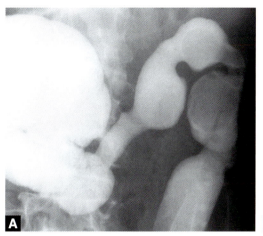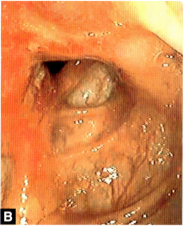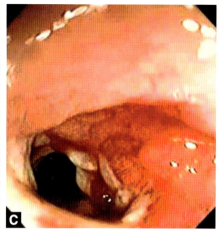

FIGURE 2.4.6 **Postischemic colonic stricture.** BE image **(A)** shows multiple smooth strictures centered on the splenic flexure region from prior ischemia. Optical colonoscopy images **(B** and **C)** from two different patients show focal luminal narrowing in the ascending **(B)** and sigmoid **(C)** colon related to prior ischemia.

2.5 Other Colitides
(Figures 2.5.1-2.5.7)

CLINICAL FEATURES

- Radiation proctocolitis can be seen after external-beam radiation therapy or brachytherapy; strictures and fistulas are feared complications.
- Neutropenic patients on chemotherapy are at increased risk for cecal inflammation ("typhlitis") of unclear etiology; the distal ileum and ascending colon are often involved as well.
- Although less appreciated than findings in the upper GI tract, use of nonsteroidal anti-inflammatory drugs (NSAIDs) can also lead to colonic pathology.
- Systemic vasculitides such as Behçet's disease can involve the colon.
- "Colonic urticaria" was originally described as an allergic reaction to medication, but similar findings can be seen with other causes of submucosal edema.
- Sarcoidosis is a rare cause of granulomatous colitis, which may mimic Crohn's disease.

IMAGING FEATURES

- Endoscopic findings of radiation proctocolitis include diffuse bleeding, irregular ulceration, and telangiectasia; radiologic imaging studies can show wall thickening or diagnose stricture or fistula formation.
- Neutropenic enterocolitis typically manifests on CT with prominent right-sided low-attenuation wall thickening.
- Imaging features of NSAID-related effects on the colon may include ulceration, inflammation, and stricture.
- At BE, an urticarial pattern of submucosal edema manifests as raised polygonal plaques in the right colon.
- Right-sided colonic wall thickening is a common incidental finding in patients with advanced cirrhosis and portal hypertension; in the absence of symptoms, it should not be mistaken for colitis.

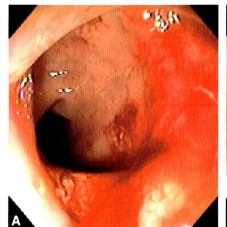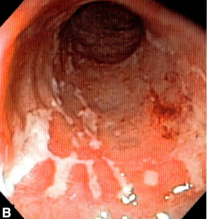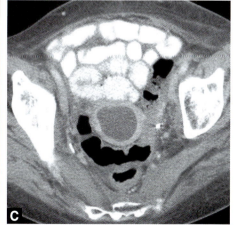

FIGURE 2.5.1 **Radiation proctocolitis.** Optical colonoscopy images **(A** and **B)** from two patients with radiation proctocolitis show diffuse bleeding **(A)** and ulceration **(B)**, respectively. Contrast-enhanced CT image **(C)** from a patient treated for cervical cancer shows moderate diffuse wall thickening of the rectosigmoid, with obscuration of fat planes. Ureteral stents are in place, and the endometrial cavity is dilated.

Illustration continued on following page

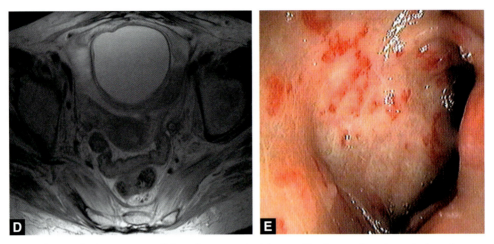

FIGURE 2.5.1 (Continued)   **Radiation proctocolitis.** Subsequent MR image **(D)** shows chronic radiation changes with fixed narrowing and mild wall thickening of the rectosigmoid. Corresponding colonoscopy image **(E)** shows multiple telangiectasias, which led to rectal bleeding.

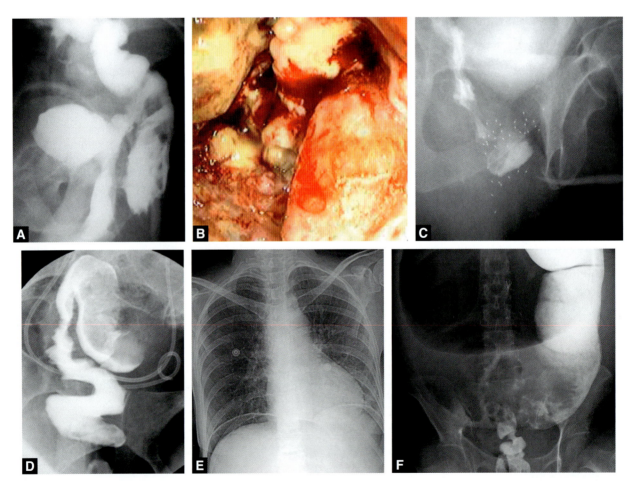

FIGURE 2.5.2   **Complications of radiation proctocolitis.** BE **(A)** and colonoscopy **(B)** images from two patients treated for cervical cancer show a complex rectovesicovaginal fistula **(A)** and friable mucosa with a rectovaginal fistula **(B)**, respectively. Image from retrograde urethrogram **(C)** from a patient who received brachytherapy for prostate cancer shows a rectourethral fistula. BE image **(D)** shows an irregular rectosigmoid radiation stricture from cervical cancer treatment. Note the impacted stool proximal to the stricture and bilateral ureteral stents. Subsequent attempt at endoscopic disimpaction resulted in frank perforation with pneumoperitoneum **(E)**. Water-soluble contrast enema **(F)** from a patient with obstructive symptoms and a history of radiation therapy for a retroperitoneal sarcoma shows long-segment irregular rectosigmoid stricturing with massive distention of the proximal colon. *(C from Pickhardt PJ, Bhalla S, Balfe DM: Acquired gastrointestinal fistulas: Classification, etiologies, and imaging evaluation. Radiology 2002; 224:9-23.)*

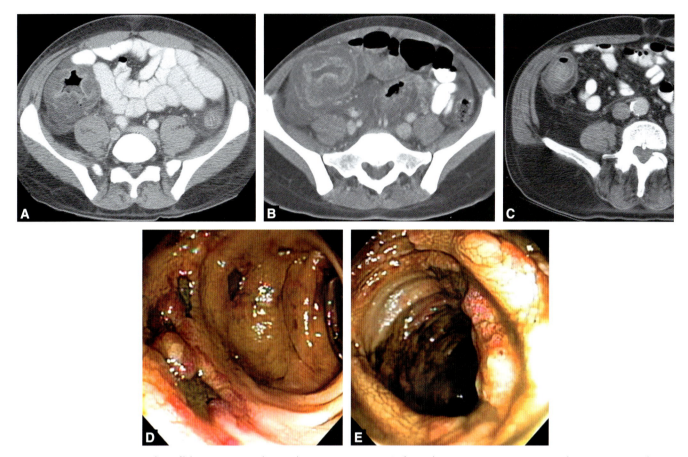

FIGURE 2.5.3 **Neutropenic colitis.** Contrast-enhanced CT images (**A** to **C**) from three neutropenic patients show prominent low-attenuation wall thickening of the right colon. Colonoscopy images (**D** and **E**) from a different patient show marked inflammation and edema of the right colonic mucosa. Areas of purplish discoloration raise concern for early necrosis.

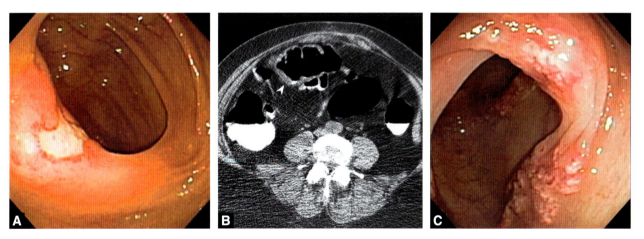

FIGURE 2.5.4 **NSAID-induced colonopathy.** Colonoscopy image (**A**) shows focal ulceration of the ileocecal valve secondary to NSAID use. Transverse 2D CTC image (**B**) shows segmental colonic wall thickening (*arrowhead*). Corresponding colonoscopy image (**C**) shows discrete plaque-like regions of mucosal inflammation. NSAID use was believed to be the most likely cause.

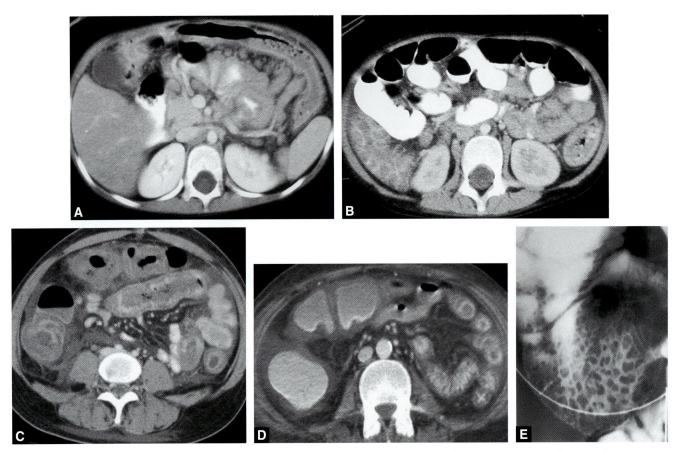

FIGURE 2.5.5 **Colonic vasculitis and "urticaria."** Contrast-enhanced CT images **(A** and **B)** from a young girl with Behçet's disease show moderate diffuse colonic wall thickening. Contrast-enhanced CT images **(C** and **D)** from two different patients with Wegener's granulomatosis show prominent small and large bowel wall thickening from vasculitis. Double-contrast BE image **(E)** from a final patient shows multiple raised polygonal plaques within the cecum representing colonic urticaria.

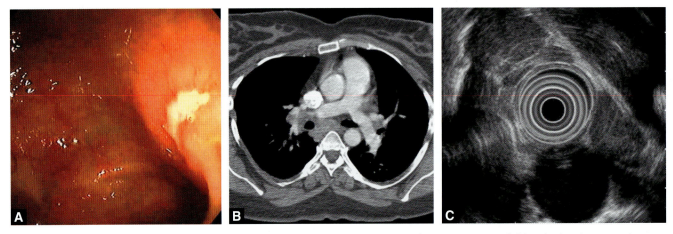

FIGURE 2.5.6 **Granulomatous colitis from sarcoidosis.** Colonoscopy image **(A)** from a patient with bloody diarrhea reveals patchy aphthoid and deep ulcerations throughout the colon. Biopsies revealed multiple noncaseating granulomas. Subsequent CT **(B)** and EUS **(C)** images show marked mediastinal and hilar lymphadenopathy. Noncaseating granulomas consistent with sarcoidosis were also found after nodal fine-needle aspiration.

Illustration continued on following page

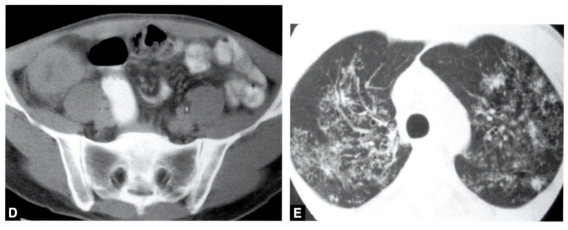

FIGURE 2.5.6 (Continued) **Granulomatous colitis from sarcoidosis.** CT image (**D**) from a second patient shows diffuse cecal wall thickening and pericolonic stranding from biopsy-proven sarcoid colitis. CT image with lung windows (**E**) from the same patient shows bilateral upper lobe reticulonodular interstitial infiltrates characteristic of sarcoidosis. Granulomatous colitis from sarcoidosis is very rare but can mimic Crohn's disease.

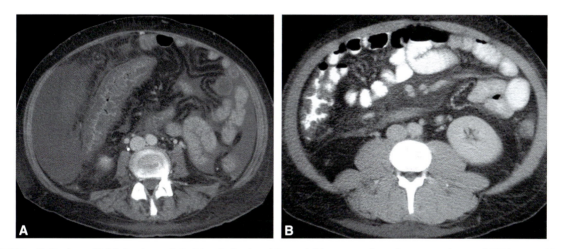

FIGURE 2.5.7 **Colonic wall thickening related to cirrhosis with portal hypertension.** Contrast-enhanced CT images (**A** and **B**) from two different patients with portal hypertension from cirrhosis show diffuse right-sided colonic wall thickening, as well as ascites (**A**) and mesenteric infiltration (**A** and **B**). Neither patient had active GI symptoms.

3. COLONIC DIVERTICULAR DISEASE

Diverticular disease of the colon is a very common acquired entity in the modern Western world, likely related to a decreased intake of dietary fiber. The spectrum of disease ranges from segmental colonic wall thickening (myochosis) to the formation of pulsion pseudodiverticula and, in some cases, diverticular perforation (diverticulitis) or a host of other potential complications.

3.1 Diverticulosis
(Figures 3.1.1-3)

CLINICAL FEATURES

- True prevalence is not known but colonic diverticula are present in over 50% of older adults in industrialized Western nations; in East Asia, right-sided diverticula are more common than left-sided diverticula.
- The sigmoid colon is involved in the majority of cases, but diverticula can be seen throughout the colon (rectal diverticula are rare).
- Most patients with diverticulosis will remain asymptomatic.

IMAGING FEATURES

- At CT, wall thickening associated with luminal narrowing and haustral foreshortening (with or without diverticula) reflects changes of myochosis from elastin deposition.
- Diverticula are an extremely common imaging finding; they are often filled with inspissated stool.
- The presence of diverticulosis can make colorectal evaluation for polyps more challenging.

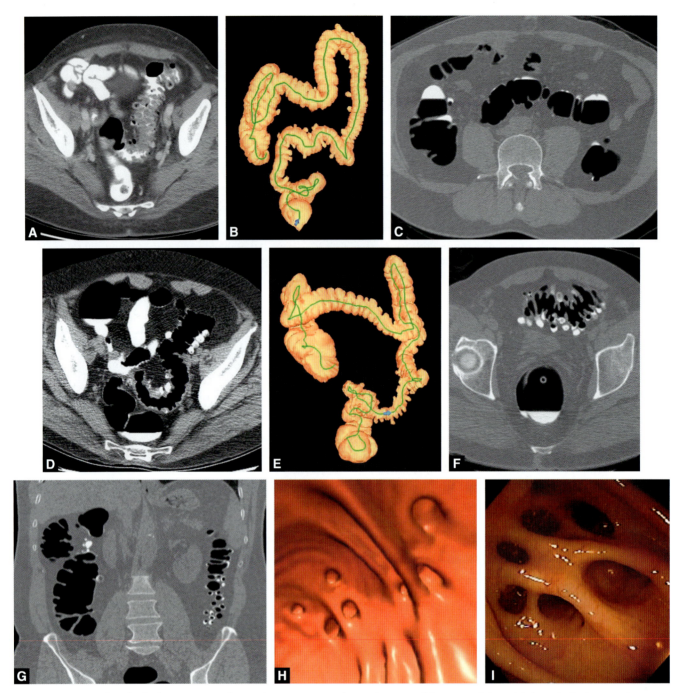

FIGURE 3.1.1 Diverticulosis. Contrast-enhanced CT image **(A)** shows the typical features of sigmoid diverticulosis: prominent fold thickening, luminal narrowing, haustral shortening, and multiple diverticula. 3D colon map **(B)** and transverse 2D **(C)** CTC images from a patient with mild diverticular disease show multiple diverticula but no significant wall thickening or luminal narrowing. Transverse 2D CTC image **(D)** from a third patient shows sigmoid diverticulosis with persistent wall thickening and luminal narrowing despite gaseous distention. 3D colon map **(E)** and transverse 2D **(F)** CTC images from a fourth patient show more advanced sigmoid diverticular disease. Coronal 2D CTC image **(G)** from a fifth patient shows multiple left- and right-sided diverticula. 3D endoluminal CTC **(H)** and colonoscopy **(I)** images from two final patients show multiple diverticula from an endoluminal perspective.

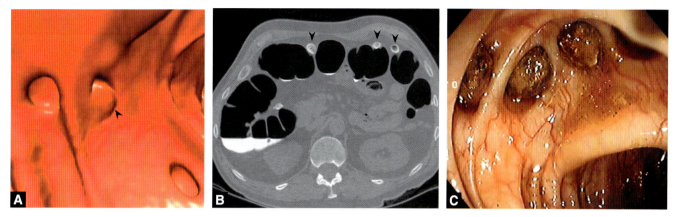

FIGURE 3.1.2 Diverticula impacted with inspissated stool. 3D endoluminal CTC image (**A**) shows several diverticula, one of which appears more polypoid due to stool filling (*arrowhead*). Transverse 2D CTC image (**B**) shows multiple stool-filled diverticula (*arrowheads*). The 2D images can easily exclude a true mucosal polyp in all cases. Colonoscopy image (**C**) from a different patient shows multiple diverticula filled with inspissated stool.

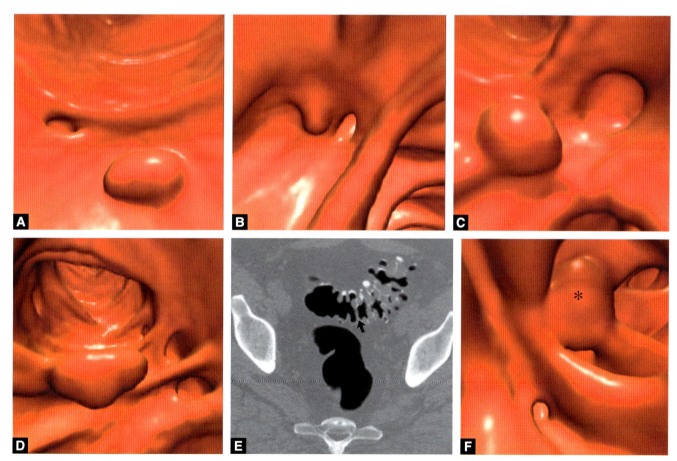

FIGURE 3.1.3 Diverticulum versus polyp at CTC. 3D endoluminal CTC images (**A** to **D**) from four different patients show diverticula adjacent to polyps. Note how easy the distinction is with appropriate volume rendering. Transverse 2D CTC image (**E**) from a different patient shows sigmoid diverticulosis, which can make 2D polyp detection very difficult. A large pedunculated adenoma is present (*arrow*), which appears similar to the adjacent thickened folds. The lesion, however, is much more conspicuous on the 3D endoluminal view (**F**, *asterisk*).

3.2 Acute Diverticulitis

(Figures 3.2.1-3.2.4)

CLINICAL FEATURES

- Acute diverticulitis represents inflammatory erosion and perforation of a diverticulum; it may occur in up to 15% of patients with known diverticulosis.
- Classic presentation consists of left lower quadrant pain, fever, and leukocytosis.
- Initial clinical management (conservative, radiologic, or surgical) hinges on disease severity.
- The great majority of cases involve the left colon (particularly the sigmoid); right-sided diverticulitis accounts for a relatively small minority of cases in the Western world.
- Presentation in younger adults (<40 years) is increasing in incidence.
- It is important to obtain follow-up in most cases to exclude the small possibility of a perforated colon cancer mimicking diverticulitis.

IMAGING FEATURES

- Because diverticulitis is an extraluminal process, CT is the imaging modality of choice for both confirming the diagnosis and evaluating for complications.
- Focal pericolonic inflammation is the CT hallmark of acute diverticulitis; associated eccentric wall thickening and additional diverticula are usually present.
- Colonoscopy is contraindicated in acute diverticulitis; findings of resolving inflammation are occasionally seen at follow up, including erythema confined to the diverticular orifice.
- Acute complications include abscesses, sinus tracts, fistulas, bowel obstruction, and peritonitis.
- CT-guided abscess drainage can greatly simplify subsequent surgical management.
- Right-sided diverticulitis can be a more challenging CT diagnosis, particularly for cecal involvement, given the wide variety of potential ileocecal inflammatory processes.
- The CT appearance of perforated colon cancer can significantly overlap with that of diverticulitis (see Figure 1.4.6).

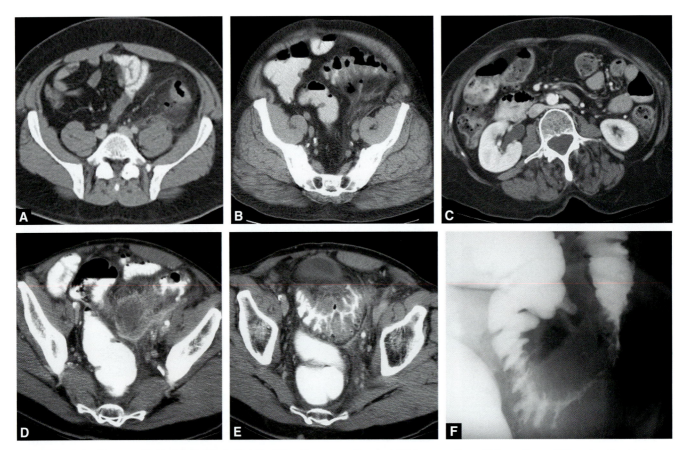

FIGURE 3.2.1 Uncomplicated left-sided diverticulitis. Contrast-enhanced CT images (**A** to **C**) from three different patients show infiltration of the pericolonic fat surrounding the sigmoid and descending colon, with focal wall thickening and a small amount of extraluminal gas contained in the mesentery (**A** and **B**). Contrast-enhanced CT images (**D** and **E**) from a fourth patient show more advanced sigmoid diverticulitis with an adjacent phlegmonous inflammatory mass. No frank abscess was present, and the patient had an uneventful recovery with conservative medical management. Contrast enema image (**F**) from a different patient shows smooth, long segment luminal narrowing with mucosal preservation.

Illustration continued on following page

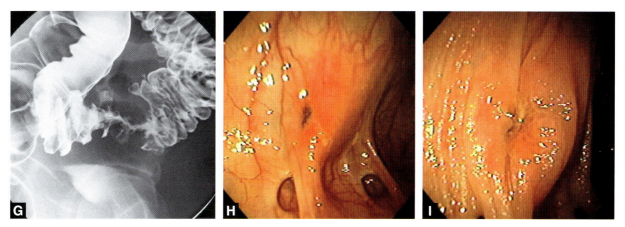

FIGURE 3.2.1 (Continued) **Uncomplicated left-sided diverticulitis.** BE image (**G**) from a different patient shows marked segmental narrowing of the sigmoid colon with mass effect but apparent preservation of the mucosa. Although enema findings are sensitive for diverticular disease, they are relatively nonspecific and clinical correlation is important. Optical colonoscopy images (**H** and **I**) from a patient who was recently treated for diverticulitis show resolving inflammation of an edematous diverticulum. Note the adjacent uninvolved diverticula.

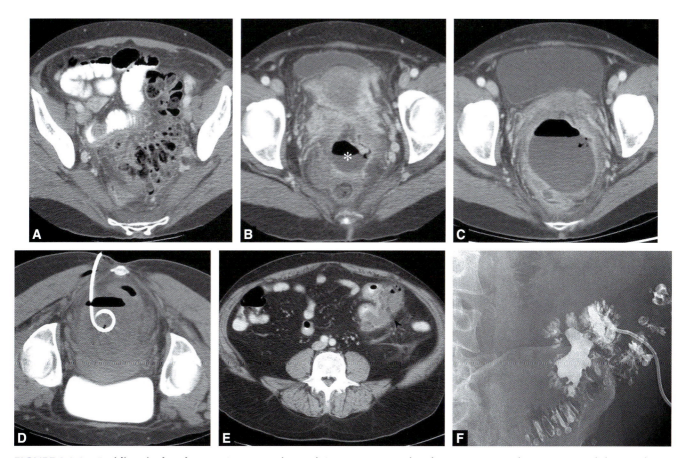

FIGURE 3.2.2 Peridiverticular abscess. Contrast-enhanced CT images (**A** and **B**) from a patient with acute sigmoid diverticulitis show severe pericolonic inflammation and a small peridiverticular abscess (**B**, *asterisk*). Follow-up CT (**C**) after conservative medical therapy shows interval increase in the abscess size, which necessitated percutaneous CT-guided drainage (**D**). Contrast-enhanced CT image (**E**) from a different patient with acute left-sided diverticulitis shows a peridiverticular abscess (*arrowhead*) contiguous with adjacent small bowel. Fluoroscopic image (**F**) from subsequent percutaneous drainage shows the abscess cavity via catheter injection. The abscess communicates with the sigmoid colon, which demonstrates advanced diverticular disease.

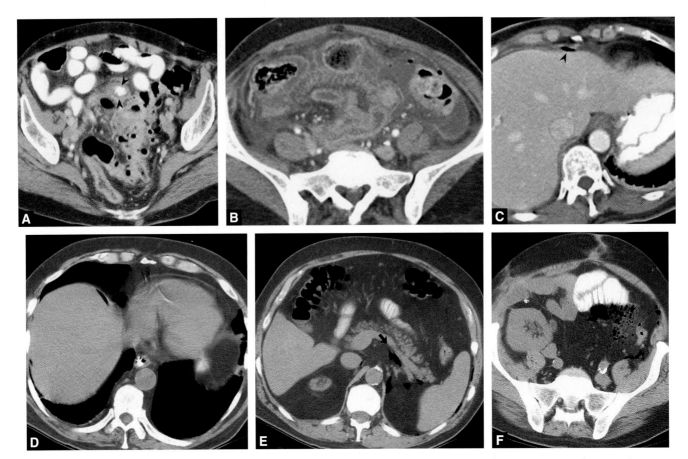

FIGURE 3.2.3   Other acute complications in diverticulitis. Contrast-enhanced CT image **(A)** from a patient with sigmoid diverticulitis shows extensive pericolonic inflammation, which narrows an adjacent contrast-filled small bowel loop (*arrowheads*), resulting in partial obstruction. Contrast-enhanced CT image **(B)** from a second patient shows diffuse peritonitis from sigmoid diverticulitis, with diffuse peritoneal thickening and moderate ascites. CT image **(C)** from a third patient with diverticulitis shows a small amount of free intraperitoneal air (*arrowhead*) anterior to the liver. CT images **(D to F)** from a renal transplant recipient show limited pneumoperitoneum **(D)**, retroperitoneal gas **(E,** *arrow*), and localized mesenteric gas **(F)** due to acute sigmoid diverticulitis. The relative paucity of pericolonic inflammatory reaction is likely related to the patient's immunosuppressed state.

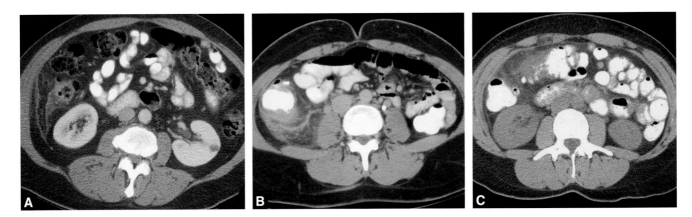

FIGURE 3.2.4   Right-sided diverticulitis. Contrast-enhanced CT images **(A and B)** from two different patients show mild **(A)** and severe **(B)** diverticulitis of the ascending colon. Other inflammatory and malignant causes are more difficult to exclude when significant wall thickening is present. CT image **(C)** from a third patient shows acute diverticulitis of the hepatic flexure with prominent wall thickening and pericolonic stranding. Multiple diverticula were present throughout the right colon.

Illustration continued on following page

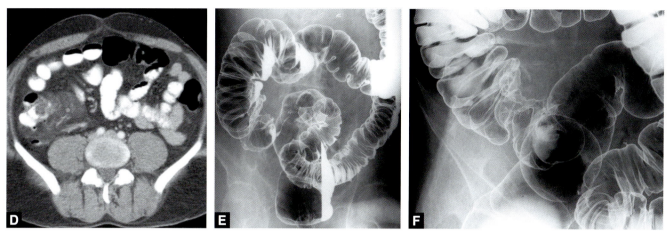

FIGURE 3.2.4 (Continued)   Right-sided diverticulitis. CT image (**D**) from a fourth patient with right lower quadrant pain shows cecal diverticulitis with extensive mesenteric infiltration. Cecal diverticula and eccentric wall thickening are present. A normal air-filled retrocecal appendix excludes appendicitis. Double-contrast BE images (**E** and **F**) from a patient with cecal diverticulitis show marked cecal irregularity with eccentric mass-like narrowing. The clinical and radiographic appearance can simulate perforated cecal carcinoma. Filling of the appendix in **E** excludes appendicitis.

3.3 Diverticular Fistulas and Strictures
(Figures 3.3.1-3.3.6)

CLINICAL FEATURES

- Fistulas resulting from diverticulitis can communicate with adjacent structures or with the GI tract itself.
- Colovesical fistulas are relatively common; delayed presentation with urinary tract infections and pneumaturia is typical.
- Most colocutaneous fistulas develop after surgical resection, but spontaneous development also occurs.
- Colonic stricture from previous diverticulitis may present as delayed obstructive symptoms.

IMAGING FEATURES

- CT is useful for the diagnosis of diverticular fistulas.
- Imaging findings of colovesical fistulas include focal bladder wall thickening, air in the bladder lumen, and contiguity with diseased sigmoid; abnormal contrast communication between structures is diagnostic.
- Localized colocolic fistulas represent subserosal communication of ruptured diverticula.
- Luminal narrowing from sigmoid diverticular disease is a common cause of incomplete colonoscopy; it is also the most common cause of inadequate segmental evaluation at CTC.
- Diverticular strictures may mimic colon cancer on imaging.

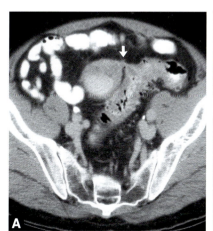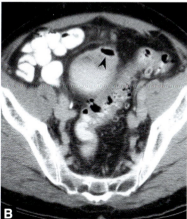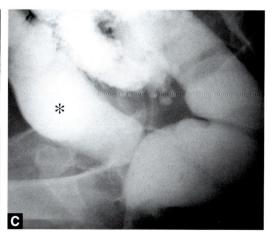

FIGURE 3.3.1   Colovesical fistulas from sigmoid diverticulitis. Contrast-enhanced CT images (**A** and **B**) show eccentric bladder wall thickening and air within the bladder lumen (**B**, *arrowhead*). Note the advanced sigmoid diverticular disease that communicates with the bladder with a tented appearance (**A**, *arrow*). BE image (**C**) from a second patient shows contrast filling of the bladder (*asterisk*) and extensive diverticulosis of the adjacent sigmoid colon. *(A and B from Pickhardt PJ, Bhalla S, Balfe DM: Acquired gastrointestinal fistulas: Classification, etiologies, and imaging evaluation. Radiology 2002; 224:9-23.)*

Illustration continued on following page

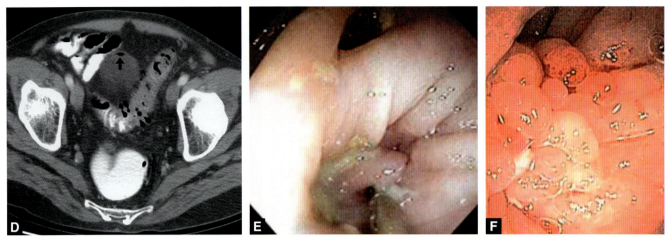

FIGURE 3.3.1 (Continued)   **Colovesical fistulas from sigmoid diverticulitis.** Contrast-enhanced CT image **(D)** from a third patient shows air within the urinary bladder (*arrow*) and adjacent sigmoid diverticular disease. Colonoscopy images **(E and F)** from two patients with colovesical fistulas demonstrate the fistula itself with surrounding mucopus in one case **(E)** and polypoid inflammatory reaction at the fistula site in the other **(F)**.

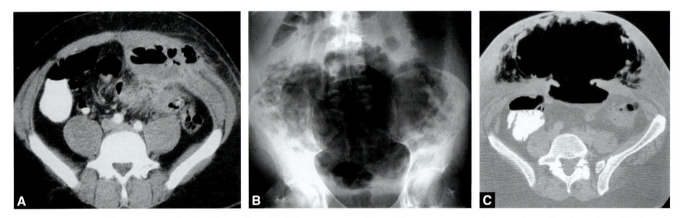

FIGURE 3.3.2   Colocutaneous fistulas from diverticulitis. Contrast-enhanced CT image **(A)** shows a large fluid- and air-filled peridiverticular abscess extending through the abdominal wall musculature. Conventional radiograph **(B)** from a different patient presenting with acute abdominal pain shows a bizarre gas collection overlying the abdomen. Subsequent CT image **(C)** with lung windows shows that the abnormal gas is primarily located subcutaneously in the anterior abdominal wall. A colocutaneous fistula from sigmoid diverticulitis was confirmed at surgery. *(A and B from Pickhardt PJ, Bhalla S, Balfe DM: Acquired gastrointestinal fistulas: Classification, etiologies, and imaging evaluation. Radiology 2002; 224:9-23.)*

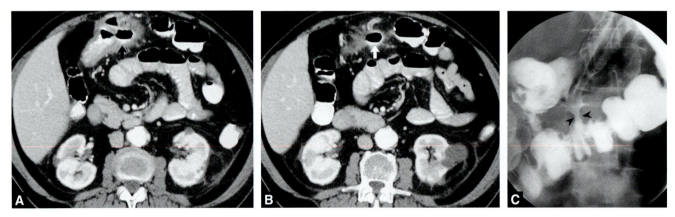

FIGURE 3.3.3   Gastrocolic fistula from diverticulitis. CT images **(A and B)** show an inflamed diverticulum of the transverse colon (*arrows*) directly communicating with the gastric antrum via the gastrocolic ligament. Image from BE **(C)** confirms the fistulous communication (*arrowheads*). *(From Pickhardt PJ, Bhalla S, Balfe DM: Acquired gastrointestinal fistulas: Classification, etiologies, and imaging evaluation. Radiology 2002; 224:9-23.)*

DIVERTICULAR FISTULAS AND STRICTURES

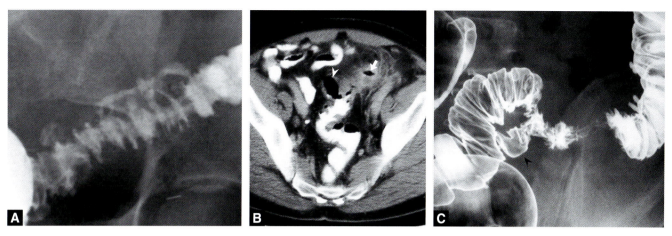

FIGURE 3.3.4 Colocolic (double-tracking) fistula. BE image **(A)** shows a localized pericolonic fistulous tract from communication of two sigmoid diverticula. Contrast-enhanced CT image **(B)** from a patient with acute sigmoid diverticulitis shows a small peridiverticular abscess (*arrow*). A large diverticulum (*arrowhead*) is present adjacent to the inflammatory process. Double-contrast BE image **(C)** performed 1 month after CT shows a long-segment sigmoid stricture fed by two contrast-filled channels. The inferior communication (*arrowhead*) resulted from fistulous communication with the large diverticulum seen on CT. The imaging findings were confirmed at subsequent surgery. (*B and C from Pickhardt PJ, Bhalla S, Balfe DM: Acquired gastrointestinal fistulas: Classification, etiologies, and imaging evaluation. Radiology 2002; 224:9-23.*)

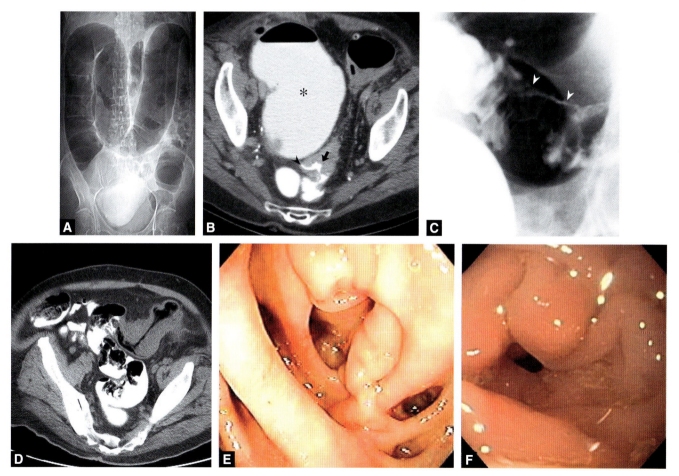

FIGURE 3.3.5 Diverticular stricture. CT scout image **(A)** shows massive colonic dilation. Transverse CT image **(B)** shows an abrupt cut-off of the rectally administered contrast (*arrow*) and a fistulous tract extending toward the serosa (*arrowhead*). Note the prominently dilated cecum filled with orally administered contrast (*asterisk*). Subsequent BE image **(C)** shows a high-grade stricture with a localized colocolic fistulous tract (*arrowheads*). CT image **(D)** from a second patient with prior bouts of diverticulitis shows focal annular wall thickening with shouldering and luminal narrowing involving the sigmoid colon. The apperance mimics colonic adenocarcinoma and required resection but was benign. Colonoscopy images **(E** and **F)** show diverticular strictures from two final patients. Identification of the true lumen can be difficult in cases with multiple large diverticula adjacent to the stricture.

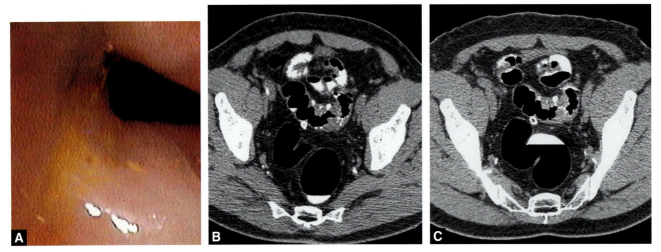

FIGURE 3.3.6 **Incomplete colonoscopy due to diverticular narrowing.** Optical colonoscopy image **(A)** shows focal luminal narrowing of the sigmoid colon due to diverticular disease, which precluded evaluation of the proximal colon. Supine **(B)** and prone **(C)** transverse 2D CTC images show irregular wall thickening and fixed luminal narrowing from advanced sigmoid diverticulosis. The proximal colon was normal.

3.4 Diverticular Hemorrhage

(Figures 3.4.1-3.4.2)

CLINICAL FEATURES

- Diverticular bleeding is a common cause of acute lower GI hemorrhage; diverticular inflammation is not a contributing factor to the onset of bleeding.
- Damage to the vasa recta within the lumen of a diverticulum is the usual cause of bleeding.
- Right-sided diverticula and angiodysplasia are the most common causes of massive lower GI bleeding in older patients; hemorrhage ceases spontaneously in approximately 80% of cases.
- Diagnostic workup depends on the stability of the patient and the rate of blood loss; rapid oral purge and urgent colonoscopy is typically the initial study performed.

IMAGING FEATURES

- Scintigraphy (^{99m}Tc–tagged red blood cell scan) can be useful for segmental localization and is more sensitive than angiography for low bleeding rates; the patient can be re-imaged hours after injection.
- Conventional angiography is useful in cases with relatively brisk, active bleeding.
- Emergent colonoscopy allows for endoscopic therapy if a bleeding site is identified; intraluminal blood and clots filling diverticula can make the offending diverticulum difficult to identify.
- The role of CT in the setting of active GI bleeding is evolving; in at least some cases, it can detect, localize, and determine the cause of bleeding.

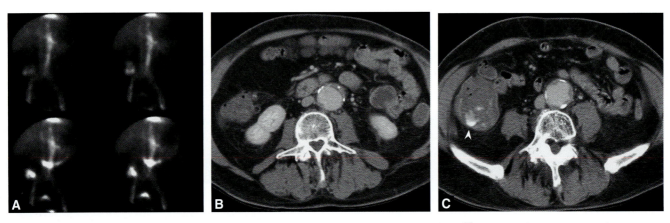

FIGURE 3.4.1 **Lower GI bleeding from diverticular hemorrhage.** Collage of images from ^{99m}Tc-tagged RBC scintigraphy **(A)** shows progressive accumulation of activity in the right lower quadrant, as well as more distal luminal activity from antegrade movement of blood. Contrast-enhanced CT images **(B** and **C)** show right-sided colonic diverticula and active extravasation of contrast **(C,** *arrowhead*) into the cecal lumen. Diverticular hemorrhage was confirmed at surgery.

Illustration continued on following page

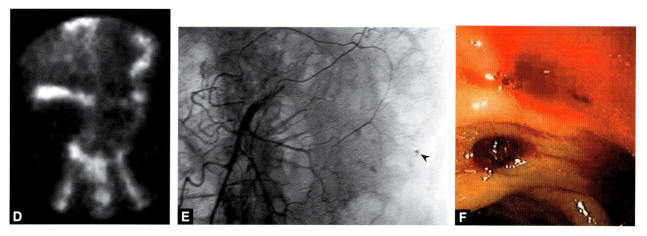

FIGURE 3.4.1 (Continued) **Lower GI bleeding from diverticular hemorrhage.** ^{99m}Tc-tagged RBC scan **(D)** from a second patient shows abundant colonic activity resulting from a bleeding right-sided diverticulum. Left-sided activity represents antegrade movement of luminal blood. Conventional mesenteric angiogram **(E)** from a third patient with lower GI bleeding shows a focus of contrast extravasation in the descending colon (*arrowhead*). Luminal blood obscured the source at colonoscopy but a bleeding diverticulum was confirmed after emergent segmental resection. Colonoscopy image **(F)** from a fourth patient shows active hemorrhage from a colonic diverticulum. Because diverticula are a common incidental finding, it is important to demonstrate the source before assuming the cause.

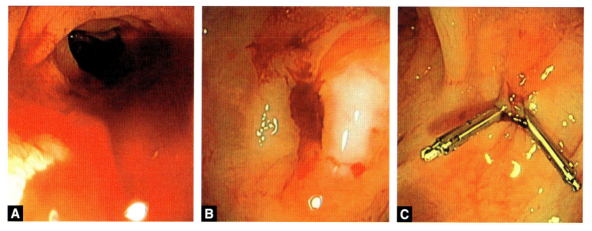

FIGURE 3.4.2 **Endoscopic treatment of diverticular hemorrhage.** Colonoscopy image **(A)** shows fresh blood in the transverse colon that obscured the visual field despite vigorous irrigation. After injection of epinephrine in the suspected site of hemorrhage, a bleeding diverticulum was identified **(B)**; note the blanching effect of the surrounding mucosa related to local vasoconstriction. Lasting hemostasis was achieved with endoscopic placement of two hemoclips **(C)**.

3.5 Giant Sigmoid Diverticulum
(Figure 3.5.1)

CLINICAL FEATURES

- This is a rare complication of diverticulitis believed to be a sequela of localized perforation with subsequent formation of a large air cavity from a ball-valve mechanism.
- Affected patients often have a history of chronic or intermittent symptoms related to diverticular disease.

IMAGING FEATURES

- Conventional abdominal radiographs demonstrate a large air-filled structure overlying the abdomen or pelvis.
- The radiographic appearance can mimic colonic volvulus, abdominal abscess, and air within the bladder.
- Evidence of additional diverticular disease is typically seen on more advanced imaging studies.
- On CT, the relationship of the air-filled structure with the colon is apparent.

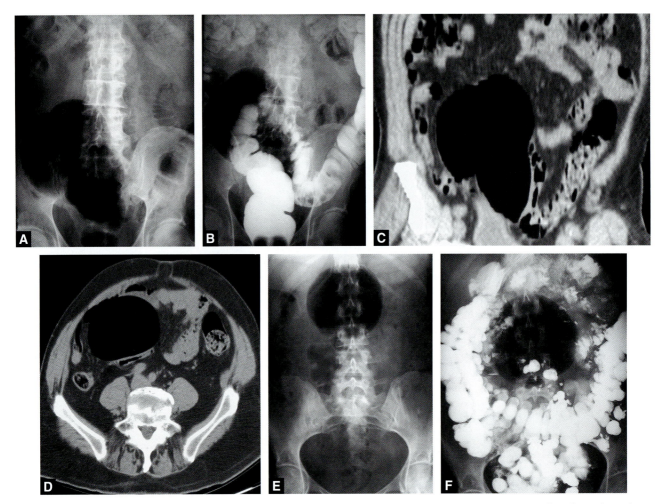

FIGURE 3.5.1 Giant sigmoid diverticulum. Abdominal radiograph **(A)** shows a large air-filled cavity extending from the pelvis. The appearance suggests colonic volvulus, but the patient was asymptomatic. BE image **(B)** shows that the dilated structure does not freely communicate with the colonic lumen, but sigmoid diverticular disease is present. Subsequent coronal **(C)** and transverse **(D)** CT images show that the air-filled structure has an imperceptible wall and appears to originate from the sigmoid colon. Abdominal radiograph **(E)** from a second patient shows a rounded air-filled collection overlying the upper abdomen in the midline. Subsequent BE **(F)** shows extensive colonic diverticulosis, but the air cyst again does not freely communicate.

4. THE APPENDIX

The vermiform appendix is a vestigial structure that serves no apparent purpose in humans yet is a common source of malady due to inflammation (appendicitis) and, rarely, appendiceal neoplasms. CT and, to a lesser extent, US have revolutionized the clinical evaluation of the appendix.

4.1 Appendicitis
(Figures 4.1.1-4.1.5)

CLINICAL FEATURES

- The lifetime risk for appendicitis is approximately 7%, with peak incidence in late teens to early 20s.
- Appendicitis remains the most common indication for emergent abdominal surgery.
- The cause is luminal obstruction leading to edema, superinfection, ischemia, and, ultimately, necrosis.
- Mortality risk for nongangrenous appendicitis is <0.1% but rises up to 5% for perforated appendicitis.
- Perforated appendicitis accounts for 20% of cases; periappendiceal abscess or phlegmon is seen in 5%.
- The classic presentation is leukocytosis associated with abdominal pain that begins in the periumbilical region and migrates to the right lower quadrant.
- Preoperative imaging can lower the negative appendectomy rate.
- Stump appendicitis in a patient with prior appendectomy is rare.

IMAGING FEATURES

- Imaging is not always indicated but is particularly useful with atypical presentations, elderly patients, young children, and women of child-bearing age.
- The appendix is retrocecal in nearly two thirds of cases and extends inferiorly over the pelvic brim in nearly one third.

- CT is accurate for appendicitis and, if the appendix is normal, can often establish an alternative diagnosis.
- Typical CT findings include diffuse mural thickening and enhancement, stranding of the periappendiceal fat, and a fluid-filled lumen; supportive findings include appendicoliths and medial cecal wall thickening.
- Graded compression sonography is particularly useful in children and young women; a noncompressible, blind-ended tubular structure >6 mm in diameter is diagnostic of appendicitis.
- CT is useful for detecting complications such as perforation, abscess formation, and bowel obstruction.
- Up to 10% to 15% of right-sided colon cancers may present with obstructive appendicitis.

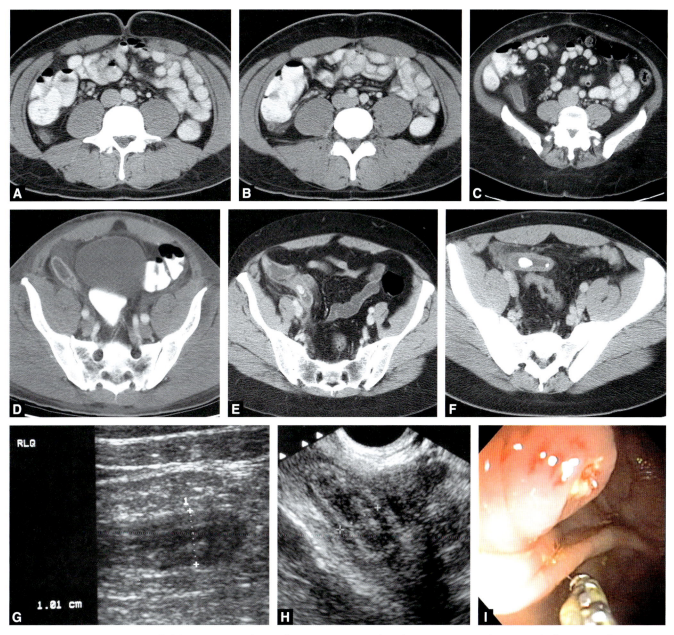

FIGURE 4.1.1 Acute appendicitis. Contrast-enhanced CT images (**A** and **B**) from a patient with acute right lower quadrant pain show a mildly dilated fluid-filled retrocecal appendix with mural enhancement and infiltration of the periappendiceal fat. Contrast-enhanced CT images (**C** to **F**) from four additional patients each show a dilated fluid-filled appendix with abnormal enhancement and periappendiceal inflammation. Luminal appendicoliths are seen in **E** and **F**. Transabdominal US image (**G**) from graded-compression study of the right lower quadrant shows a noncompressible, blind-ended tubular structure measuring 10 mm in diameter, which is diagnostic of appendicitis. Transvaginal US (**H**) from a patient with pelvic pain shows an inflamed appendix (*calipers*) as the cause. Colonoscopy image (**I**) from a final patient shows an edematous appendiceal orifice with an appendicolith visible in the center.

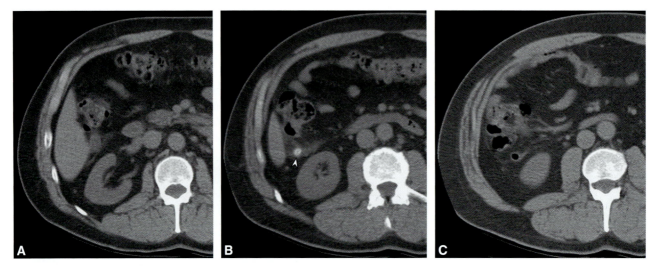

FIGURE 4.1.2 Tip appendicitis. Noncontrast CT images **(A** to **C)** performed to evaluate for suspected urolithiasis in a patient with right-sided pain shows "tip appendicitis" involving a retrocecal appendix; note the appendicolith (**B**, *arrowhead*) at the point of occlusion and infiltration of the periappendiceal fat. The caudal image **(C)** shows a normal air-filled appendix closer to its base.

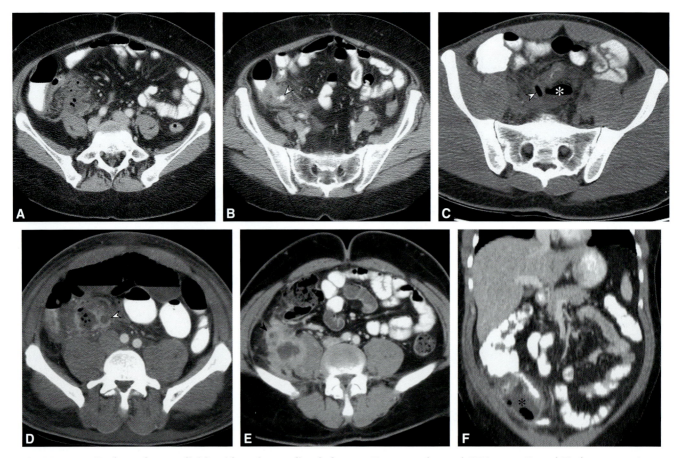

FIGURE 4.1.3 Perforated appendicitis with periappendiceal abscess. Contrast-enhanced CT images **(A** and **B)** show extensive mesenteric inflammatory changes medial to the ileocecal region **(A)**, with extraluminal fluid and gas bubbles in the center of the phlegmon. Marked periappendiceal inflammation and appendicoliths (**B**, *arrowhead*) are present adjacent to the thickened medial cecal wall. This developing abscess has not yet matured into a well-defined drainable collection. Contrast-enhanced CT image **(C)** from a second patient shows an air-filled but thick-walled appendix (*arrowhead*) leading into an abscess cavity (*asterisk*). The surrounding mesenteric fat is inflamed. Note how the presence of air within the appendiceal lumen does not by itself exclude appendicitis in this case. Contrast-enhanced CT images **(D** and **E)** from two different patients show perforated appendicitis (*arrowheads*) with pronounced periappendiceal inflammation and abscess formation. Coronal CT image **(F)** from a final patient shows mass effect on the contrast-filled ileocecal region by a complex periappendiceal abscess (*asterisk*).

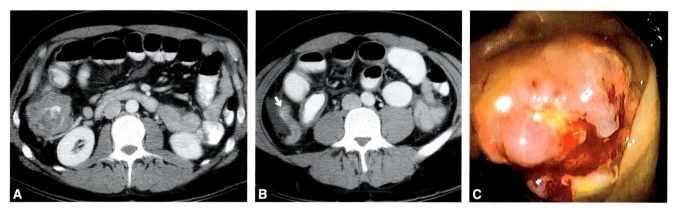

FIGURE 4.1.4 Colon cancer presenting with obstructive appendicitis. Contrast-enhanced CT images (**A** and **B**) from a patient with acute right lower quadrant pain show findings of acute appendicitis (**B**, *arrow*), but luminal obstruction in this case was due to a large cecal adenocarcinoma (**A**). Colon cancer covering the appedicael orifice was confirmed at colonoscopy (**C**).

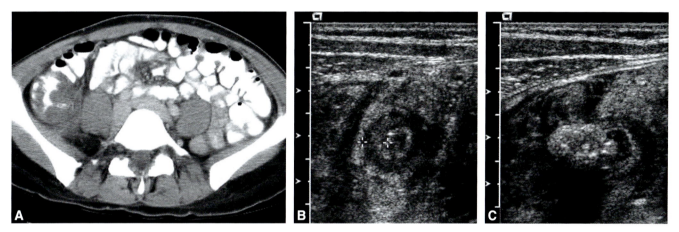

FIGURE 4.1.5 Stump appendicitis. Contrast-enhanced CT image (**A**) from a symptomatic patient with a history of laparoscopic appendectomy 3 years earlier shows marked eccentric wall thickening of the medial cecal wall with surrounding inflammation. The findings are centered on the region of the appendiceal stump, where a subtle focal density is present. Transverse (**B**) and longitudinal (**C**) US images show an abnormally thickened appendiceal stump (*calipers*) with a shadowing appendicolith impacted at the orifice.

4.2 Appendiceal Tumors
(Figures 4.2.1-4.2.7)

CLINICAL FEATURES

- Primary appendiceal neoplasms are uncommon.
- Mucoceles resulting from mucinous cystic neoplasms are often detected incidentally on imaging studies.
- Mucoceles may also present as a palpable mass or with intussusception (see also section 5.2), superinfection, or torsion.
- Pseudomyxoma peritonei is a rare complication related to rupture of a mucinous cystadenocarcinoma.
- Although carcinoid tumor is the most common primary tumor of the appendix, it is usually small and asymptomatic.
- Other primary neoplasms are rare and most often present as obstructive appendicitis.

IMAGING FEATURES

- Mucoceles from mucinous adenomas cause smooth, broad-based impressions at luminal examination; cross-sectional studies (especially CT) are more accurate for the diagnosis.
- Mural calcification of a mucocele due to a mucinous neoplasm is relatively common; prominent soft tissue suggests malignancy.
- Colonic-type adenocarcinoma of the appendix is rare and generally manifests as a soft tissue mass (not a mucocele).
- Appendiceal carcinoids are typically small and not identified at preoperative imaging; symptoms from obstructive appendicitis and metastatic spread are rare.
- Primary appendiceal lymphoma typically results in prominent vermiform enlargement of the appendix.
- An inverted appendiceal stump may mimic a colonic polyp at endoluminal evaluation.

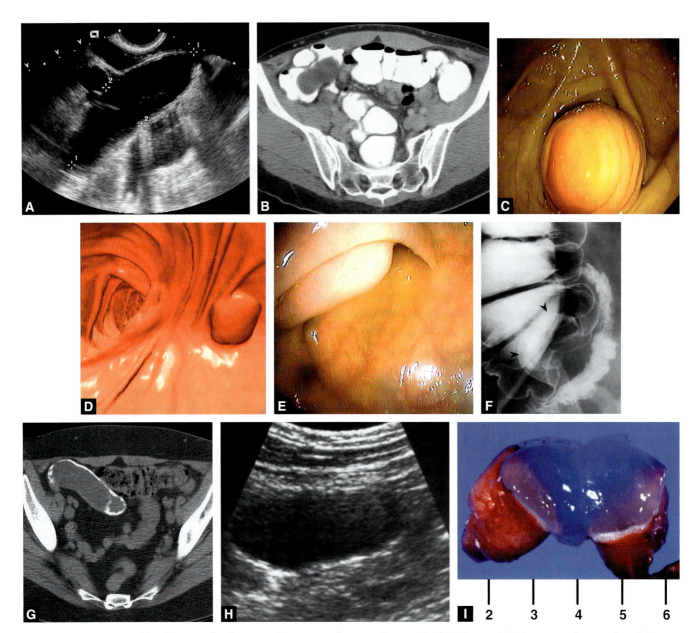

FIGURE 4.2.1 Appendiceal mucoceles from mucinous cystadenoma. Transvaginal US image (**A**) shows an elongated ovoid cystic lesion in the right adnexal region, which was confirmed to represent a mucocele of the appendix at CT (**B**) and colonoscopy (**C**). 3D endoluminal CTC image (**D**) viewed from the cecum from a second patient shows a rounded, 3-cm lesion at the appendiceal orifice. Note the adjacent ileocecal valve. 2D CTC images confirmed a mucocele of the appendix (not shown). Image from colonoscopy (**E**) performed the same day shows only the bulging at the appendiceal orifice. Double-contrast BE image (**F**) from a third patient shows a smooth, broad-based filling defect (*arrowheads*) at the expected location of the appendix. CT image (**G**) from a fourth patient shows a grossly dilated appendix with extensive mural calcification. Transabdominal US image (**H**) from a final patient shows an elongated cystic structure in the right lower quadrant. The surgical specimen (**I**) in this case demonstrates mucinous contents of the lesion.

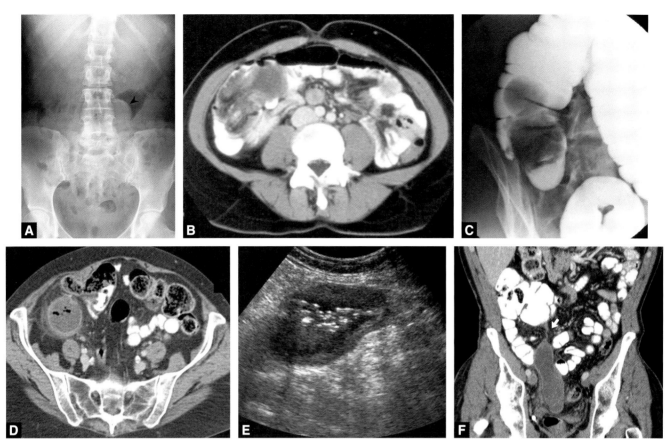

FIGURE 4.2.2 **Acute presentation of appendiceal mucoceles.** Conventional radiograph (A) shows a rounded mass projecting into the distal transverse colon with a subtle rim of calcification (*arrowhead*). Contrast-enhanced CT (B) and BE (C) images confirm intussusception due to an appendiceal mucocele, which has been partially reduced back to the ascending colon. Contrast-enhanced CT (D) and US (E) images from a second patient show a thick-walled mucocele with internal gas bubbles and surrounding inflammatory changes. Superinfection of a mucinous cystadenocarcinoma was found at surgery. Curved reformatted coronal CT image (F) from a third patient shows a large mucocele that has twisted on the pedicle (*arrow*) connecting it to the cecum. Note the surrounding inflammation. A torsed mucocele was confirmed at surgery. *(A to C from Pickhardt PJ, Levy AD, Rohrmann CA, Kende AI: Primary neoplasms of the appendix: Radiologic spectrum of disease with pathologic correlation. Radiographics 2003; 23:645-662.)*

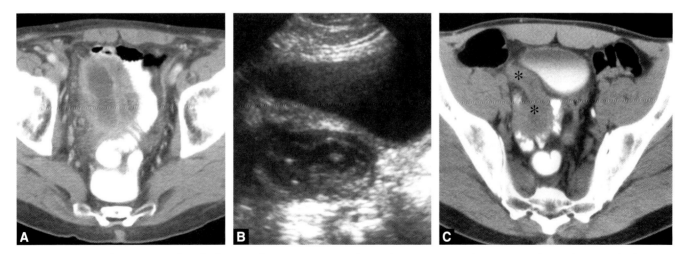

FIGURE 4.2.3 **Primary appendiceal adenocarcinoma.** Contrast-enhanced CT image (A) shows a complex, enhancing thick-walled mucocele from mucinous cystadenocarcinoma. Invasion of adjacent structures is suggested. Transabdominal US image (B) from a second patient shows a similar-appearing complex thick-walled mucocele posterior to the bladder, which also proved to be from mucinous cystadenocarcinoma. Contrast-enhanced CT image (C) from a third patient shows marked soft tissue thickening of the appendix (*asterisks*) with a bulbous mass projecting from its distal aspect. This proved to be a colonic-type adenocarcinoma of the appendix, which is much less common than mucinous tumors.

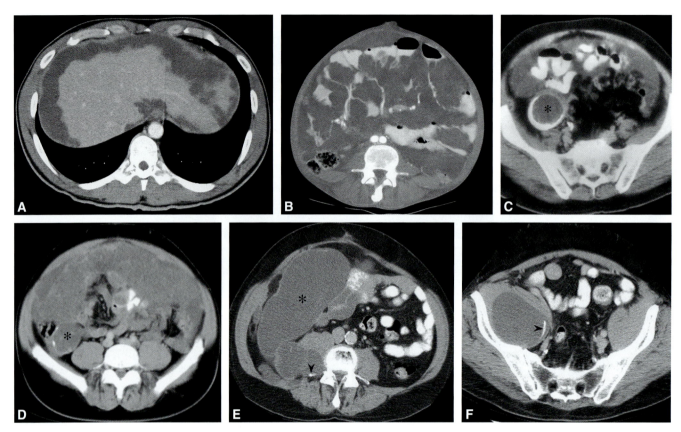

FIGURE 4.2.4 **Pseudomyxoma peritonei and retroperitonei (from mucinous adenocarcinoma).** Contrast-enhanced CT image (**A**) shows scalloping of the liver by complex loculated low-attenuation fluid collections. Similar mucinous material with mass effect was present throughout the peritoneal cavity. Contrast-enhanced CT image (**B**) from a second patient shows loculated low-attenuation peritoneal collections distending the abdomen. CT images (**C** and **D**) from two different patients show nonspecific findings of peritoneal carcinomatosis, but the persistence of rim calcified appendiceal mucoceles (*asterisks*) indicates the underlying cause. Contrast-enhanced CT images (**E** and **F**) from a final patient show a massive appendiceal mucocele (**E**, *asterisk*) with retroperitoneal extension (pseudomyxoma retroperitonei) of loculated collections behind the psoas and iliacus muscles. Note areas of rim calcification (**E**, **F**, *arrowheads*).

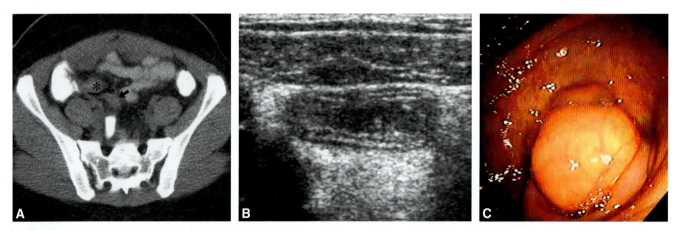

FIGURE 4.2.5 **Carcinoid tumor of the appendix.** CT image (**A**) shows diffuse thickening of the appendix (*asterisk*) from infiltration by carcinoid tumor. Direct mesenteric spread is present (*arrow*), which is extremely rare for appendiceal carcinoid tumors. US image (**B**) from a second patient shows a dilated appendix with wall thickening due to obstruction from a carcinoid tumor involving the base. Most carcinoid tumors involve the distal appendix and do not cause obstructive appendicitis. Colonoscopy image (**C**) from a third patient shows another carcinoid tumor involving the base of the appendix.

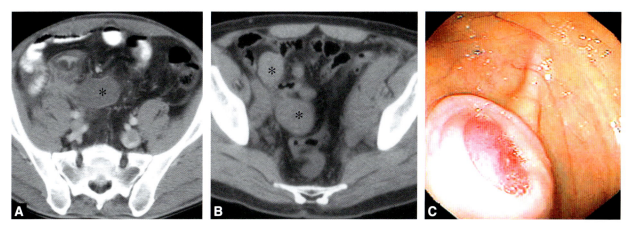

FIGURE 4.2.6 Non-Hodgkin's lymphoma of the appendix. Contrast-enhanced CT image (**A**) from a patient with suspected appendicitis shows prominent low-attenuation enlargement of the appendix (*asterisk*), with infiltration of the adjacent fat. Diffuse lymphomatous infiltration with secondary appendicitis was confirmed at surgery. CT image (**B**) from a second patient shows massive soft tissue enlargement of the appendix (*asterisks*), which is curved but maintains its vermiform shape. Colonoscopy image (**C**) from a third patient shows bulbous enlargement at the appendiceal base with abnormal mucosa protruding from the orifice; the entire appendix was enlarged by lymphoma.

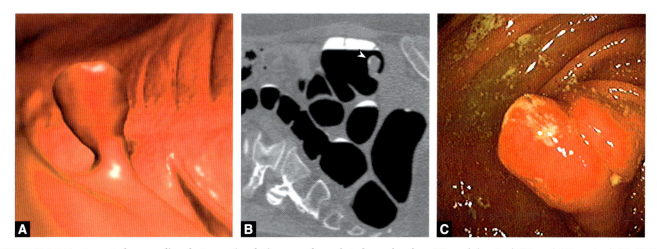

FIGURE 4.2.7 Inverted appendiceal stump simulating a pedunculated cecal polyp. 3D endoluminal (**A**) and 2D sagittal (**B**) CTC images show a pedunculated cecal lesion (**B**, *arrowhead*) that proved to be an inverted appendiceal stump at colonoscopy (**C**).

5. OTHER COLORECTAL CONDITIONS

5.1 Anorectal Disease
(Figures 5.1.1-5.1.10)

CLINICAL FEATURES

- Evaluation of the anorectum can include visual inspection, digital examination, anoscopy, and both rigid and flexible endoscopy.
- Internal hemorrhoids and rectal varices are covered in section 5.3.
- A spectrum of entities can be seen in the setting of rectal mucosal prolapse, including solitary rectal ulcer syndrome, colitis cystica profunda, and inflammatory cloacogenic polyp.
- Disease entities associated with rectal mucosal prolapse have a varied presentation, ranging from incidental endoscopic detection to symptoms including hematochezia, tenesmus, and rectal pain.
- Colitis cystica profunda is a rare disease characterized by dilated mucin-filled submucosal rectal cysts.
- Anal fissures are longitudinal splits in the anoderm and are usually posterior; chronic fissures can lead to hypertrophied anal papillae at the dentate line proximally and tender skin tags at the anal verge distally.
- Perianal fistulas can be characterized as intersphincteric, trans-sphincteric, and translevator; preoperative imaging is sometimes used as a road map to guide surgical intervention.
- Condylomata acuminata (anal warts) are caused by the human papillomavirus, which is usually sexually transmitted; the disease tends to be more aggressive in immunocompromised patients (e.g., those with AIDS).
- Retrorectal cystic hamartomas, or tailgut cysts, may be asymptomatic or present as rectal bleeding or pain with defecation.
- Retained rectal foreign bodies may be classified as low lying and high lying; high-lying objects impacted for more than 24 hours often require laparotomy.

IMAGING FEATURES

- Solitary rectal ulcer syndrome is somewhat of a misnomer, because multiple ulcers or no ulcers may also be present; a polypoid and even villous-like appearance is seen in about 25% of cases.
- Localized colitis cystica profunda manifests as a low submucosal mass due to dilated mucin-filled glands.
- Hypertrophied anal papillae are characterized by their location at the dentate line and their pale appearance; low rectal adenomatous polyps should not be dismissed as anal papillae.
- Inflammatory cloacogenic polyps are also located at the dentate line but appear erythematous and friable.
- Perianal fistulas can be demonstrated by multiple imaging modalities.
- The extent of large condylomas can be assessed at endoscopy and cross-sectional imaging.
- Retrorectal cystic hamartomas manifest as complex cystic lesions in the presacral space.
- Abdominal radiographs are useful for directing the appropriate management of a suspected rectal foreign body.

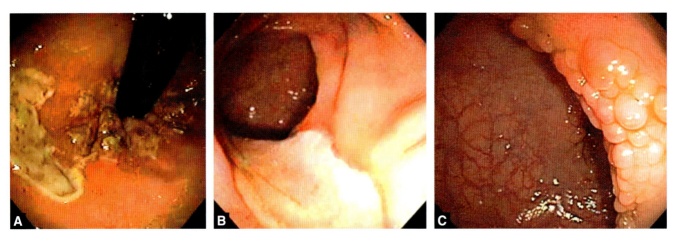

FIGURE 5.1.1 Solitary rectal ulcer syndrome. Colonoscopy images (**A** and **B**) from two different patients show large solitary rectal ulcers. These are classically found along the anterior rectal wall. Colonoscopy image (**C**) from a third patient shows a villous-like polypoid lesion on a rectal fold, mimicking an adenomatous lesion. Diagnosis was confirmed by histopathology.

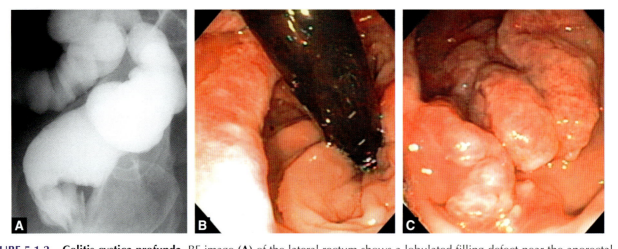

FIGURE 5.1.2 Colitis cystica profunda. BE image (**A**) of the lateral rectum shows a lobulated filling defect near the anorectal junction from dilated mucin-filled submucosal glands. Colonoscopy images (**B** and **C**) from a second patient show irregularly thickened rectal folds.

Illustration continued on following page

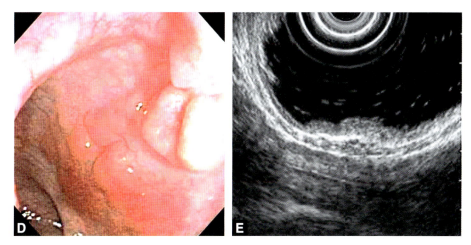

FIGURE 5.1.2 (Continued) **Colitis cystica profunda.** Colonoscopy image **(D)** from a third patient shows a multilobulated rectal lesion just proximal to the dentate line. TRUS of the lesion **(E)** shows thickening of the mucosal layer with subtle tiny cystic areas within the submucosal layer. Obvious cystic spaces may not always be present on endosonography.

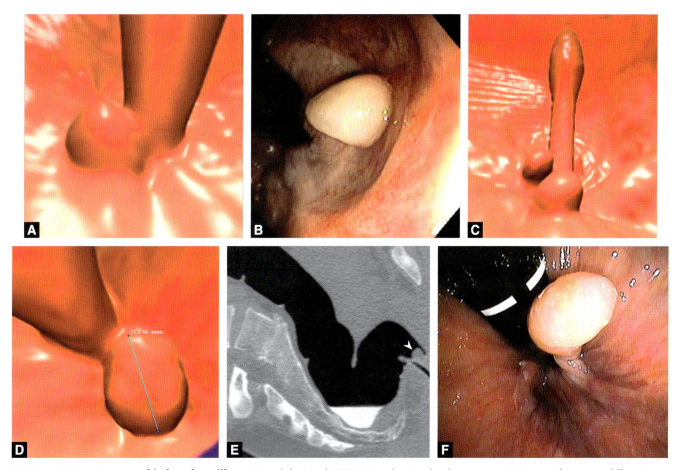

FIGURE 5.1.3 **Hypertrophied anal papillae.** 3D endoluminal CTC **(A)** and optical colonoscopy **(B)** images from two different patients show anal papillae at the dentate line, adjacent to the rectal catheter **(A)** and colonoscope **(B)**, respectively. 3D endoluminal CTC image **(C)** from a third patient shows two anal papillae next to the rectal catheter at the anorectal junction. 3D endoluminal CTC **(D)**, sagittal 2D CTC **(E)**, and colonoscopy **(F)** images show a large hypertrophied anal papilla **(E,** *arrowhead*), which appears pedunculated at colonoscopy.

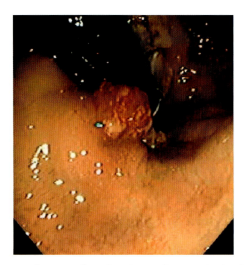

FIGURE 5.1.4 **Inflammatory cloacogenic polyp.** Image from optical colonoscopy shows a small erythematous polyp at the anorectal junction. Note the hemorrhagic mucosa and overlying exudate.

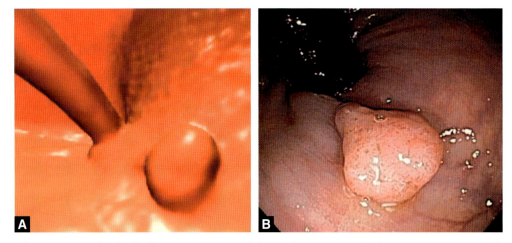

FIGURE 5.1.5 **Adenomatous polyp in the low rectum.** 3D endoluminal CTC **(A)** and colonoscopy **(B)** images show a large rectal adenoma with a characteristic cerebriform appearance at colonoscopy. Note how the lesion is slightly removed from the dentate line at the anorectal junction.

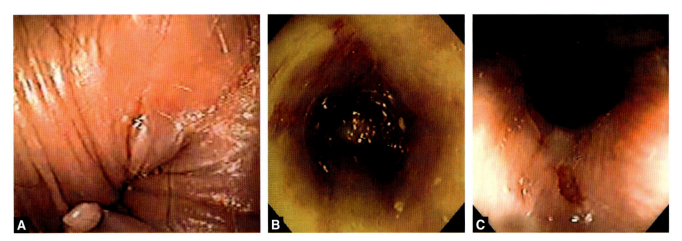

FIGURE 5.1.6 **Anal fissures.** External **(A)** and endoanal **(B** and **C)** views from optical colonoscopy in three patients show longitudinal anal fissures. The skin tag in **A** is a common associated finding.

ANORECTAL DISEASE

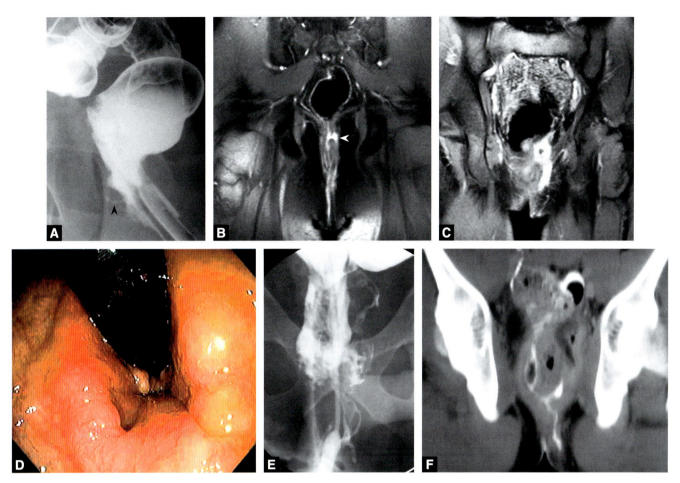

FIGURE 5.1.7 Perianal fistulas. BE image **(A)** and post-contrast coronal MR image **(B)** from two patients with Crohn's disease show transsphincteric perianal fistulas (*arrowheads*). Postcontrast coronal MR image **(C)** and colonoscopy **(D)** images from two additional Crohn's patients show translevator fistulas. Fluoroscopic **(E)** and thick-section coronal CT **(F)** images from a patient with repair for Hirschsprung's disease as a child show a complex postoperative translevator fistula that encircles the anorectum. *(B from Pickhardt PJ, Bhalla S, Balfe DM: Acquired gastrointestinal fistulas: Classification, etiologies, and imaging evaluation. Radiology 2002; 224:9-23.)*

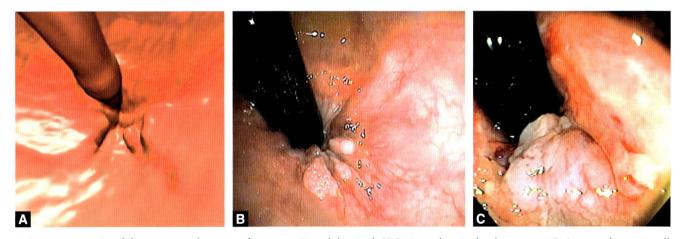

FIGURE 5.1.8 Condylomata acuminata (anal warts). 3D endoluminal CTC **(A)** and optical colonoscopy **(B)** images show a small condyloma at the anorectal junction. Colonoscopy image **(C)** from a second patient shows a larger condyloma.

Illustration continued on following page

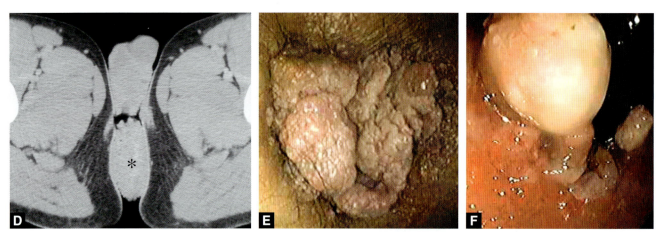

FIGURE 5.1.8 (Continued) **Condylomata acuminata (anal warts).** CT image **(D)** from a patient with AIDS shows a large fungating mass extending from the anus (*asterisk*). External **(E)** and retroflexed rectal **(F)** images from colonoscopy from another AIDS patient show a large verrucous lesion with a prominent rectal component.

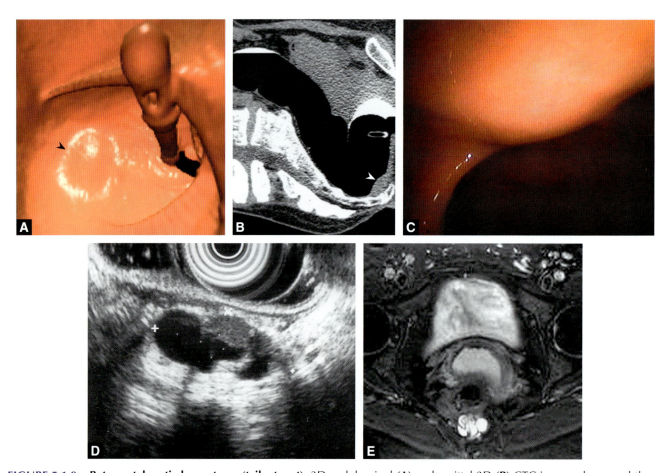

FIGURE 5.1.9 **Retrorectal cystic hamartoma (tailgut cyst).** 3D endoluminal **(A)** and sagittal 2D **(B)** CTC images show a subtle luminal impression (*arrowheads*) on the posterior rectum from a submucosal or presacral lesion. The lesion was initially missed at colonoscopy, but a subtle bulge was confirmed on subsequent flexible sigmoidoscopy **(C)**. The lesion has a complex cystic and solid appearance at both TRUS **(D)** and T2-weighted MR **(E)** imaging and proved to be a retrorectal cystic hamartoma after surgical resection.

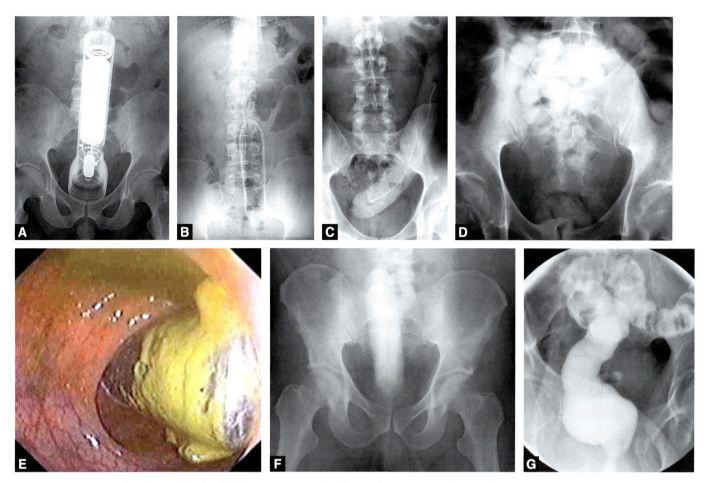

FIGURE 5.1.10 Retained rectal foreign bodies. Conventional radiographs (**A** to **D**) and optical colonoscopy (**E**) from five different patients show retained rectal foreign bodies that came to medical attention, some of which required open surgical intervention. The rounded intraluminal densities in **D** represent multiple cocaine packets, and the object in **E** is a roll-on deodorant canister. Conventional radiograph (**F**) from a sixth patient shows a rectal foreign body of rubber density. Rectal perforation after endoanal removal was confirmed on contrast enema (**G**); note the extraluminal air and contrast extending from the left lateral rectal wall.

5.2 Intussusception
(Figures 5.2.1-5.2.4)

CLINICAL FEATURES

- Intussusception represents invagination or telescoping of one segment of bowel into another.
- Obstructive symptoms are the usual presentation, including abdominal pain, nausea, and vomiting.
- In young children (roughly age 3 months to 3 years), intussusception is commonly ileocolic and idiopathic; fluoroscopic enema reduction is often successful.
- In older children and adults, a pathologic lead point must be suspected with intussusception involving the colon.
- Enema reduction is rarely indicated for adult intussusception because surgical resection is generally necessary.

IMAGING FEATURES

- Reduction of idiopathic ileocolic intussusception in children can be done with air or contrast enemas.
- Intussusception can be suggested on radiographs and confirmed on US or enema, but CT is generally superior for evaluation in adults.
- Identification of mesenteric fat and vessels projecting within a bowel loop is diagnostic of intussusception at CT.
- At contrast fluoroscopy, a "coiled-spring" appearance is classic; at US, a target appearance in the short axis and a "pseudokidney" appearance in the long axis are typical.

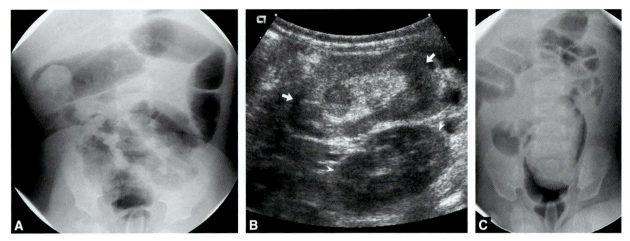

FIGURE 5.2.1 Idiopathic ileocolic intussusception in young children. Fluoroscopic image (**A**) during successful pneumatic reduction of intussusception shows a rounded filling defect at the hepatic flexure, which was easily reduced without recurrence. Longitudinal US image (**B**) from a second child shows the "pseudokidney" appearance of intussusception (*arrows*), with central echogenic mesenteric fat simulating renal sinus and thickened hypoechoic bowel wall simulating renal cortex. Note the actual right kidney (*arrowheads*) posteriorly. Fluoroscopic image (**C**) from attempted air reduction in a third child shows the intussusceptum extending well into the rectum. The intussusception was irreducible and required ileocecal resection.

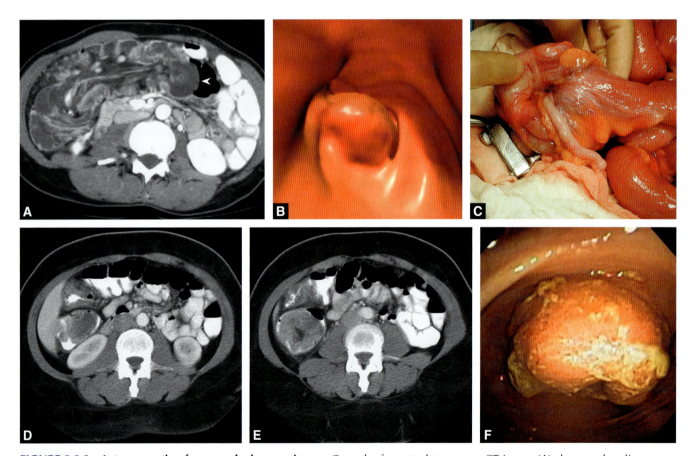

FIGURE 5.2.2 Intussusception from cecal adenocarcinoma. Curved reformatted transverse CT image (**A**) shows colocolic intussusception with mesenteric fat and vessels drawn into the transverse colon. Note the rounded lead mass (*arrowhead*), which can also be demonstrated on a 3D endoluminal view (**B**). At surgery, the intussusception (**C**) proved to be due to primary cecal adenocarcinoma. CT (**D** and **E**) and colonoscopy (**F**) images from two different patients show additional examples of cecal adenocarcinoma acting as a lead mass for intussusception. Note the colonic wall thickening at the hepatic flexure distal to the intussusceptum at CT.

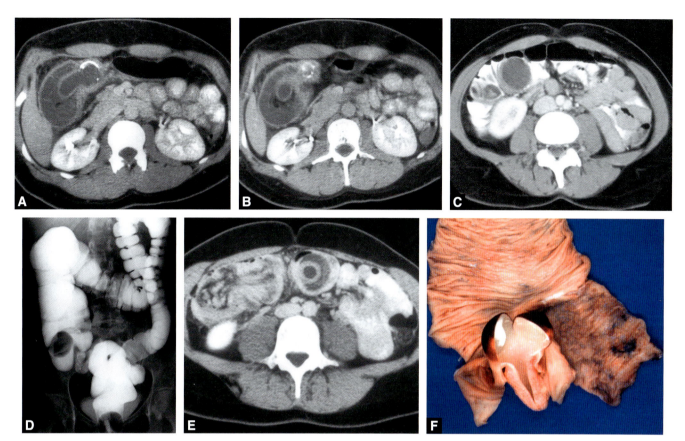

FIGURE 5.2.3 Intussusception from appendiceal mucoceles (mucinous adenomas). Contrast-enhanced CT images (**A** and **B**) show intussusception from a mucocele that can be identified by the presence of curvilinear mural calcification. Contrast-enhanced CT (**C**) and BE (**D**) images from a second patient show a large mucocele that had extended to the transverse colon at CT presentation but was reduced back to the cecum at fluoroscopy before surgery. Contrast-enhanced CT (**E**) and surgical specimen (**F**) images from a third patient show another mucocele that presented as intussusception to the transverse colon.

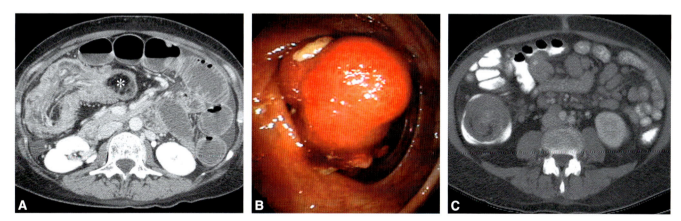

FIGURE 5.2.4 Intussusception from other pathologic lead points. Contrast-enhanced CT image (**A**) shows bowel obstruction due to colocolic intussusception resulting from a colonic lipoma (*asterisk*). Optical colonoscopy image (**B**) from a second patient shows another colonic lipoma acting as the lead point for intussusception. The usual pale yellow appearance is absent due to mucosal edema and erythema. Contrast-enhanced CT image (**C**) from a third patient shows intussusception from ileocecal lymphoma, which is specifically suggested by the presence of extensive abdominal lymphadenopathy.

Illustration continued on following page

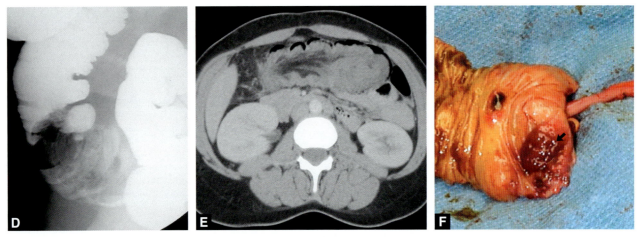

FIGURE 5.2.4 (Continued)   **Intussusception from other pathologic lead points.** BE image **(D)** from a fourth patient shows an intraluminal filling defect with a "coiled spring" appearance due to contrast within the intussuscipiens that outlines the intussusceptum. The lead point in this case was bowel involvement by post-transplantation lymphoproliferative disorder. Contrast-enhanced CT image **(E)** from a final patient shows colocolic intussusception, which at surgery **(F)** proved to be due to a cecal hematoma (*arrow*) related to cocaine use. Note the adjacent ileocecal valve and appendix in the surgical specimen.

5.3 Vascular Lesions

(Figures 5.3.1-5.3.7)

CLINICAL FEATURES

- Angiodysplasia (vascular ectasia or telangiectasia) of the colon is predominantly a right-sided entity that is usually seen in elderly patients, either as an incidental finding or as a source of bleeding.
- Multiple telangiectasias can be seen with certain syndromes or after radiation.
- Dieulafoy-type lesions may present as massive acute arterial hemorrhage.
- Hemangiomas can be solitary, multifocal, or diffuse (hemangiomatosis).
- Cavernous hemangiomas of the colon may be associated with diffuse GI or multisystem hemangiomatosis syndromes.
- Internal hemorrhoids originate above the dentate line and may present as bleeding or prolapse.
- External hemorrhoids are visible at the anal verge and are covered with squamous epithelium; although they do not bleed, they may present as pain related to thrombosis or irritation.
- Rectal varices are associated with portal hypertension, whereas internal hemorrhoids are not; colonic varices beyond the rectum are uncommon.

IMAGING FEATURES

- Vascular ectasia of the colon has a variety of appearances at optical colonoscopy and angiography; brisk bleeding after attempted endoscopic cautery suggests that the lesion is a potential source of blood loss.
- As with diverticular hemorrhage, scintigraphy, angiography, CT angiography, and colonoscopy can all play a role in massive bleeding due to angiodysplasia.
- Dieulafoy lesions manifest as a protruding submucosal vessel with normal surrounding mucosa.
- The presence of phleboliths at radiologic imaging can suggest hemangioma or hemangiomatosis.
- Internal hemorrhoids and varices can be seen at radiologic and endoscopic evaluation.

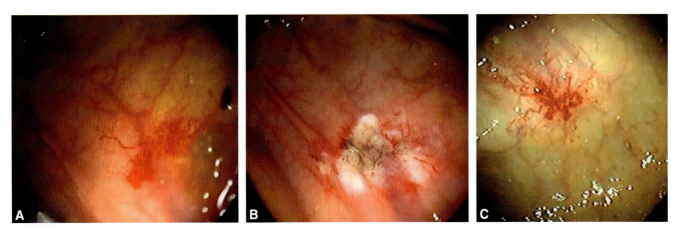

FIGURE 5.3.1   **Colonic angiodysplasia (vascular ectasia).** Colonoscopy images before **(A)** and after **(B)** bipolar electrocoagulation show a radiating cluster of ectatic vessels in the right colon typical of angiodysplasia. Colonoscopy image **(C)** from a second patient shows angiodysplasia that bled briskly upon attempted cauterization **(D)**.

Illustration continued on following page

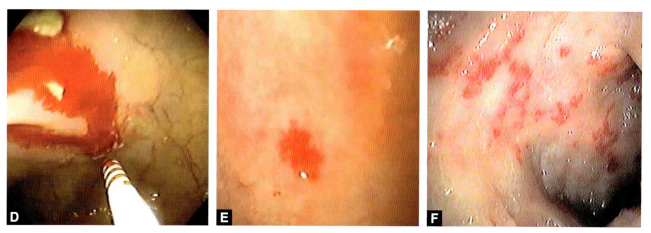

FIGURE 5.3.1 (Continued) **Colonic angiodysplasia (vascular ectasia).** Colonoscopy image **(E)** from a patient with CREST syndrome shows a small telangiectasia similar to the cutaneous lesions seen in these patients. Colonoscopy image **(F)** from a patient with a history of prior pelvic radiation and intermittent rectal bleeding shows multiple rectal telangiectasias.

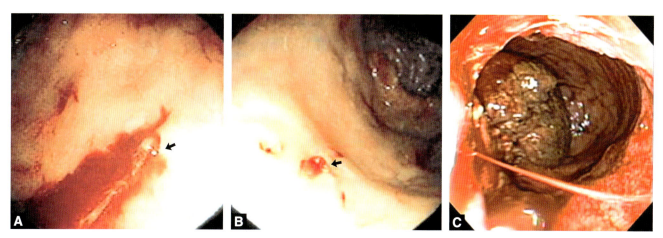

FIGURE 5.3.2 **Rectal Dieulafoy lesion.** Colonoscopy image **(A)** shows active arterial bleeding (*arrow*) near the anal verge that, after treatment with hypertonic saline/epinephrine injection **(B)** revealed a protuberant, visible vessel without surrounding mucosal ulceration (*arrow*). Colonoscopy image **(C)** from an unprepped patient with hematochezia and hemodynamic instability shows active arterial bleeding from another rectal Dieulafoy lesion. Only 5% of Dieulafoy lesions are located in the large intestine and they represent a rare cause of lower GI bleeding. *(A and B from Meister TE, et al: Endoscopic management of rectal Dieulafoy-like lesions. Gastrointest Endosc 1998; 48:302-305.)*

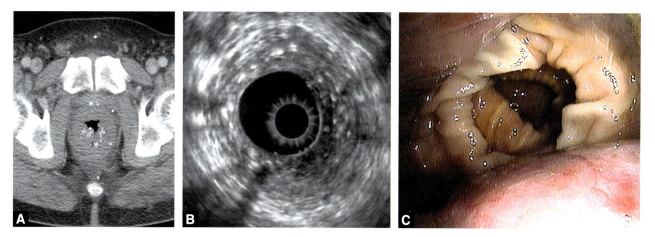

FIGURE 5.3.3 **Colorectal hemangiomatosis.** Contrast-enhanced CT image **(A)** from a patient with Klippel-Trenaunay-Weber syndrome shows circumferential rectal wall thickening associated with multiple calcified phleboliths from hemangiomatosis. Correlative EUS image **(B)** shows rectal wall thickening and multiple echogenic foci representing phleboliths. Colonoscopy image **(C)** shows broad-based submucosal rectal masses with a reddish hue.

Illustration continued on following page

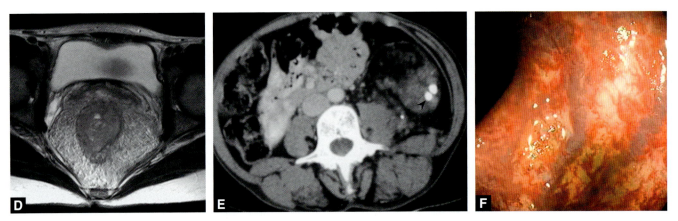

FIGURE 5.3.3 (Continued)   Colorectal hemangiomatosis. MR image (D) from a patient with rectal hemangiomatosis shows extensive circumferential rectal and perirectal infiltration. Contrast-enhanced CT (E) and colonoscopy (F) images from two patients with Klippel-Trenaunay-Weber syndrome show findings of diffuse colonic hemangiomas, with colonic and pericolonic soft tissue infiltration and phleboliths (*arrowhead*) at CT (E) and extensive engorged varicosities and vascular malformations involving the rectum and distal sigmoid colon at colonoscopy (F).

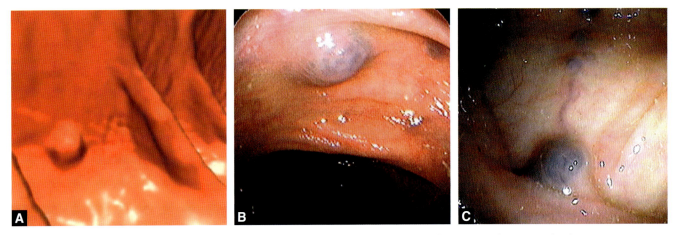

FIGURE 5.3.4   Venous hemangiomas (vascular blebs). 3D endoluminal CTC (A) and corresponding optical colonoscopy (B) images show a smooth poylpoid lesion, which has a characteristic bluish hue at endoscopy. Other similar vascular blebs were seen. Colonoscopy image (C) from a second patient shows multiple such blebs. These are typically incidental findings without clinical significance.

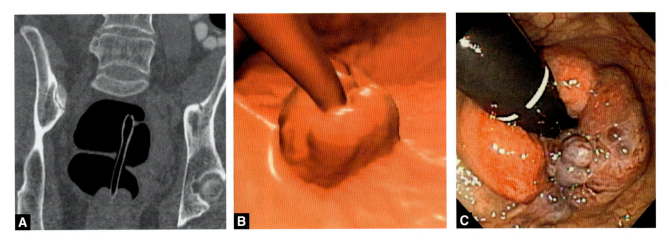

FIGURE 5.3.5   Hemorrhoids. Coronal 2D CTC (A), 3D endoluminal CTC (B) and corresponding colonoscopy (C) images show internal hemorrhoids that form a circumferential mass that encircles the rectal catheter and colonoscope.

Illustration continued on following page

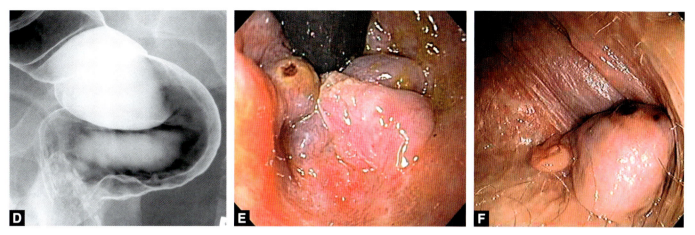

FIGURE 5.3.5 *(Continued)* **Hemorrhoids.** Double-contrast BE image **(D)** from a second patient shows a smooth lobulated filling defect from internal hemorrhoids near the anorectal junction. Colonoscopy image **(E)** from a third patient shows an eschar on an internal hemorrhoid, suggestive of recent bleeding. External image **(F)** from a final patient shows a prominent thrombosed external hemorrhoid.

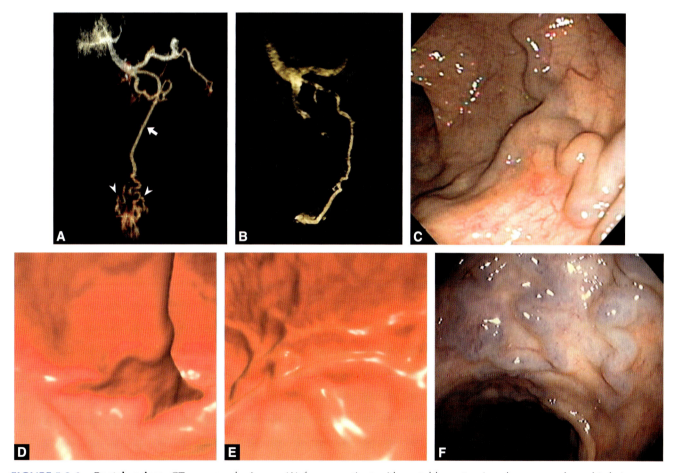

FIGURE 5.3.6 **Rectal varices.** CT venography image **(A)** from a patient with portal hypertension shows an enlarged inferior mesenteric vein (*arrow*) leading to prominent rectal varices (*arrowheads*). MR venography **(B)** from a second patient shows similar inferior mesenteric vein enlargement and rectal varices. Colonoscopy image **(C)** from this patient shows dilated, tortuous submucosal rectal varices. 3D endoluminal CTC **(D** and **E)** and colonoscopy **(F)** images from three different patients show tortuous submucosal rectal veins.

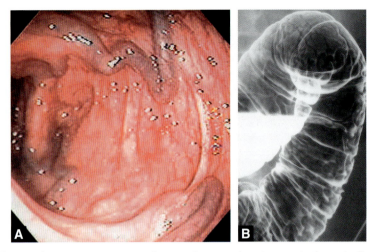

FIGURE 5.3.7 Colonic varices. Colonoscopy image **(A)** shows submucosal varices at the hepatic flexure from venous congestion related to a carcinoid tumor. Double-contrast BE image **(B)** from a second patient shows tortuous submucosal veins centered on the splenic flexure, which were idiopathic in this case.

5.4 Colonic Volvulus

(Figures 5.4.1-5.4.3)

CLINICAL FEATURES

- Colonic volvulus can result in vascular compromise if prolonged and twisted greater than 360 degrees.
- Frequency of segmental colonic involvement is as follows: sigmoid > cecal > transverse > splenic flexure.
- Redundancy and excessive mobility of the involved segment are the major risk factors; a strong association exists between sigmoid volvulus and chronic disabling neurologic and psychiatric conditions.
- Colonic volvulus most often presents as abdominal pain, distention, and constipation.
- Colonoscopic decompression can temporize the acute condition, often avoiding the need for emergent surgery.

IMAGING FEATURES

- Abdominal radiographs are often suggestive of both sigmoid and cecal volvulus.
- The classic radiographic appearance of sigmoid volvulus consists of a "coffee bean" appearance to the dilated air-filled sigmoid colon, which is often oriented toward the right upper quadrant.
- The typical radiographic appearance of cecal volvulus consists of a markedly dilated cecum pointing toward the left upper quadrant.
- "Beaking" of the contrast column near the rectosigmoid junction confirms sigmoid volvulus at contrast enema.
- CT is now generally preferred to more rapidly evaluate for suspected cecal volvulus; sigmoid volvulus can also be efficiently diagnosed by CT.

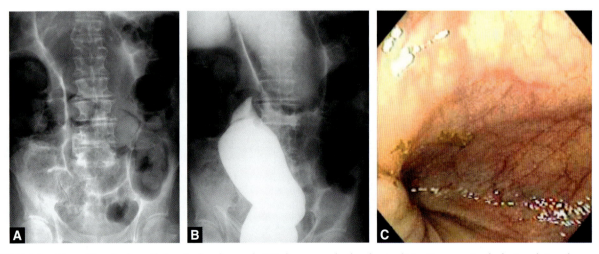

FIGURE 5.4.1 Sigmoid volvulus. Abdominal radiograph **(A)** shows marked colonic distention, particularly involving the gas-filled sigmoid colon centrally. Subsequent BE image **(B)** shows the classic beak sign as the column of rectal contrast reaches the point of sigmoid volvulus. Colonoscopy image **(C)** from a second patient shows luminal occlusion from sigmoid volvulus.

Illustration continued on following page

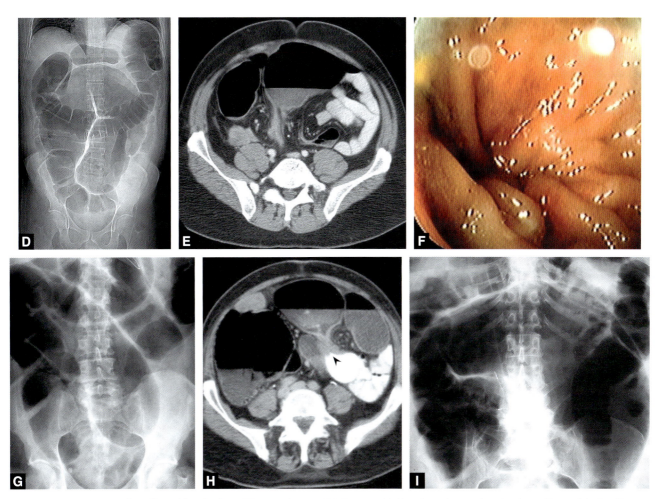

FIGURE 5.4.1 (Continued) **Sigmoid volvulus.** CT scout image **(D)** from a third patient shows the classic radiographic "coffee bean" appearance to the massively dilated sigmoid colon. Proximal colonic obstruction is also present. Corresponding CT image **(E)** shows the region of sigmoid twist. Conventional colonoscopy **(F)** performed for decompression confirms the diagnosis. The patient eventually underwent successful sigmoid resection for recurrent volvulus. Abdominal radiograph **(G)** from a fourth patient shows prominent dilatation of an elongated sigmoid colon. Contrast-enhanced CT image **(H)** with rectal contrast shows the distal point of volvulus (*arrowhead*), which prevents contrast from entering the dilated proximal sigmoid. Abdominal radiograph **(I)** from a final patient shows a massively distended sigmoid colon with a coffee bean appearance occupying the majority of the abdomen. An inferior vena cava filter is incidentally noted.

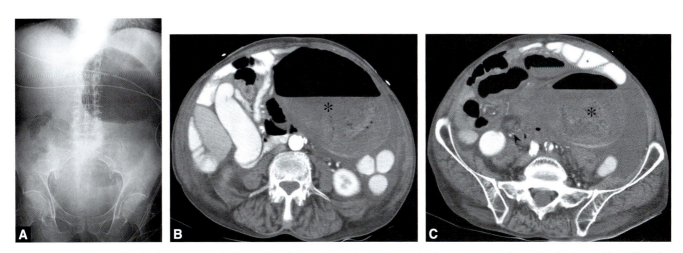

FIGURE 5.4.2 **Cecal volvulus.** Supine abdominal radiograph **(A)** shows the typical appearance of cecal volvulus, with a dilated air-filled cecum projecting toward the left upper quadrant. CT images **(B** and **C)** show a markedly dilated cecum displaced to the left abdomen (*asterisks*). Note the surrounding free fluid, obstruction of dilated contrast-filled small bowel loops, and site of mesenteric twist (*arrowhead*) of the redundant supporting ligament.

Illustration continued on following page

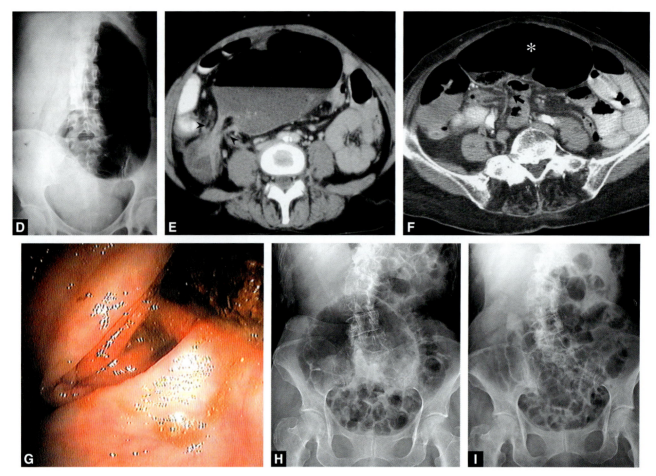

FIGURE 5.4.2 (Continued) **Cecal volvulus.** Abdominal radiograph (**D**) from a second patient shows a massively dilated air-filled cecum projecting over the left abdomen. Corresponding CT image (**E**) shows the dilated air- and fluid-filled cecum distal to the point of volvulus (*arrowheads*). CT image (**F**) from a third patient with an abrupt onset of abdominal pain shows a dilated air-filled cecum (*asterisk*) and crossing mesenteric vessels (*arrow*) related to volvulus. The diagnosis of early cecal volvulus was confirmed at colonoscopy (**G**), where a clear-cut twist was seen at the level of the ascending colon. Patchy erythema without ulceration or dark ischemia was noted within the dilated cecum after endoscopic decompression. Abdominal radiographs before (**H**) and after (**I**) colonoscopy show interval decompression of the dilated cecum. Emergent surgery was averted in this elderly woman.

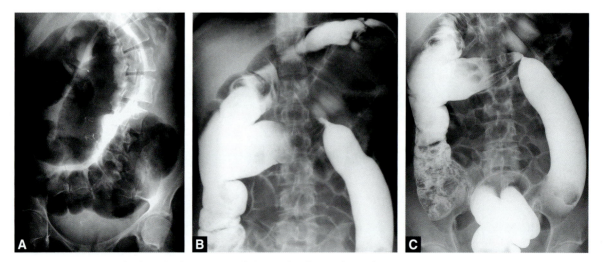

FIGURE 5.4.3 **Transverse colonic volvulus.** Supine abdominal radiograph (**A**) from a patient with underlying scoliosis shows prominent distention of the proximal colon, including an unusual configuration of the transverse colon due to volvulus of this segment. BE images (**B** and **C**) from a second patient show beaking of the contrast column at the splenic flexure, leading to a redundant and dilated transverse colon. Intermittent or incomplete volvulus of the transverse colon allows for passage of some contrast to the right colon.

5.5 Endometriosis

(Figures 5.5.1-5.5.2)

CLINICAL FEATURES

- Endometriosis refers to the presence of ectopic endometrial tissue outside the uterine cavity.
- Symptomatic GI involvement is relatively uncommon; the rectosigmoid region is by far the most common site, followed by the distal ileum and appendix.
- The process begins as serosal implantation on the bowel wall, with variable intramural extension.
- Symptoms, if present, often mimic IBS; hematochezia can be seen with deeply penetrating lesions.

IMAGING FEATURES

- The radiographic features of rectosigmoid involvement range from a focal submucosal mass to an irregular process that closely mimics invasive malignancy.
- At endoluminal imaging, endometriosis typically appears as an extrinsic or submucosal mass lesion; cross-sectional imaging modalities better define the full extent of the lesion.

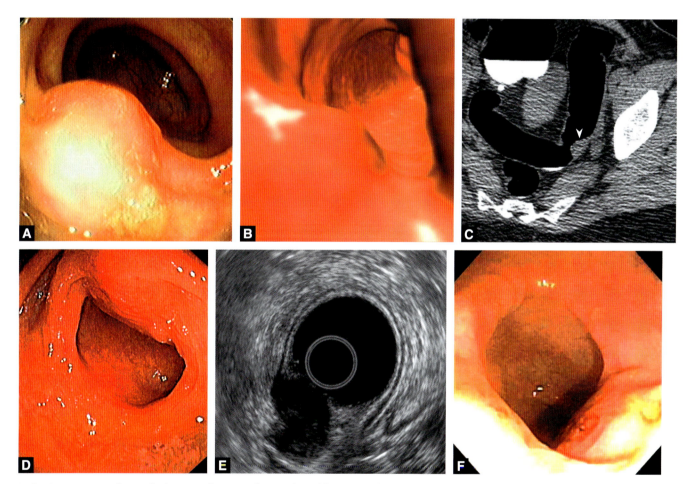

FIGURE 5.5.1 Endometriosis as a submucosal rectosigmoid mass. Colonoscopy image (**A**) shows a smooth, broad-based impression believed to represent a submucosal mass. CTC was performed for further evaluation, which again demonstrates luminal impression on the 3D endoluminal view (**B**). The transverse 2D images (**C**), however, provide additional information on the nature and extent of this soft tissue lesion (*arrowhead*) from endometriosis. Colonoscopy image (**D**) from a second patient shows another broad-based submucosal impression. On TRUS (**E**), a heterogeneous hypoechoic mass is seen invading through the submucosa and into the muscularis propria. Colonoscopy image (**F**) from a third patient with endometriosis shows a submucosal mass with overlying mucosal ulceration.

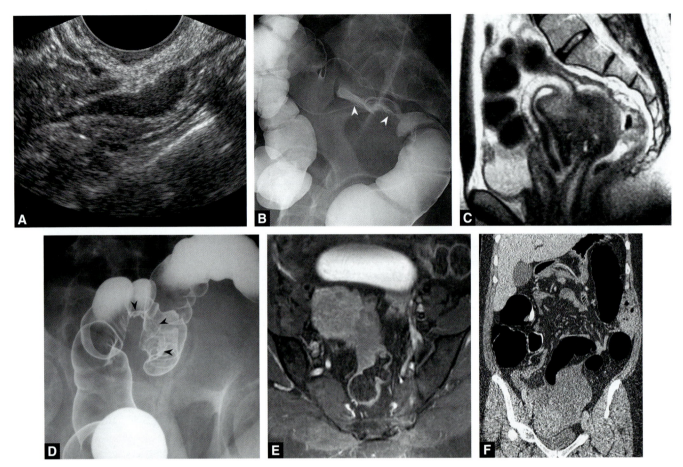

FIGURE 5.5.2 Endometriosis mimicking invasive cancer. Longitudinal transvaginal US image (**A**) from a symptomatic young woman shows a broad-based hypoechoic serosal mass that appears to thicken the muscularis propria layer of the anterior rectal wall. Lateral rectal view (**B**) from double-contrast BE shows irregular eccentric narrowing (*arrowheads*) involving the anterior rectal wall. Sagittal T2-weighted MR image (**C**) shows a low-signal mass centered in the rectovaginal cul-de-sac, associated with a retroflexed uterus. Double-contrast BE image (**D**) from a young woman with rectal bleeding shows fixed eccentric luminal narrowing of the sigmoid colon (*arrowheads*) from the serosa-based process. Contrast-enhanced fat-suppressed MR image (**E**) from a third woman shows massive asymmetrical wall thickening of the rectosigmoid colon. Coronal 2D contrast-enhanced CTC image (**F**) from a patient referred for a suspected submucosal cecal mass at optical colonoscopy shows an extensive peritoneum-based soft tissue mass, which proved to be endometriosis at surgery.

5.6 Pneumatosis Coli
(Figures 5.6.1-5.6.2)

CLINICAL FEATURES

- Primary pneumatosis is a benign condition that typically affects the left colon and consists of submucosal and/or subserosal cystic air collections (termed pneumatosis cystoides intestinalis).
- Secondary pneumatosis is most commonly associated with severe ischemia and necrosis; the gas tends to have a more linear configuration.
- Iatrogenic causes of colonic pneumatosis are typically self-limited in the absence of frank perforation.
- Correlation with the patient's status is critical to avoid misinterpretation of clinical significance.

IMAGING FEATURES

- Benign pneumatosis cystoides is often an incidental imaging finding and manifests as a striking cluster of air cysts in the left colon; the endoluminal appearance at colonoscopy and 3D CTC simulates polyposis.
- At CT, pneumatosis related to ischemia is associated with other findings of vascular compromise; mesenteric and portal venous gas can be an ominous sign in these patients.
- Secondary pneumatosis related to conditions other than necrosis also tends to have a linear appearance.

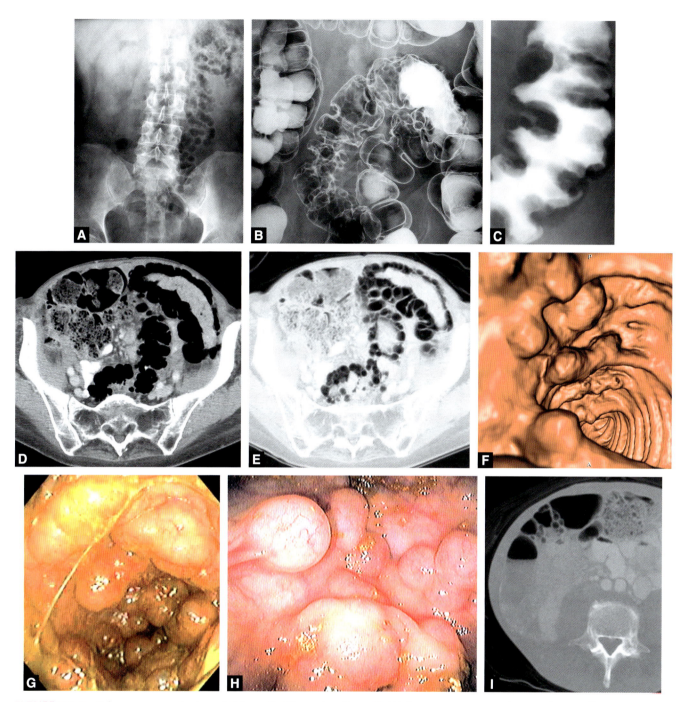

FIGURE 5.6.1 **Primary pneumatosis cystoides coli.** BE scout radiograph (**A**) from an asymptomatic man shows a linear arrangement of air-filled cystic structures in the left abdomen. Double-contrast BE image (**B**) shows that the air cysts are located within the wall of the sigmoid colon, which give a scalloped or polyposis appearance to the lumen. BE image (**C**) from a second patient shows extensive cystic pneumatosis. CT images with soft tissue (**D**) and lung (**E**) windows from a third asymptomatic patient show innumerable air-filled cysts associated with the wall of the left colon. 3D endoluminal CTC (**F**) and colonoscopy (**G**) images from two different patients show the endoluminal appearance of pneumatosis cystoides. Colonoscopy image (**H**) from a final patient shows multiple rounded submucosal lesions in the right colon, which were confirmed to be air filled at subsequent CT (**I**).

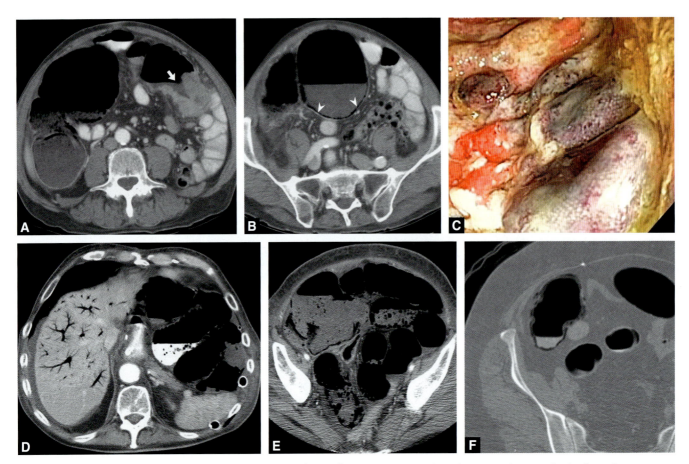

FIGURE 5.6.2 Secondary pneumatosis coli. Contrast-enhanced CT images (**A** and **B**) show prominent colonic distention proximal to an obstructing primary cancer (**A**, *arrow*). Ischemia of the proximal colon is indicated by the presence of linear pneumatosis involving the cecal wall (**B**, *arrowheads*). Colonoscopy image (**C**) from a patient with severe colonic ischemia shows raised areas from pneumatosis with overlying purplish mucosa. This endoscopic appearance is of concern for gangrene and necrosis, requiring surgical intervention. Contrast-enhanced CT images (**D** and **E**) from a patient who had recently undergone esophagectomy show extensive portal venous gas and pneumatosis throughout the small and large intestine. Emergent laparotomy showed nonsurvivable necrosis of nearly the entire gut. Transverse 2D image (**F**) from screening CTC shows linear pneumatosis involving the right colon without gas beyond the bowel wall. The patient remained asymptomatic and no treatment was necessary. This represents a rare incidental finding at CTC that should not be mistaken for perforation.

5.7 Colonic Hernias
(Figures 5.7.1-5.7.4)

CLINICAL FEATURES

- Due to the large caliber of the colon and retroperitoneal fixation of the ascending and descending portions, colonic herniation is much less common than small bowel herniation.
- Left inguinal herniation of the sigmoid colon is most common; a variety of other external and internal hernias can rarely be seen.

IMAGING FEATURES

- Although BE can demonstrate colonic hernias, CT generally provides more diagnostic information overall.
- Sigmoid inguinal herniation can be problematic at both optical colonoscopy and CTC; incarceration of the colonoscope and perforation have been reported.

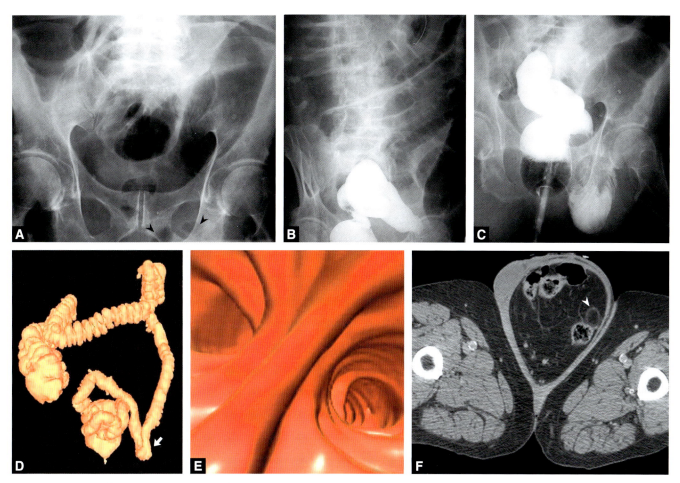

FIGURE 5.7.1 Left inguinal herniation of sigmoid colon. Pelvic radiograph (**A**) from a patient with obstructive symptoms shows dilated bowel and abnormal gas overlying the left inguinal region (*arrowheads*). Subsequent BE images (**B** and **C**) show distal bowel obstruction secondary to inguinal herniation of the sigmoid colon. Note the right colonic thumbprinting suggestive of ischemia. CTC 3D colon map (**D**) from a patient in whom colonoscopy was incomplete due to inguinal herniation of the sigmoid colon (*arrow*). 3D endoluminal CTC image (**E**) from the vantage of the hernia sac shows that the afferent and efferent limbs are well-distended for CTC evaluation. CT image (**F**) from a third patient shows a giant left inguinal hernia that contains sigmoid colon and abundant fat. Note the additional findings of epiploic appendagitis (*arrowhead*).

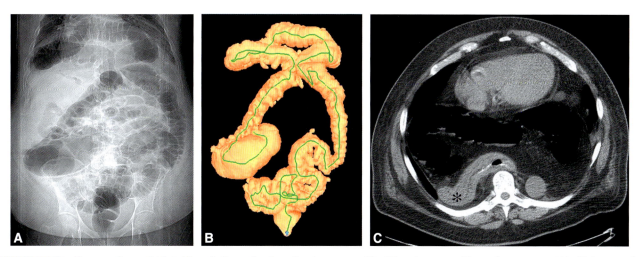

FIGURE 5.7.2 Paraesophageal hiatal herniation of colon. Supine scout (**A**), 3D colon map (**B**), and transverse 2D (**C**) images for CTC from a patient with recent incomplete colonoscopy show a large paraesophageal hernia containing the entire transverse colon, as well as the stomach (*asterisk*). Colonic herniation was the reason for failure to reach the cecum at colonoscopy.

Illustration continued on following page

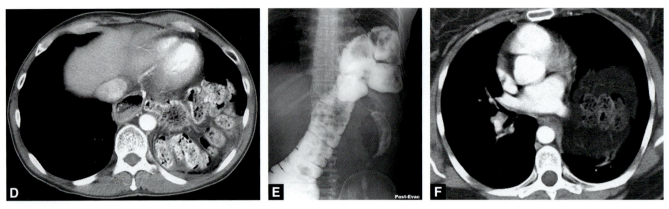

FIGURE 5.7.2 (Continued) **Paraesophageal hiatal herniation of colon.** Contrast-enhanced CT image **(D)** from a symptomatic patient status post–laparoscopic esophagectomy shows suspected hiatal herniation of the splenic flexure, which was confirmed on subsequent BE **(E)**. Note partial obstruction of contrast on this postevacuation image. Contrast-enhanced CT image **(F)** from a third patient shows asymptomatic paraesophageal herniation of abdominal fat and colon.

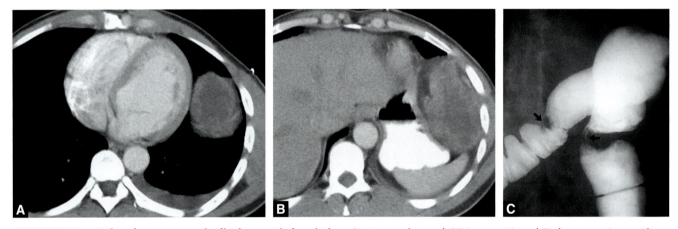

FIGURE 5.7.3 **Delayed post-traumatic diaphragmatic herniation.** Contrast-enhanced CT images **(A** and **B)** from a patient with prior blunt abdominal trauma show diaphragmatic herniation of the splenic flexure, which demonstrates wall thickening and decreased enhancement from vascular compromise. A small left pleural effusion is also present. BE image **(C)** from a second patient shows diaphragmatic herniation of the splenic flexure related to prior trauma, with extrinsic impression of the lumina at the hernia site (*arrows*).

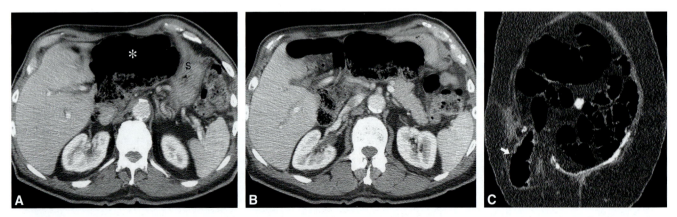

FIGURE 5.7.4 **Other colonic hernias.** Contrast-enhanced CT images **(A** and **B)** from a patient with abrupt onset of epigastric pain show herniation of dilated stool-filled colon **(A**, *asterisk*) into the lesser sac via the foramen of Winslow. Note the lateral displacement of the stomach (S) and mesenteric fat and vessels extending between the portal vein and inferior vena cava (foramen of Winslow). Coronal 2D CTC image **(C)** from a patient with prior incomplete colonoscopy shows parastomal herniation of the cecum (*arrow*) at the site of ileal loop urinary diversion.

Illustration continued on following page

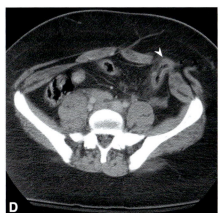 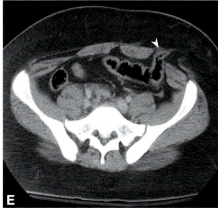 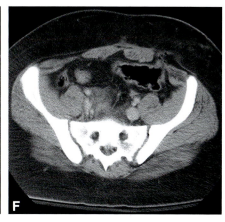

FIGURE 5.7.4 (Continued) **Other colonic hernias.** Contrast-enhanced CT images (**D** to **F**) from a patient with a bicycle handlebar injury to the left lower quadrant show traumatic avulsion of the abdominal wall muscles with herniation of sigmoid colon (**D**, **E**, *arrowheads*). Focal sigmoid wall thickening associated with extraluminal gas bubbles and surrounding inflammatory changes are of concern for focal perforation, which was confirmed at surgery.

5.8 Complications of Colonoscopy

(Figures 5.8.1-5.8.4)

CLINICAL FEATURES

- Reported rates of significant complications at conventional optical colonoscopy range from 1% to 5%.
- Perforation rates are approximately 0.1% for diagnostic colonoscopy and up to 0.4% for therapeutic colonoscopy.
- Other notable complications include hemorrhage and postpolypectomy syndromes.

IMAGING FEATURES

- Although pneumoperitoneum can be identified on conventional radiography (particularly with upright or lateral decubitus views), CT can better assess for suspected complications after colonoscopy.
- Extraluminal gas resulting from colonoscopic perforation is often extraperitoneal, which may be missed on conventional radiographs.
- CT can also evaluate for intramural hematoma, hemoperitoneum, and abscess formation.
- Scintigraphy and angiography may rarely be indicated for persistent bleeding.

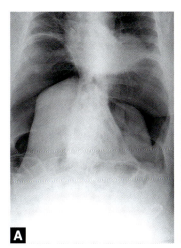 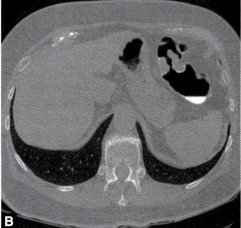 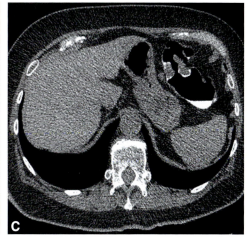

FIGURE 5.8.1 **Colonic perforation at screening colonoscopy.** Upright conventional radiograph (**A**) shows massive pneumoperitoneum from perforation at screening colonoscopy; only the rectosigmoid region was evaluated. Emergent sigmoid colectomy was performed. The patient eventually underwent CTC to complete colonic evaluation; transverse 2D CTC images with polyp (**B**) and soft tissue (**C**) windows show an annular constricting mass at the hepatic flexure.

Illustration continued on following page

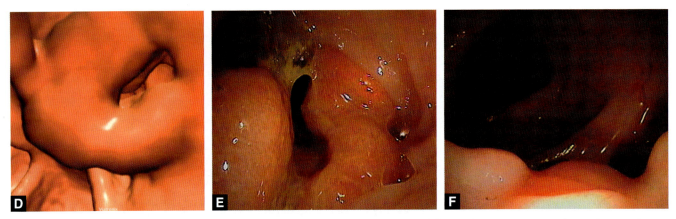

FIGURE 5.8.1 (Continued) **Colonic perforation at screening colonoscopy.** 3D endoluminal CTC image **(D)** shows the annular constricting mass. Subsequent colonoscopy confirmed the primary cancer **(E)** and also demonstrated the anastomotic site from the prior sigmoid resection **(F)**.

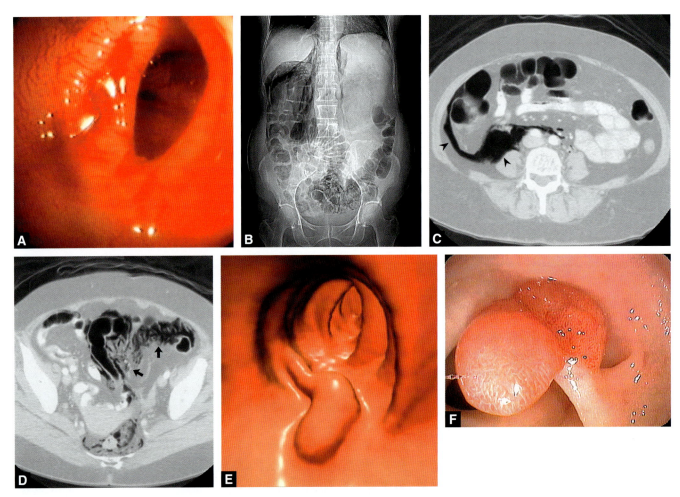

FIGURE 5.8.2 **Colonic perforation at screening colonoscopy.** Colonoscopy image **(A)** from an asymptomatic patient undergoing screening shows a wide-mouth sigmoid diverticulum through which mesenteric fat was directly visible. Scout **(B)** and CT **(C and D)** images show extensive extraluminal gas that extends from the sigmoid mesentery **(D,** *arrows*) into retroperitoneal and extraperitoneal fascial planes **(C,** *arrowheads*). There was no free peritoneal air. 3D endoluminal CTC image **(E)** from a study performed several months after recovery shows a large pedunculated polyp in the sigmoid colon proximal to the point of previous perforation. An advanced adenoma was confirmed and removed at repeat colonoscopy **(F)**.

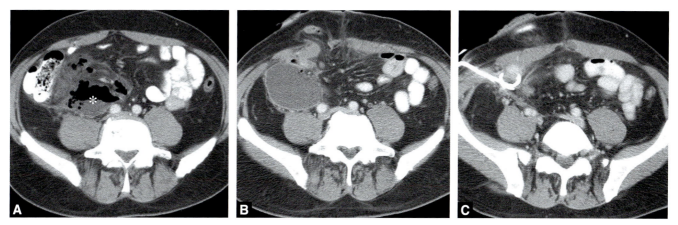

FIGURE 5.8.3 Colonoscopic perforation presenting as delayed abscess formation. Contrast-enhanced CT (**A**) performed 1 week after a negative screening colonoscopy for persistent pain, fever, and leukocytosis shows an abdominal abscess (*asterisk*) adjacent to the right colon. Follow-up CT (**B**) after right hemicolectomy shows a recurrent abscess collection adjacent to the ileostomy, which required percutaneous drainage (**C**).

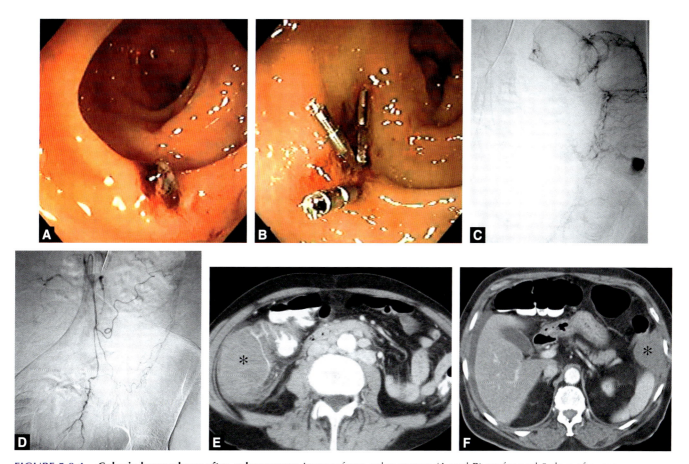

FIGURE 5.8.4 Colonic hemorrhage after colonoscopy. Images from colonoscopy (**A** and **B**) performed 8 days after snare polypectomy show an ulcer with adherent clot and oozing (**A**). The clot was removed and the site was irrigated, revealing an underlying visible vessel. Hemostasis was achieved utilizing the placement of hemoclips (**B**). Catheter angiography image (**C**) from a patient with persistent bleeding after colonoscopic polypectomy shows a dense focus of contrast extravasation within the descending colon. Angiogram of the inferior mesenteric artery after pitressin administration (**D**) shows resolution of bleeding. Contrast-enhanced CT image (**E**) from a third patient shows a large contained intramural hematoma (*asterisk*) involving the ascending colon from recent colonoscopic biopsy. Retroperitoneal lymphadenopathy is present. Contrast-enhanced CT image (**F**) from a different patient after colonoscopic polypectomy shows moderate hemoperitoneum with higher-attenuation blood adjacent to the splenic flexure (*asterisk*) indicating the site of bleeding ("sentinel clot" sign). The perihepatic blood appears closer to fluid attenuation.

5.9 Epiploic Appendagitis
(Figures 5.9.1-5.9.2)

CLINICAL FEATURES

- Epiploic appendagitis is a self-limited condition that results from torsion or thrombosis of one of the fatty appendages projecting off the colonic serosa.
- Clinical presentation can closely mimic diverticulitis or appendicitis.

IMAGING FEATURES

- CT is diagnostic and prevents unnecessary intervention in symptomatic patients.
- Normal epiploic appendages are indistinguishable from adjacent intra-abdominal fat on CT but are easily detectable when inflamed; rarely, evidence of prior appendagitis is seen as an incidental finding.
- On US, the inflamed epiploic appendage appears as an ovoid, hyperechoic mass adjacent to the colon that corresponds to the area of pain.

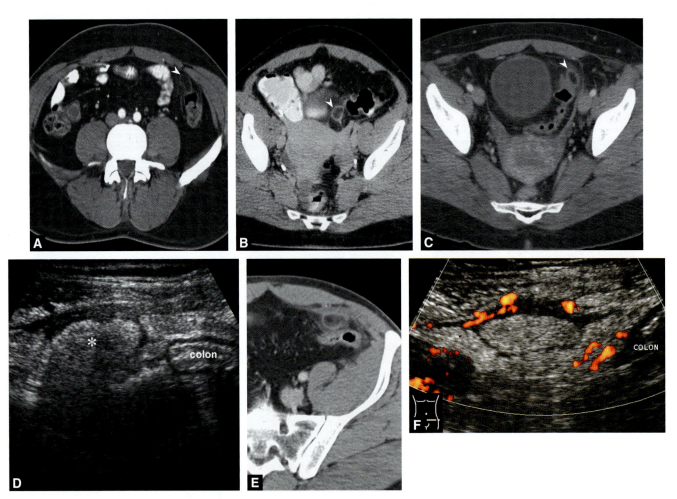

FIGURE 5.9.1 **Epiploic appendagitis.** Contrast-enhanced CT images **(A to C)** from three patients with acute abdominal pain show ovoid fatty structures (*arrowheads*) extending off the serosa of the left colon with rim thickening and infiltration of the surrounding fat. The CT findings are diagnostic of epiploic appendagitis. Transabdominal US image **(D)** from a fourth symptomatic patient shows an ovoid echogenic focus (*asterisk*) extending off the sigmoid colon that corresponded to the area of pain. The diagnosis of epiploic appendagitis is confirmed on CT **(E)**. Transabdominal US image **(F)** from a final patient with epiploic appendagitis shows increased blood flow on power Doppler surrounding the echogenic mass.

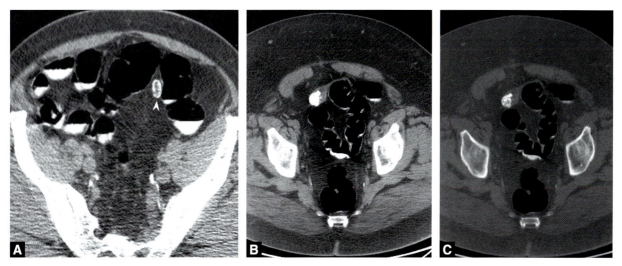

FIGURE 5.9.2 **Incidental detection of old healed epiploic appendagitis.** Transverse 2D CTC image (**A**) from an asymptomatic patient shows evidence of old epiploic appendagitis (*arrowhead*), with dystrophic calcification from fat necrosis. Transverse 2D CTC images with soft tissue (**B**) and bone (**C**) windows from another asymptomatic patient show a complex ovoid structure extending off the sigmoid serosa containing coarse calcification as well as soft tissue and fatty components.

5.10 Melanosis Coli
(Figures 5.10.1-5.10.2)

CLINICAL FEATURES

- Melanosis coli is a brownish discoloration of the colonic mucosa due to accumulation of pigment within macrophages in the lamina propria; it is generally regarded as harmless and reversible.
- The term "pseudomelanosis" may be more appropriate because the pigment has been found to be lipofuscin and not melanin in the benign form.
- True generalized melanosis is a rare paraneoplastic syndrome associated with melanoma that portends a dismal prognosis.

IMAGING FEATURES

- The brownish appearance to the colonic mucosa at endoscopy has no radiographic correlate.
- Mucosal crypts may be nonmelanotic and easily recognized.
- True melanosis related to melanoma manifests as scattered macular black-pigmented lesions.

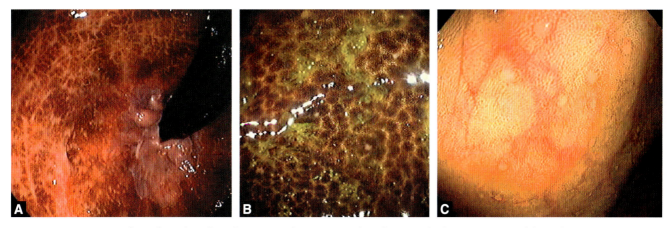

FIGURE 5.10.1 **(Pseudo)melanosis coli.** Colonoscopy images (**A** and **B**) show marked pigmentation of the colonic mucosa. Note the relative sparing below the dentate line. Colonoscopy image (**C**) from a second patient shows multiple lymphoid follicles that are more conspicuous due to the mild pigmentation of the surrounding mucosa.

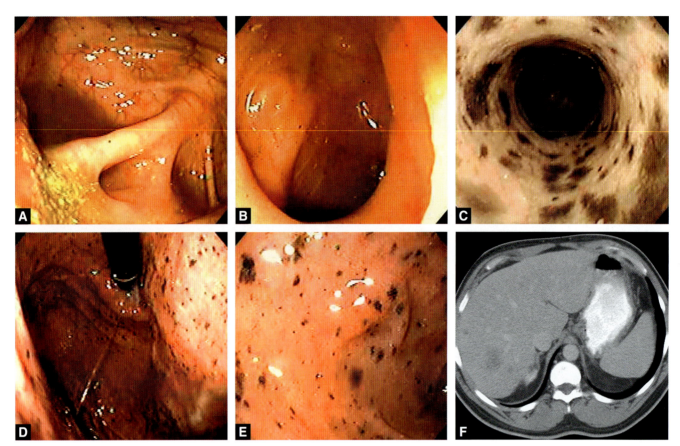

FIGURE 5.10.2 Panenteric melanosis from malignant melanoma. Colonoscopy image **(A)** from a patient with worsening abdominal symptoms shows tiny pigmented foci scattered throughout the mucosa. The ileum was similarly involved **(B)**. The findings were more pronounced at EGD, with dark macules throughout the esophagus **(C)**, stomach **(D)**, and duodenum **(E)**. No GI malignancy was found, but subtle hepatic lesions were seen on CT **(F)**. The patient died of progressive multiorgan system failure within a week of endoscopy. Melanoma involving the nail bed of the right thumb was identified as the primary site at autopsy.

CHAPTER 6

THE BILIARY SYSTEM

Peter J. Chase, MD • Perry J. Pickhardt, MD

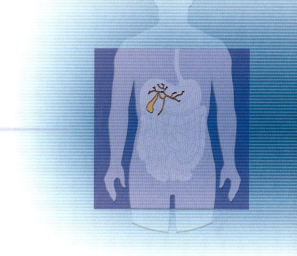

1. **BILIARY TUMORS**
   1.1 Cholangiocarcinoma
   1.2 Gallbladder Carcinoma
   1.3 Periampullary Tumors
   1.4 Metastatic Disease
   1.5 Other Biliary Tumors
2. **BILIARY CALCULI**
   2.1 Cholelithiasis
   2.2 Choledocholithiasis
   2.3 Mirizzi's Syndrome
   2.4 Biliary-Enteric Fistulas
3. **INFLAMMATORY DISEASES**
   3.1 Cholecystitis
   3.2 Primary Sclerosing Cholangitis
   3.3 Ascending Cholangitis
   3.4 Recurrent Pyogenic Cholangitis
   3.5 AIDS Cholangiopathy
4. **OTHER BILIARY CONDITIONS**
   4.1 Choledochal Cysts
   4.2 Caroli's Disease
   4.3 Adenomyomatosis
   4.4 Porcelain Gallbladder
   4.5 Biliary Leak
   4.6 Other Causes of Stricture and Obstruction
   4.7 Hemobilia

Evaluation of biliary disease often requires significant interaction between radiologists and gastroenterologists. US and CT provide simple noninvasive means for initial evaluation of the gallbladder and biliary tree. More detailed evaluation of the biliary system can be performed using a variety of techniques, including noninvasive MR cholangiopancreatography (MRCP) or more invasive approaches such as endoscopic ultrasonography (EUS), endoscopic retrograde cholangiopancreatography (ERCP), and percutaneous transhepatic cholangiography (PTC). The invasive studies allow for diagnostic evaluation as well as therapeutic interventions. Best practice combines the complementary expertise of both specialties to optimize patient care. In this chapter the discussion focuses on biliary tumors, inflammatory diseases of the biliary tree, biliary calculi, and a host of other biliary conditions.

1. BILIARY TUMORS

Most biliary neoplasms are malignant; however, they are often asymptomatic early in the course of disease and have an insidious onset of symptoms. This frequently results in diagnosis at a late stage when surgical resection is not possible. Benign tumors occur but often cannot be reliably distinguished from malignant tumors and generally require surgical resection. CT and US are typically the initial imaging studies performed, with additional evaluation of the biliary tree provided by MRCP and/or ERCP.

1.1 Cholangiocarcinoma
(Figures 1.1.1-1.1.5)

CLINICAL FEATURES

- Cholangiocarcinomas are classified as distal (common bile duct involvement), central (hilar and perihilar; Klatskin), or intrahepatic (peripheral); peripheral cholangiocarcinoma is covered in Chapter 8.
- Most tumors (60% or more) are located in the central region, defined as the level of the common hepatic duct within 2 cm of the right and left hepatic duct confluence; the majority involve the confluence.
- Average age at diagnosis is approximately 65 years; typical presentation includes gradual onset of painless jaundice, weight loss, and intermittent epigastric pain.
- Tumors may be exophytic, infiltrative, or polypoid; most central and distal tumors are infiltrative.
- Major risk factors include primary sclerosing cholangitis (PSC) (often in the setting of inflammatory bowel disease), chronic stasis (e.g., choledochal cysts and Caroli's disease), and liver fluke infestation.
- Tumor spread is primarily via lymphatics and direct extension; hematogenous metastases are rare.

- Outcome is related to tumor stage and location, with peripheral intrahepatic and distal tumors having a better prognosis than central tumors; overall survival is poor due to late presentation.

IMAGING FEATURES

- Cross-sectional imaging typically demonstrates biliary ductal dilatation proximal to the obstructing mass.
- Central tumors tend to be infiltrative and subtle on imaging but may have an exophytic component; delayed enhancement of the tumor can be identified in some cases (also see Chapter 8).
- Cholangiography most often demonstrates a high-grade stricture with upstream dilatation; extrahepatic primary lesions can have an intraluminal polypoid appearance.
- The Bismuth classification is often used to classify hilar and perihilar tumors based on the level of ductal obstruction, which has prognostic significance and guides surgical resection vs. palliative drainage.
- Cholangiocarcinoma of the distal common bile duct may be classified as a periampullary carcinoma.
- Dominant strictures in the setting of PSC should raise suspicion for the development of cholangiocarcinoma.
- ERCP can provide tissue sampling and allow placement of a biliary stent to relieve obstruction.
- MRCP can be used as a "road map" for Klatskin tumors to optimize stent placement for biliary drainage; this can also minimize contrast injection and bacterial seeding of poorly drained segments.
- Distant metastatic disease is uncommon at cross-sectional imaging.

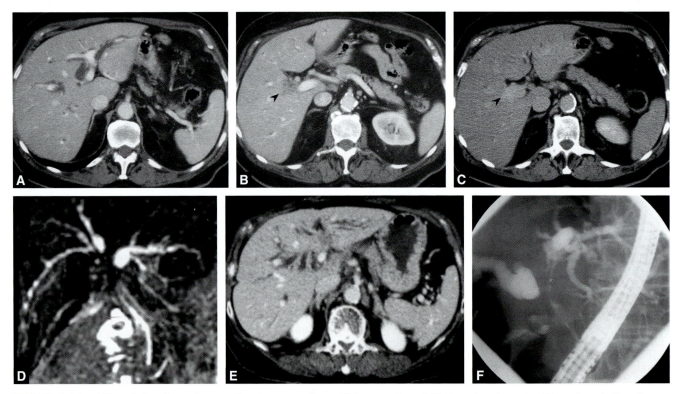

FIGURE 1.1.1 Hilar cholangiocarcinoma. Portal venous phase CT images (**A** and **B**) show intrahepatic biliary ductal dilatation with abrupt termination related to subtle hilar low attenuation (**B**, *arrowhead*). A 12-minute delayed image (**C**) shows increased enhancement in the hilar region (*arrowhead*) relative to the hepatic parenchyma. MRCP image (**D**) shows malignant obstruction of both the left and right main ducts with involvement of the right secondary intrahepatic ducts (Bismuth IIIA). Note the beaded appearance of the dilated intrahepatic ducts from underlying PSC. Contrast-enhanced CT (**E**) and ERCP (**F**) images from a second patient show an abrupt cut-off of dilated intrahepatic bile ducts from a hilar cholangiocarcinoma involving the secondary intrahepatic ducts bilaterally (Bismuth IV); the infiltrative tumor itself is quite subtle on CT.

Illustration continued on following page

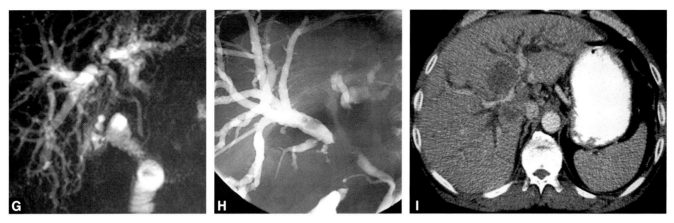

FIGURE 1.1.1 (Continued) **Hilar cholangiocarcinoma.** Corresponding MRCP **(G)** and ERCP **(H)** images from a different patient show an additional example of a Bismuth IV tumor. The left intrahepatic system is not well visualized in **(H)** due to almost complete obstruction of the left main duct, leading to underfilling with contrast. Contrast-enhanced CT image **(I)** from a final patient shows a hilar cholangiocarcinoma with a prominent exophytic component; note the biliary obstruction and vascular encasement from the tumor.

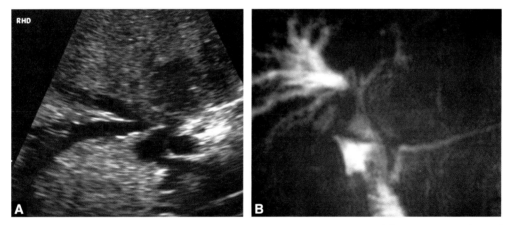

FIGURE 1.1.2 **Focal hilar cholangiocarcinoma.** US **(A)** and MRCP **(B)** images from two different patients show obstruction of the right hepatic ducts from cholangiocarcinoma, with sparing of the left ductal system.

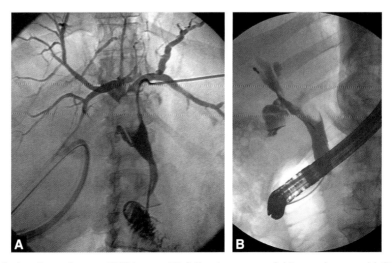

FIGURE 1.1.3 **Polypoid cholangiocarcinoma.** PTC image **(A)** following successful internal-external biliary drainage shows a large polypoid filling defect involving the common hepatic duct with extension to the hilum. ERCP image **(B)** from a second patient shows an elongated intraluminal polypoid mass involving the extrahepatic duct. Gallstones are incidentally noted.

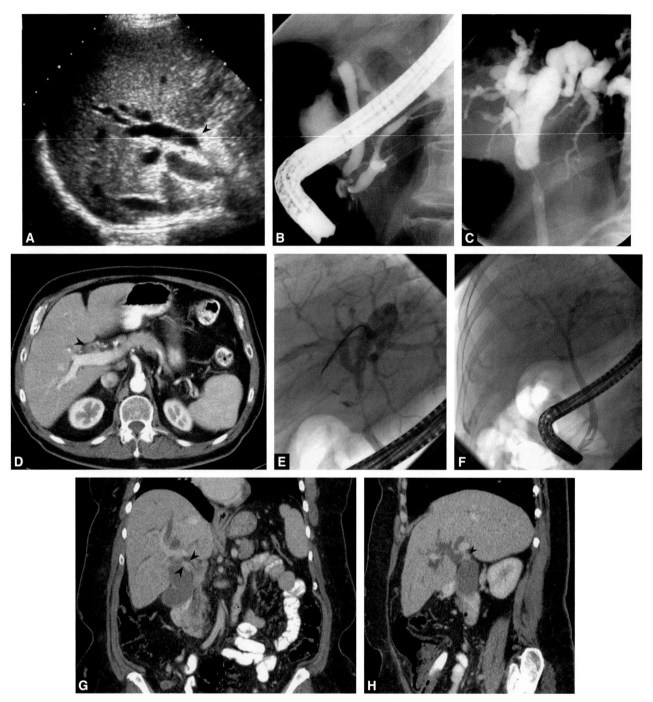

FIGURE 1.1.4 Perihilar cholangiocarcinoma. US image **(A)** from a patient with painless jaundice shows biliary obstruction with abrupt extrahepatic ductal termination (*arrowhead*). Subsequent ERCP image **(B)** of the distal biliary tree shows a normal-caliber common bile duct with an abrupt "shelf" in the common hepatic duct. Further contrast injection **(C)** reveals a high-grade malignant stricture of the common hepatic duct approaching but not involving the markedly dilated intrahepatic system (Bismuth I). Contrast-enhanced CT image **(D)** from a second patient with a Bismuth I tumor shows circumferential wall thickening of the common hepatic duct (*arrowhead*). Intrahepatic biliary ductal dilatation was present on other sections (not shown). Subsequent ERCP image **(E)** shows a 2-cm stricture of the common hepatic duct with proximal intrahepatic ductal dilatation. Note the cholecystectomy clips. Plastic biliary stents were placed across the stricture into the left and right main intrahepatic ducts for drainage **(F)**. Coronal **(G)** and sagittal **(H)** contrast-enhanced CT images from a third patient show focal segmental soft tissue thickening (*arrowheads*) involving the extrahepatic duct near the level of cystic duct insertion, which causes proximal obstruction of the gallbladder and bile ducts.

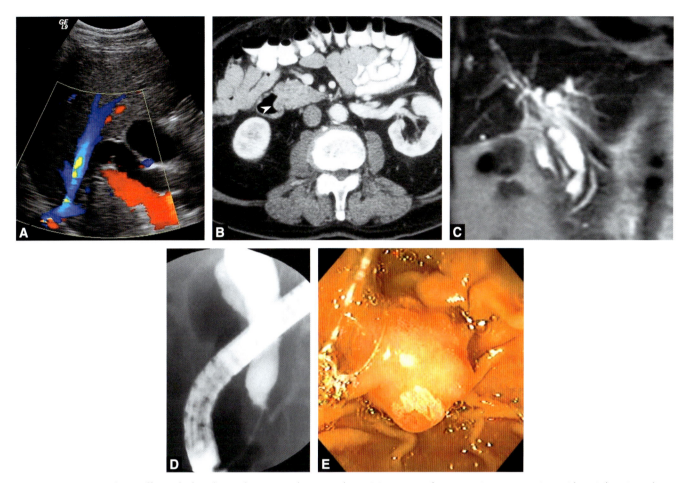

FIGURE 1.1.5 Periampullary cholangiocarcinoma. Color Doppler US image **(A)** from a patient presenting with painless jaundice shows prominent biliary ductal dilatation, which extends down to the common bile duct. Contrast-enhanced CT image **(B)** shows soft tissue fullness in the ampullary region (*arrowhead*), which could be a normal finding in the absence of obstruction. MRCP **(C)** and ERCP **(D)** images show biliary dilatation proximal to an abrupt termination in the distal common bile duct. Endoscopic image **(E)** shows corresponding soft tissue fullness at the major papilla, which proved to be a periampullary cholangiocarcinoma.

1.2 Gallbladder Carcinoma
(Figures 1.2.1-1.2.2)

CLINICAL FEATURES

- The great majority of primary gallbladder malignancies are adenocarcinomas; squamous cell carcinomas and other histologic subtypes are rare.
- Elderly women are most often affected and typically present with chronic right upper quadrant pain and elevated levels of liver enzymes; clinical symptoms overlap those of biliary calculi.
- Risk factors include obesity, female gender, cholelithiasis, chronic cholecystitis, porcelain gallbladder, gallbladder polyps, anomalous pancreaticobiliary union, familial polyposis, and PSC.
- Tumors are most often infiltrative with diffuse gallbladder wall thickening or replacement; polypoid growth is a less common growth pattern.
- Most patients have unresectable disease at the time of presentation, and survival is poor.

IMAGING FEATURES

- US and CT may demonstrate a heterogeneous polypoid mass, irregular focal or diffuse gallbladder wall thickening, direct liver invasion, or complete replacement of the gallbladder.
- The imaging findings overlap with chronic cholecystitis; gallstones are present in up to 85% of cases.
- CT is more accurate for identifying metastatic disease, which most often involves contiguous invasion of the liver, hepatoduodenal ligament, regional lymph nodes, and the peritoneum.
- Cholangiography may demonstrate a stricture in the midportion of the extrahepatic bile duct.
- Porcelain gallbladder may be the initial imaging finding (see section 4.4).

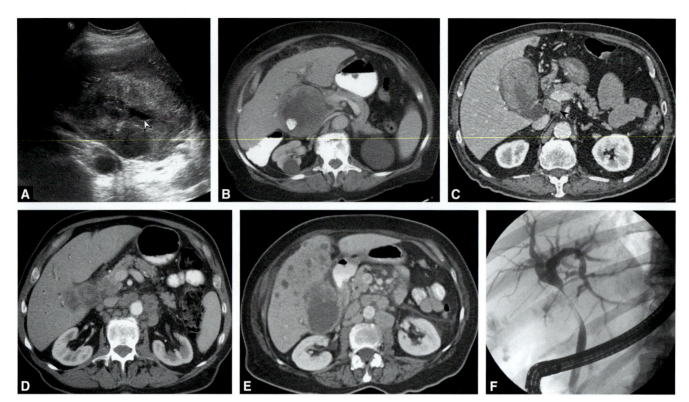

FIGURE 1.2.1 Gallbladder adenocarcinoma. US (**A**) and CT (**B**) images show massive diffuse gallbladder wall thickening, which is heterogeneous and nearly obliterates the lumen on US (**A**, *arrowhead*). Associated cholelithiasis is seen on CT. Contrast-enhanced CT image (**C**) from a second patient shows marked irregular gallbladder wall thickening. An enlarged foramen of Winslow node is seen adjacent to the gallbladder (*arrowhead*). Contrast-enhanced CT images (**D** and **E**) from two additional patients show eccentric gallbladder masses associated with marked lymphadenopathy that extends into the retroperitoneum. Multiple liver metastases are present in **E**. ERCP image (**F**) from a final patient shows tapered long-segment narrowing of the extrahepatic bile duct related to local extension of gallbladder carcinoma.

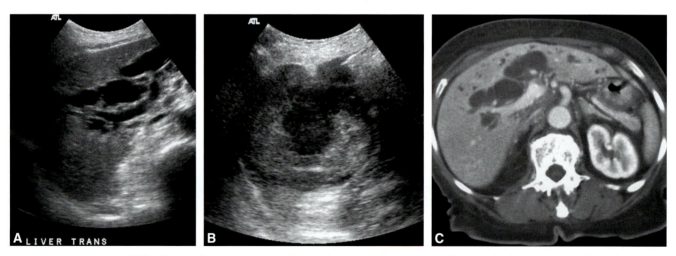

FIGURE 1.2.2 Rare gallbladder carcinomas. US (**A** and **B**) and CT (**C** and **D**) images show marked intrahepatic biliary ductal dilation and massive eccentric heterogeneous gallbladder wall thickening, which proved to be a primary squamous cell carcinoma.

Illustration continued on following page

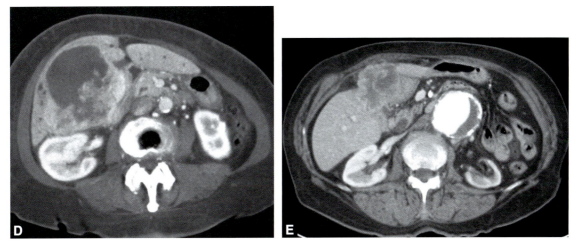

FIGURE 1.2.2 (Continued) **Rare gallbladder carcinomas.** CT image **(E)** from a different patient shows a heterogeneously enhancing gallbladder mass that proved to be a primary neuroendocrine carcinoma. An abdominal aortic aneurysm and left renal atrophy are incidentally noted.

1.3 Periampullary Tumors
(Figures 1.3.1-1.3.5)

CLINICAL FEATURES

- Periampullary tumors (<2 cm from the ampulla) may arise from the ampulla itself, the duodenum, the pancreatic head, or the distal common bile duct.
- Determining the precise origin is sometimes difficult, owing to the close proximity of these structures.
- The most common malignant tumor type is adenocarcinoma; there is likely an adenoma-carcinoma progression that is analogous to that seen in the colon.
- Risk factors of primary ampullary carcinoma include familial adenomatous polyposis and Peutz-Jeghers syndrome.
- Patients may present with obstructive jaundice, weight loss, abdominal pain, and, less commonly, occult or overt GI bleeding.
- Early symptomatology often leads to a higher successful resection rate, either by local excision or pancreaticoduodenectomy (Whipple procedure).

IMAGING FEATURES

- Imaging often demonstrates dilatation of both the biliary tree as well as the pancreatic duct ("double duct sign") with abrupt termination at the level of the mass.
- Due to location and early ductal obstruction, masses are often small and even difficult to visualize by CT or routine US; EUS is an accurate tool for detection and staging of most periampullary tumors.
- Primary ampullary neoplasia can range in endoscopic appearance from nodular overlying mucosa to a large fungating mass with loss of anatomic landmarks.
- MRCP can provide useful preoperative imaging assessment for intraductal tumor extension and local excision.
- ERCP allows for direct visualization of the mass as well as palliative biliary drainage if unresectable.

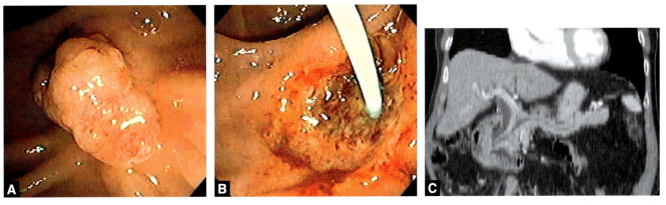

FIGURE 1.3.1 **Ampullary adenoma.** Endoscopic image **(A)** shows an enlarged, nodular ampulla. EUS (not shown) demonstrated involvement limited to the mucosal layer, and a snare papillectomy was therefore performed. Endoscopic image **(B)** 2 days after resection shows a large ulcer with no residual adenoma present. Note the pancreatic stent in place. Coronal curved reformatted CT image **(C)** from a different patient shows a soft tissue mass in the ampullary region resulting in biliary and pancreatic ductal dilatation.

Illustration continued on following page

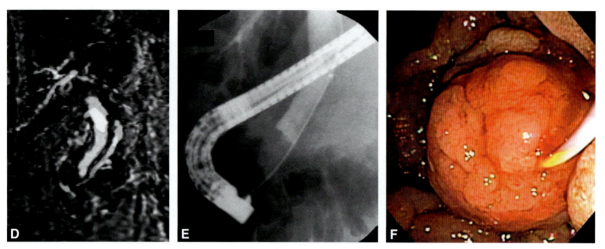

FIGURE 1.3.1 (Continued) **Ampullary adenoma.** MRCP **(D)**, ERCP **(E)**, and endoscopic **(F)** images show biliary and pancreatic ductal obstruction from the lobulated ampullary mass. Extension of the mass into the bile duct appears as a "shelf" in both the MRCP and ERCP images. Histologic examination after pancreaticoduodenectomy revealed a benign adenoma without evidence of malignancy.

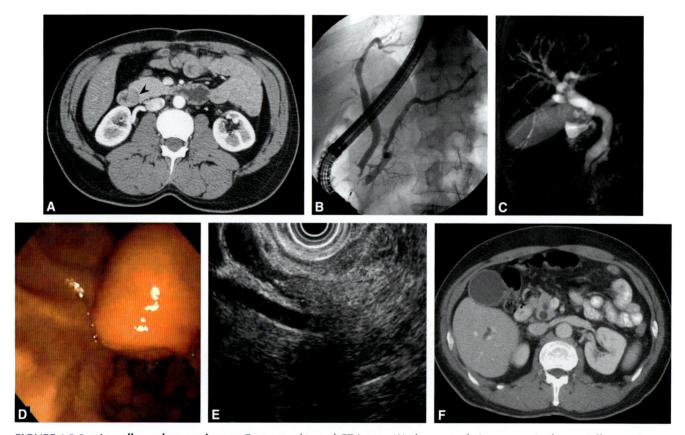

FIGURE 1.3.2 **Ampullary adenocarcinoma.** Contrast-enhanced CT image **(A)** shows a soft tissue mass in the ampullary region (*arrowhead*). At ERCP **(B)**, irregular periampullary filling defects are appreciated, leading to obstruction of the dilated biliary and pancreatic ducts. MRCP **(C)** image from a second patient shows biliary and pancreatic ductal dilation due to an ampullary soft tissue mass; the ampulla appears markedly enlarged at endoscopy **(D)**. EUS image **(E)** shows an irregular mass with tumor extension into the bile duct. Contrast-enhanced CT image **(F)** from a third patient shows prominent biliary and pancreatic ductal dilatation.

Illustration continued on following page

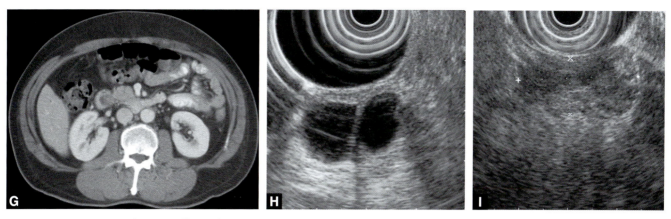

FIGURE 1.3.2 (Continued) **Ampullary adenocarcinoma.** CT image **(G)** inferior to **F** shows an obstructing ampullary mass bulging into the duodenal lumen. EUS images **(H** and **I)** further demonstrate the marked biliary and pancreatic ductal dilatation **(H)** caused by an ovoid, heterogeneous ampullary soft tissue mass invading into the pancreatic head **(I,** *calipers*).

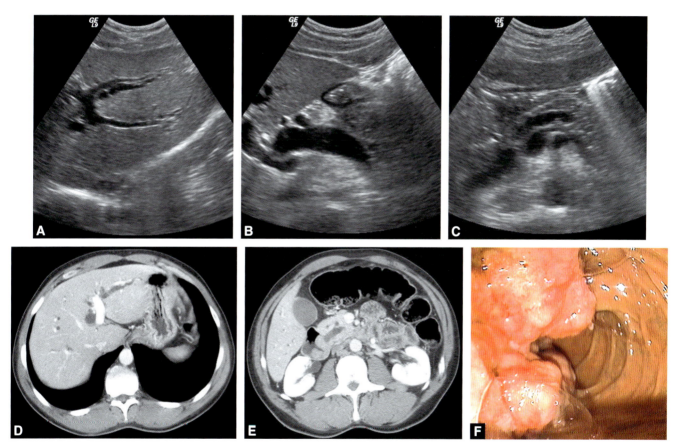

FIGURE 1.3.3 **Periampullary tumor (duodenal villous adenoma).** US images **(A to C)** show marked dilation of the biliary tree and main pancreatic duct. Corresponding CT images **(D** and **E)** show similar findings, as well as a large intraluminal duodenal soft tissue mass involving the medial wall. EGD image **(F)** confirms a duodenal mucosal mass, which proved to be a villous adenoma.

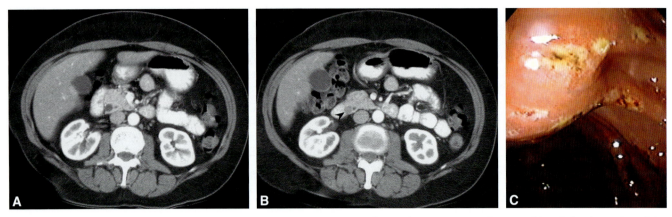

FIGURE 1.3.4 **Periampullary tumor (cholangiocarcinoma).** Contrast-enhanced CT image **(A)** shows a dilated distal common bile duct. On a more inferior image **(B)**, the offending small periampullary soft tissue mass (*arrowhead*) is seen, and it appears as a bulging ampulla at endoscopy **(C)**.

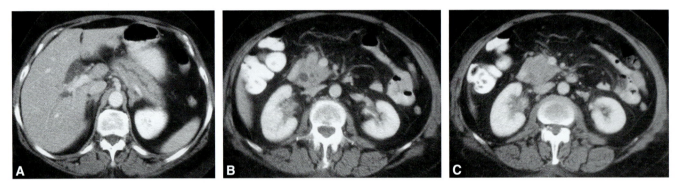

FIGURE 1.3.5 **Periampullary tumor (pancreatic adenocarcinoma).** Contrast-enhanced CT images **(A to C)** show biliary and pancreatic ductal dilatation, which abruptly ends at an ill-defined soft tissue mass within the pancreatic head **(C)**. Endoscopic brushings were nondiagnostic, but pancreatic adenocarcinoma was confirmed by CT-guided biopsy.

1.4 Metastatic Disease
(Figures 1.4.1-1.4.5)

CLINICAL FEATURES

- Hematogenous metastatic disease to the gallbladder and biliary tree is relatively rare; biliary obstruction related to extrinsic metastatic tumor or periportal lymphadenopathy is more common.
- Symptoms are similar to primary tumors and include jaundice, weight loss, and right upper quadrant pain.
- Biliary symptoms in a patient with a history of prior malignancy should raise suspicion.
- Hepatic and pancreatic primaries may spread to the biliary tree by direct invasion.
- Hematogenous spread to the gallbladder is most often seen with melanoma, sarcomas, and lung cancer; colon cancer has a predilection for metastasizing to the bile ducts.

IMAGING FEATURES

- Metastases to the gallbladder and bile ducts are often difficult to distinguish from primary tumors; clinical history of malignancy and presence of extrabiliary metastatic disease are important clues.
- Gallbladder metastases typically appear as polypoid masses.
- Hematogenous biliary tree metastases often appear as intraluminal polypoid masses, whereas extrinsic lesions give rise to strictures; both can result in biliary obstruction.
- Although pancreatic head adenocarcinoma does not represent metastatic disease, it is a common secondary cause of malignant biliary obstruction.

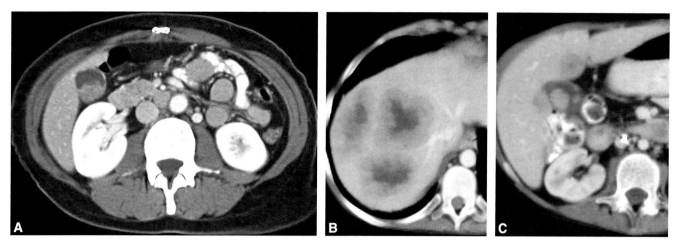

FIGURE 1.4.1 Gallbladder metastases. Contrast-enhanced CT image (**A**) shows a soft tissue mass within the gallbladder from metastatic melanoma. Contrast-enhanced CT images (**B** and **C**) from a child show multiple large, heterogeneous hepatic masses (**B**) and multiple polypoid soft tissue lesions in the gallbladder (**C**) from an aggressive metastatic post-transplant sarcoma.

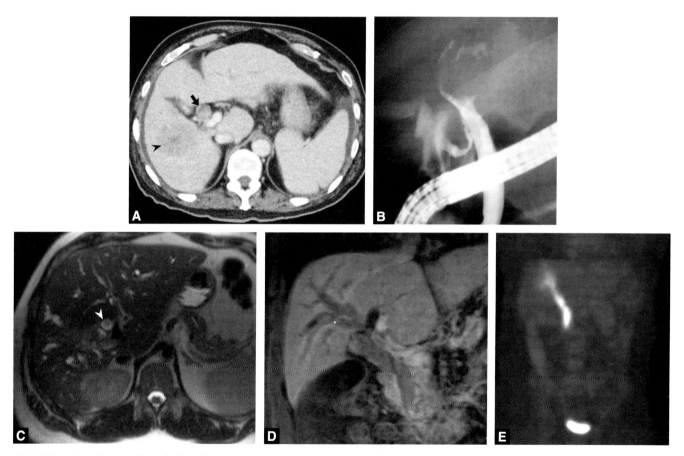

FIGURE 1.4.2 Metastatic colonic adenocarcinoma. Contrast-enhanced CT image (**A**) shows focal heterogeneous soft tissue expansion of the common hepatic duct (*arrow*), as well as a subtle hepatic mass (*arrowhead*). Image from subsequent ERCP (**B**) shows a rounded intraluminal mass in the common hepatic duct. T2-weighted (**C**) and post-contrast minimum intensity projection (**D**) MR images from a different patient show intraluminal soft tissue (*arrowhead*) extending along the entire extrahepatic bile duct and into the right intrahepatic ducts. Subsequent FDG-PET study (**E**) shows hypermetabolic activity corresponding to the abnormal biliary soft tissue, consistent with metastatic disease.

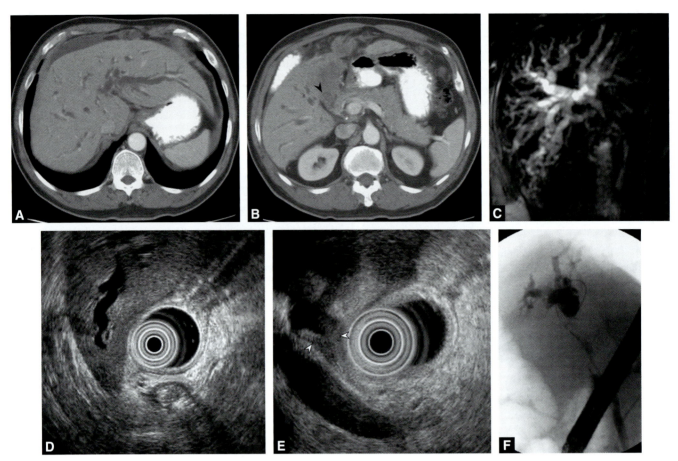

FIGURE 1.4.3 **Metastatic colonic adenocarcinoma.** Contrast-enhanced CT images (**A** and **B**) show marked intrahepatic biliary ductal dilatation leading to an intraluminal biliary soft tissue lesion (**B**, *arrowhead*). Note also adjacent hepatic parenchymal low attenuation. MRCP (**C**) and EUS (**D** and **E**) images again demonstrate the intrahepatic biliary dilatation; the obstructing heterogeneous perihilar mass is also seen at EUS (**E**, *arrowheads*). Note the portal vein adjacent to the mass. ERCP image (**F**) shows a tight common hepatic duct stricture extending to the hilum. A metallic stent was subsequently placed for palliative drainage.

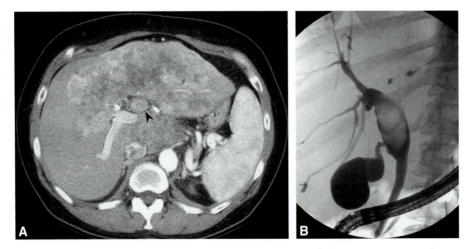

FIGURE 1.4.4 **Direct biliary extension of hepatocellular carcinoma.** Late arterial phase CT image (**A**) from a patient with cirrhosis shows a large, heterogeneous hypervascular mass involving the left hepatic and caudate lobes. Note also the enhancing soft tissue within an expanded common hepatic duct (*arrowhead*), which has a polypoid intraluminal appearance at ERCP (**B**).

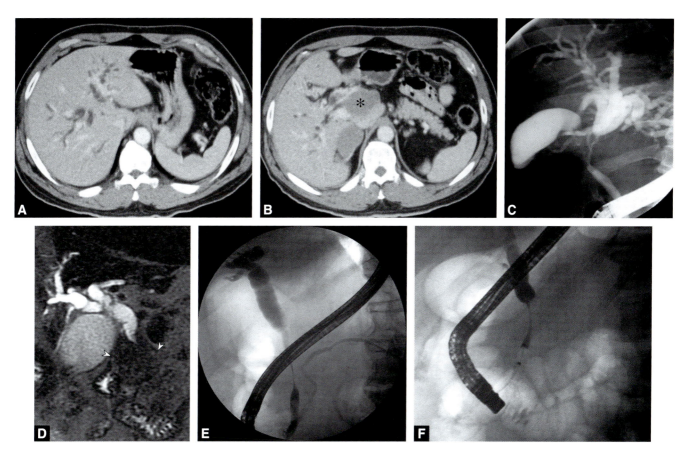

FIGURE 1.4.5 Biliary obstruction from extrinsic malignancy. Contrast-enhanced CT images (**A** and **B**) from a patient with metastatic melanoma show a bulky periportal soft tissue mass (**B**, *asterisk*), which causes upstream biliary obstruction. A right adrenal metastasis is also evident. Corresponding ERCP image (**C**) shows extrahepatic ductal narrowing and proximal dilatation secondary to extrinsic compression from the adjacent mass. MRCP (**D**) and ERCP (**E**) images from a patient with non-Hodgkin's lymphoma show biliary obstruction related to a bulky nodal mass (**D**, *arrowheads*) centered in the hepatoduodenal ligament. ERCP image (**F**) from a patient with pancreatic adenocarcinoma involving the pancreatic head shows long-segment narrowing of the distal common bile duct.

1.5 Other Biliary Tumors

(Figures 1.5.1-1.5.6)

CLINICAL FEATURES

- Biliary cystadenoma and cystadenocarcinoma are rare cystic neoplasms usually involving the intrahepatic bile ducts; they usually present in middle-aged women with abdominal pain and distention.
- Noncystic biliary adenomas may occur in the gallbladder or extrahepatic bile ducts; they are most often asymptomatic, incidental findings but can be associated with periampullary carcinoma.
- Biliary intraductal papillary mucinous neoplasms (IPMN) are rare mucin-hypersecreting tumors analogous to pancreatic IPMN.
- Granular cell tumors are benign neoplasms of Schwann cell origin; most often they affect black women 30 to 40 years of age; they usually present as painless jaundice due to obstruction of the extrahepatic ducts.
- The majority of gallbladder polyps are non-neoplastic cholesterol polyps, and only a small percentage are adenomas; polyps >1 cm are often removed, given the increased potential for neoplasm and malignancy.
- Primary biliary tract malignant melanoma is rare and requires exclusion of primary cutaneous or ocular disease.
- Other rare benign bile duct tumors include fibromas, hamartomas, neuromas, lipomas, and heterotopic pancreatic rests.

IMAGING FEATURES

- In general, it is difficult to distinguish benign from malignant biliary neoplasms by imaging.
- Biliary cystadenomas manifest as multiseptated cystic masses within the liver; the presence of mural nodules and thickened septations is suggestive of cystadenocarcinoma but not diagnostic.
- Biliary IPMN appear as filling defects within dilated ducts on cholangiography, often due to both tumor and thick intraductal mucus; one may see a gaping papillary orifice with extruding mucus on endoscopy.
- Adenomas of the extrahepatic bile ducts are seen as small, smooth filling defects on cholangiography.
- Gallbladder adenomas are best seen by US as a solid, nonshadowing polypoid mass but are difficult to distinguish from cholesterol polyps; subcentimeter polyps can generally be followed with US or ignored if diminutive.

- Primary melanoma of the biliary tree typically manifests as extensive or multifocal intraluminal soft tissue masses, which often expand the ductal lumen.
- Granular cell tumors are small and may be difficult to directly detect by CT or US, but proximal biliary dilatation is usually present; cholangiography typically shows a smooth, short-segment stricture.

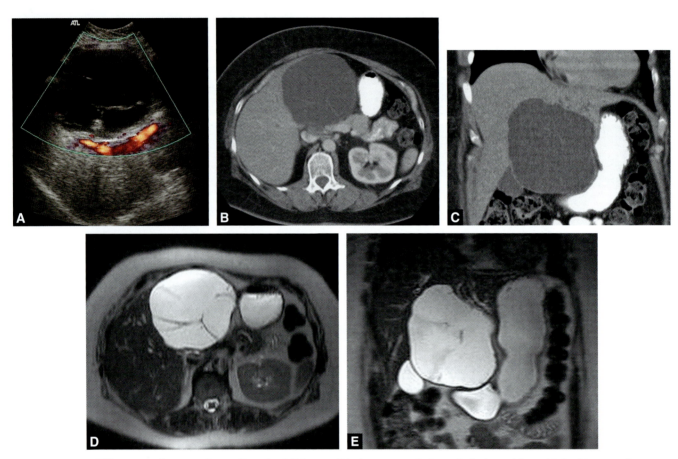

FIGURE 1.5.1 **Biliary cystadenoma.** Power Doppler US image **(A)** shows a cystic hepatic lesion with multiple thin septations. Transverse **(B)** and coronal **(C)** CT images show the location of the large cystic lesion relative to the gallbladder and stomach, but the internal septations are more subtle as compared with US. Transverse **(D)** and coronal **(E)** T2-weighted MR images clearly show both the tumor location and internal septations.

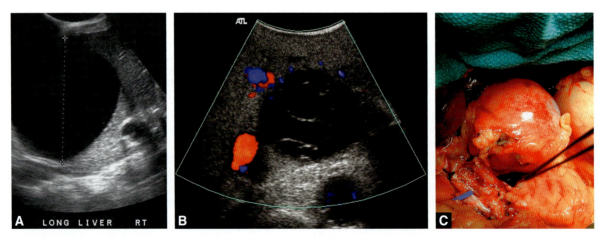

FIGURE 1.5.2 **Biliary cystadenoma.** US image **(A)** shows a large, relatively simple-appearing intrahepatic cyst, which proved to be a biliary cystadenoma. Color Doppler US image **(B)** from a second patient shows a more complex multiseptated cystic lesion, which is a more typical appearance. The lesion was well encapsulated at surgical resection **(C)**.

Illustration continued on following page

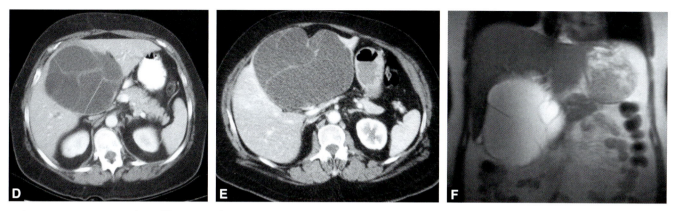

FIGURE 1.5.2 (Continued)   **Biliary cystadenoma.** Transverse CT (**D** and **E**) and coronal T2-weighted MR (**F**) images from three different patients show typical biliary cystadenomas with multiple thin internal septations.

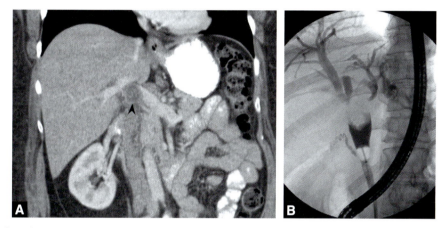

FIGURE 1.5.3   **Intraductal mucinous biliary neoplasm.** Contrast-enhanced coronal CT image (**A**) shows expansion of the common hepatic duct by a heterogeneous low-attenuation mass (*arrowhead*). Image from subsequent ERCP (**B**) shows a large smooth filling defect expanding the common hepatic duct and extending into the left hepatic duct. The small filling defects seen in the left intrahepatic system and distal common bile duct are secondary to thick intraluminal mucus secreted by the tumor.

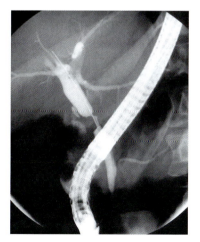

FIGURE 1.5.4   **Granular cell tumor.** ERCP image from a young woman who presented with painless jaundice shows a short-segment high-grade stricture of the extrahepatic bile duct. The remainder of the biliary tree appears normal.

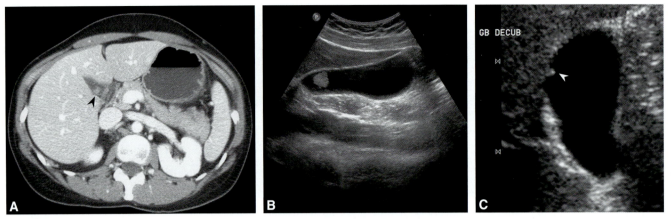

FIGURE 1.5.5 **Gallbladder polyps.** Contrast-enhanced CT image **(A)** shows a soft tissue density lesion (*arrowhead*) near the gallbladder neck. Upright longitudinal image from subsequent US **(B)** shows a nonmobile, nonshadowing 1-cm homogeneous soft tissue polyp within the gallbladder, which proved to be an adenoma. US image **(C)** from a different patient shows a fixed 3-mm gallbladder lesion (*arrowhead*) that represents a small cholesterol polyp.

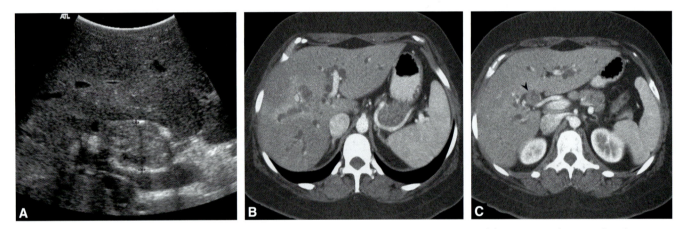

FIGURE 1.5.6 **Primary biliary tract melanoma.** US image **(A)** shows prominent expansion of the common hepatic duct by heterogeneous echogenic soft tissue (*calipers*). Corresponding contrast-enhanced CT images **(B** and **C)** show massive intrahepatic biliary ductal dilatation proximal to the enhancing intraductal enhancing soft tissue mass (**C**, *arrowhead*).

2. BILIARY CALCULI

Biliary calculi, particularly gallstones, are a common condition in most Western populations. Although most cases amount to no real clinical significance, an impressive array of symptomatic conditions and complications are possible and must be recognized.

2.1 Cholelithiasis

(Figures 2.1.1-2.1.4)

CLINICAL FEATURES

- Gallstones are very common, occurring in approximately 10% of the adult population and increasing in prevalence with age; women have a twofold to threefold higher risk of developing gallstones.
- Other risk factors include obesity, hemolysis, rapid weight loss, total parenteral nutrition, ileal resection or disease (e.g., Crohn's disease), pregnancy, certain drugs (e.g., estrogen), and genetic factors.
- Most calculi are composed primarily of cholesterol; pigment stones are associated with hemolytic disorders (black) or ascending cholangitis (brown).
- Most patients are asymptomatic; biliary colic usually manifests as postprandial right upper quadrant pain that is steady, has a gradual onset, and lasts over a number of hours.
- Laboratory tests are typically normal unless there is a complication such as cholecystitis, choledocholithiasis, or cholangitis.
- Treatment is generally unnecessary unless there are recurrent symptoms or complications develop.

IMAGING FEATURES

- US is the diagnostic imaging modality of choice; gallstones are echogenic, produce posterior acoustic shadowing, and move with changes in patient position (unless impacted).
- If the gallbladder is entirely filled with one large stone or multiple stones, a "wall-echo-shadow complex" (WES sign) may be seen.
- Radiographic detection requires a significant calcific component, present in only about 15% of cases.

- CT is somewhat less sensitive than US but much more sensitive than conventional radiography; stone attenuation can be less than, greater than, or equal to fluid density and is often mixed.
- Gallstones generally appear as signal void defects at MR.
- Calculi appear as lucent filling defects on cholangiography and oral cholecystography (which is now only rarely performed).
- Biliary sludge usually appears as nonshadowing dependent debris at US; it occasionally demonstrates a tumefactive appearance.
- Dropped gallstones from laparoscopic cholecystectomy may be identified at CT.

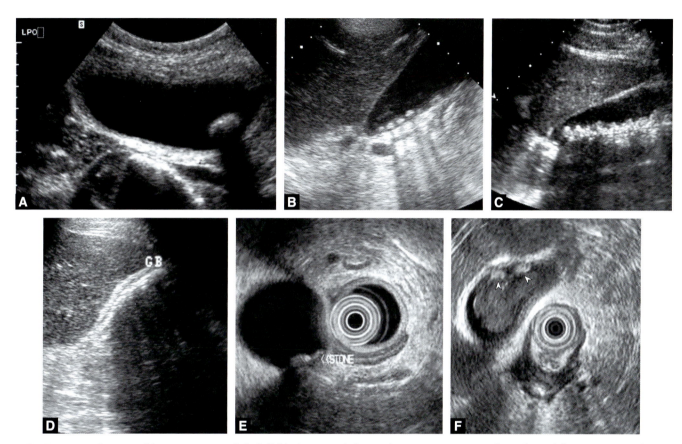

FIGURE 2.1.1 Sonographic appearance of cholelithiasis. Transabdominal US images (**A** to **C**) from three different patients show a single large echogenic shadowing stone (**A**) and multiple smaller calculi (**B** and **C**). Transabdominal US image (**D**) from a fourth patient shows the wall-echo-shadow complex (WES sign) from a single large stone, with alternating echogenic layer from the gallbladder wall, hypoechoic layer from a thin layer of bile, and echogenic shadowing layer from the stone itself. EUS images (**E** and **F**) from two different patients show a solitary echogenic calculus in one case (**E**) and multiple echogenic shadowing stones (**F**, *arrowheads*) adjacent to nonshadowing tumefactive sludge in the other case (**F**).

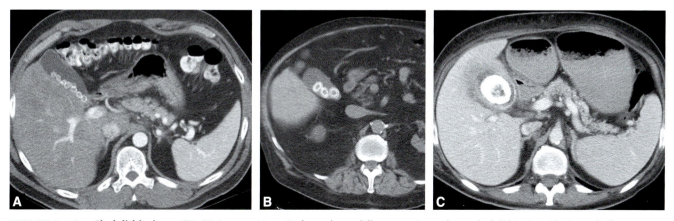

FIGURE 2.1.2 Cholelithiasis on CT. CT images (**A** to **C**) from three different patients show cholelithiasis with rim calcification (**A**), lamellated calcific appearance (**B**), and dense calcification with early gallbladder wall calcification (**C**).

Illustration continued on following page

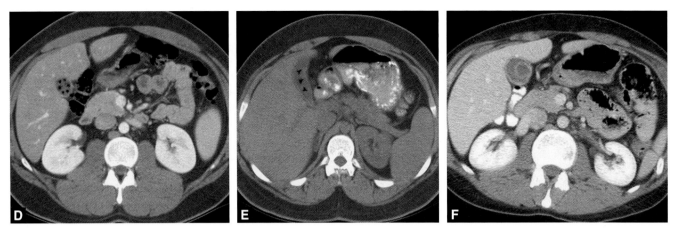

FIGURE 2.1.2 (Continued) **Cholelithiasis on CT.** CT images (**D** to **F**) from three additional patients show low attenuation with central gas density (**D**), internal gas density with a "Mercedes-Benz" appearance (**E**), and fluid attenuation that would render the stone undetectable if not for the soft tissue density rim (**F**).

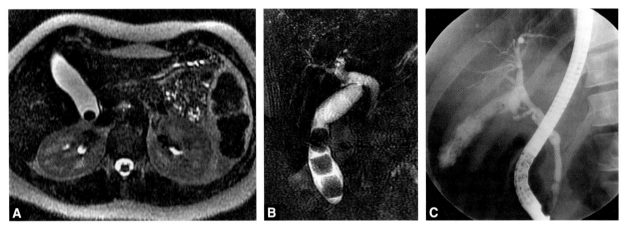

FIGURE 2.1.3 **Cholelithiasis on MRCP and ERCP.** Transverse T2-weighted MR image (**A**) shows a typical rounded signal void calculus within the fluid-filled gallbladder. MRCP image (**B**) from a second patient shows three large faceted gallstones appearing as low-signal filling defects. ERCP image (**C**) from a third patient shows innumerable rounded filling defects from small stones within the gallbladder. Small calculi are generally best seen during early gallbladder filling and may be obscured with more complete filling.

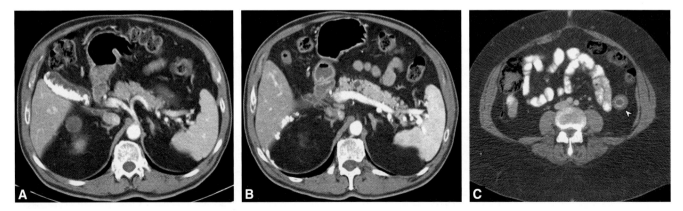

FIGURE 2.1.4 **Dropped gallstones from laparoscopic cholecystectomy.** Preoperative CT image (**A**) shows multiple dense stones lying dependently within the gallbladder. CT image after cholecystectomy (**B**) shows multiple intraperitoneal stones within the hepatorenal fossa. Postoperative CT image (**C**) from a different patient shows a predominantly low-density lamellated intraperitoneal stone (*arrowhead*). Most dropped stones are right sided, with variable amounts of surrounding inflammation.

2.2 Choledocholithiasis
(Figures 2.2.1-2.2.5)

CLINICAL FEATURES

- Choledocholithiasis refers to the presence of stones within the common bile duct.
- Although usually associated with cholelithiasis, it may arise de novo or after cholecystectomy.
- Of patients with cholelithiasis, approximately 15% have choledocholithiasis; of patients with choledocholithiasis, 95% have or have had cholelithiasis.
- Symptoms generally depend on the degree of obstruction, ranging from an asymptomatic state to high-grade obstruction with acute pain and jaundice.
- Unlike cholelithiasis, even asymptomatic common duct stones generally warrant intervention for removal due to feared complications such as pancreatitis and ascending cholangitis (see section 3.3).
- Strictures, stasis, and infection are risk factors for development.

IMAGING FEATURES

- US is often the initial imaging study, and detection of biliary ductal dilation is a suggestive finding; ductal fibrosis may result in a normal duct size in up to 25% of patients with choledocholithiasis.
- US can detect the majority of ductal stones utilizing current imaging techniques; distal common duct stones may be more difficult to visualize secondary to overlying bowel gas.
- Sensitivity of detection with CT depends on stone composition and degree of ductal dilatation; the presence of a crescent of bile outlining a common duct stone is a useful finding.
- Cholangiography with MRCP is highly sensitive (>85%) for ductal stones but may miss smaller calculi—EUS is also highly sensitive (95%), allows for detection of small ductal stones and sludge, and represents a less invasive alternative for ductal evaluation compared with ERCP and PTC.
- ERCP and PTC are both highly sensitive (95%) and also therapeutic, allowing for stone removal and drainage of the biliary tree; PTC is generally performed after ERCP failure.
- At endoscopy, a bulging papilla often signifies impacted distal common duct stones; depending on the underlying cause, stones may appear yellow/green (cholesterol) or pigmented (black or brown).

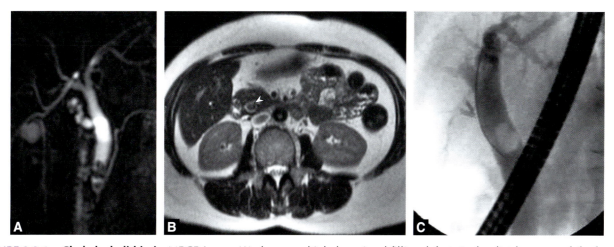

FIGURE 2.2.1 Choledocholithiasis. MRCP image **(A)** shows multiple low-signal filling defects in the distal common bile duct with moderate proximal ductal dilatation. Transverse T2-weighted MR image **(B)** demonstrates one of the stones as a rounded signal void within the dilated common bile duct (*arrowhead*). ERCP **(C)** demonstrates the largest of the stones. All were successfully extracted during the procedure.

Illustration continued on following page

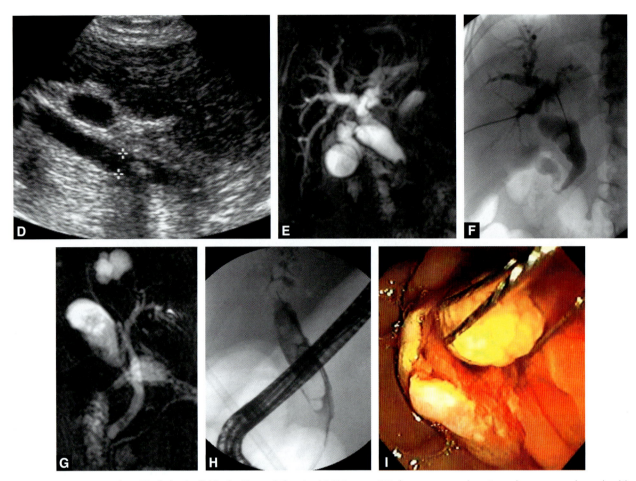

FIGURE 2.2.1 (Continued)   **Choledocholithiasis.** Transabdominal US image (**D**) from a second patient shows a moderately dilated common bile duct (*calipers*) associated with an echogenic shadowing stone. MRCP image (**E**) from a third patient demonstrates massive dilatation of the biliary tree proximal to an abrupt cut-off at a rounded low-signal filling defect in the distal common bile duct. PTC image (**F**) after a failed ERCP confirms the presence of a mobile 15-mm calculus. MRCP image (**G**) from a fourth patient shows two low-signal filling defects in the distal common duct. Gallstones and a large hepatic cyst are also demonstrated. Fluoroscopic (**H**) and endoscopic (**I**) images during ERCP from different patients show common duct stones that were captured and subsequently extracted with a biliary basket.

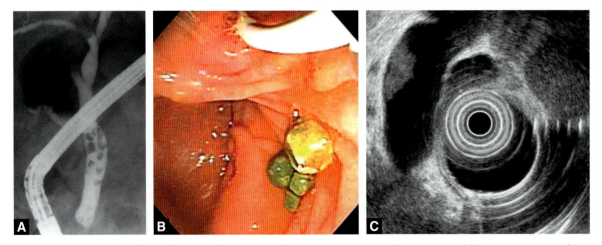

FIGURE 2.2.2   **Choledocholithiasis.** Fluoroscopic (**A**) and endoscopic (**B**) images during ERCP with stone extraction show numerous small polygonal calculi. The green color is consistent with cholesterol stones. EUS image (**C**) from a second patient shows nonshadowing tumefactive sludge in a dilated common duct.

Illustration continued on following page

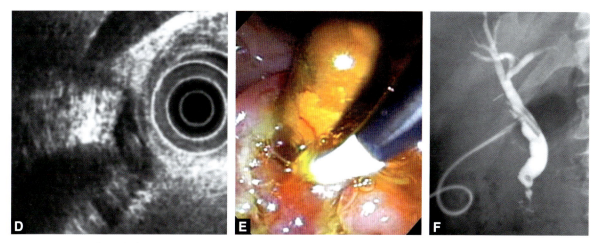

FIGURE 2.2.2 (Continued) **Choledocholithiasis.** EUS image (**D**) in a third patient shows an echogenic shadowing common duct stone, and correlative endoscopic image (**E**) demonstrates the stone during removal. Image from a T-tube cholangiogram (**F**) in a patient after open cholecystectomy shows a retained stone in the distal common duct.

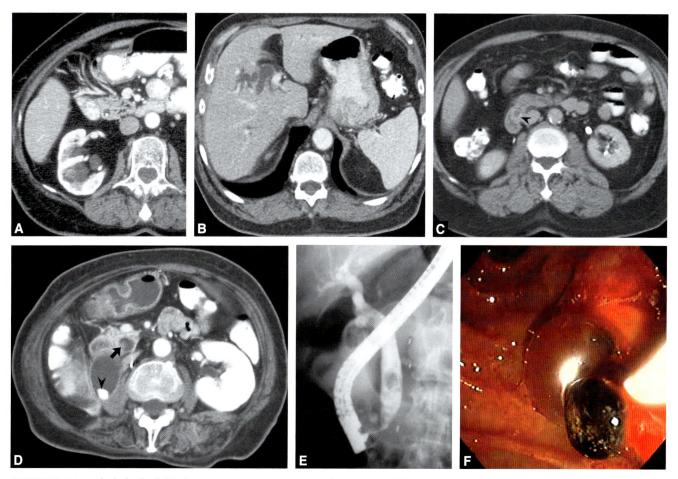

FIGURE 2.2.3 **Choledocholithiasis on CT.** CT images (**A** to **F**) from three different patients show a small calcified stone within a mildly dilated distal common bile duct (**A**), proximal biliary obstruction (**B**) secondary to a subtle rim calcified stone (**C**, *arrowhead*) with a crescent of surrounding bile, and a slightly dense common duct stone (**D**, *arrow*); a dense gallstone is also present (*arrowhead*). ERCP image (**E**) from the third case demonstrates the common duct stone before removal and endoscopic appearance (**F**) after extraction with a retrieval balloon.

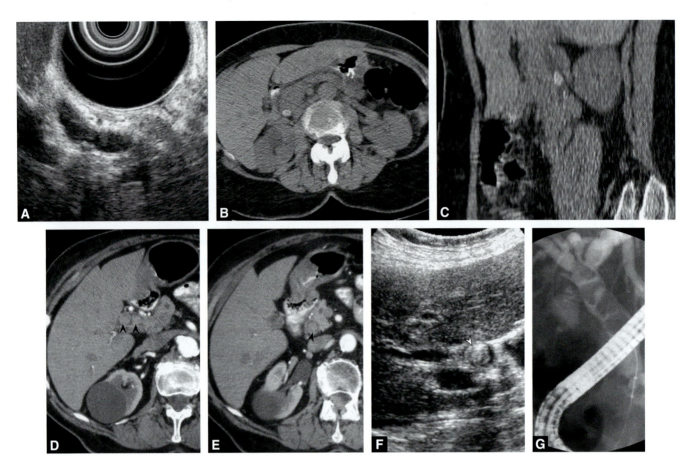

FIGURE 2.2.4 **Asymptomatic choledocholithiasis.** EUS image (**A**) shows a 3-mm echogenic shadowing common duct stone that was incidentally detected. Noncontrast transverse (**B**) and sagittal (**C**) CT images from screening CT colonography show an incidental distal common duct stone. Contrast-enhanced CT images (**D** and **E**) from a third patient show multiple large soft tissue–density stones (*arrowheads*) surrounded by a thin layer of bile, which was an unsuspected incidental finding. Serum bilirubin was within normal limits. Choledocholithiasis was confirmed on US (**F**, *arrowhead*) and ERCP (**G**).

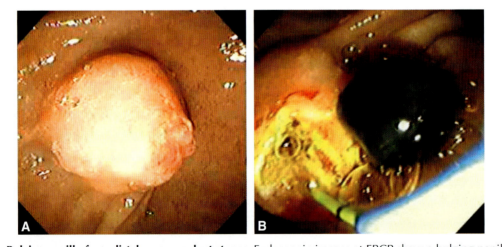

FIGURE 2.2.5 **Bulging papilla from distal common duct stones.** Endoscopic images at ERCP show a bulging papilla (**A**) from a large pigmented calculus (**B**).

Illustration continued on following page

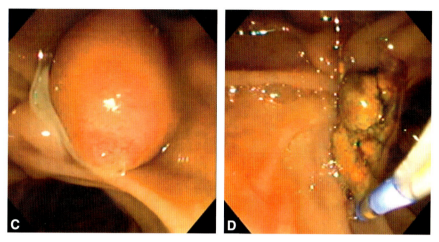

FIGURE 2.2.5 (Continued) **Bulging papilla from distal common duct stones.** Endoscopic images at ERCP (**C** and **D**) from a patient with ascending cholangitis show a bulging papilla with draining pus (**C**) and subsequent removal of a large brown pigmented stone (**D**).

2.3 Mirizzi's Syndrome
(Figures 2.3.1-2.3.3)

CLINICAL FEATURES

- Mirizzi's syndrome is a complication of cholelithiasis in which an impacted cystic duct stone causes extrinsic compression of the common hepatic duct, resulting in biliary obstruction.
- In some cases, the stone may fistulize into the bile duct, which complicates surgery.
- A long cystic duct with a low medial insertion and common sheath with the common hepatic duct is purportedly a predisposing factor.
- Treatment usually requires open cholecystectomy, although endoscopic stenting with laparoscopy has also been utilized.

IMAGING FEATURES

- US can demonstrate the impacted stone in the gallbladder neck region and the proximal biliary ductal dilation, but definitive diagnosis is difficult; specific CT diagnosis is also challenging.
- Cholangiography classically demonstrates smooth eccentric narrowing and obstruction of the common hepatic duct due to extrinsic compression from the impacted cystic duct stone.

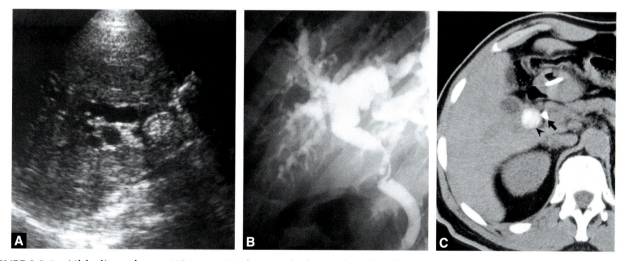

FIGURE 2.3.1 **Mirizzi's syndrome.** US image (**A**) shows a shadowing lamellated stone and dilatation of the proximal biliary tree, suggesting possible Mirizzi's syndrome versus choledocholithiasis. The diagnosis of Mirizzi's syndrome is confirmed at cholangiography (**B**), where eccentric narrowing of the common hepatic duct by the large cystic duct stone is shown to cause upstream biliary obstruction. CT image (**C**) after stenting shows the dense cystic duct stone (*arrowhead*) adjacent to the stented common duct (*arrow*).

THE BILIARY SYSTEM

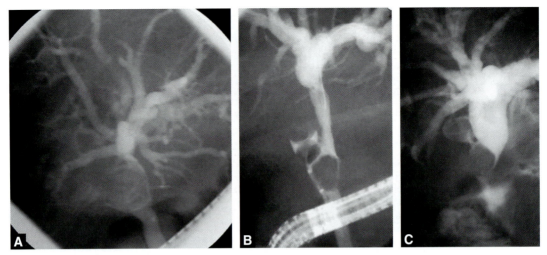

FIGURE 2.3.2 Mirizzi's syndrome. ERCP image (**A**) shows a large lamellated cystic duct stone causing extrinsic obstruction of the common hepatic duct. ERCP image from a second patient (**B**) shows multiple cystic duct stones with the most distal at the cystic duct insertion causing main duct obstruction. PTC image from a third patient (**C**) shows massive proximal biliary ductal dilatation with tapered narrowing due to extrinsic compression from a large cystic duct stone.

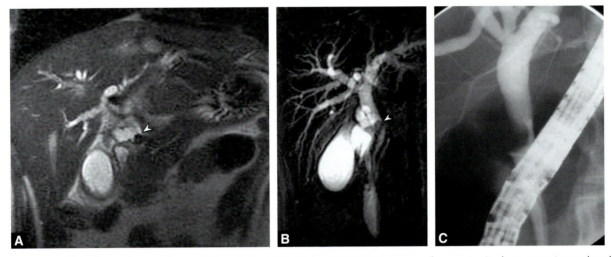

FIGURE 2.3.3 Mirizzi's syndrome. Coronal T2-weighted MR (**A**) and MRCP (**B**) images show a cystic duct stone (*arrowheads*) causing moderate biliary obstruction. The eccentric filling defect from the cystic duct stone was confirmed at subsequent ERCP (**C**).

2.4 Biliary-Enteric Fistulas
(Figures 2.4.1-2.4.6)

CLINICAL FEATURES

- Biliary-enteric fistulas usually result from a stone eroding into the bowel; a cholecystoduodenal fistula related to chronic cholecystitis is the most common type.
- Less common fistulas include cholecystocolic and choledochoduodenal types.
- Infrequent causes of biliary-enteric fistulas include peptic ulcer disease, malignancy, and prior surgery.
- Most stones pass without obstruction or complication; mechanical bowel obstruction caused by an ectopic stone is referred to as "gallstone ileus" (ileus from Latin meaning "obstruction").
- Bouveret's syndrome is a special subset of gallstone ileus in which a large stone causes duodenal or gastric outlet obstruction.
- Cholangitis is rarely present because the biliary tree remains decompressed.

IMAGING FEATURES

- The diagnosis of a biliary-enteric fistula can be suggested by the presence of unsuspected pneumobilia on imaging.
- Barium and endoscopic evaluation can directly demonstrate most biliary-enteric fistulas.
- The classic radiographic findings of gallstone ileus consist of pneumobilia, small bowel obstruction, and calcified ectopic gallstone (Rigler's triad); CT is much more sensitive for this triad and diagnosis.
- Obstructing stones tend to be large (usually >2.5 cm).
- The findings in Bouveret's syndrome are those of gallstone ileus located at the duodenal bulb/pyloric level; a dilated stomach may be present on imaging secondary to gastric outlet obstruction.

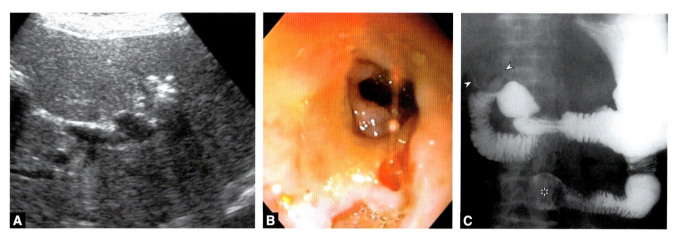

FIGURE 2.4.1 Cholecystoduodenal fistula. US image **(A)** from a patient with a cholecystoduodenal fistula shows bright echogenic foci with "dirty" posterior shadowing from pneumobilia. EGD image **(B)** from a second patient directly demonstrates a cholecystoduodenal fistula. Barium UGI image **(C)** from a third patient shows oral contrast extending through a cholecystoduodenal fistula to outline a large stone within the gallbladder (*arrowheads*). An ectopic gallstone (*asterisk*) is present within the proximal jejunum, causing a partial small bowel obstruction ("gallstone ileus").

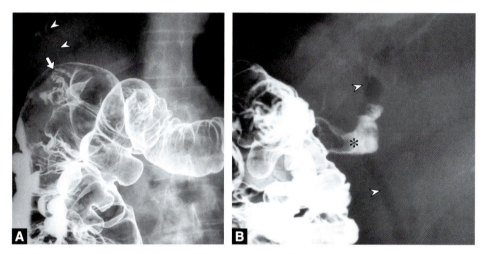

FIGURE 2.4.2 Cholecystocolic fistula. Radiograph from air-contrast BE **(A)** shows unsuspected extraluminal contrast within the biliary tree (*arrowheads*). Note the contrast opacifying the cystic duct (*arrow*) and gallbladder. Oblique radiograph **(B)** profiling the offending cholecystocolic fistula shows barium within the gallbladder (*asterisk*) and air within the bile ducts (*arrowheads*).

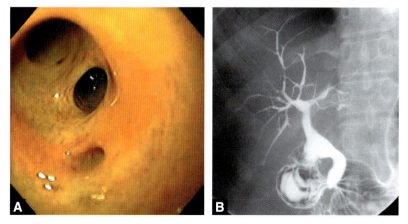

FIGURE 2.4.3 Choledochoduodenal fistula. EGD image **(A)** from a patient with recurrent cholangitis demonstrates endoluminal views of the common hepatic duct and cystic duct through a fistulous communication with the duodenal bulb. The large communication is further demonstrated on barium UGI examination **(B)**. This choledochoduodenal fistula was of uncertain etiology.

Illustration continued on following page

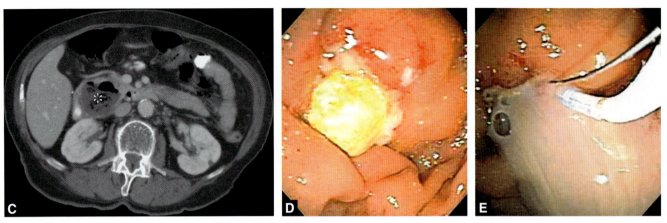

FIGURE 2.4.3 *(Continued)* **Choledochoduodenal fistula.** Contrast-enhanced CT image (**C**) from a different patient shows a large periduodenal abscess (*asterisk*), which at endoscopy (**D**) was found to be due to a common duct stone that had eroded directly into the duodenum. Note the drainage of pus into the duodenum after removal of the stone (**E**).

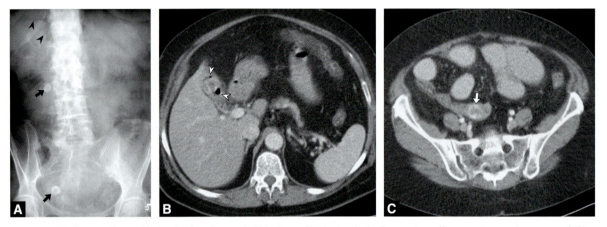

FIGURE 2.4.4 **Gallstone ileus.** Abdominal radiograph (**A**) shows Rigler's triad of ectopic gallstones (*arrows*), pneumobilia (*arrowheads*), and an obstructive bowel gas pattern. Contrast-enhanced CT images (**B** and **C**) from a second patient show the CT equivalent of Rigler's triad, with gas bubbles in the gallbladder (**B**, *arrowheads*) adjacent to a large, faintly rim-calcified stone, and small bowel obstruction caused by a second ectopic calculus (**C**, *arrow*) within the distal ileum. *(A from Pickhardt PJ, Bhalla S, Balfe DM: Acquired gastrointestinal fistulas: Classification, etiologies, and imaging evaluation. Radiology 2002; 224:9-23.)*

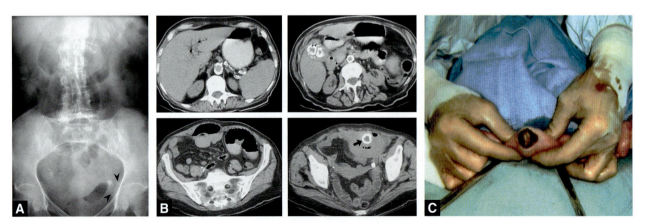

FIGURE 2.4.5 **Gallstone ileus.** Abdominal radiograph (**A**) shows rim calcified gallstones in the right upper quadrant and a subtle but similar-appearing ectopic gallstone in the left lower quadrant (*arrowheads*). Vascular calcifications are also present, including a prominent phlebolith adjacent to the ectopic calculus. The bowel gas pattern appears nonobstructive. Collage of images from subsequent CT (**B**) shows the ectopic gallstone (*arrow*), pneumobilia (which may be present in retrospect on radiography), and high-grade small bowel obstruction. Note also the other gallstones and vascular calcification that were seen on radiography. Rigler's triad is much more obvious on CT. The obstructing ectopic gallstone was removed by enterotomy (**C**). *(B from Pickhardt PJ, Bhalla S, Balfe DM: Acquired gastrointestinal fistulas: Classification, etiologies, and imaging evaluation. Radiology 2002; 224:9-23.)*

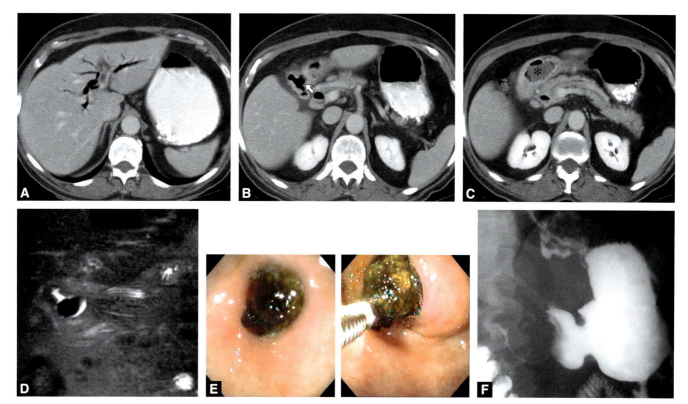

FIGURE 2.4.6 Bouveret's syndrome. Contrast-enhanced CT images (**A** to **C**) show air throughout the central biliary tree, including the common duct and gallbladder. A cholecystoduodenal fistula is present (**B**, *arrow*), which leads to a large, low-attenuation ectopic stone (**C**, *asterisk*) that is impacted in the duodenal bulb. Coronal MRCP image (**D**) shows the low-signal duodenal stone. Note the fluid-filled fistula connecting the duodenal bulb with the contracted gallbladder. EGD images (**E**) show the impacted stone obturating the pyloric channel and causing gastric outlet obstruction. Barium UGI image (**F**) from a second patient shows a large, rounded filling defect within the duodenal bulb. Note the thin layer of oral contrast extending into the gallbladder. (*A to C from Pickhardt PJ, Friedland JA, Hruza DS, Fisher AJ: Bouveret's syndrome: CT, MRCP, and endoscopic findings. AJR 2003; 180:1033-1035.*)

3. INFLAMMATORY DISEASES

Inflammatory conditions of the gallbladder and biliary tree include a host of noninfectious and infectious causes. Acute cholecystitis remains a common indication for abdominal surgery. In general, both the clinical evaluation of the biliary tree for suspected inflammatory disease and its subsequent management often require a collaborative effort that employs both radiologic and endoscopic techniques.

3.1 Cholecystitis
(Figures 3.1.1-3.1.7)

CLINICAL FEATURES

- In 90% or more of cases, acute cholecystitis is caused by stone impaction in the cystic duct causing luminal obstruction; secondary bacterial infection occurs in approximately 50% of cases.
- Common signs and symptoms include right upper quadrant tenderness, nausea, low-grade fever, mild leukocytosis, and mildly elevated liver enzyme levels.
- The majority of patients have had previous episodes of biliary colic, but the duration of symptoms without remitting (>6 hours) and the intensity of pain often alert patients to seek medical attention.
- Marked leukocytosis, high fever with chills, and jaundice must raise suspicion for concurrent ascending cholangitis from choledocholithiasis.
- Many cases spontaneously resolve without immediate surgical treatment, but approximately 10% are complicated by gangrene, perforation, or emphysematous cholecystitis.
- Emphysematous cholecystitis most often occurs in the elderly diabetic patient and indicates a severe infection with gas-forming organisms; the significant risk for perforation warrants emergent surgery.
- Acalculous cholecystitis is less common and typically seen in the critical care setting; diagnosis can be difficult owing to overlap with secondary causes of gallbladder wall thickening (e.g., hypoalbuminemia).
- Percutaneous cholecystostomy or needle aspiration can be performed as a temporizing measure before more definitive management in poor operative candidates.
- The term "chronic cholecystitis" is sometimes used when imaging findings of cholecystitis relate to absent or chronic intermittent symptoms of biliary colic; gallbladder wall calcification may be seen.
- Xanthogranulomatous cholecystitis is a rare chronic inflammatory disorder of uncertain etiology; it is often difficult to differentiate from malignancy at imaging and surgery.

IMAGING FEATURES

- US is the most appropriate initial imaging test; the triad of cholelithiasis, wall thickening (>3 mm), and pain with transducer pressure over the gallbladder (sonographic Murphy's sign) is generally diagnostic.
- CT can also demonstrate the typical findings of acute cholecystitis but is most useful for detecting complications such as gangrenous or emphysematous cholecystitis.
- Imaging findings in chronic cholecystitis of irregular wall thickening and cholelithiasis can mimic gallbladder carcinoma.
- Acalculous cholecystitis usually manifests as a hydropic gallbladder with diffuse wall thickening; luminal sludge is a common finding.
- Other causes of gallbladder wall thickening (e.g., adjacent inflammation from acute hepatitis) can mimic primary cholecystitis.
- Cholescintigraphy with ^{99m}Tc-labeled iminodiacetic acid analogues demonstrates nonvisualization of the gallbladder due to cystic duct obstruction; this test is highly sensitive and moderately specific for the diagnosis.
- Gangrenous cholecystitis and gallbladder perforation manifest on US and CT with mural discontinuity, loculated pericholecystic fluid collections, and intraluminal membranes.
- Emphysematous cholecystitis appears echogenic with indistinct ("dirty") shadowing on US, which can be confirmed on CT (or radiography); the abnormal gas may be located within the wall or lumen.
- Imaging features of xanthogranulomatous cholecystitis include irregular wall thickening with ill-defined borders and cystic intramural or pericholecystic collections.

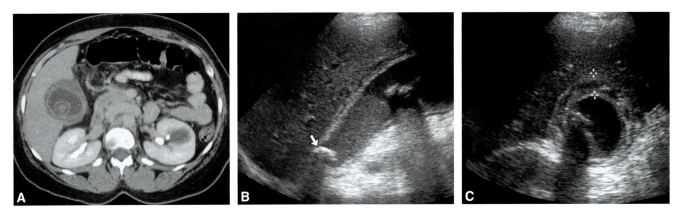

FIGURE 3.1.1 Acute calculous cholecystitis. Contrast-enhanced CT image (**A**) shows diffuse gallbladder wall thickening with low-attenuation intramural edema, a lamellated low-attenuation gallstone, and infiltration of the pericholecystic fat, all compatible with cholecystitis. Longitudinal (**B**) and transverse (**C**) US views of the gallbladder demonstrate the prominent wall thickening (**C**, *calipers*), echogenic shadowing stones, and nonshadowing sludge. The impacted shadowing calculus at the gallbladder neck (**B**, *arrow*) represents the cause of luminal obstruction. Sonographic Murphy's sign was present.

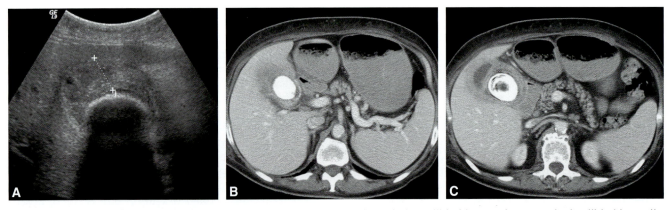

FIGURE 3.1.2 Chronic calculous cholecystitis. Transverse US image through the gallbladder (**A**) shows marked gallbladder wall thickening over 2 cm (calipers) around a large stone, giving a wall-echo-shadow complex (WES sign). Gallbladder carcinoma was a preoperative concern given the degree of soft tissue wall thickening. Images from contrast-enhanced CT (**B** and **C**) show the large calcified stone and irregular gallbladder wall thickening, including early changes of porcelain gallbladder. Chronic inflammation without tumor was found after open cholecystectomy.

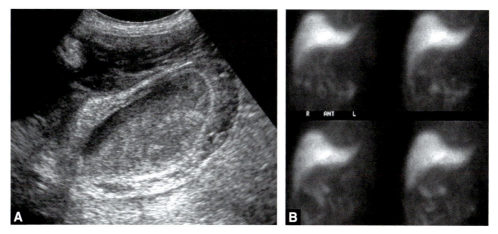

FIGURE 3.1.3 Acalculous cholecystitis. Longitudinal US image through the gallbladder (**A**) shows marked diffuse gallbladder wall thickening associated with a dilated, sludge-filled lumen. Collage of images from hepatobiliary scintigraphy (**B**) show no evidence of gallbladder filling, which is a sensitive but relatively nonspecific finding for acalculous cholecystitis in the critically ill patient setting.

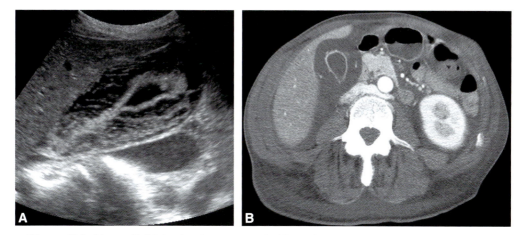

FIGURE 3.1.4 Diffuse gallbladder wall thickening from acute viral hepatitis. US (**A**) and CT (**B**) images show massive diffuse gallbladder wall thickening, which has a striated appearance on US. The low-attenuation intramural edema deep to the enhancing mucosa on CT is often mistaken for pericholecystic fluid. The degree of diffuse gallbladder wall thickening in acute viral hepatitis is often quite prominent.

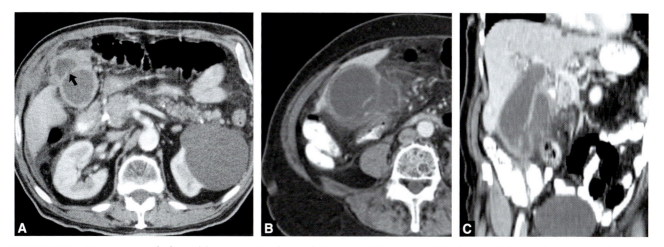

FIGURE 3.1.5 Gangrenous cholecystitis. Contrast-enhanced CT image (**A**) shows gallbladder wall thickening with focal discontinuity (*arrow*) leading to a pericholecystic abscess. Extensive peritoneal inflammatory changes related to the perforation are present. Transverse (**B**) and coronal (**C**) CT images from a second patient show another case of gangrenous cholecystitis with focal wall disruption, large medial pericholecystic abscess, and infiltration of the surrounding fat.

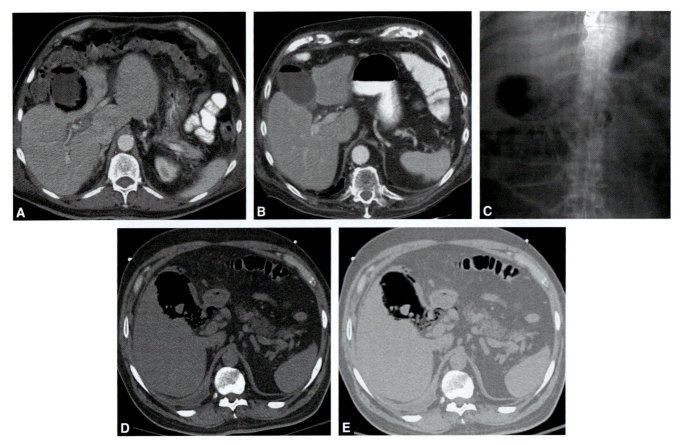

FIGURE 3.1.6 **Emphysematous cholecystitis.** Contrast-enhanced CT images (**A** and **B**) from two patients with emphysematous cholecystitis show gas within the gallbladder wall (**A**) and gallbladder lumen (**B**). Abdominal radiograph (**C**), CT with soft tissue window (**D**), and CT with lung window (**E**) show extensive luminal and intramural gas related to a gas-forming clostridial infection. Intraluminal debris likely represents cholelithiasis and possibly sloughed membranes.

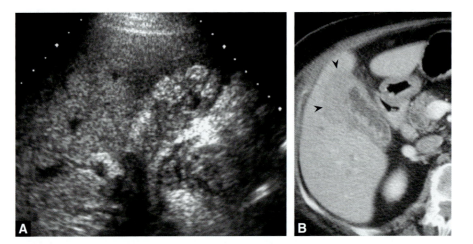

FIGURE 3.1.7 **Xanthogranulomatous cholecystitis.** Longitudinal US (**A**) and transverse CT (**B**) images show heterogeneous gallbladder wall thickening with an indistinct liver margin and mass-like infiltration of the inflammatory process in the fundal region (*arrowheads*).

Illustration continued on following page

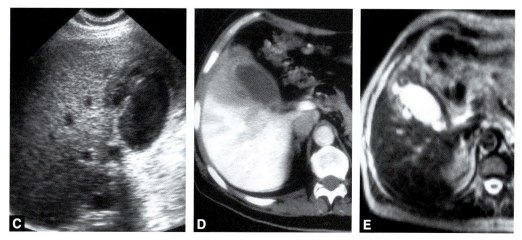

FIGURE 3.1.7 (Continued)   **Xanthogranulomatous cholecystitis.** Longitudinal US image (**C**) from a different patient shows complex focal pericholecystic collections from extension of the inflammatory process. CT image (**D**) shows decreased hepatic parenchymal enhancement around the gallbladder fossa with loss of the gallbladder wall interface. T2-weighted MR image (**E**) shows the foci of pericholecystic fluid to a better degree.

3.2 Primary Sclerosing Cholangitis
(Figures 3.2.1-3.2.5)

CLINICAL FEATURES

- Primary sclerosing cholangitis (PSC) is a chronic idiopathic disease characterized by fibrosis and inflammation of the biliary tree.
- Diagnosis is made based on cholangiographic findings in the appropriate clinical setting.
- Approximately 80% of patients with PSC have inflammatory bowel disease (ulcerative colitis >> Crohn's disease); conversely, PSC is seen in <5% of all patients with inflammatory bowel disease.
- Other demographic characteristics include male predominance and relatively young age at onset (< 45 years).
- Common symptoms include right upper quadrant pain, jaundice, and pruritus; up to 50% of patients are clinically asymptomatic with cholestasis on laboratory evaluation.
- Main complications include fat malabsorption, biliary calculi, secondary biliary cirrhosis, and cholangiocarcinoma; marked weight loss should raise the suspicion of cholangiocarcinoma.
- Patients with PSC and IBD have a markedly increased risk of developing colonic adenocarcinoma and require yearly colonoscopic surveillance for development of dysplasia.
- PSC is slowly progressive, with a mean survival of 12 years from diagnosis; liver transplantation is the only known effective treatment, but PSC may recur after transplantation in a small subset of patients.
- Exclusion of secondary causes of sclerosing cholangitis is important; these include choledocholithiasis, recurrent bacterial cholangitis, atypical infections, medication-induced changes, and biliary neoplasms.
- PSC-like biliary changes can also be associated with other idiopathic fibrosing conditions, such as retroperitoneal fibrosis and autoimmune (sclerosing) pancreatitis.

IMAGING FEATURES

- Cholangiography demonstrates multiple segmental biliary strictures with intervening ducts of normal or mildly dilated caliber, which give the classic beaded appearance.
- Other variable cholangiographic findings include diverticula, mural irregularity, and peripheral ductal pruning.
- The intrahepatic and hilar ducts are almost always involved; larger extrahepatic ducts may be spared in 10% to 20% of cases.
- Cholangiocarcinoma should be suspected in the setting of a dominant focal stricture (see section 1.1); a polypoid intraluminal mass is a less common manifestation of cholangiocarcinoma.
- MRCP now allows for a noninvasive diagnosis in some cases without risking complications such as ascending cholangitis secondary to bacterial seeding of poorly drained segments.
- Despite complication risks, ERCP remains an important diagnostic tool and can sample dominant strictures for cholangiocarcinoma.
- CT can show ductal wall thickening and areas of skip dilatation but is most useful in assessing for complications such as cirrhosis and malignancy.

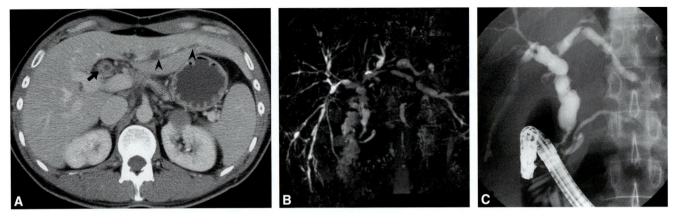

FIGURE 3.2.1 Primary sclerosing cholangitis. Contrast-enhanced CT image **(A)** shows irregular left intrahepatic biliary ductal dilatation (*arrowheads*) and segmental wall thickening of the extrahepatic duct (*arrow*). MRCP **(B)** and ERCP **(C)** images show multifocal strictures and irregularity involving both intrahepatic and extrahepatic ducts. Note how the peripheral intrahepatic ducts are better depicted on MRCP because contrast opacification is not needed.

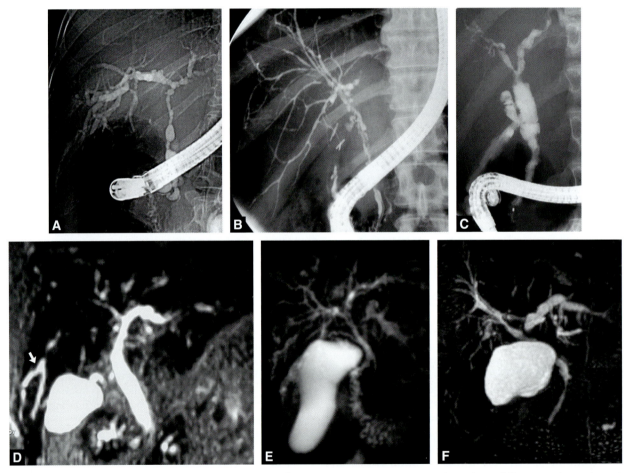

FIGURE 3.2.2 Primary sclerosing cholangitis on ERCP and MRCP. ERCP images **(A to C)** from three different patients show the classic beaded appearance from multifocal strictures **(A)**, diffuse irregular ductal diminution and diverticular outpouchings of the extrahepatic duct **(B)**, and mucosal irregularity of the central biliary tree with marked peripheral pruning **(C)**. MRCP images **(D to F)** from three different patients show multifocal intrahepatic strictures and dilatation **(D,** *arrow*) with relative sparing of the extrahepatic duct **(D)**, diffuse irregularity to the entire biliary tree **(E)**, and intrahepatic ductal dilatation and irregularity with a dominant left hepatic duct stricture **(F)**.

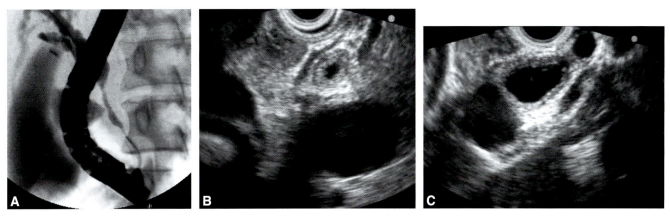

FIGURE 3.2.3 Primary sclerosing cholangitis on EUS. ERCP image (**A**) shows long-segment narrowing of the distal common duct associated with upstream dilatation. EUS images (**B** and **C**) show circumferential mural thickening of the extrahepatic duct wall, both at (**B**) and above (**C**) the stricture.

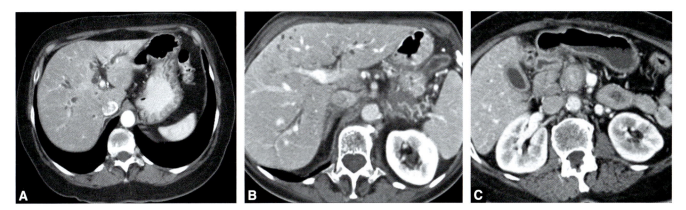

FIGURE 3.2.4 Primary sclerosing cholangitis on CT. Contrast-enhanced CT images (**A** and **B**) from two different patients show skip areas of intrahepatic biliary ductal dilatation related to multifocal strictures. Contrast-enhanced CT image (**C**) from a third patient shows diffuse gallbladder wall thickening related to underlying PSC.

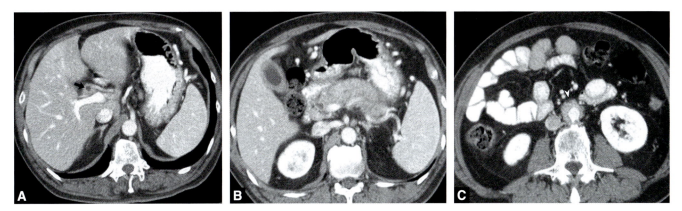

FIGURE 3.2.5 Autoimmune pancreatitis with involvement of the biliary tree and retroperitoneum. Contrast-enhanced CT images (**A** to **C**) show circumferential wall thickening of the extrahepatic bile duct (**A**, *arrow*) and gallbladder (**B**), suggestive of PSC. However, diffuse pancreatic enlargement with decreased parenchymal enhancement and a periaortic rind of soft issue (**C**, *arrowhead*) are also present, suggestive of autoimmune pancreatitis generally and retroperitoneal fibrosis, respectively. Unlike PSC, sclerosing cholangitis associated with autoimmune pancreatitis generally improves with corticosteroids.

3.3 Ascending Cholangitis

(Figures 3.3.1-3.3.2)

CLINICAL FEATURES

- Ascending cholangitis occurs when infected bile and pus are present in an obstructed bile duct; choledocholithiasis is the underlying etiology in >80% of cases.
- Neoplastic obstruction of the bile duct rarely presents with ascending cholangitis and usually only after biliary intervention (e.g., obstruction of a previously placed stent for drainage).
- Charcot's triad of right upper quadrant pain, jaundice, and fever is the classic presentation but only occurs in 50% to 70% of patients; one may also see altered mental status and hypotension.
- Infection is usually polymicrobial; blood cultures are usually positive.
- Empiric use of antibiotics is usually sufficient to control the infection as a temporizing measure before drainage; emergent biliary decompression may be required if initial conservative measures fail.

IMAGING FEATURES

- Initial imaging with CT or US is used to assess for the presence and possible cause of biliary obstruction.
- Radiologic imaging is similar to choledocholithiasis; cross-sectional imaging can appear normal in some patients with ascending cholangitis.
- ERCP is both diagnostic and therapeutic, with endoscopic visualization of stones and pus on decompression; PTC is generally reserved for cases with unsuccessful ERCP.
- MRCP has little or no role in patients presenting with a high clinical suspicion for ascending cholangitis.
- Chronic cholangitis may cause multifocal strictures resembling the imaging appearance of PSC.

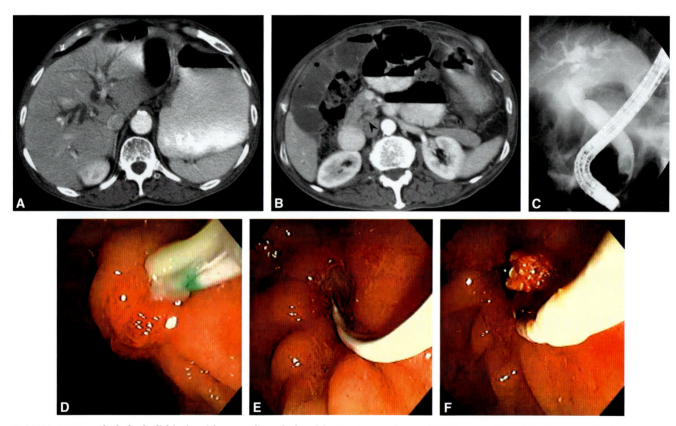

FIGURE 3.3.1 Choledocholithiasis with ascending cholangitis. Contrast-enhanced CT images (**A** and **B**) from a patient presenting with fever and jaundice show prominent biliary ductal dilation secondary to choledocholithiasis manifesting as an intraluminal soft tissue density (**B**, *arrowhead*) with a surrounding crescent of bile. Filling defects within the distal common bile duct are confirmed at therapeutic ERCP (**C**). Endoscopic images at ERCP (**D** to **F**) from a second patient with ascending cholangitis show pus extruding from the major papilla upon cannulation with a sphincterotome (**D**). A sphincterotomy was performed to open the biliary orifice (**E**). Note the white internal fibers of the cut biliary sphincter. Successful stone removal was subsequently performed utilizing a retrieval balloon (**F**).

Illustration continued on following page

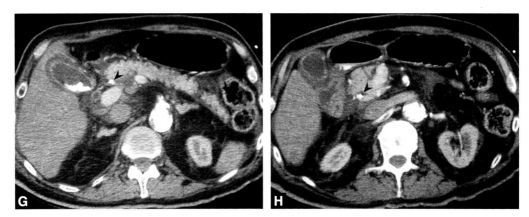

FIGURE 3.3.1 (Continued)   **Choledocholithiasis with ascending cholangitis.** Contrast-enhanced CT images (**G** and **H**) from a third patient show cholelithiasis and gallbladder wall thickening suggestive of cholecystitis. However, dense calculi are also seen within the extrahepatic duct (*arrowheads*) with associated inflammatory changes surrounding the adjacent duodenum and pancreatic head related to severe bacterial cholangitis.

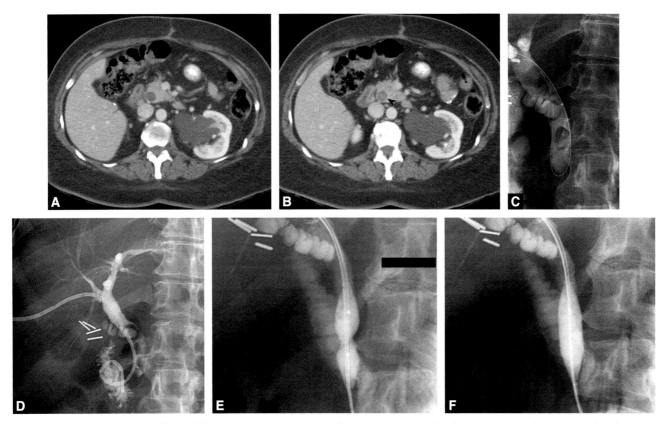

FIGURE 3.3.2   PTC for ascending cholangitis. Contrast-enhanced CT images (**A** and **B**) from a patient who had previously undergone gastric bypass surgery show a dilated common bile duct and relatively subtle choledocholithiasis (**B**, *arrowhead*). Given the postsurgical anatomy, a percutaneous transhepatic approach was necessary to access the biliary tree. Images from PTC (**C** to **F**) show choledocholithiasis (**C**) due to an underlying benign stricture. The stones were removed percutaneously and the biliary tree was drained via internal-external catheter placement (**D**). Balloon dilatation of the stricture was performed during PTC at a later date (**E** and **F**).

3.4 Recurrent Pyogenic Cholangitis

(Figure 3.4.1-3.4.2)

CLINICAL FEATURES

- Recurrent pyogenic cholangitis (RPC) was previously referred to as "oriental cholangiohepatitis" because of its almost exclusive presence within Southeast Asia.
- RPC is characterized by formation of pigmented stones within the intrahepatic bile ducts, biliary strictures, and recurrent bacterial cholangitis.
- It most commonly presents in the third and fourth decades of life with equal gender distribution.
- Clinical symptoms are similar to those of ascending cholangitis but are characterized by multiple intermittent recurrences.
- The etiology is unknown, but parasitic infestation with the liver fluke *Clonorchis sinensis* is often associated and has been identified as a possible cause.
- Acute complications include sepsis, hepatic abscess, and pancreatitis; chronic complications include secondary biliary cirrhosis and cholangiocarcinoma.
- Treatment involves antibiotics for acute cholangitis, evaluation for parasitic infection, and endoscopic biliary drainage and stone clearance; partial hepatectomy may be required in refractory cases.

IMAGING FEATURES

- US can demonstrate dilated intrahepatic ducts, echogenic ductal stones or sludge, and complications such as intrahepatic abscesses; pneumobilia from prior interventions can limit sonographic assessment.
- CT and MR provide a more comprehensive assessment for anatomic distribution and complications.
- The left lateral lobe of the liver is usually the most severely affected area, often with significant atrophy.
- Cholangiography demonstrates stones and strictures usually involving the larger intrahepatic ducts and hilar confluence; dilated central intrahepatic ducts with abrupt tapering of peripheral ducts is common.
- ERCP allows for both diagnosis and intervention; MRCP can provide noninvasive surveillance.

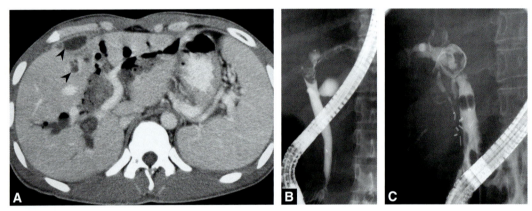

FIGURE 3.4.1 RPC. Contrast-enhanced CT image (**A**) from a patient with an acute exacerbation of RPC shows massive dilatation of the central biliary tree filled with multiple large, pigmented stones that are of slightly increased attenuation compared with the fluid attenuation of bile. Pneumobilia is likely related to prior sphincterotomy and not an acute infectious complication. Rim-enhancing fluid collections (*arrowheads*) represent acute intrahepatic and perihepatic abscesses. ERCP images (**B** and **C**) from two different patients with RPC show irregular hilar filling defects representing pigmented calculi. Luminal contour irregularity is more pronounced in the last case.

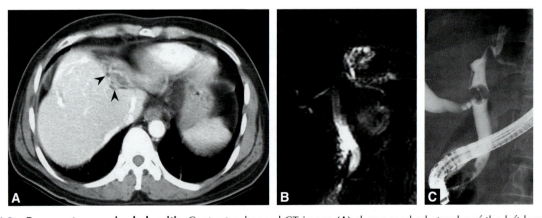

FIGURE 3.4.2 Recurrent pyogenic cholangitis. Contrast-enhanced CT image (**A**) shows marked atrophy of the left hepatic lobe (*arrowheads*) with associated segmental intrahepatic biliary ductal dilatation. Areas of intraluminal increased attenuation suggest calculi, which are confirmed on subsequent MRCP (**B**) and ERCP (**C**). Both **B** and **C** also demonstrate a left main hepatic duct stricture that is contributing to the pathology. The remainder of the intrahepatic biliary tree is not well depicted on these images. Note the filling defect in **C** at the level of the cystic duct insertion is a retrieval balloon and not a stone.

3.5 AIDS Cholangiopathy
(Figure 3.5.1)

CLINICAL FEATURES

- This secondary cholangitis often resembles PSC with superimposed papillary stenosis.
- It is likely due to opportunistic infection by *Cryptosporidium*, cytomegalovirus (CMV), or both.
- Presentation typically involves right upper quadrant pain with marked elevation of alkaline phosphatase.
- It generally is not associated with shortened survival.
- Incidence has markedly decreased with the widespread use of highly active antiretroviral therapy (HAART).

IMAGING FEATURES

- CT and US can detect biliary abnormalities, including dilatation and ductal wall thickening in the majority of patients; however, a normal examination does not exclude the diagnosis.
- The gallbladder wall is often grossly thickened.
- Cholangiographic imaging features resemble those of PSC, papillary stenosis (with common bile duct dilatation), or both.
- ERCP and sphincterotomy with or without stent placement relieves symptoms in most patients.

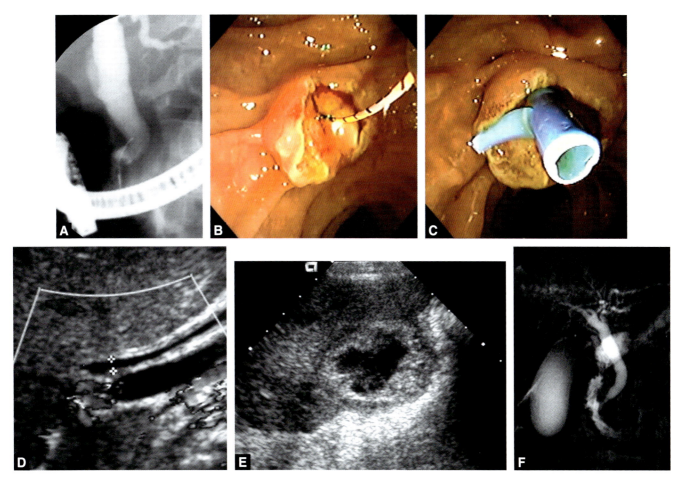

FIGURE 3.5.1 AIDS cholangiopathy. ERCP image (**A**) shows biliary ductal dilatation related to papillary stenosis. The common bile duct measures approximately 11 mm. Subsequent endoscopic images demonstrates successful sphincterotomy (**B**) and stent placement (**C**). Images from subsequent US (**D** and **E**) show decompression of the extrahepatic duct with a normal luminal caliber (**D**, calipers) but diffuse biliary wall thickening and marked irregular gallbladder wall thickening (**E**). MRCP image (**F**) from a different patient shows the classic findings of AIDS cholangiopathy with diffuse dilatation from papillary stenosis and multifocal irregularity of the intrahepatic ducts simulating PSC.

4. OTHER BILIARY CONDITIONS

4.1 Choledochal Cysts
(Figures 4.1.1-4.1.4)

CLINICAL FEATURES

- Choledochal cysts are congenital cystic dilatations of the biliary tree; potential causes include congenital muscle wall weakness and an anomalous pancreaticobiliary junction.
- Most patients present in early childhood, often with jaundice, vomiting, and failure to thrive; adults may present with recurrent cholangitis, pancreatitis, or as an incidental imaging finding.
- Choledochal cysts are classified by the Todani system (types I to V) based on the pattern of involvement of the intrahepatic and extrahepatic biliary tree.
- Complications include cholangitis, stone formation, secondary biliary cirrhosis, and cholangiocarcinoma; biliary stasis contributes to the development of stones and malignancy.
- An anomalous pancreaticobiliary union is found in up to 90% of patients; biliary reflux of pancreatic enzymes may contribute to both cyst formation and the increased risk of cholangiocarcinoma.
- Treatment of extrahepatic disease usually consists of surgical excision of the cyst with choledochojejunostomy to avoid the development of complications.

IMAGING FEATURES

- Because US is often the initial modality for biliary imaging, most choledochal cysts are detected with this modality as prominent cystic dilatation of a portion of the biliary tree.
- Cholangiography with MRCP or ERCP can best define the areas of involvement and is required to delineate ductal anatomy prior to surgical treatment.
- Type I is the most common form (80% to 90%) and manifests as segmental or diffuse fusiform dilatation of the extrahepatic duct.
- Type II is rare and represents a true diverticulum anywhere in the extrahepatic duct.
- Type III is referred to as a choledochocele and is characterized by cystic dilatation of the ampullary portion of the common bile duct.
- Type IVa consists of multiple fusiform intrahepatic and extrahepatic cysts; Type IVb consists of multiple extrahepatic cysts without intrahepatic cysts.
- Type V represents Caroli's disease with cystic dilatation of only the intrahepatic ducts (see next section).
- An anomalous pancreaticobiliary union manifests as a long common channel located outside the duodenal wall.

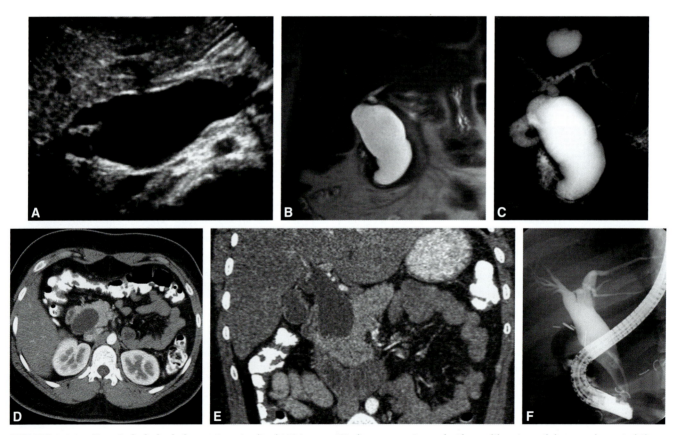

FIGURE 4.1.1 Type I choledochal cyst. Longitudinal US image **(A)** shows prominent fusiform dilatation of the extrahepatic bile duct. T2-weighted MR **(B)** and MRCP **(C)** images from a second patient show similar dilatation of the entire extrahepatic duct. The MRCP image also demonstrates lack of intrahepatic involvement and a simple hepatic cyst. Transverse **(D)** and coronal **(E)** contrast-enhanced CT images from a third patient show another typical type I choledochal cyst. ERCP image **(F)** from a final patient shows findings that are similar to the other cases. The slight prominence of the left and right hepatic ducts near their confluence seen in some of these cases should not be considered as separate intrahepatic involvement (i.e., type IVa disease).

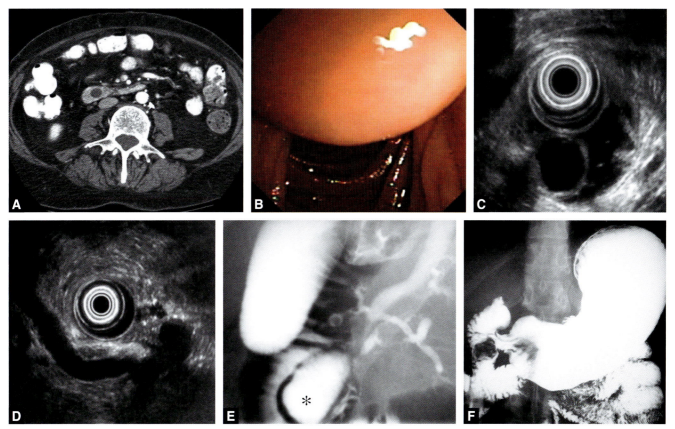

FIGURE 4.1.2 Type III choledochal cyst (choledochocele). Contrast-enhanced CT image **(A)** shows a well-defined cystic lesion projecting within the lumen of the duodenum at the level of the major papilla. At EGD **(B)**, the lesion appears as a smooth submucosal mass bulging from the major papilla. The cystic nature is confirmed at EUS **(C)**, which also demonstrates continuity with the common bile duct **(D)**. Cholangiography is not needed for confirmation in this case. ERCP image **(E)** from a second patient shows contrast filling of a choledochocele (*asterisk*). Note the surrounding uniform linear lucency that represents the combined cyst and duodenal walls. Barium UGI image **(F)** from a third patient shows a polypoid filling defect involving the second portion of the duodenum. Although the fluoroscopic findings are nonspecific, further workup confirmed a large choledochocele in this case.

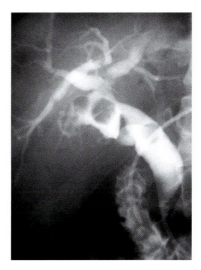

FIGURE 4.1.3 Type II choledochal cyst. Cholangiogram obtained from contrast injection of a nasobiliary catheter demonstrates a large irregular diverticular outpouching extending off the common hepatic duct. Filling defects within this type II choledochal cyst represent calculi resulting from stasis.

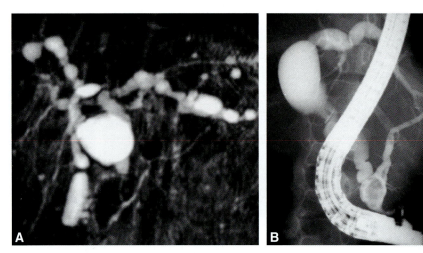

FIGURE 4.1.4 **Type IVa choledochal cyst.** MRCP image **(A)** shows multiple areas of cystic dilatation involving the intrahepatic and extrahepatic ducts. ERCP image **(B)** from a different patient also shows dilatation of both intrahepatic and extrahepatic ducts, as well as an abnormal pancreaticobiliary union that is dilated and contains stones or sludge.

4.2 Caroli's Disease
(Figures 4.2.1-4.2.3)

CLINICAL FEATURES

- Multifocal, saccular or segmental dilatation of the intrahepatic bile ducts; it is also classified as a type V choledochal cyst (Todani classification).
- Pathogenesis is related to incomplete embryologic remodeling of the biliary ductal plate with subsequent inflammation and segmental dilatation.
- The "pure" form only includes the above described intrahepatic duct abnormalities; the term Caroli's syndrome is reserved for patients with associated congenital hepatic fibrosis.
- Duct abnormalities usually involve the liver diffusely but may be segmental or lobar.
- Renal tubular ectasia and polycystic renal disease are often seen with the syndromic form.
- Complications include biliary stones, recurrent cholangitis, hepatic abscess, and cholangiocarcinoma.
- Patients having associated congenital hepatic fibrosis may present with hepatosplenomegaly and esophageal varices.
- Medical and endoscopic therapy have variable success rates; hepatic resection in lobar disease and liver transplantation in diffuse disease are surgical options in patients with frequent complications.

IMAGING FEATURES

- CT, US, and MR demonstrate multiple intrahepatic cystic areas that connect with the biliary tree.
- The "central dot" sign (although more often eccentric) is a characteristic cross-sectional imaging finding that represents the portal vascular bundle surrounded by the ductal plate.
- Imaging findings of renal tubular ectasia, discrete renal cysts, or hepatic fibrosis may coexist.
- Cholangiography can confirm the biliary nature of the cystic areas and assess for complications such as stones and strictures.
- Hepatobiliary scintigraphy can show retained activity corresponding to biliary cysts, but MRCP with biliary contrast agents may now be used for noninvasive diagnosis.

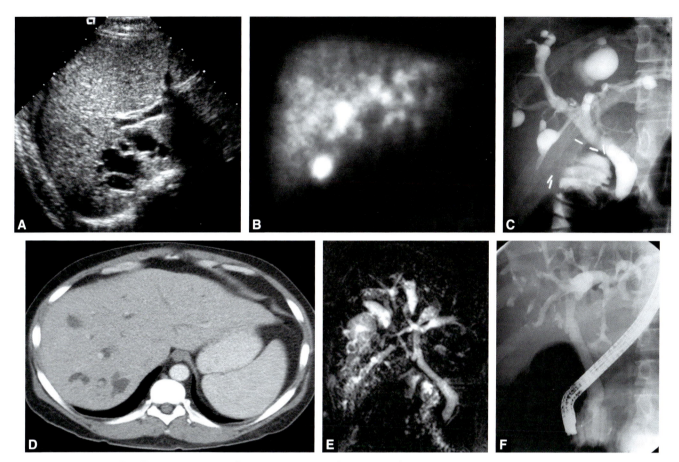

FIGURE 4.2.1 Caroli's disease. Transverse liver US image (**A**) shows several large cystic lesions within the posterior segment of the right hepatic lobe. Note the small echogenic foci projecting within these cystic areas, which represent portal vessels and are essentially pathognomonic for the diagnosis. Delayed image from subsequent hepatobiliary scintigraphy (**B**) shows foci of increased activity corresponding to accumulation of the tracer within the areas of cystic biliary dilatation. Conventional cholangiogram (**C**) from a second patient shows multiple well-defined areas of intrahepatic cystic dilatation with sparing of the extrahepatic bile duct. Contrast-enhanced CT image (**D**) from a third patient shows multiple intrahepatic cystic lesions, which have an elongated appearance on MRCP (**E**) and ERCP (**F**). Note how the enhancing portal venous branches are closely associated with the cysts on CT.

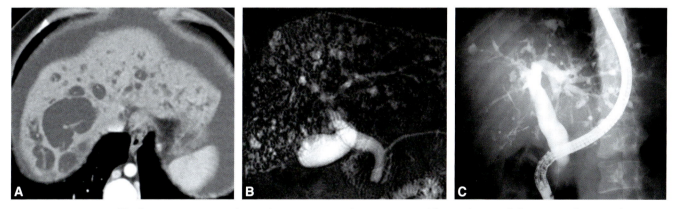

FIGURE 4.2.2 Caroli's disease. Contrast-enhanced CT image (**A**) shows innumerable intrahepatic biliary cystic lesions of varying size but with typical associated vascular bundles coursing through them. Ascites may be related to portal hypertension from hepatic fibrosis. MRCP (**B**) and ERCP (**C**) images from two different patients show diffuse involvement with small intrahepatic biliary cystic foci.

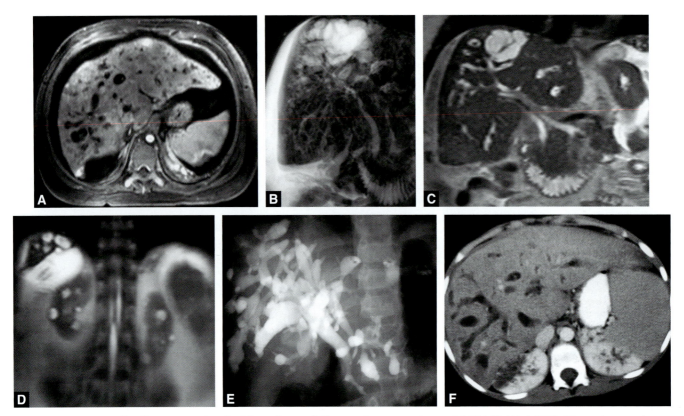

FIGURE 4.2.3 Caroli's disease associated with cystic renal disease. Contrast-enhanced SGE MR (**A**), MRCP (**B**), and coronal T2-weighted MR (**C** and **D**) images show findings of Caroli's disease, hepatic disease with ascites, and cystic renal disease. ERCP (**E**) and contrast-enhanced CT (**F**) images from a different patient also show findings of extensive Caroli's and cystic renal disease.

4.3 Adenomyomatosis
(Figures 4.3.1-4.3.3)

CLINICAL FEATURES

- Adenomyomatosis is a benign, asymptomatic condition found incidentally on imaging studies characterized by mucosal overgrowth, muscular wall thickening, and intramural diverticula (Rokitansky-Aschoff sinuses); cholelithiasis is found in over half of patients with adenomyomatosis.
- Distribution may be diffuse, focal (fundal), or segmental (annular).
- In the past, cholesterolosis and adenomyomatosis were referred to as "hyperplastic cholecystosis."
- No treatment is necessary, but cholecystectomy is often performed for cases in which carcinoma or cholecystitis cannot be excluded.

IMAGING FEATURES

- US findings include focal or diffuse gallbladder wall thickening; intramural diverticula or sinuses may be directly seen or give rise to a "comet-tail" artifact related to echogenic debris within the sinuses.
- CT and MR can also show wall thickening; the Rokitansky-Aschoff sinuses are best seen as outpouchings on cholangiographic imaging such as MRCP, ERCP, or oral cholecystography.
- Focal fundal adenomyomatosis may have a mass-like appearance on cross-sectional imaging.
- The segmental (annular) form usually results in an hourglass appearance to the gallbladder.

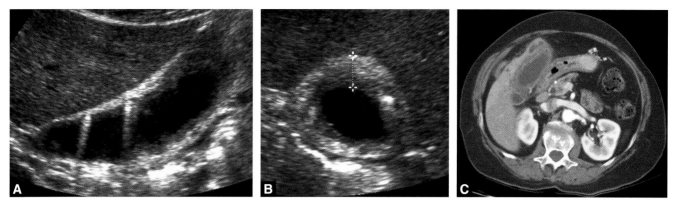

FIGURE 4.3.1 Diffuse form of adenomyomatosis. Longitudinal (**A**) and transverse (**B**) US images of the gallbladder show diffuse wall thickening and scattered heterogeneous intramural foci representing Rokitansky-Aschoff sinuses, some of which demonstrate "comet-tail" artifact from echogenic internal debris. Contrast-enhanced CT image (**C**) from a different patient shows diffuse gallbladder wall thickening punctuated by multiple scattered intramural cysts. Symptoms suggestive of acute cholecystitis are generally absent in such cases.

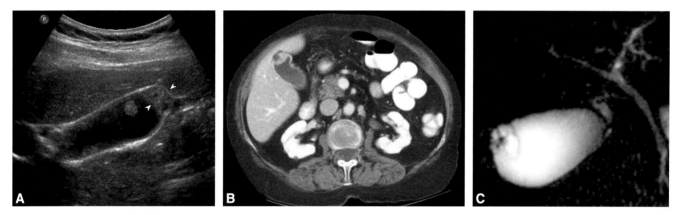

FIGURE 4.3.2 Focal (fundal) form of adenomyomatosis. Longitudinal US image (**A**) of the gallbladder shows focal crescentic wall thickening (*arrowheads*) and intramural cystic foci (sinuses) located at the gallbladder fundus. The patient also has a large, adherent nonshadowing polyp. Contrast-enhanced CT image (**B**) from a second patient shows heterogeneous solid and cystic gallbladder wall thickening confined to the fundus. MRCP image (**C**) from a third patient shows focal irregularity of the gallbladder fundus, typical of focal adenomyomatosis.

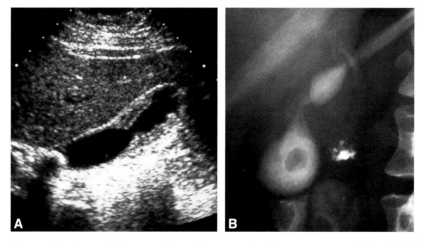

FIGURE 4.3.3 Segmental (annular) form of adenomyomatosis. Longitudinal US image (**A**) of the gallbladder shows circumferential segmental wall thickening involving the body of the gallbladder, which gives rise to an hourglass appearance to the lumen. Spot film from an oral cholecystogram (**B**) in a different patient shows annular narrowing of the gallbladder body from segmental adenomyomatosis, as well as cholelithiasis. Oral cholecystography is now only rarely performed.

4.4 Porcelain Gallbladder
(Figure 4.4.1)

CLINICAL FEATURES

- Porcelain gallbladder refers to mural calcification caused by chronic inflammation.
- Gallstones are frequently present in the setting of porcelain gallbladder.
- Porcelain gallbladder is seen predominately in the adult female population.
- Its significance is primarily related to the association with gallbladder carcinoma (precise risk not known but reportedly as high as 25%).
- Prophylactic cholecystectomy is generally indicated unless the patient is a high surgical risk.

IMAGING FEATURES

- Conventional radiographs show diffuse or discontinuous curvilinear calcification conforming to the shape of the gallbladder.
- On US, porcelain gallbladder manifests as a bright echogenic curvilinear surface with dense posterior shadowing; it must be distinguished from the WES sign and emphysematous cholecystitis, which can appear similar on US.
- CT is the best imaging modality for detection and characterization, as well as for evaluating for superimposed carcinoma; it is useful for confirming cases suspected on US.

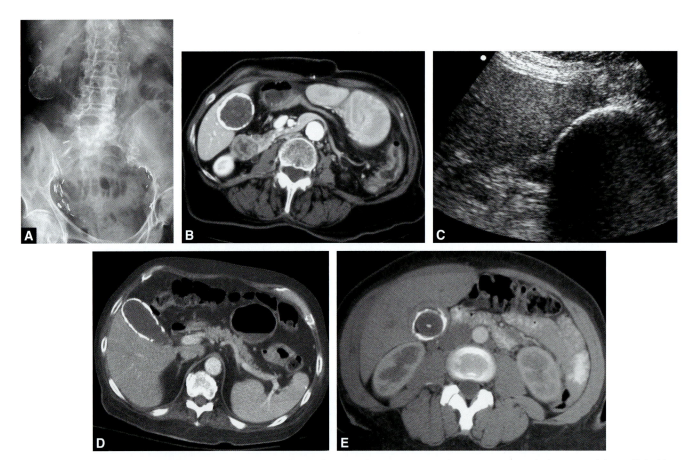

FIGURE 4.4.1 Porcelain gallbladder. Abdominal radiograph **(A)** and CT image **(B)** show extensive calcification of the gallbladder wall. US image **(C)** from a different patient shows an echogenic curvilinear surface with dense posterior shadowing in the expected region of the gallbladder. The WES sign of cholelithiasis and emphysematous cholecystitis can have a fairly similar US appearance. Contrast-enhanced CT images **(D** and **E)** show porcelain gallbladder in two additional patients. A large calculus with a central calcific focus occupies the gallbladder lumen in the last case.

4.5 Biliary Leak

(Figures 4.5.1-4.5.5)

CLINICAL FEATURES

- Most injuries to the biliary tree resulting in subsequent bile leakage are iatrogenic.
- Common locations of iatrogenic leak after cholecystectomy include the cystic duct stump and ducts of Luschka (small accessory ducts that drain directly into the gallbladder); both are usually self-limited.
- Unrecognized aberrant ductal anatomy, often related to the right posterior branch, can lead to iatrogenic injury at cholecystectomy.
- Extravasated bile initially disperses freely throughout the peritoneal cavity; collections that loculate over time are referred to as bilomas.
- Symptoms may include right upper quadrant pain, jaundice, fever, and leukocytosis; symptoms can be due to peritoneal irritation or superimposed infection.
- Treatment includes temporary placement of a biliary stent to facilitate preferential flow of bile into the duodenum; bridging the site of the bile leak with the stent is advantageous.

IMAGING FEATURES

- A small amount of perihepatic fluid can be a normal finding after cholecystectomy; biliary leak can be suggested when CT or US shows increasing peritoneal fluid over time.
- CT and US can readily demonstrate peritoneal fluid but are not specific for confirming biliary leak; encapsulation of fluid is suggestive of a biloma after cholecystectomy.
- Hepatobiliary scintigraphy is sensitive for detecting the presence of an active bile leak but is poor for localization; MR with biliary-excreted contrast agents can precisely define leaks.
- Direct cholangiography (intraoperative, T-tube, or ERCP) can detect and localize contrast extravasation.
- ERCP allows for nasobiliary drainage, sphincterotomy, and stenting in the setting of a biliary leak.

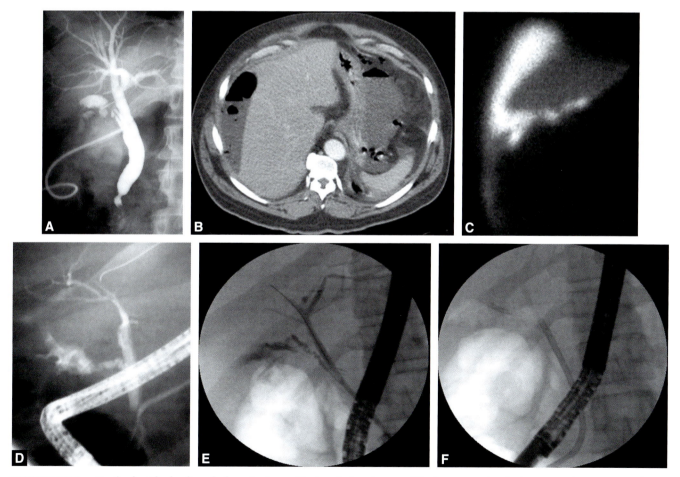

FIGURE 4.5.1 Cystic duct leak after cholecystectomy. T-tube cholangiogram **(A)** shows extraluminal contrast from a cystic duct stump leak. Contrast-enhanced CT image **(B)** from a second patient with a recent cholecystectomy shows multiple intraperitoneal collections containing fluid and gas. Subsequent hepatobiliary scintigraphy **(C)** shows tracer activity within the perihepatic fluid and tracking down the right paracolic gutter, which confirms a biliary leak but cannot localize the exact site. The leak was shown to be at the cystic duct stump at ERCP **(D)**. ERCP images **(E** and **F)** from a third patient show a cystic duct leak **(E)**, with subsequent placement of a biliary stent that bridges the cystic duct insertion **(F)**. The stent was removed 6 weeks later, and repeat cholangiogram (not shown) showed resolution of the leak.

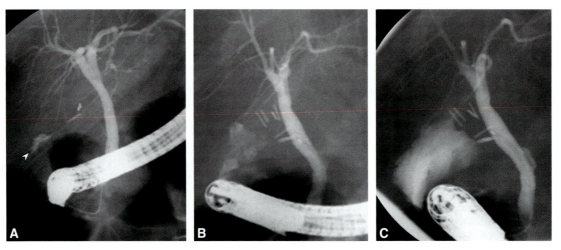

FIGURE 4.5.2 **Ducts of Luschka leak after cholecystectomy.** ERCP image (**A**) shows contrast leakage (*arrowhead*) into the gallbladder fossa via communicating intrahepatic ducts of Luschka. ERCP images (**B** and **C**) from a different patient show a similar leak. Localizing the site of leakage can be more difficult on delayed images as the extraluminal contrast accumulates (**C**).

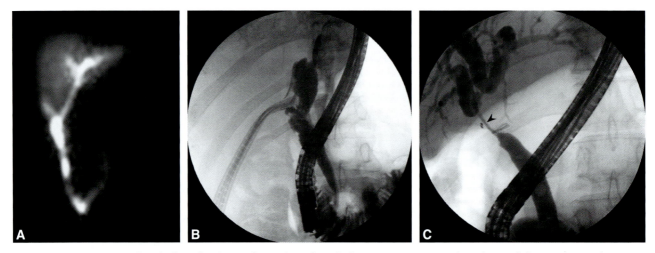

FIGURE 4.5.3 **Common duct leak and stricture formation after cholecystectomy.** Image from hepatobiliary scintigraphy (**A**) demonstrates intraperitoneal activity from a biliary leak. ERCP image (**B**) shows prominent subhepatic leakage of contrast without opacification of the proximal bile ducts. Subsequent ERCP image (**C**) after healing shows a high-grade common duct stricture (*arrowhead*) related to fibrosis at the site of injury.

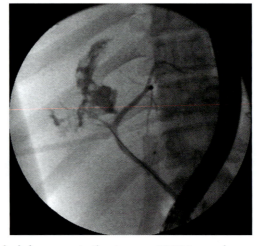

FIGURE 4.5.4 **Biliary leak from penetrating trauma.** ERCP image from a patient with a shrapnel injury to the liver shows extraluminal contrast secondary to a disruption of the right main intrahepatic duct.

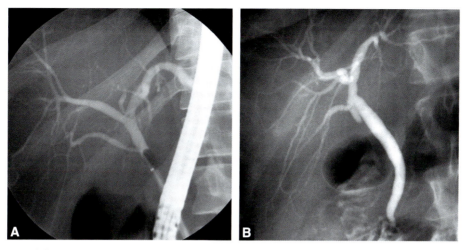

FIGURE 4.5.5 Aberrant biliary anatomy. ERCP images (**A** and **B**) from two different patients demonstrate the variable anatomy involving the right posterior duct, with low insertion into the common hepatic duct (**A**) and high insertion of the cystic duct into the right posterior branch (**B**).

4.6 Other Causes of Stricture and Obstruction

(Figures 4.6.1-4.6.6)

CLINICAL FEATURES

- In addition to the neoplasms, stones, and inflammatory conditions previously discussed, other conditions may occasionally result in biliary obstruction.
- Iatrogenic postoperative strictures of the extrahepatic duct are rare but tend to occur when the cystic duct is ligated at or near its insertion; presentation is often delayed until fibrosis causes significant obstruction.
- Both acute and chronic pancreatitis can cause clinically significant compromise of the extrahepatic duct.
- Ischemic and anastomotic strictures in the setting of liver transplantation are covered in Chapter 8.
- Portal biliopathy refers to extrinsic compression from dilated portal collaterals and/or ischemic strictures related to portal hypertension and extrahepatic venous occlusion.

IMAGING FEATURES

- Common duct strictures after cholecystectomy manifest on imaging with proximal biliary obstruction and little or no excretion on scintigraphy; the stricture can be confirmed on cholangiography.
- Biliary compromise from pancreatitis can result from compression due to adjacent inflammation or pseudocyst or from chronic inflammation leading to common bile duct stricture formation.
- Portal biliopathy can mimic PSC at cholangiography, but the areas of narrowing often appear smoother; cross-sectional imaging demonstrates the underlying portal vein occlusion.
- Other benign causes of biliary stricture and obstruction can mimic malignancy or other more common inflammatory conditions.

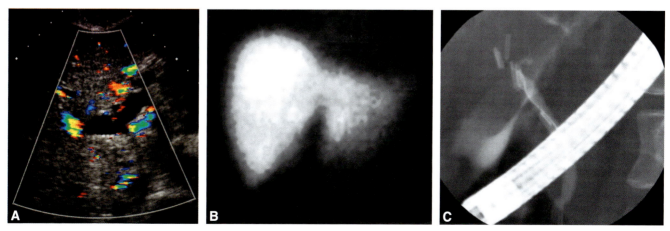

FIGURE 4.6.1 Common duct stricture from injury at cholecystectomy. Color Doppler US image (**A**) shows significant intrahepatic biliary ductal dilatation. Delayed image from subsequent hepatobiliary scintigraphy (**B**) shows no biliary excretion of the radiotracer. ERCP image (**C**) shows abrupt cut-off of the contrast column at the level of the cholecystectomy clips. Note the leakage of contrast without visualization of the proximal ducts.

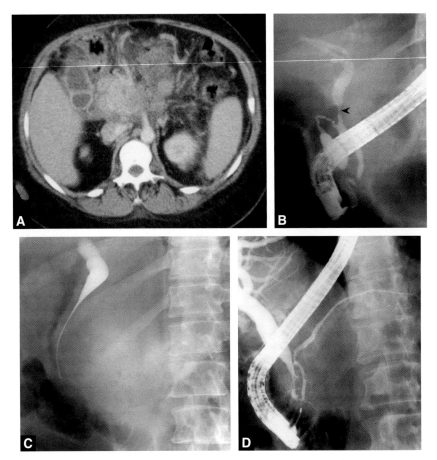

FIGURE 4.6.2 **Biliary compromise from pancreatitis.** Contrast-enhanced CT image **(A)** shows extensive pancreatic and peripancreatic inflammatory changes. Subsequent ERCP **(B)** shows extrinsic narrowing of the common hepatic duct (*arrowhead*) with proximal dilatation related to the surrounding inflammation from acute pancreatitis. ERCP image **(C)** from a second patient shows long-segment narrowing and lateral displacement of the common bile duct from a large pancreatic pseudocyst. The adjacent duodenal lumen is also compromised. ERCP image **(D)** from a patient with chronic pancreatitis shows a distal common bile duct stricture with proximal dilatation. Mild pancreatic ductal changes of chronic pancreatitis are also present.

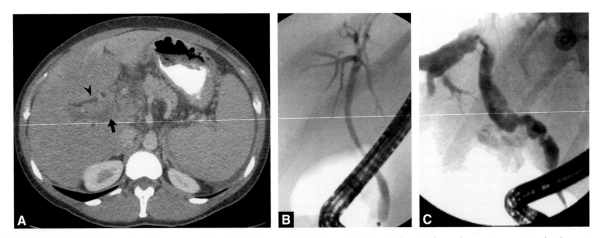

FIGURE 4.6.3 **Portal biliopathy.** Contrast-enhanced CT image **(A)** shows right portal vein thrombosis (*arrow*) and adjacent intrahepatic biliary ductal dilatation (*arrowhead*). ERCP image **(B)** shows smooth narrowing of the extrahepatic duct. ERCP image **(C)** from a second patient shows marked ectasia, caliber irregularities, and angulation of the common bile and hepatic ducts. Note multiple filling defects from choledocholithiasis.

Illustration continued on following page

OTHER CAUSES OF STRICTURE AND OBSTRUCTION 377

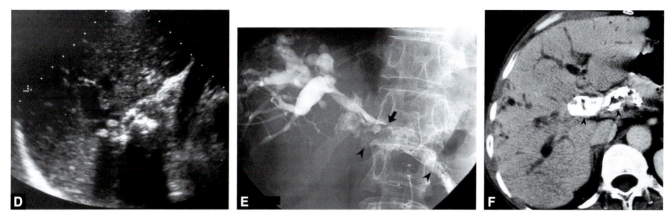

FIGURE 4.6.3 (Continued)   **Portal biliopathy.** US image **(D)** from a third patient shows dilated intrahepatic bile ducts proximal to echogenic shadowing foci, suggestive of choledocholithiasis. However, images from subsequent PTC **(E)** and CT **(F)** show dense portal vein calcification (*arrowheads*) that leads to a secondary biliary stricture (**E**, *arrow*). *(D to F from Pickhardt PJ, Balfe DM: Portal vein calcification and associated biliary stricture in idiopathic portal hypertension (Banti's syndrome). Abdom Imaging 1998; 23:180-182.)*

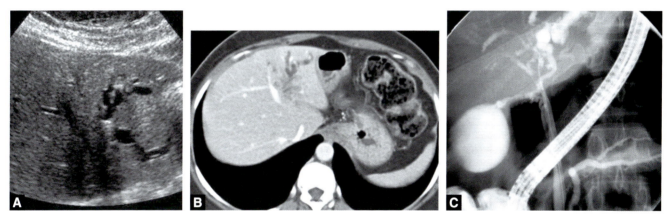

FIGURE 4.6.4   **Biliary stricture from sarcoidosis.** US image **(A)** shows segmental intrahepatic biliary ductal dilatation proximal to an ill-defined region with acoustic shadowing. Contrast-enhanced CT **(B)** shows similar findings with segmental biliary obstruction proximal to an area of decreased attenuation. ERCP **(C)** demonstrates a central stricture with segmental left hepatic dilatation; sarcoidosis was confirmed on biopsy.

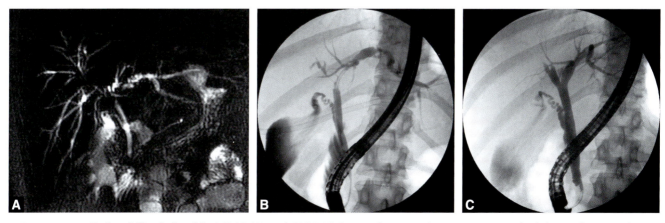

FIGURE 4.6.5   **Eosinophilic cholangitis.** MRCP **(A)** and ERCP **(B)** images from a patient presenting with abdominal pain and obstructive jaundice show cholangiographic findings suggestive of primary sclerosing cholangitis. Peripheral eosinophilia was present on laboratory evaluation. Follow-up ERCP **(C)** after corticosteroid treatment shows resolution of the biliary abnormalities.

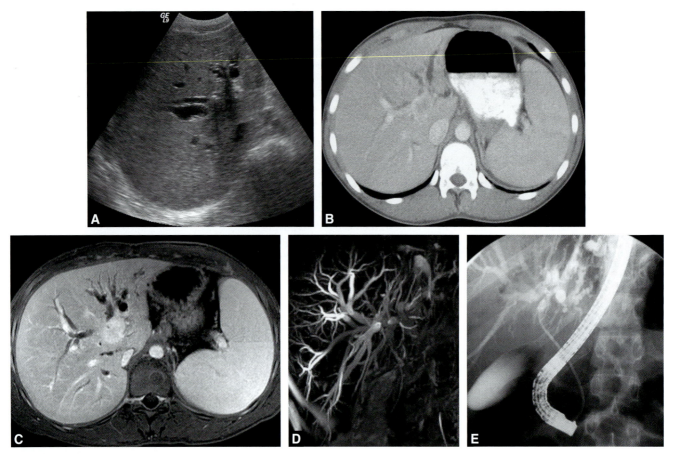

FIGURE 4.6.6 Biliary obstruction from hepatic inflammatory pseudotumor (myofibroblastic tumor). US (**A**), CT (**B**), and MR (**C**) images show intrahepatic biliary ductal dilatation secondary to an ill-defined mass in the hilar region, worrisome for malignancy. Hilar obstruction is well demonstrated on MRCP (**D**) and ERCP (**E**). Although percutaneous biopsy suggested an inflammatory pseudotumor, liver transplantation was deemed necessary due to the location of the mass. Inflammatory pseudotumor was confirmed in the explanted liver.

4.7 Hemobilia
(Figures 4.7.1-4.7.3)

CLINICAL FEATURES

- Hemobilia, or hemorrhage into the biliary tract, is most often due to blunt or iatrogenic trauma; less common causes include mycotic aneurysm, hepatic abscess, and neoplastic disease.
- Hemobilia often presents as jaundice, right upper quadrant pain, and melena and/or hematemesis.
- Clinical diagnosis can be difficult and mortality tends to be high.

IMAGING FEATURES

- Diagnosis is usually made at endoscopy with blood seen coming from the ampulla of Vater.
- CT angiography may be useful for localizing the source of active bleeding.
- Conservative treatment and maintaining biliary patency may be adequate therapy in patients with minor bleeding episodes.
- The preferred treatment option in active bleeding is selective arterial embolization; surgical ligation is usually performed in situations when angiographic techniques have failed to achieve hemostasis.

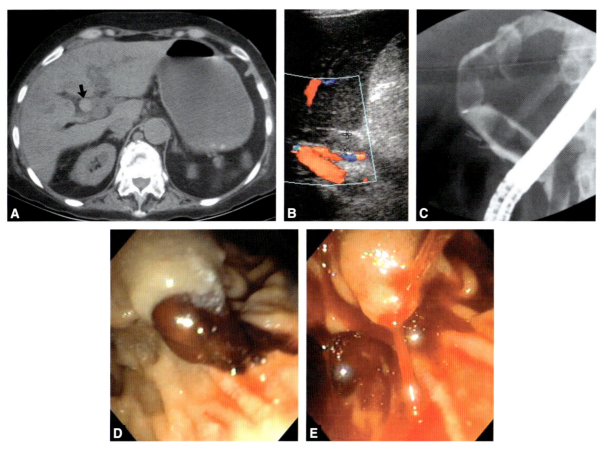

FIGURE 4.7.1 Hemobilia related to liver biopsy. Noncontrast CT image **(A)** shows high-attenuation material expanding the extrahepatic bile duct (*arrow*) worrisome for recent hemorrhage. Color Doppler US image **(B)** shows intraluminal material expanding the extrahepatic duct, which appears as a long cast-like filling defect at ERCP **(C)**. Endoscopic images show clot extruding from the major papilla **(D)**, followed by acute bleeding **(E)** after clot removal.

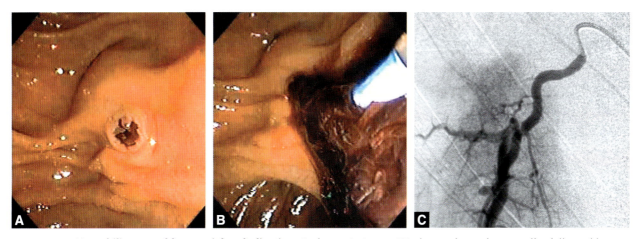

FIGURE 4.7.2 Hemobilia treated by arterial embolization. Endoscopic image **(A)** shows clot at the ampulla, followed by more extensive clot draining into the duodenum **(B)** after endoscopic manipulation with a sphincterotome during ERCP. Image from selective hepatic arterial angiogram **(C)** shows early venous filling and parenchymal extravasation. The arteriovenous fistula leading to hemobilia was caused by a liver biopsy. The fistula was treated by endovascular coil embolization.

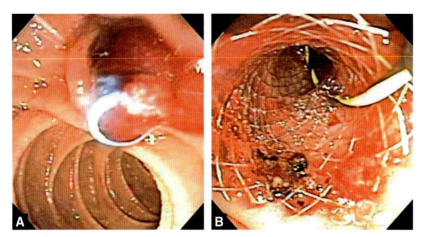

FIGURE 4.7.3 **Hemobilia treated with endoscopic stent placement.** Endoscopic image **(A)** shows blood draining from a plastic biliary stent that was previously placed for unresectable pancreatic adenocarcinoma invading the common bile duct. ERCP confirmed multiple filling defects consistent with intraductal clot (not shown). This was treated with balloon-assisted clot removal and endoscopic placement of a covered metallic stent to tamponade the friable tumor and maintain biliary patency **(B)**.

CHAPTER 7

THE PANCREAS

Andrew D. Lee, MD • Perry J. Pickhardt, MD

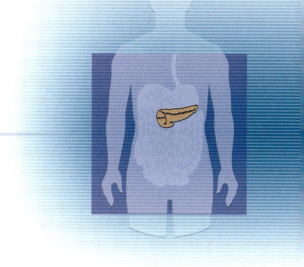

1. **PANCREATIC NEOPLASMS**
   1.1 Ductal Adenocarcinoma
   1.2 Mucinous Cystic Neoplasms
   1.3 Intraductal Papillary Mucinous Neoplasm
   1.4 Serous Cystadenoma
   1.5 Islet Cell Tumors
   1.6 Solid-Pseudopapillary Tumor
   1.7 Metastatic Disease
   1.8 Other Pancreatic Neoplasms

2. **PANCREATITIS**
   2.1 Acute Pancreatitis
   2.2 Chronic Pancreatitis
   2.3 Pancreatic Pseudocysts
   2.4 Autoimmune Pancreatitis

3. **OTHER PANCREATIC CONDITIONS**
   3.1 Pancreas Divisum
   3.2 Annular Pancreas
   3.3 Simple Pancreatic Cysts
   3.4 Pancreatic Trauma

Located in the anterior pararenal space of the retroperitoneum, the pancreas occupies an anatomic location that is relatively inaccessible by clinical examination. The combined use of CT, MR, US, ERCP, and EUS has revolutionized pancreatic evaluation. These complementary imaging modalities provide key information that guides clinical management for a diverse array of pancreatic diseases. Earlier diagnosis of pancreatitis and pancreatic ductal adenocarcinoma can lead to an improved clinical outcome. In this chapter the clinical and imaging features of a variety of pancreatic diseases, including neoplasms, inflammatory conditions, and a host of other pancreatic conditions, are discussed.

1. PANCREATIC NEOPLASMS

The classic differential diagnostic approach to pancreatic neoplasms begins with classifying a mass as solid or cystic. However, the overlapping of clinical and imaging features of the various tumors often precludes definitive characterization, making histopathologic diagnosis necessary in many cases. Regardless, the great majority of pancreatic neoplasms encountered in clinical practice are ductal adenocarcinomas, which continue to carry an ominous prognosis. In addition to ductal adenocarcinoma, the features of other less common pancreatic neoplasms, such as mucinous cystic neoplasms, serous cystadenomas, and islet cell tumors are discussed.

1.1 Ductal Adenocarcinoma
(Figures 1.1.1-1.1.7)

CLINICAL FEATURES
- Ductal adenocarcinoma accounts for the vast majority of pancreatic neoplasms.
- Although representing only 2% to 3% of all cancers in the United States, it is the fourth leading cause of cancer death, which reflects the dismal prognosis.
- It most often affects older patients, typically those 60 to 80 years old.
- Reported risk factors include cigarette smoking, diabetes mellitus, and various heritable syndromes.
- Early signs and symptoms include abdominal pain, jaundice, weight loss, nausea, and anorexia.
- Obstructive jaundice may be associated with a large, palpable, nontender gallbladder (Courvoisier's sign).
- Patients may rarely present with a migratory thrombophlebitis (Trousseau's sign).
- CA 19-9 is a nonspecific tumor marker, but it is elevated in 90% of cases.
- Greater than 60% of adenocarcinomas originate in the pancreatic head, with the remainder affecting the body and tail of the organ.
- The propensity for early invasion of local structures often prevents resectability, even for small tumors; vascular, lymphatic, and perineural spread is common.

- Regional lymph nodes, liver, and peritoneum are the most common sites of more distant metastatic spread.

IMAGING FEATURES

- US is often the initial imaging study in patients with jaundice and can confirm biliary ductal dilatation; if visualized, the primary tumor is hypoechoic and ill defined.
- Contrast-enhanced CT and MR are the initial imaging studies of choice for a suspected mass; ductal adenocarcinoma generally manifests as a hypovascular infiltrative mass.
- Tumors in the head of the pancreas often demonstrate both biliary and pancreatic ductal dilatation ("double duct sign").
- Obstructing tumors may result in pancreatitis and pseudocyst formation, resulting in overlap of imaging findings with bland pancreatitis.
- CT, MR, and EUS can assess for resectability; negative predictors include vascular encasement, invasion of local organs, lymphadenopathy, and hematogenous metastases.
- EUS is sensitive for the detection of small tumors, vascular involvement, and early lymph node metastases, in addition to providing a means for tissue sampling.
- MRCP or ERCP can depict the level and degree of biliary and pancreatic ductal obstruction.
- ERCP allows for palliative biliary stenting and brush cytology of strictures, although the diagnostic yield is relatively low (30% to 40%).

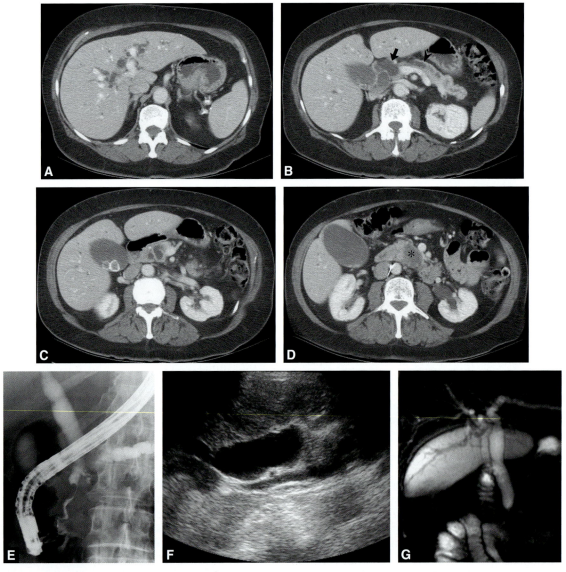

FIGURE 1.1.1 Pancreatic head ductal adenocarcinoma. Contrast-enhanced CT images (**A** to **D**) show marked biliary and pancreatic ductal dilatation ("double duct sign"). The gallbladder is also distended. The dilated common bile duct (**B**, *arrow*) and main pancreatic duct (**B**, *arrowhead*) are abruptly cut off by an ill-defined low-attenuation pancreatic head mass (**D**, *asterisk*). ERCP image (**E**) shows an eccentric obstructing filling defect in the distal common bile duct and again demonstrates the double duct sign. US (**F**) and MRCP (**G**) images from different patients show prominent extrahepatic biliary ductal dilatation with an abrupt cut-off from adenocarcinoma of the pancreatic head. Massive enlargement of the gallbladder on MRCP is the imaging correlate of Courvoisier's sign.

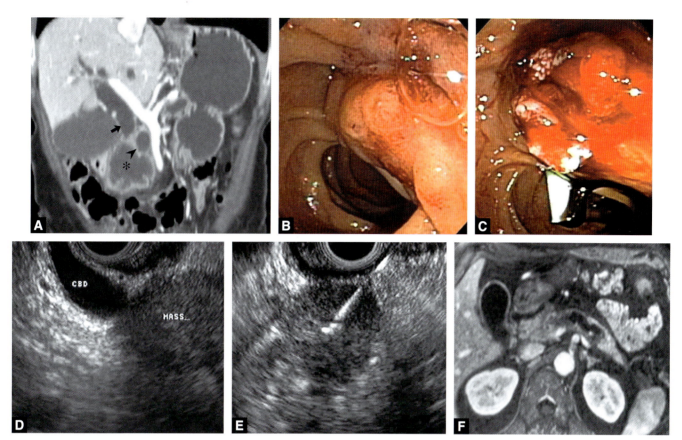

FIGURE 1.1.2 Pancreatic head ductal adenocarcinoma. Coronal reformatted CT image (**A**) shows a large low-attenuation pancreatic head mass (*asterisk*) causing both biliary (*arrow*) and pancreatic (*arrowhead*) ductal obstruction (double duct sign). Endoscopic images before (**B**) and after (**C**) biliary stent placement show the tumor invading the duodenum. EUS image (**D**) from a different patient shows a large hypoechoic mass resulting in biliary obstruction, which was successfully sampled under EUS-guided fine-needle aspiration (**E**). Contrast-enhanced fat-suppressed SGE MR image (**F**) from a third patient shows marked dilatation of the main pancreatic duct with an abrupt cut-off due to an infiltrative low-signal mass involving the pancreatic head and neck.

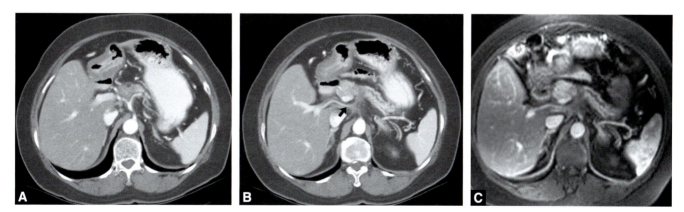

FIGURE 1.1.3 Ductal adenocarcinoma of the pancreatic body. Contrast-enhanced CT images (**A** and **B**) show an infiltrative low-attenuation mass involving the pancreatic body that causes pancreatic ductal obstruction and extends posteriorly into the peripancreatic fat, with encasement of the celiac axis and replaced right hepatic artery (**B**, *arrow*). Note the small pseudocyst superior to the dilated pancreatic duct. Contrast-enhanced fat-suppressed SGE MR image (**C**) shows similar findings.

Illustration continued on following page

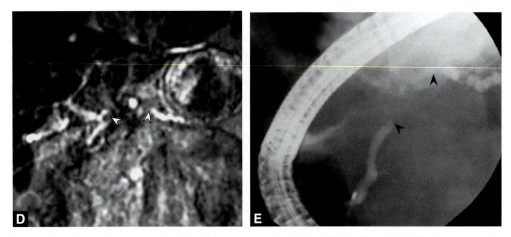

FIGURE 1.1.3 *(Continued)* **Ductal adenocarcinoma of the pancreatic body.** MRCP **(D)** and ERCP **(E)** images show segmental occlusion of the main pancreatic duct (*arrowheads*). The small pseudocyst seen in **A** is also demonstrated on MRCP **(D)**.

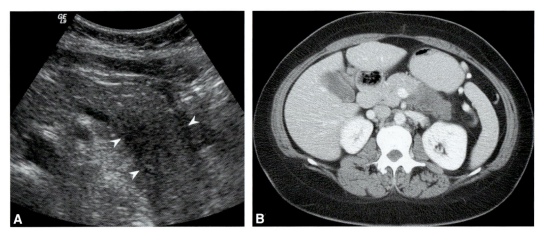

FIGURE 1.1.4 **Ductal adenocarcinoma of the pancreatic tail.** Transabdominal US image **(A)** shows a subtle decrease in echogenicity of the pancreatic tail (*arrowheads*) relative to the pancreatic body. Contrast-enhanced CT **(B)** shows diffusely decreased attenuation involving the pancreatic tail from the infiltrating tumor.

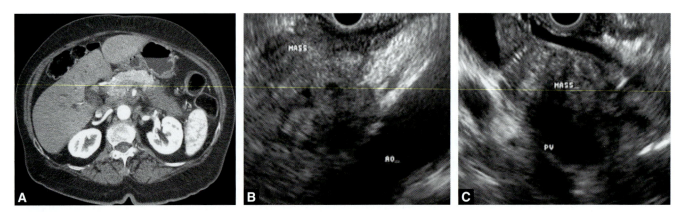

FIGURE 1.1.5 **Ductal adenocarcinoma with vascular invasion.** Contrast-enhanced CT image **(A)** shows an infiltrative low-attenuation mass involving the pancreatic tail, with direct posterior extension of soft tissue that encases the superior mesenteric artery and contacts the aorta. EUS image **(B)** from a second patient shows a hypoechoic, heterogeneous soft tissue mass with irregular borders extending to and abutting the aorta (AO). EUS image **(C)** from a third patient shows a hypoechoic mass with broad contact and loss of interface with the portal vein (PV).

Illustration continued on following page

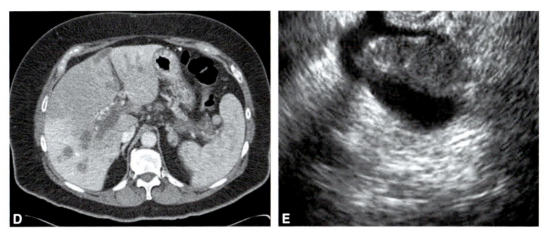

FIGURE 1.1.5 (Continued)   **Ductal adenocarcinoma with vascular invasion.** Contrast-enhanced CT image **(D)** from a fourth patient shows extensive portal vein tumor thrombosis. EUS image **(E)** from a final patient shows a hypoechoic mass with direct extension into the portal vein.

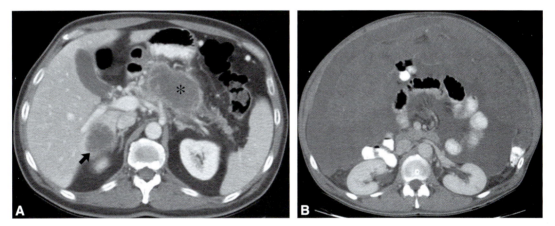

FIGURE 1.1.6   **Metastatic ductal adenocarcinoma.** Contrast-enhanced CT image **(A)** shows a large primary lesion (*asterisk*) involving the pancreatic body, as well as a low-attenuation hepatic lesion (*arrow*) from hematogenous spread. CT image **(B)** from a second patient shows extensive peritoneal carcinomatosis, with malignant ascites and thick omental caking.

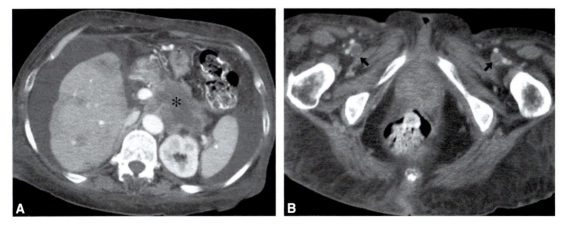

FIGURE 1.1.7   **Trousseau's sign in ductal adenocarcinoma.** Contrast-enhanced CT image **(A)** shows the pancreatic primary lesion (*asterisk*) with evidence of direct vascular invasion, hepatic metastases, and peritoneal carcinomatosis. A more caudal CT image **(B)** shows deep venous thrombosis involving the common femoral veins (*arrows*).

1.2 Mucinous Cystic Neoplasms

(Figures 1.2.1-1.2.2)

CLINICAL FEATURES

- Mucinous cystic neoplasm (MCN) is characteristically a macrocystic tumor.
- Intraductal papillary mucinous neoplasm (IPMN), a subset of MCN, is covered in the next section.
- MCNs are all regarded as at least potentially malignant (cystadenoma or cystadenocarcinoma).
- These tumors are most often diagnosed in middle-aged women, 40 to 60 years old.
- They may present as epigastric pain or fullness; weight loss and jaundice are of concern for malignant MCN.
- After complete resection, prognosis is more favorable compared with ductal adenocarcinoma.

IMAGING FEATURES

- Imaging features include large tumor size (often >10 cm), single or multiple large mucin-containing cysts (generally >2 cm), and thickened septations (with focal calcification in 15% to 20%).
- The propensity is for involvement of the pancreatic body and tail.
- Lack of ductal communication helps distinguish peripheral MCN from IPMN.
- CT and MR can demonstrate enhancement of the cyst walls and septations.
- Both transabdominal US and EUS can effectively depict the cystic and solid tumor components.
- PET may be useful for preoperative distinction of benign versus malignant status.
- Mural nodules are of concern for malignancy.
- A unilocular MCN may be initially misdiagnosed as a pancreatic pseudocyst; image-guided cyst aspiration with fluid analysis for amylase and tumor markers may help distinguish between the two.

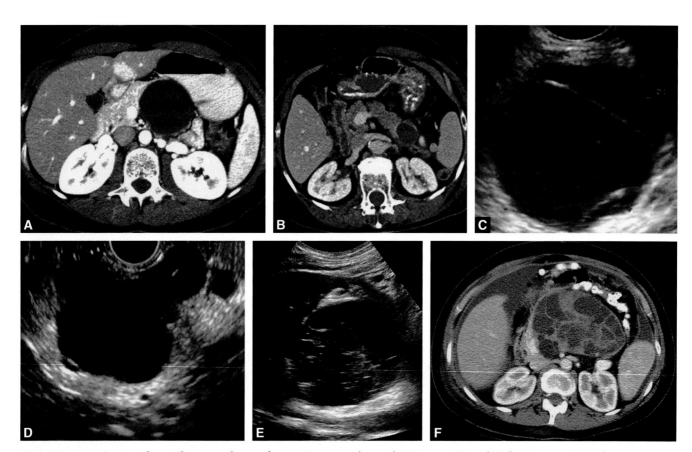

FIGURE 1.2.1 Pancreatic mucinous cystic neoplasms. Contrast-enhanced CT images (**A** and **B**) from two patients show pancreatic cystic lesions that demonstrate a relatively simple unilocular appearance, which can be mistaken for non-neoplastic disease. EUS images (**C** and **D**) from two different patients show more complex cystic lesions. Internal septations are often more conspicuous at sonographic evaluation. Transabdominal US (**E**) and CT (**F**) images from another patient show a large malignant multilocular cystic pancreatic tumor with a more prominent soft tissue component. Peritoneal carcinomatosis is present.

Illustration continued on following page

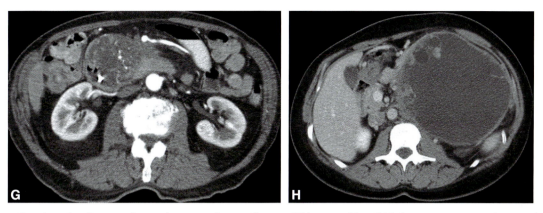

FIGURE 1.2.1 (Continued) **Pancreatic mucinous cystic neoplasms.** CT images (**G** and **H**) from two more patients with malignant MCN show complex cystic masses with septal calcification (**G**) and mural nodules (**H**).

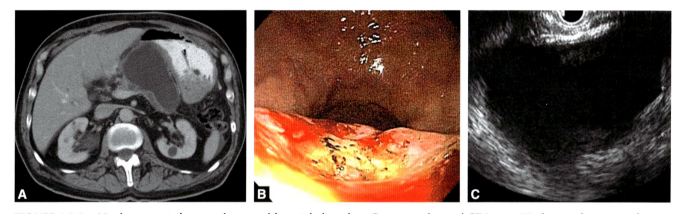

FIGURE 1.2.2 Mucinous cystadenocarcinoma with gastric invasion. Contrast-enhanced CT image (**A**) shows a large complex pancreatic cystic lesion with mass effect upon the stomach. EGD image (**B**) shows gastric mucosal ulceration related to invasion by the mass. EUS image (**C**) re-demonstrates the large complex cystic mass. Note the focal wall thickening suggestive of a malignancy.

1.3 Intraductal Papillary Mucinous Neoplasm
(Figures 1.3.1-1.3.4)

CLINICAL FEATURES

- Intraductal papillary mucinous neoplasm (IPMN) is a distinct subset of MCN that is being recognized with increasing frequency.
- IPMN was previously referred to by many other names, including duct ectatic mucinous cystadenoma (or cystadenocarcinoma), intraductal mucin-hypersecreting tumor, and intraductal papillary tumor.
- It is characterized by papillary tumor growth and mucin production within the main pancreatic duct, side branches, or both.
- Owing to presumed malignant or premalignant behavior, surgical resection is often considered the treatment of choice.
- Older adults are typically affected, with a slight predilection for males (unlike other cystic pancreatic neoplasms, which predominate in females).
- The clinical picture may resemble that of relapsing or chronic pancreatitis.
- Prognosis is generally favorable in the absence of invasive carcinoma.

IMAGING FEATURES

- Imaging features differ for main duct versus side branch involvement.
- ERCP features of main duct IPMN include a bulging or gaping papilla with extruding mucus, a dilated main pancreatic duct, and intraductal filling defects representing mucin or tumor.
- The imaging appearance of main duct IPMN can mimic chronic pancreatitis.
- Branch duct IPMN most often involves the uncinate process.
- Demonstrating communication of a multicystic lesion with the ductal system is key for diagnosis of branch duct IPMN; MRCP and ERCP may be useful in this regard.
- CT and MR features of invasive carcinoma in IPMN can include marked dilatation of the main pancreatic duct, diffuse or multifocal disease, mural nodules, or a solid mass.
- EUS characteristics include marked ductal dilation, mural nodules, and large irregularly septated cysts; tumors originating from side branches may appear as small clusters of cysts.

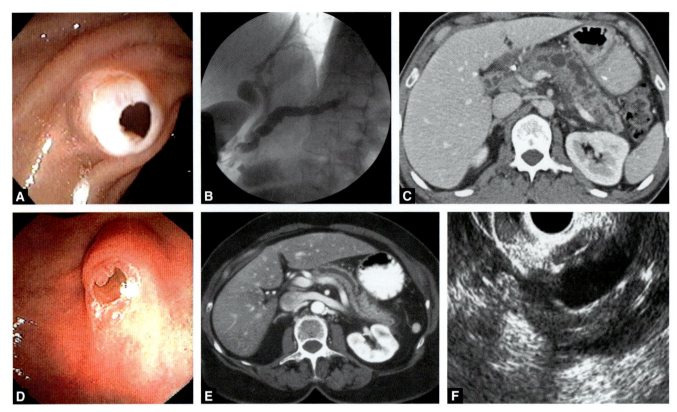

FIGURE 1.3.1 Main duct IPMN. Endoscopic image (A) shows a bulging major papilla with a gaping orifice filled with clear mucin. Corresponding ERCP image (B) shows dilatation of the main pancreatic duct. Contrast-enhanced CT image (C) from a different patient shows extensive pancreatic ductal dilatation with relative parenchymal preservation. Endoscopic image (D) from a third patient shows mucin extruding from a prominent papilla; contrast-enhanced CT image (E) shows a dilated main pancreatic duct. EUS image (F) from a final patient shows marked ductal dilatation.

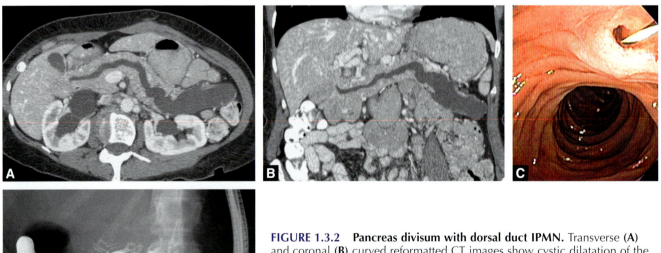

FIGURE 1.3.2 Pancreas divisum with dorsal duct IPMN. Transverse (A) and coronal (B) curved reformatted CT images show cystic dilatation of the entire dorsal duct in a patient with pancreas divisum (note how the dilated duct drains to the minor papilla). Endoscopic image (C) shows cannulation of the dilated minor papilla orifice. ERCP image (D) after injection via the minor papilla shows a massively dilated dorsal duct. The filling defects in the pancreatic tail represent intraluminal mucin. No invasive carcinoma was found at distal pancreatectomy.

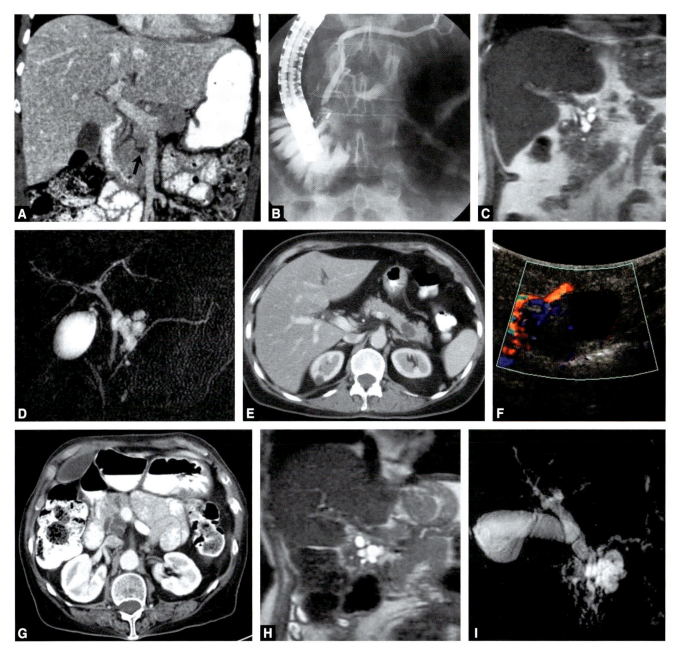

FIGURE 1.3.3 Side branch IPMN. Coronal reformatted CT image (**A**) shows cystic dilatation of a single side branch in the pancreatic head (*arrow*). On subsequent ERCP (**B**), contrast opacifies the same dilated side branch. Coronal T2-weighted SSFSE MR image (**C**) from a second patient shows a cluster of cystic lesions in the pancreatic head, which on MRCP (**D**) appears as a branching multicystic structure that communicates with, but does not directly involve, the main pancreatic duct. Contrast-enhanced CT (**E**) and intraoperative US (**F**) images from a third patient show a more nonspecific cystic lesion involving the pancreatic tail. Contrast-enhanced CT (**G**), T2-weighted MR (**H**), and MRCP (**I**) images from a final patient show a multicystic-appearing side branch IPMN involving the uncinate process.

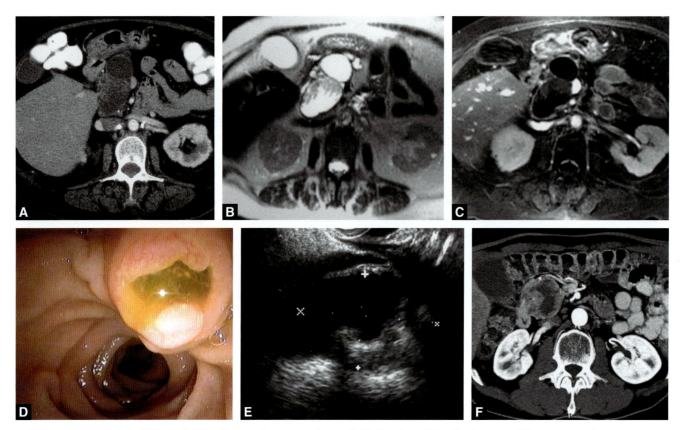

FIGURE 1.3.4 IPMN with invasive carcinoma. Contrast-enhanced CT (**A**), T2-weighted MR (**B**), and fat-suppressed contrast-enhanced SGE MR (**C**) images show a complex cystic and solid lesion occupying the pancreatic head. Enhancement of the soft tissue component is best depicted on the contrast-enhanced MR image (**C**). Endoscopic image (**D**) from a second patient shows a prominently bulging major papilla with abundant mucus. Corresponding EUS image (**E**) shows a massively dilated pancreatic duct and a solid mural nodule. Contrast-enhanced CT image (**F**) from a third patient shows a complex solid and cystic pancreatic head mass.

1.4 Serous Cystadenoma

(Figures 1.4.1-1.4.4)

CLINICAL FEATURES

- This benign lesion is also referred to as microcystic adenoma, but rare oligocystic macrocystic variants exist.
- Most of these tumors occur in middle-aged to elderly female patients; it is also associated with von Hippel-Lindau disease.
- Clinical presentation is often nonspecific; many lesions are detected incidentally at imaging.
- Tumors are primarily composed of multiple small glycogen-rich cysts separated by fibrous septa.
- Surgical resection may be performed in select cases where tumor mass effect results in obstructive jaundice, pancreatic insufficiency, or gastric outlet obstruction.

IMAGING FEATURES

- Tumor size varies from small to very large; there is no clear site predilection between the head, body, and tail.
- CT and MR show a lobulated, multicystic mass with a lacy or reticular pattern of septal enhancement.
- A central stellate scar with or without dystrophic calcification is characteristic.
- Individual cysts are generally <2 cm in diameter.
- Macrocystic and oligocystic variants may be difficult to distinguish from mucinous cystic neoplasm.
- US can usually resolve the individual cysts, but the lesion may appear hyperechoic if cysts are tiny.
- EUS may allow for better characterization of individual cysts due to a close proximity with the lesion.

SEROUS CYSTADENOMA

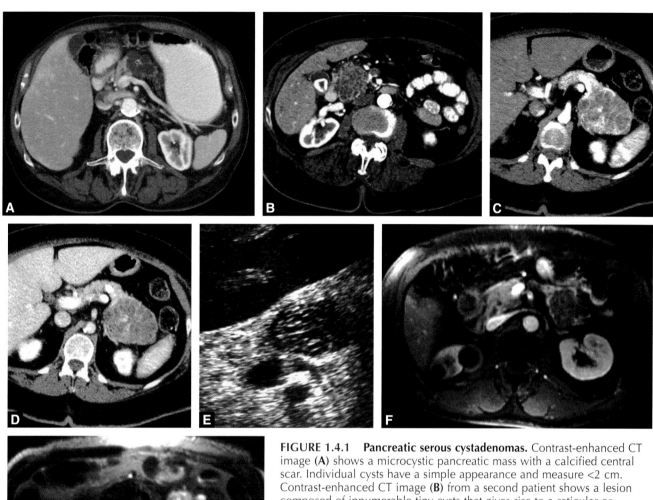

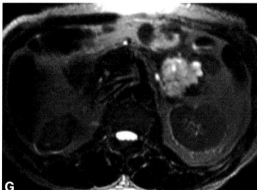

FIGURE 1.4.1 Pancreatic serous cystadenomas. Contrast-enhanced CT image (**A**) shows a microcystic pancreatic mass with a calcified central scar. Individual cysts have a simple appearance and measure <2 cm. Contrast-enhanced CT image (**B**) from a second patient shows a lesion composed of innumerable tiny cysts that gives rise to a reticular or honeycomb appearance from septal enhancement. An incidental rim calcified gallstone is present. Arterial (**C**) and portal venous (**D**) phase CT images from a third patient show a microcystic pancreatic tail lesion that demonstrates lacy septal enhancement that is more conspicuous on the earlier phase. Magnified image from transabdominal US (**E**) from a fourth patient shows a microcystic pancreatic mass that demonstrates a somewhat echogenic appearance from the multiple septal interfaces. Fat-suppressed contrast-enhanced SGE (**F**) and T2-weighted (**G**) MR images from a final patient show a microcystic lesion in the pancreatic tail.

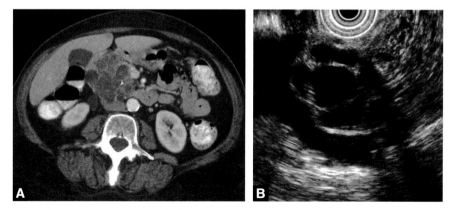

FIGURE 1.4.2 Serous cystadenomas: CT-EUS correlation. Contrast-enhanced CT image (**A**) shows a large microcystic pancreatic head mass with a punctuate focus of calcification. Corresponding EUS image (**B**) shows a portion of the mass with multiple discrete thin-walled cysts that compress the portal vein.

Illustration continued on following page

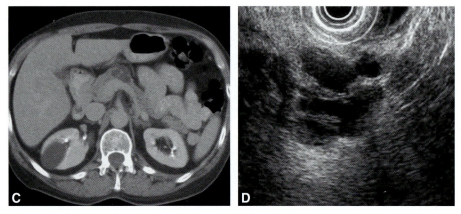

FIGURE 1.4.2 (Continued) **Serous cystadenomas: CT-EUS correlation.** Contrast-enhanced CT image (**C**) from a different patient shows another typical serous cystadenoma. Corresponding EUS image (**D**) again demonstrates the multicystic nature of the lesion.

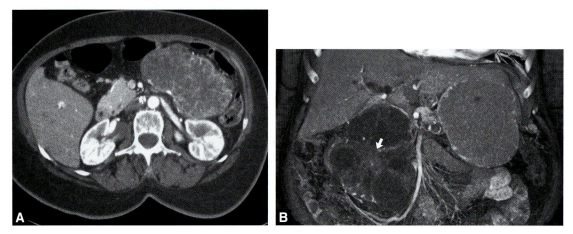

FIGURE 1.4.3 **Large serous cystadenomas.** Contrast-enhanced CT image (**A**) shows a large microcystic-appearing serous cystadenoma involving the pancreatic body and tail. Volume-rendered coronal CT image (**B**) from a second patient shows a large serous cystadenoma of the pancreatic head. Note the central scar (*arrow*) and mass effect on the mesenteric vessels.

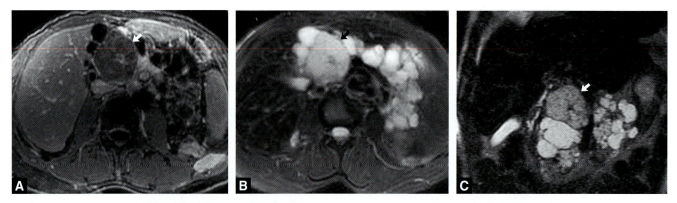

FIGURE 1.4.4 **Serous cystadenoma in von Hippel-Lindau disease.** Transverse contrast-enhanced SGE (**A**), transverse T2-weighted (**B**), and coronal T2-weighted (**C**) MR images show multiple simple cysts throughout the pancreas, as well as a serous cystadenoma (*arrows*), which demonstrates a central scar and signal characteristics that are distinct from the simple cysts.

1.5 Islet Cell Tumors

(Figures 1.5.1-1.5.7)

CLINICAL FEATURES

- These uncommon neoplasms arise from the neuroendocrine cells of pancreatic islets.
- Islet cell tumors may be sporadic or associated with syndromes such as multiple endocrine neoplasia (MEN) type-1 and von Hippel-Lindau disease.
- Hyperfunctioning (syndromic) tumors cause symptoms related to oversecretion of an active hormone and tend to be small in size at presentation.
- The remainder are considered nonhyperfunctioning (nonsyndromic) and tend to be larger at presentation.
- Insulinomas are the most common islet cell tumor (75% to 80% of hyperfunctioning tumors) and are predominately benign (>90%); patients present with hypoglycemia during exercise and fasting.
- Gastrinomas are the second most common type, are associated with MEN-1 in 40%, and are malignant in 60% of cases (less often in sporadic cases); patients often present with Zollinger-Ellison syndrome.
- Nonfunctional tumors are the third most common type, with malignant transformation occurring in 80% or more of cases.
- Rare islet cell tumors include VIPoma (associated with WDHA syndrome), glucagonoma (associated with cutaneous necrolytic migratory erythema), and somatostatinoma; these tumors are often malignant.

IMAGING FEATURES

- Most hyperfunctioning islet cell tumors are <4 cm (insulinomas are usually <2 cm), whereas most nonhyperfunctioning tumors are much larger (often >10 cm).
- On CT and MR, small islet cell tumors typically show enhancement during the arterial phase (i.e., hypervascular); large tumors are more heterogeneous and often demonstrate areas of cystic necrosis.
- Calcification is seen in 20% to 25% of cases on CT.
- At US, small islet cell tumors appear hypoechoic; EUS and intraoperative US are useful in the detection of small hyperfunctioning tumors.
- A cystic appearance is more common with larger tumors but is occasionally seen with smaller tumors.
- In patients with MEN-1, additional findings of the underlying syndrome may be present.
- Octreotide scintigraphy is a fairly specific test for detection and staging of islet cell tumors.
- Insulinomas occur anywhere in the pancreas; calcifications are uncommon but suggestive of malignancy.
- Gastrinomas are multifocal and metastatic in >50% of cases; most arise within the "gastrinoma triangle," involving the pancreatic head, second to third portion of the duodenum, distal stomach, and peripancreatic nodes.
- Metastatic disease most often affects the liver and peri–pancreatic nodes; liver lesions are typically hypervascular on CT and MR and have a target appearance at US (with a hypoechoic outer rim).
- A splenule (accessory spleen) adjacent to or within the pancreatic tail can mimic an islet cell tumor.

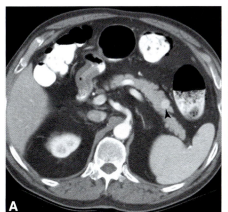 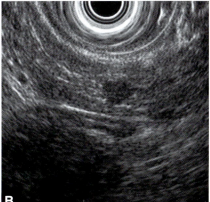 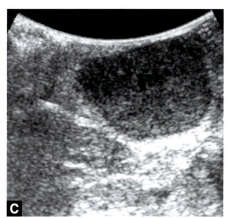

FIGURE 1.5.1 Islet cell tumors (insulinomas). Contrast-enhanced CT image **(A)** shows a small rounded hypervascular lesion (*arrowhead*) involving the pancreatic tail. EUS **(B)** and intraoperative US **(C)** images from two different patients show well-defined rounded hypoechoic pancreatic lesions.

Illustration continued on following page

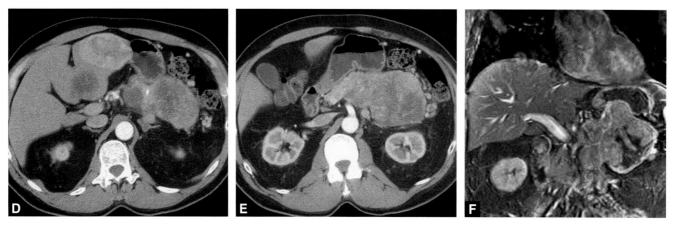

FIGURE 1.5.1 *(Continued)* **Islet cell tumors (insulinomas).** Contrast-enhanced CT **(D** and **E)** and MR **(F)** images in a patient presenting with symptomatic hypoglycemia show a large heterogeneously enhancing pancreatic tail mass. Liver metastases confirm the malignant nature in this atypical case of insulinoma.

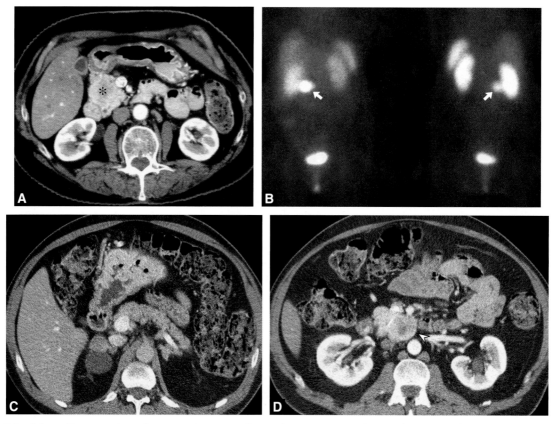

FIGURE 1.5.2 Islet cell tumors (gastrinomas). Contrast-enhanced CT image **(A)** shows a hypervascular mass (*asterisk*) that expands the pancreatic head. Mild gastric wall thickening is present from hypergastrinemia. Anterior and posterior views from octreotide scintigraphy **(B)** show uptake within the pancreatic mass (*arrows*) and physiologic uptake elsewhere without evidence of metastatic disease. Contrast-enhanced CT images **(C** and **D)** from a patient with malignant gastrinoma show hypervascular peripancreatic lymphadenopathy (**D**, *arrowhead*) and prominent gastric wall thickening. The primary tumor could not be found, which is not uncommon with small gastrinomas.

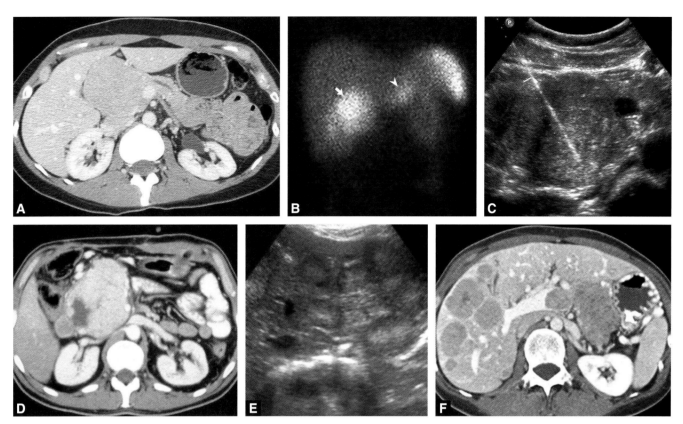

FIGURE 1.5.3 Nonhyperfunctioning (nonsyndromic) islet cell tumors. Contrast-enhanced CT image **(A)** shows a large rounded enhancing pancreatic mass, which is causing mild dilatation of the pancreatic duct. Octreotide imaging **(B)** shows uptake in the lesion (*arrow*), as well as a second smaller lesion (*arrowhead*) that also proved to be a nonhyperfunctioning islet cell tumor. Diagnosis was made by US-guided biopsy **(C)**. Contrast-enhanced CT image **(D)** from a second patient shows a large hypervascular pancreatic head mass with an area of cystic change. US image **(E)** from a third patient shows multiple hepatic "target" lesions with a hypoechoic outer rim, indicative of metastatic disease. Contrast-enhanced CT image **(F)** in this case shows both the hepatic metastases and the primary pancreatic tumor, which demonstrates direct venous extension to the portosplenic confluence.

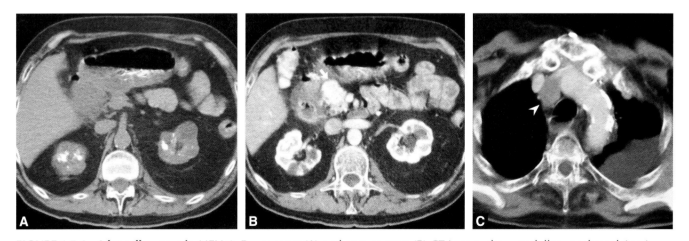

FIGURE 1.5.4 Islet cell tumors in MEN-1. Pre-contrast **(A)** and post-contrast **(B)** CT images show medullary nephrocalcinosis related to hyperparathyroidism and a briskly hypervascular pancreatic lesion (**B**, *arrow*), which proved to be an insulinoma. Thoracic CT image **(C)** shows a mediastinal parathyroid adenoma (*arrowhead*) adjacent to the aortic arch. The left pleural effusion was related to a thymic carcinoid tumor.

Illustration continued on following page

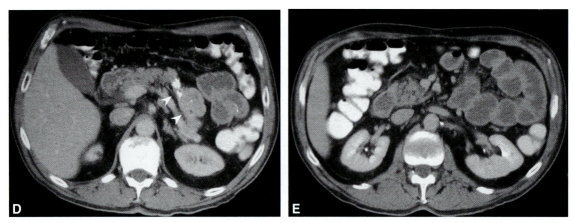

FIGURE 1.5.4 (Continued)   **Islet cell tumors in MEN-1.** Contrast-enhanced CT images (**D** and **E**) from a patient with MEN-1 and secretory diarrhea show a complex pancreatic tail mass (*arrowheads*) with coarse calcification, which proved to be a VIPoma. Note the watery small bowel contents resulting from the hypersecretory state. Bilateral adrenal enlargement related to a pituitary adenoma was seen better at other levels.

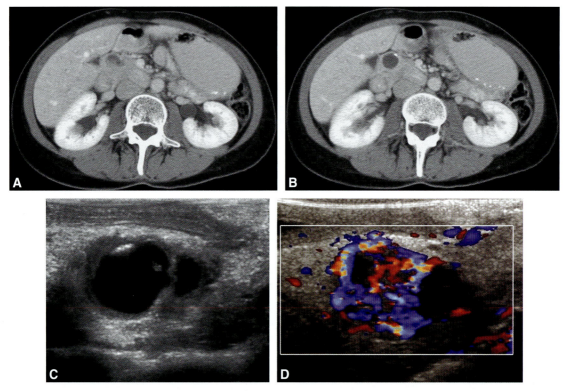

FIGURE 1.5.5 **Cystic islet cell tumor.** Contrast-enhanced CT images (**A** and **B**) show a complex cystic pancreatic mass with soft tissue and calcific components. Intraoperative US images (**C** and **D**) again demonstrate the complex cystic lesion and show prominent vascularity on color Doppler evaluation (**D**).

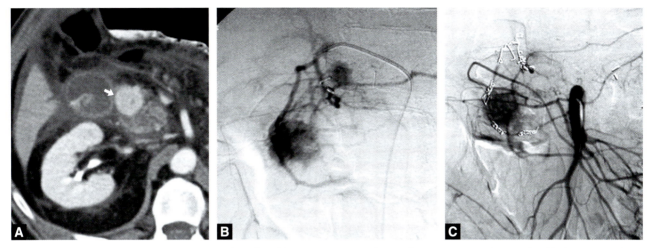

FIGURE 1.5.6 **Islet cell tumor in von-Hippel Lindau disease.** Contrast-enhanced CT image (**A**) shows a briskly hypervascular gastrinoma (*arrow*) from a patient who presented with bleeding duodenal ulcers from hypergastrinemia (Zollinger-Ellison syndrome). Invasive angiogram (**B**) with selective gastroduodenal artery injection shows two hypervascular gastrinomas within the pancreas. Subsequent selective injection of the superior mesenteric artery (**C**) after gastroduodenal artery embolization shows that the larger lesion remains vascularized.

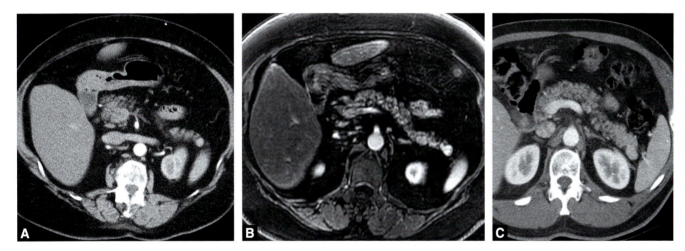

FIGURE 1.5.7 **Splenules simulating islet cell tumors.** Arterial phase CT (**A**) and MR (**B**) images show a small rounded hypervascular soft tissue nodule within the pancreatic tail that matches splenic enhancement. Contrast-enhanced CT image (**C**) from a different patient shows another case of accessory spleen within the pancreatic tail.

1.6 Solid-Pseudopapillary Tumor

(Figure 1.6.1)

CLINICAL FEATURES

- This rare low-grade tumor is also known as solid and papillary epithelial neoplasm (SPEN).
- It mostly affects younger women (<35 years old) and has a predilection for African-Americans and Asians.
- Clinical presentation is often nonspecific; many patients are asymptomatic at detection.
- Clinical laboratory tests and tumor markers are typically negative.
- Most tumors exhibit benign behavior, but approximately 15% are malignant.
- Prognosis is good after surgical resection, with only rare cases of recurrence and metastases.

IMAGING FEATURES

- The average size of these large tumors is approximately 10 cm at presentation.
- They are most commonly located in the pancreatic body and tail.
- On CT, US, and MR, these tumors typically appear as encapsulated, lobulated masses with both solid and cystic components; smaller tumors may appear completely solid.
- Cyst formation results from hemorrhagic degeneration; cysts often have thick walls and mural nodules.
- The hypovascular appearance on arterial-phase CT or MR helps to distinguish them from islet cell tumors.
- Dystrophic calcifications are an uncommon feature.

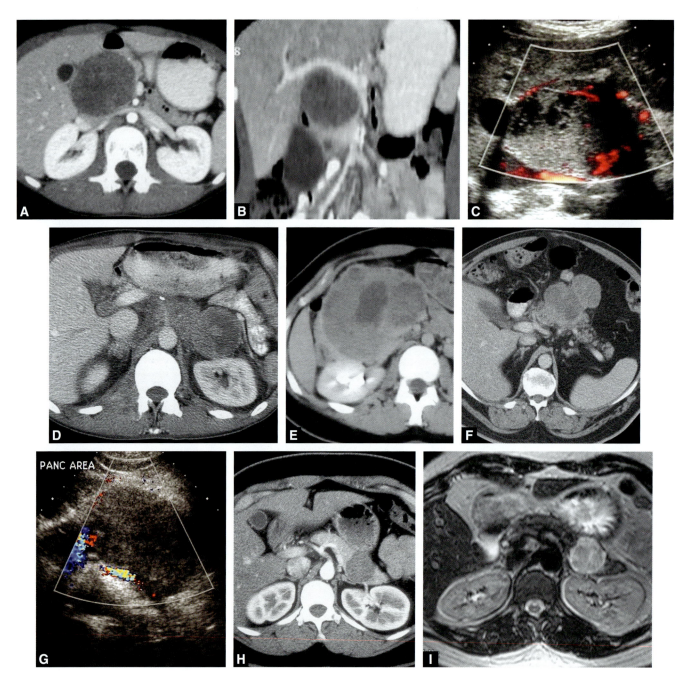

FIGURE 1.6.1 **Solid-pseudopapillary tumor.** Contrast-enhanced transverse (**A**) and coronal (**B**) CT images show a large heterogeneous low-attenuation pancreatic mass. The smaller cystic components are better depicted on US (**C**). Contrast-enhanced CT images (**D** to **F**) from three different patients show a complex solid and cystic mass with a mural nodule (**D**), a complex cystic mass with varying attenuation due to hemorrhage (**E**), and a lobulated solid mass (**F**). US image (**G**) from one patient and contrast-enhanced CT (**H**) and T2-weighted MR (**I**) images from another patient show predominantly solid pancreatic lesions.

1.7 Metastatic Disease

(Figures 1.7.1-1.7.3)

CLINICAL FEATURES

- Metastatic disease to the pancreas is a rare clinical manifestation of malignancy.
- The most common primary tumor with hematogenous spread to the pancreas is renal cell carcinoma.
- Less common hematogenous metastases include melanoma, lung cancer, and sarcomas, among others.
- Direct invasion by primary cancers of the stomach, colon, and duodenum is also seen.

IMAGING FEATURES

- Pancreatic metastases have a variable appearance on contrast-enhanced CT and MR.
- Hematogenous metastases from hypervascular primary tumors, particularly renal cell carcinoma, demonstrate prominent arterial phase enhancement.
- Hypovascular metastases can simulate pancreatic ductal adenocarcinoma if solitary.
- Depending on tumor location, biliary or pancreatic ductal dilatation from obstruction may be seen.

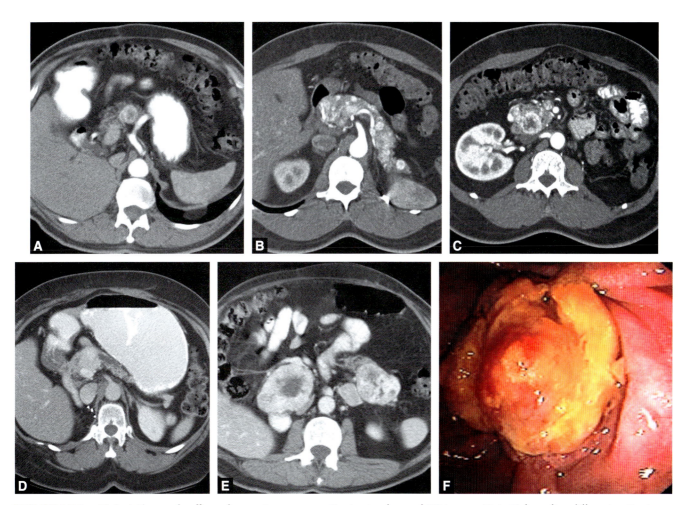

FIGURE 1.7.1 Metastatic renal cell carcinoma to pancreas. Contrast-enhanced CT images (**A** to **E**) from five different patients show hypervascular pancreatic lesions from metastatic renal cell carcinoma. In one case (**D**), a metastatic lesion causes pancreatic ductal dilatation. EGD image (**F**) from a final patient shows a large metastatic lesion involving the periampullary region.

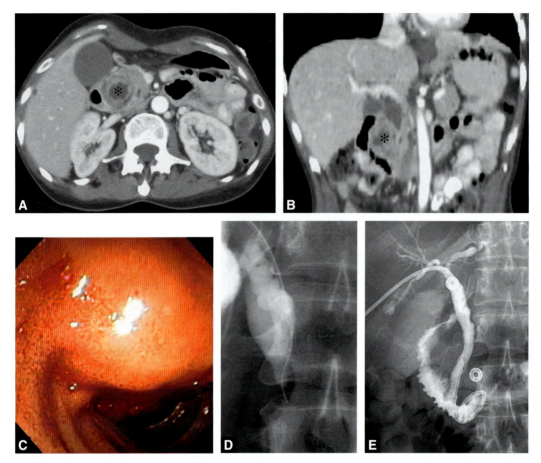

FIGURE 1.7.2 Biliary obstruction from metastatic lung cancer to pancreas. Transverse (**A**) and curved coronal (**B**) contrast-enhanced CT images show a large heterogeneous mass (*asterisks*) involving the pancreatic head causing biliary obstruction. EGD image (**C**) shows smooth external compression of the duodenum from the mass; endoscopic attempts at biliary decompression were unsuccessful. Images from percutaneous transhepatic cholangiography (PTC) show the level of biliary obstruction (**D**) and placement of a biliary drainage catheter (**E**) beyond the obstruction.

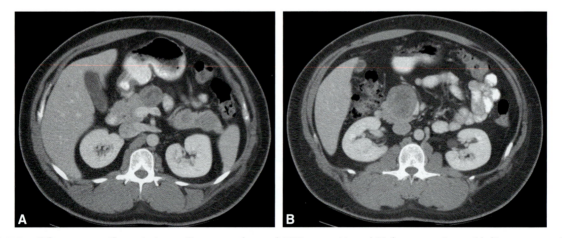

FIGURE 1.7.3 Other pancreatic metastases. Contrast-enhanced CT images (**A** and **B**) from a patient with liposarcoma show multifocal low attenuation pancreatic metastases.

Illustration continued on following page

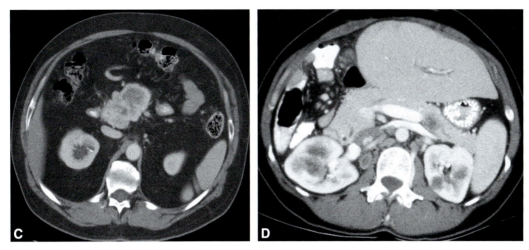

FIGURE 1.7.3 *(Continued)* **Other pancreatic metastases.** Contrast-enhanced CT images (**C** and **D**) from two different patients show metastatic lesions to the pancreas from meningeal hemangiopericytoma (**C**) and colonic adenocarcinoma (**D**). In the last case, metastatic colon cancer also involves the kidneys and retroperitoneal lymph nodes; partial hepatectomy was previously performed for metastatic disease.

1.8 Other Pancreatic Neoplasms
(Figures 1.8.1-1.8.7)

CLINICAL FEATURES

- Primary pancreatic lymphoma is far less common than direct spread by peripancreatic lymphadenopathy.
- Pancreatic and other extranodal forms of lymphoma are more common in the setting of immunocompromise, such as in patients with AIDS and organ transplantation (post-transplantation lymphoproliferative disorder [PTLD]).
- Other lymphoproliferative disorders, such as leukemia and multiple myeloma, can rarely affect the pancreas.
- Pancreatic acinar cell carcinoma is a rare exocrine neoplasm seen in elderly patients that portends a poor prognosis; systemic fat necrosis from elevated serum lipase can result in panniculitis.
- Small cell carcinoma of the pancreas is extremely rare but aggressive, usually affecting the elderly.
- Pancreaticoblastoma is rare but is the most common primary pancreatic tumor in children (< 8 years old).
- Pancreatic lipomas are uncommon benign tumors that are generally of no clinical significance.

IMAGING FEATURES

- Pancreatic lymphoma can manifest as multifocal or diffuse disease on cross-sectional imaging; most suspected cases are likely the result of spread via peripancreatic lymphadenopathy.
- AIDS-related lymphoma and PTLD should be suspected with pancreatic masses in the appropriate clinical setting.
- Lymphoproliferative diseases generally appear hypoechoic on US.
- Acinar cell carcinoma tends to be a large lobulated mass with central necrosis, occasionally with calcifications; metastatic disease is often present.
- Small cell carcinoma is typically an ill-defined low-attenuation tumor on CT; metastatic findings are common at presentation.
- Pancreaticoblastomas are large lobulated masses with variable amounts of necrosis, hemorrhage, and calcification; metastatic disease carries a poor prognosis, but most tumors are surgically resectable.
- Pancreatic lipomas demonstrate fat attenuation at CT; some suspected cases may simply represent peripancreatic fat insinuating between parenchymal lobules.

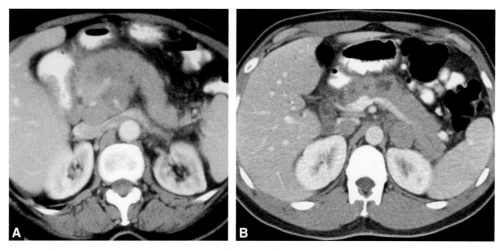

FIGURE 1.8.1 Pancreatic lymphoma. Contrast-enhanced CT image **(A)** shows ill-defined enlargement of the pancreatic head and neck region by lymphomatous tumor infiltration. Contrast-enhanced CT image **(B)** from a second patient shows more discrete low-attenuation foci of pancreatic involvement, as well as peripancreatic lymphadenopathy.

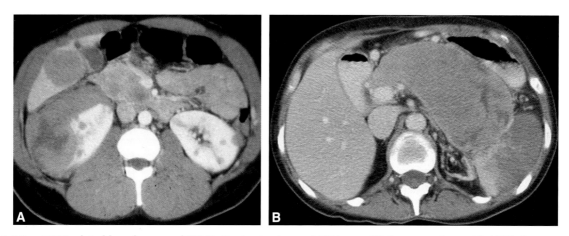

FIGURE 1.8.2 AIDS-related lymphoma and PTLD. Contrast-enhanced CT image **(A)** from a patient with AIDS shows lymphomatous involvement of the pancreatic head, kidneys, and liver. Contrast-enhanced CT image **(B)** from a renal transplant recipient shows massive enlargement of the pancreatic body and tail by PTLD, with associated subtotal splenic infarction related to splenic vein compromise. Note the atrophic native left kidney.

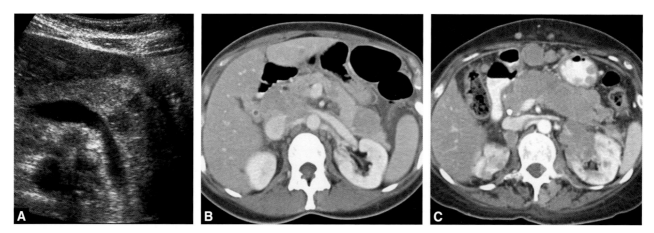

FIGURE 1.8.3 Other lymphoproliferative disorders. US image **(A)** shows two small hypoechoic foci within the pancreatic body from acute lymphoblastic leukemia. Corresponding CT image **(B)** shows the subtle pancreatic body lesions, as well as more bulky disease within the pancreatic tail and peripancreatic tissues. Contrast-enhanced CT image **(C)** from a patient with multiple myeloma shows extensive extramedullary involvement of the pancreas, as well as the peritoneum, retroperitoneum, kidneys, stomach, and subcutaneous fat.

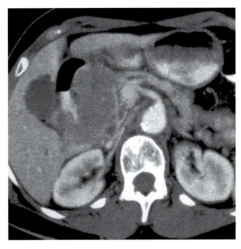

FIGURE 1.8.4 Pancreatic acinar cell carcinoma. Contrast-enhanced CT image shows a large, irregular, low-attenuation mass involving the pancreatic head.

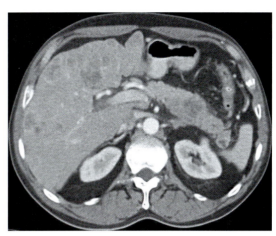

FIGURE 1.8.5 Pancreatic small cell carcinoma. Contrast-enhanced CT image shows an ill-defined low-attenuation mass within the pancreatic tail. Low-attenuation liver lesions represent metastatic disease from the pancreatic primary tumor.

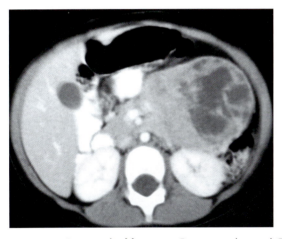

FIGURE 1.8.6 Pancreaticoblastoma. Contrast-enhanced CT image from an infant shows a large, complex, solid and cystic tumor extending off the pancreatic tail.

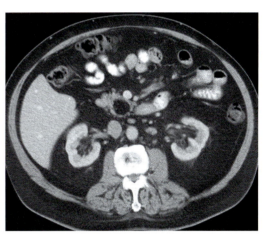

FIGURE 1.8.7 Pancreatic lipoma. Contrast-enhanced CT image shows a well-defined fat-containing lesion within the pancreatic head.

2. PANCREATITIS

The clinical diagnosis of pancreatitis can be challenging owing to its varied clinical manifestations. Delayed diagnosis or underestimation of disease severity can result in significant morbidity and mortality. The widespread use of contrast-enhanced CT has aided in the earlier diagnosis and triage of pancreatitis, resulting in improved clinical management of the disease, particularly for severe cases. The classification of pancreatitis into acute and chronic types is not simply a description of disease chronicity; rather, these two distinct entities have relatively little clinical overlap. This section will cover the clinical and imaging features of acute pancreatitis, chronic pancreatitis, pancreatic pseudocysts (common to both acute and chronic pancreatitis), and other inflammatory conditions of the pancreas.

2.1 Acute Pancreatitis

(Figures 2.1.1-2.1.7)

CLINICAL FEATURES

- In the United States, alcohol and biliary calculi account for 70% to 90% of acute pancreatitis.
- Less common causes include trauma, ERCP, mass effect from tumor, congenital anomalies, infection, medications, and metabolic disorders; in about 10% of cases, no identifiable cause is found.
- Clinical presentation can vary from vague abdominal pain and nausea to severe distress with shock and sepsis.
- The Ranson score, Acute Physiology and Chronic Health Evaluation (APACHE) II score, and Multi Organ System Score (MOSS) instruments estimate severity of disease to predict clinical outcome.

- The majority of cases represent mild edematous pancreatitis, which responds well to supportive care.
- The more feared diagnosis of necrotizing pancreatitis often requires intensive care and is associated with a mortality rate that exceeds 20%.
- Local complications include (peri)pancreatic fluid collections, abscess, pseudocysts, biliary obstruction, hemorrhage, bowel obstruction, venous thrombosis, and arterial pseudoaneurysm.
- Systemic complications include multiorgan system failure, renal failure, acute respiratory distress syndrome (ARDS), and sepsis, among others.

IMAGING FEATURES

- Suspected mild or uncomplicated pancreatitis is a clinical diagnosis; imaging is generally not indicated and can be normal.
- CT is the imaging modality of choice for suspected severe or complicated disease.
- Distinguishing between edematous and necrotizing pancreatitis is critical for management and prognosis.
- Typical CT findings of edematous pancreatitis include enlargement of the gland with preserved parenchymal enhancement and infiltration of the peripancreatic fat by inflammatory exudate.
- US findings of acute pancreatitis are more subtle; in the acute setting, this study is usually performed to evaluate for gallstones, which can suggest the underlying etiology.
- The peripancreatic inflammatory process typically dissects along retroperitoneal fascial planes; the anterior pararenal spaces and lesser peritoneal sac are common locations for exudate and fluid collections.
- Some peripancreatic fluid collections will evolve into pseudocysts, whereas others will completely resolve; large volume pancreatic ascites is uncommon.
- Necrotizing pancreatitis manifests on CT as areas of absent parenchymal enhancement, the degree of which correlates with clinical outcome.
- Abscess from superinfection of pancreatic necrosis or peripancreatic fluid should be suspected with clinical deterioration or gas bubbles on CT; needle aspiration may be necessary for confirmation.
- Pseudoaneurysm from erosion of a vessel wall by surrounding inflammatory exudate or adjacent pseudocyst is readily detected at CT; splenic and gastroduodenal arteries are most often affected.
- Venous thrombosis affecting the splenic or superior mesenteric veins is another vascular complication seen on contrast-enhanced CT.

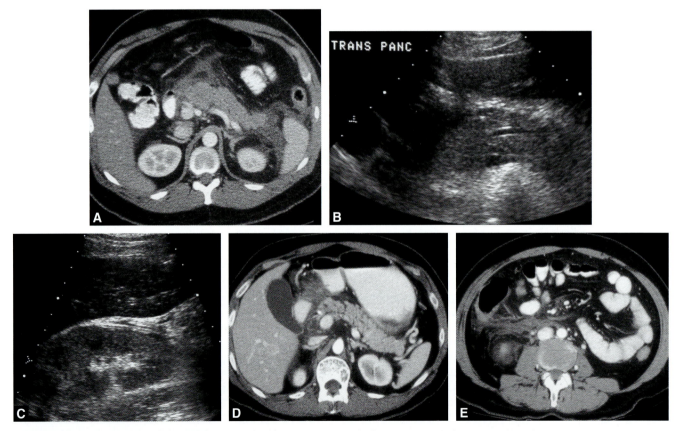

FIGURE 2.1.1 Edematous (interstitial) pancreatitis. Contrast-enhanced CT image (**A**) shows prominent peripancreatic inflammatory exudate with preserved enhancement of the pancreatic parenchyma. US image (**B**) from a second patient shows a slightly enlarged and hypoechoic appearing pancreas, with prominence of the main pancreatic duct. Imaging over the right flank (**C**) shows fluid tracking within the anterior pararenal space adjacent to the kidney, a common finding in acute pancreatitis. Contrast-enhanced CT images (**D** and **E**) from a third patient show peripancreatic inflammatory changes that extend inferiorly along the right anterior pararenal space, similar to the previous case. No evidence of pancreatic necrosis is present.

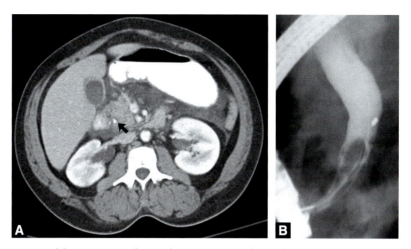

FIGURE 2.1.2 Gallstone pancreatitis. Contrast-enhanced CT image **(A)** shows findings of severe edematous pancreatitis with extensive peripancreatic inflammation. Note the dense gallstone (*arrow*) within the distal common bile duct, which reflects the underlying cause of pancreatitis. ERCP image **(B)** from a second patient with gallstone pancreatitis shows endoscopic removal of a common duct stone utilizing a retrieval basket.

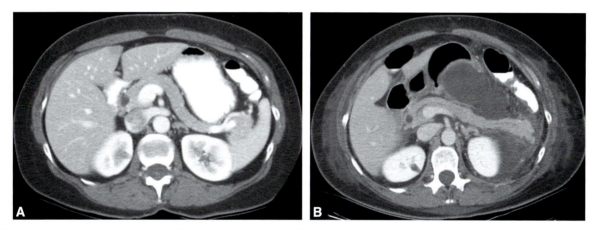

FIGURE 2.1.3 ERCP-induced pancreatitis. Contrast-enhanced CT images obtained before **(A)** and after **(B)** ERCP examination show the interval development of severe edematous pancreatitis. The large peripancreatic fluid collection within the lesser sac imparts mass effect upon the stomach. Subcutaneous inflammatory exudate and hemorrhage seen in bilateral flanks may give rise to the Grey-Turner sign on physical examination.

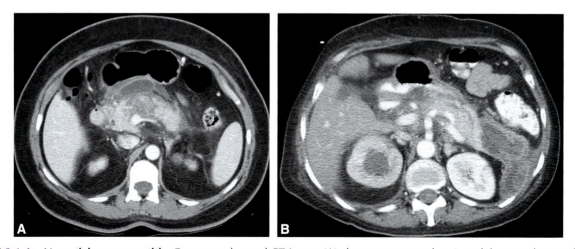

FIGURE 2.1.4 Necrotizing pancreatitis. Contrast-enhanced CT image **(A)** shows a segmental region of decreased parenchymal enhancement in the pancreatic body and neck, associated with peripancreatic inflammatory changes. Contrast-enhanced CT **(B)** from a second patient shows extensive peripancreatic exudate with necrosis involving the pancreatic tail. Right-sided hydronephrosis is present due to inflammation tracking along retroperitoneal fascial planes.

Illustration continued on following page

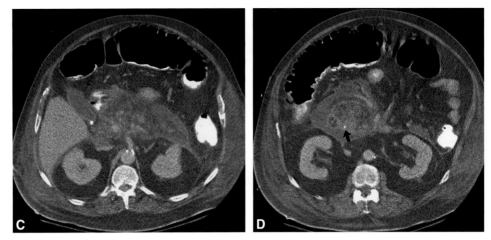

FIGURE 2.1.4 (Continued) **Necrotizing pancreatitis.** Contrast-enhanced CT images (**C** and **D**) from a third patient show extensive pancreatic and peripancreatic inflammation. The appearance of patchy pancreatic enhancement is due in part to underlying fatty involution, as well as superimposed necrosis. Note dense stones within the gallbladder and common bile duct (*arrow*) in this case of necrotizing gallstone pancreatitis.

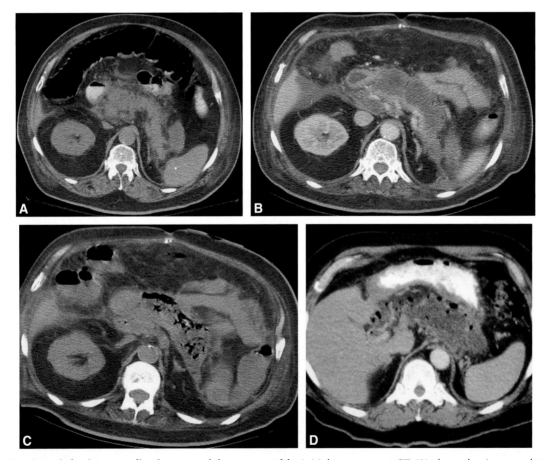

FIGURE 2.1.5 **Superinfection complicating necrotizing pancreatitis.** Initial noncontrast CT (**A**) shows haziness and stranding of the peripancreatic fat, consistent with acute pancreatitis. Evaluation for pancreatic necrosis is generally not possible without IV contrast. Follow-up CT with IV contrast (**B**) shows extensive pancreatic necrosis and overall worsening of peripancreatic inflammation and fluid. Subsequent noncontrast CT (**C**) obtained after rapid deterioration of the patient's condition shows interval development of mottled gas throughout the necrotic gland from intervening superinfection. Contrast-enhanced CT image (**D**) from another patient with declining clinical status in the setting of necrotizing pancreatitis shows gas bubbles throughout the poorly enhancing gland, which was a new finding not seen on the previous CT (*not shown*).

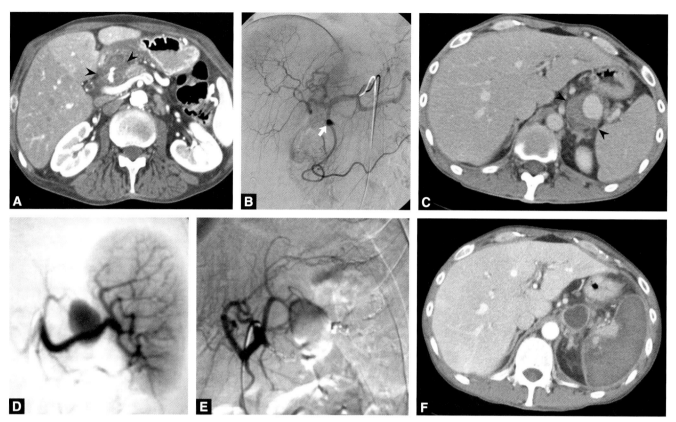

FIGURE 2.1.6 Pseudoaneurysms from pancreatitis. CT image (**A**) obtained during the arterial phase shows a large pseudoaneurysm (*arrowheads*) with prominent luminal thrombus involving the gastroduodenal artery related to local inflammation from pancreatitis. The gastroduodenal artery pseudoaneurysm was confirmed at invasive angiography (**B**, *arrow*) and treated. Note how the lesion appears smaller at angiography because the thrombus is not imaged. Contrast-enhanced CT image (**C**) from another patient with pancreatitis shows a large pseudoaneurysm involving the splenic artery (*arrowheads*), which was confirmed at invasive angiography (**D**) and treated with embolization (**E**) both proximal and distal to the pseudoaneurysm. Subsequent CT image (**F**) shows complete thrombosis of the pseudoaneurysm, as well as subtotal infarction of the spleen.

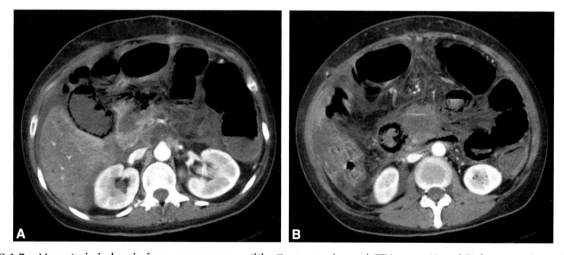

FIGURE 2.1.7 Mesenteric ischemia from severe pancreatitis. Contrast-enhanced CT images (**A** and **B**) from a patient with severe necrotizing pancreatitis show extensive pneumatosis and portomesenteric venous gas, indicating advanced mesenteric ischemia related to inflammatory occlusion of the superior mesenteric vessels.

2.2 Chronic Pancreatitis

(Figures 2.2.1-2.2.5)

CLINICAL FEATURES

- Progressive pancreatic inflammation leads to irreversible impairment of pancreatic function.
- This is a clinically distinct entity from acute pancreatitis, which only rarely progresses to chronic pancreatitis.
- Alcohol abuse is the primary cause; other causes include hyperlipidemia, hypercalcemia, and hereditary factors.
- Patients typically present with epigastric pain that is often accompanied by weight loss.
- Exocrine and endocrine dysfunction can lead to malabsorption with steatorrhea and insulin-dependent diabetes, respectively.

IMAGING FEATURES

- Abdominal radiographs may be diagnostic by showing punctate dystrophic calcifications that are focal or diffuse throughout the gland.
- CT may demonstrate an atrophic pancreas with a dilated and beaded appearance to the main pancreatic duct; dystrophic calcifications are present in the majority of cases.
- As with acute pancreatitis, pseudocysts are a common associated finding.
- EUS is more sensitive than transabdominal US for detecting characteristic findings, such as ductal dilatation, duct wall changes, or parenchymal findings such as lobularity or hyperechoic foci.
- ERCP and MRCP may show an irregularly dilated pancreatic duct, as well as side branch ectasia.
- Both pancreatic duct and distal common bile duct strictures may be seen.
- Exclusion of superimposed ductal adenocarcinoma in the setting of chronic pancreatitis can be difficult, because there is significant overlap in imaging findings.
- Vascular complications include splenic vein thrombosis and pseudoaneurysm formation.
- Pancreatic fistulas can result in ascites and pleural effusions; ERCP can be useful for localization.
- Occasionally, CT findings of acute-on-chronic pancreatitis will be seen.

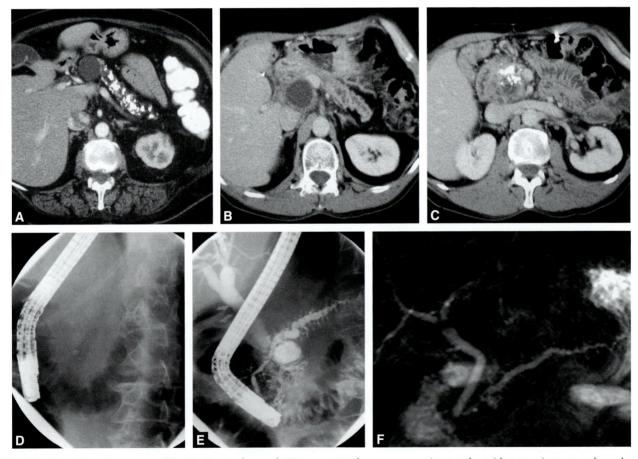

FIGURE 2.2.1 Chronic pancreatitis. Contrast-enhanced CT image (**A**) shows pancreatic atrophy with extensive parenchymal calcification and a well-defined pseudocyst. CT images from a second patient (**B** and **C**) show irregular pancreatic ductal dilatation with a beaded appearance, parenchymal atrophy, pseudocyst formation, and coarse pancreatic head calcifications. ERCP images (**D** and **E**) from a third patient show subtle pancreatic head calcifications (**D**) and irregular pancreatic ductal dilatation (**E**) with side branch ectasia and a small communicating pseudocyst. MRCP image (**F**) from a fourth patient shows a prominent main pancreatic duct with mild side branch ectasia and focal inflammatory stricture in the pancreatic head. Apparent cut-off of the biliary tree near the hilum is due to crossing hepatic vessels.

Illustration continued on following page

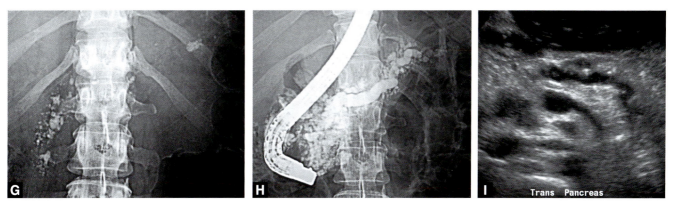

FIGURE 2.2.1 (Continued) **Chronic pancreatitis.** Scout radiograph **(G)** before ERCP from a fifth patient shows coarse calcifications distributed along the expected course of the pancreas. Subsequent ERCP image **(H)** shows massive dilatation of the pancreatic ductal system. Transabdominal US image **(I)** from a final patient shows an irregularly dilated main pancreatic duct and parenchymal heterogeneity with echogenic foci corresponding to calcifications, which were better seen on CT (*not shown*).

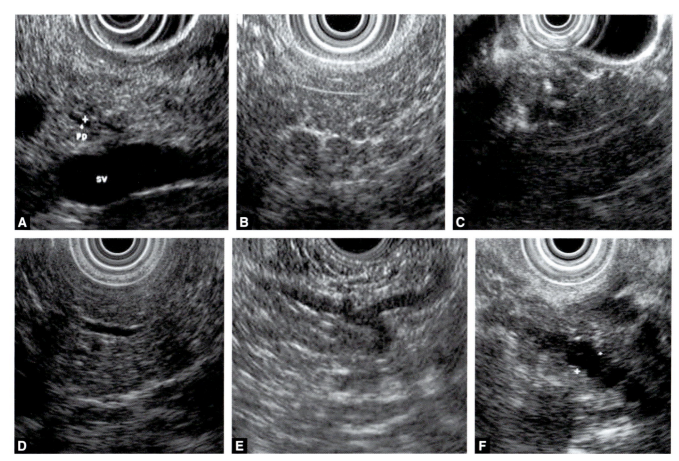

FIGURE 2.2.2 **EUS evaluation of chronic pancreatitis.** Multiple EUS images from different patients demonstrate the various characteristic changes of the pancreas that may be identified by endosonography. EUS of the normal pancreatic body **(A)** shows a homogeneous, finely granular parenchymal appearance, referred to as "salt and pepper." The main pancreatic duct is small without evidence of visible side branches. Parenchymal changes seen with chronic pancreatitis include lobulation with a mixed echogenic parenchyma **(B)** and multiple shadowing hyperechoic foci from calcifications **(C)**. Ductal changes include hyperechoic duct walls **(D)**, dilated secondary branches off the main duct **(E)**, and a dilated duct with irregular contours **(F)**. Also note the irregular outer margins of the pancreas in the last image, which is also a common finding.

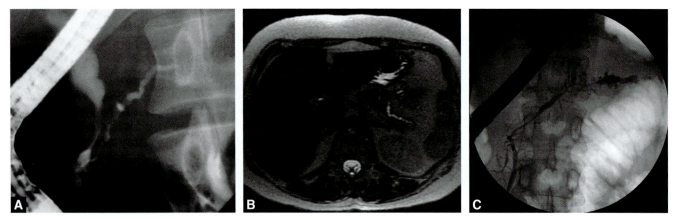

FIGURE 2.2.3 Ductal strictures in chronic pancreatitis. ERCP image (A) shows narrowing of both the main pancreatic and distal common bile ducts, an appearance that can simulate malignancy. T2-weighted MRCP image (B) from another patient shows focal ductal dilatation in the pancreatic tail. Subsequent ERCP image (C) shows an irregular long-segment inflammatory stricture with upstream ductal dilatation.

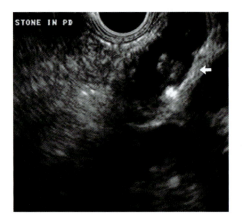

FIGURE 2.2.4 Ductal calculus in chronic pancreatitis. EUS image shows a stone (*arrow*) within an irregularly dilated main pancreatic duct.

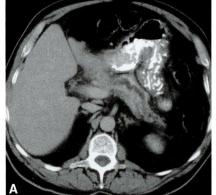 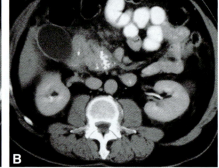

FIGURE 2.2.5 Acute-on-chronic pancreatitis. Contrast-enhanced CT images from a patient with abdominal pain show peripancreatic soft tissue infiltration from acute inflammation superimposed upon changes of underlying chronic pancreatitis, including ductal dilatation (A) and parenchymal calcification (B).

2.3 Pancreatic Pseudocysts
(Figures 2.3.1-2.3.8)

CLINICAL FEATURES

- Pseudocysts are organized fluid collections of pancreatic secretions surrounded by a fibrous rim of granulation tissue.
- These develop over a 4- to 6-week interval from acute fluid collections due to pancreatitis.
- Pseudocysts are reported to occur most commonly in alcoholic pancreatitis, but other causes include trauma, choledocholithiasis, and pancreatic carcinoma.
- Many pseudocysts demonstrate communication with the pancreatic duct.
- Symptoms are generally related to size and location of the pseudocyst; they may cause pain, nausea/vomiting, early satiety (from gastric or duodenal compromise), or jaundice (from biliary obstruction).
- Pseudocysts may rupture and cause ascites or peritonitis; superinfection results in abscess formation.
- Erosion into vessels can lead to pseudoaneurysm or massive hemorrhage.
- Management of symptomatic pseudocysts includes percutaneous, surgical, and endoscopic approaches to drainage.

IMAGING FEATURES

- Pseudocysts are most often located in a pancreatic or peripancreatic location but can dissect along any accessible fascial plane, ligament, or mesentery.
- On cross-sectional imaging, pseudocysts appear as well-defined rounded or ovoid fluid collections.
- Increased attenuation or heterogeneity of the fluid can suggest infection or hemorrhage; other findings such as rupture or change in size are easily detected on serial CT examinations.

- ERCP may demonstrate communication of the pancreatic duct with the pseudocyst; associated duct disruption or dominant stricture can sometimes be identified and treated with a bridging pancreatic stent.
- Endoscopy may show smooth luminal narrowing in the stomach or duodenum from mass effect.
- In a patient with a cystic pancreatic lesion but no documented history of pancreatitis, other causes such as mucinous cystic neoplasm should also be considered.

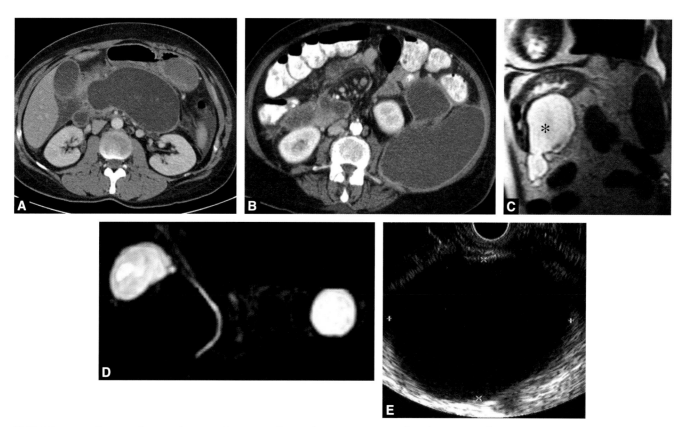

FIGURE 2.3.1 **Pancreatic pseudocysts.** Contrast-enhanced CT images (**A** and **B**) from two different patients show large well-defined pseudocysts in the lesser sac (**A**) and left pararenal space (**B**). Sagittal T2-weighted SSFSE MR image (**C**) from a third patient shows a large pseudocyst (*asterisk*) centered in the lesser sac with mass effect upon the stomach. MRCP image (**D**) from a fourth patient shows a pseudocyst in the pancreatic tail region; the biliary tree is normal. EUS image (**E**) from a final patient shows a large anechoic pseudocyst.

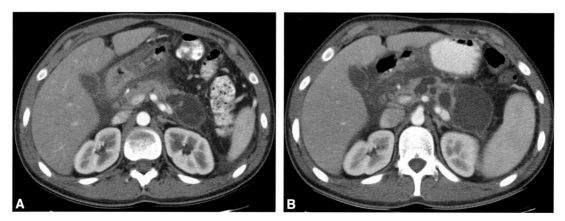

FIGURE 2.3.2 **Evolution of pancreatic pseudocysts.** Initial contrast-enhanced CT study (**A**) from a patient with acute pancreatitis shows extensive peripancreatic inflammation and a loculated fluid collection in the pancreatic tail region. Over time, multiple loculated collections increased in size and evolved into pseudocysts (**B**).

Illustration continued on following page

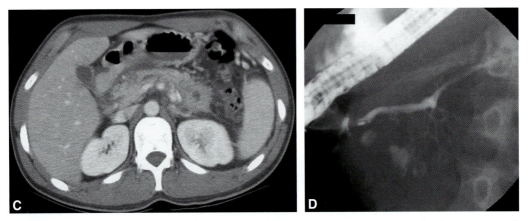

FIGURE 2.3.2 (Continued) **Evolution of pancreatic pseudocysts.** These pseudocysts largely resolved over time without intervention (**C**). ERCP image (**D**) shows small residual communicating pseudocysts in the pancreatic head region.

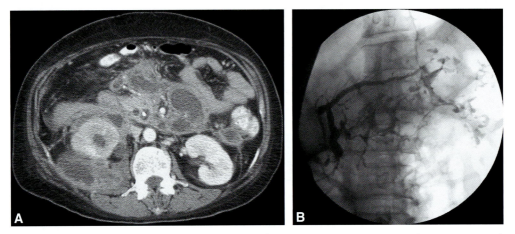

FIGURE 2.3.3 **Severe pancreatitis with multiple communicating collections.** Contrast-enhanced CT image (**A**) shows extensive inflammation involving the pancreas and extending along bilateral retroperitoneal fascial planes, including multiple loculated fluid collections. Note the right-sided hydronephrosis and delayed nephrogram related to partial obstruction from the inflammatory exudate. ERCP image (**B**) shows communication with multiple irregular peripancreatic collections.

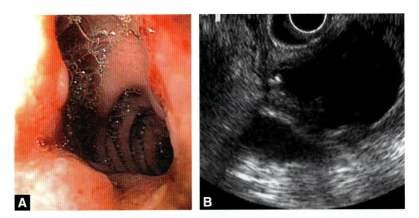

FIGURE 2.3.4 **Periduodenal pancreatic pseudocysts.** EGD image (**A**) shows duodenal luminal compromise and mucosal inflammation related to extrinsic compression by pseudocysts. The full extent of the fluid collections is better assessed by EUS (**B**).

Illustration continued on following page

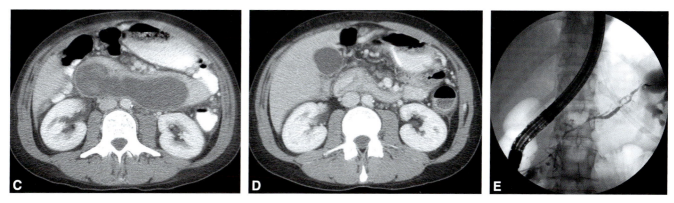

FIGURE 2.3.4 (Continued)   **Periduodenal pancreatic pseudocysts.** Contrast-enhanced CT image (**C**) from a different patient shows a large, complex elongated pseudocyst that follows the course of the duodenum and causes significant luminal compromise. Short-interval follow-up CT (**D**) shows complete resolution of this fluid collection, possibly related to spontaneous decompression into the duodenal lumen, since all other pseudocysts in this case demonstrated interval increase in size (*not shown*). ERCP image (**E**) shows strictures and ectasia related to chronic pancreatitis, as well as communication with another pseudocyst off the pancreatic tail.

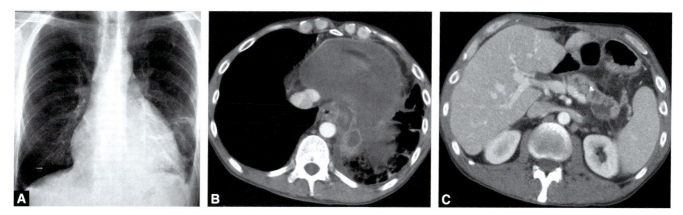

FIGURE 2.3.5   **Pericardial pancreatic pseudocyst.** Frontal chest radiograph (**A**) shows enlargement of the cardiac silhouette. Contrast-enhanced CT images (**B** and **C**) show that the radiographic findings are due to pericardial extension of a pancreatic pseudocyst. Note the calcified intraductal calculus in the pancreatic tail.

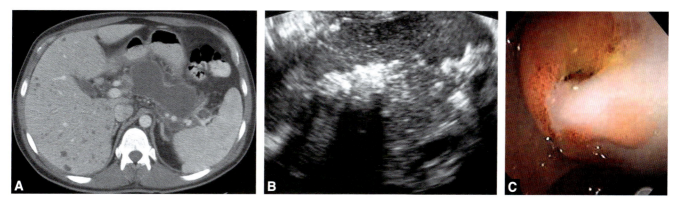

FIGURE 2.3.6   **Superinfected pancreatic pseudocyst.** Contrast-enhanced CT image (**A**) from a patient with severe necrotizing pancreatitis shows a large complex fluid collection that largely replaces the pancreas. The multiple cystic liver lesions represent biopsy-proven benign biliary hamartomas (von Meyenberg complexes). EUS image (**B**) obtained after the patient's condition rapidly deteriorated better demonstrates the complex nature of the fluid, which has transformed into an abscess. The echogenic shadowing foci deep to the complex fluid may represent gas bubbles, since no calcification was present on CT. Frank pus was seen emanating from the major papilla at endoscopy (**C**). Note the clear bile emanating from the top of the papilla, confirming that the pus is draining from the pancreatic duct.

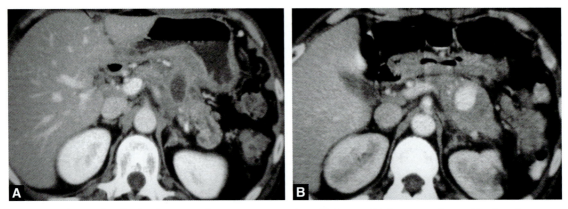

FIGURE 2.3.7 **Pseudocyst developing into pseudoaneurysm.** Baseline CT image **(A)** from a patient with chronic pancreatitis shows a well-defined pseudocyst near the junction of the pancreatic body and tail. Follow-up CT image **(B)** shows brisk filling of this collection by IV contrast, consistent with pseudoaneurysm formation.

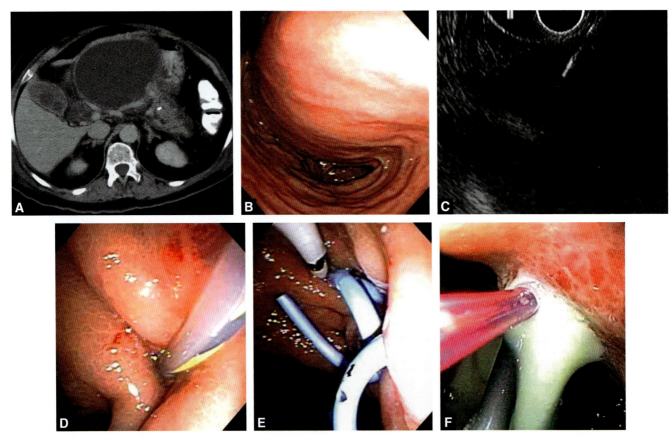

FIGURE 2.3.8 **Endoscopic drainage of pancreatic pseudocysts.** Contrast-enhanced CT image **(A)** shows a large pseudocyst extending into the lesser sac, with significant mass effect upon the stomach. Pancreatic calcification and low-attenuation lamellated gallstones are incidentally noted. EGD image **(B)** shows the luminal compromise of the stomach caused by the adjacent pseudocyst. EUS image **(C)** shows needle placement into the fluid collection to aspirate and examine the cyst fluid before transgastric drainage. A needle knife papillotome is subsequently used to create a fistula between the gastric lumen and pseudocyst **(D)**. Balloon dilatation of the tract is performed over a guidewire, and two double-pigtail stents are placed to maintain patency of the cyst-gastrostomy for adequate drainage **(E)**. EGD image from a different patient undergoing the same procedure shows pus extruding from the fistula indicating the development of an abscess **(F)**. Endoscopic drainage of pancreatic abscesses has a high failure rate and usually requires surgical treatment.

Illustration continued on following page

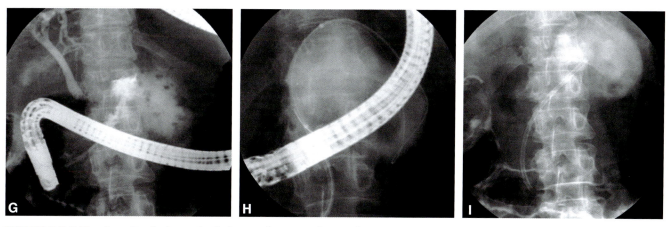

FIGURE 2.3.8 (Continued) **Endoscopic drainage of pancreatic pseudocysts.** ERCP images (**G** to **I**) from a different patient show contrast opacification of a large pseudocyst (**G**), with subsequent wire (**H**) and stent (**I**) placement for transpapillary drainage. This technique is most successful in pseudocysts communicating with the main duct in the pancreatic head or proximal body.

2.4 Autoimmune Pancreatitis
(Figures 2.4.1-2.4.2)

CLINICAL FEATURES

- Autoimmune pancreatitis, also known as lymphoplasmacytic sclerosing pancreatitis, fibrosing pancreatitis, or nonalcoholic duct-destructive pancreatitis, is a fibrosclerotic condition that is being increasingly recognized.
- Autoimmune pancreatitis is often associated with other fibrosing entities, such as sclerosing cholangitis and retroperitoneal fibrosis; it usually presents with mild abdominal symptoms.
- Serum IgG4 is usually elevated.
- Corticosteroid treatment in autoimmune pancreatitis has been effective for both pancreatic and extrapancreatic disease.
- Inflammatory pseudotumor of the pancreas is a related condition or atypical variant of autoimmune pancreatitis.

IMAGING FEATURES

- On CT and MR, autoimmune pancreatitis manifests as focal or diffuse pancreatic enlargement with decreased parenchymal enhancement; a surrounding capsule-like rim may be seen.
- Autoimmune pancreatitis can often mimic ductal adenocarcinoma; unlike typical chronic pancreatitis, calcifications, peripancreatic fluid collections, and pseudocysts are generally not seen.
- Associated findings such as bile duct changes similar to PSC or retroperitoneal fibrosis should suggest the diagnosis of autoimmune pancreatitis; renal involvement is occasionally seen.
- Inflammatory pseudotumor is usually indistinguishable from malignancy on imaging.

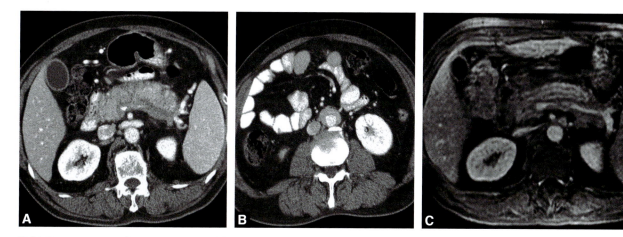

FIGURE 2.4.1 **Autoimmune pancreatitis.** Contrast-enhanced CT image (**A**) shows diffuse pancreatic enlargement with decreased enhancement and a low-attenuation capsule-like rim surrounding the pancreas. A more caudal CT image (**B**) shows a rind of periaortic soft tissue from coexisting retroperitoneal fibrosis. Contrast-enhanced fat-suppressed SGE MR image (**C**) again demonstrates decreased pancreatic enhancement and a surrounding rind of low signal.

Illustration continued on following page

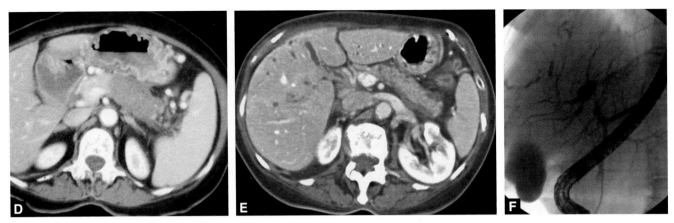

FIGURE 2.4.1 *(Continued)* **Autoimmune pancreatitis.** Contrast-enhanced CT image **(D)** from a second patient shows diffuse low-attenuation enlargement of the pancreatic body and tail, with sparing of the pancreatic head and neck. The appearance closely mimics that of ductal adenocarcinoma. Contrast-enhanced CT image **(E)** from a third patient shows pancreatic findings that are similar to the first case. Note also the irregular wall thickening of the extrahepatic bile duct and scattered intrahepatic biliary dilatation, which are due to coexisting PSC-like changes and better shown at cholangiography **(F)**.

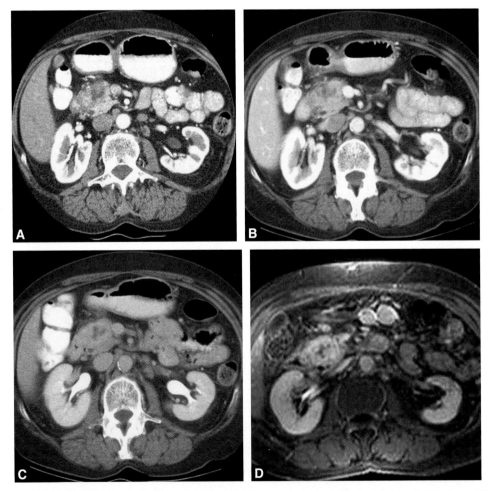

FIGURE 2.4.2 Pancreatic inflammatory pseudotumor. Arterial **(A)**, portal venous **(B)**, and delayed **(C)** phase CT images show a heterogeneous pancreatic head mass with both early and late peripheral enhancement and a persistent area of central low attenuation. Contrast-enhanced fat-suppressed SGE MR image **(D)** shows similar findings. It is imperative to exclude malignancy in such cases.

3. OTHER PANCREATIC CONDITIONS

3.1 Pancreas Divisum
(Figures 3.2.1-3.2.2)

CLINICAL FEATURES

- This common anatomic variant (4% to 10% of adults) results from a lack of normal fusion between the dorsal and ventral pancreatic anlagen during development; most cases remain clinically silent.
- A short ductal system from the pancreatic head and uncinate process drains via the major papilla, and the dorsal duct from the entire body and tail is drained via the minor papilla.
- Patients with recurrent idiopathic pancreatitis have pancreas divisum in up to 25% of cases; often the minor papilla is stenotic, thus impeding the flow of pancreatic body and tail secretions.
- Treatment consists of endoscopic sphincterotomy of the minor papilla with temporary pancreatic stent placement; surgical sphincteroplasty has also been performed for therapy.

IMAGING FEATURES

- ERCP is the imaging modality of choice for confident diagnosis or confirmation of pancreas divisum; MRCP can provide noninvasive diagnosis when indicated.
- CT can suggest the diagnosis when the dorsal duct is well visualized to the minor papilla without ventral communication; the pancreatic head may have an elongated apperance.
- During ERCP, cannulation and injection at the major papilla demonstrates a short ventral pancreatic duct within the pancreatic head that does not cross midline; in one third of cases, the ventral duct is absent.
- Cannulation of the minor papilla and injection of the dorsal duct (of Santorini) opacifies the entire body and tail region, without communication with the ventral duct (of Wirsung).
- Imaging findings of associated pancreatitis may be seen involving the dorsal anlage.
- Cystic bulging at the minor papilla, the so-called santorinicele, can suggest the diagnosis.

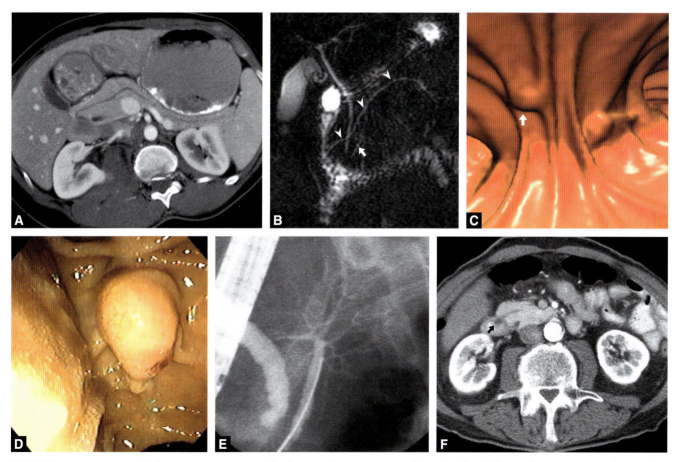

FIGURE 3.1.1 Pancreas divisum. Transverse curved reformatted CT image **(A)** shows the dorsal duct (of Santorini) extending to the minor papilla without communication with the ventral system. MRCP image **(B)** from a second patient noninvasively demonstrates the separated dorsal (*arrowheads*) and ventral (*arrow*) ducts. 3D endoluminal image **(C)** from CT "virtual EGD" study shows a slightly prominent minor papilla (*arrow*) above the normal-appearing major papilla. EGD image **(D)** from a different patient shows a bulging minor papilla (santorinicele). ERCP image **(E)** after injection of the ventral ductal system demonstrates abrupt arboreal termination. Note acinarization from aggressive contrast injection. Contrast-enhanced CT image **(F)** in a final patient shows a prominent dorsal duct leading to a santorinicele at the minor papilla (*arrow*). Visual separation of the primary pancreatic ductal system from the common bile duct is the key to quick recognition of pancreas divisum on cross-sectional imaging.

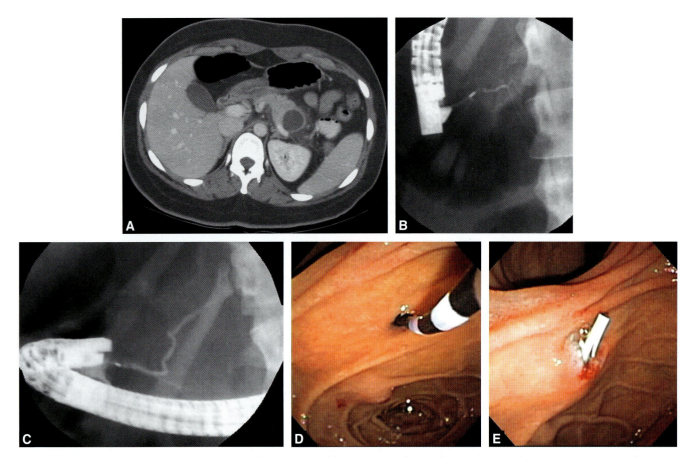

FIGURE 3.1.2 Pancreas divisum with "idiopathic" pancreatitis. Contrast-enhanced CT image **(A)** from a young woman shows inflammatory peripancreatic stranding and a developing pseudocyst involving the pancreatic tail. ERCP image **(B)** after cannulation of the major papilla shows a diminutive ventral duct, whereas injection through the minor papilla **(C)** opacifies the entire dorsal duct draining the pancreatic body and tail. EGD images show sphincterotomy **(D)** and stent placement **(E)** at the minor papilla.

3.2 Annular Pancreas

(Figures 3.2.1-3.2.2)

CLINICAL FEATURES

- In this rare developmental anomaly, a band of pancreatic tissue originates from the ventral anlage and encircles the second portion of the duodenum.
- Symptoms may occur in the neonatal period or later in life.
- Neonatal symptoms typically relate to duodenal obstruction; the disorder may be associated with duodenal atresia or stenosis, gastrointestinal malrotation, and cardiac anomalies.
- Nonspecific delayed presentation may include pain, nausea, and/or vomiting; symptoms may be related to peptic ulceration, recurrent pancreatitis, or duodenal stenosis.

IMAGING FEATURES

- Neonatal radiographs and US demonstrate gastric and proximal duodenal dilatation, the so-called double-bubble sign.
- Barium UGI studies show extrinsic ring-like stenosis at the second portion of the duodenum; periampullary duodenal ulcers may occasionally be seen.
- CT demonstrates soft tissue encircling the second portion of the duodenum that matches the attenuation of pancreatic parenchyma; proximal duodenal dilatation may be present.
- ERCP is often diagnostic because contrast injection of the major papilla will show a small duct encircling the duodenum; the main pancreatic duct in the body and tail is usually normal.
- MRCP may also demonstrate the duct encircling the duodenum; the cuff of pancreatic tissue surrounding the duodenum can be confirmed on other MR sequences.

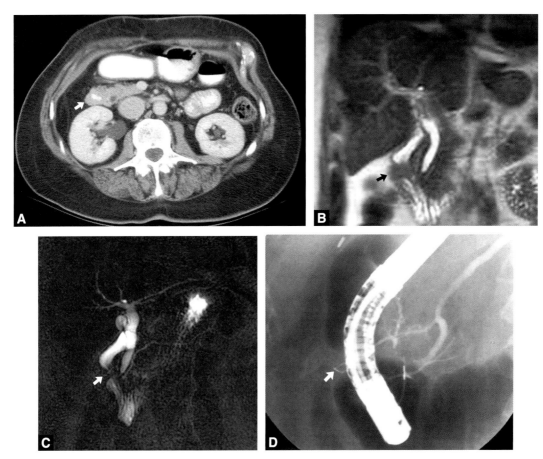

FIGURE 3.2.1 Annular pancreas. Contrast-enhanced CT image **(A)** shows a cuff of soft tissue (*arrow*) surrounding the contrast-filled duodenum that closely matches the appearance of the inseparable adjacent pancreatic head tissue. Coronal T2-weighted SSFSE MR image **(B)** again demonstrates the cuff of soft tissue (*arrow*) around the second portion of duodenum. MRCP image **(C)** shows a subtle duct (*arrow*) encircling the duodenum at the point of annular constriction. ERCP image **(D)** clearly shows the abnormal duct (*arrow*) encircling the endoscope within the focally narrowed portion of duodenum.

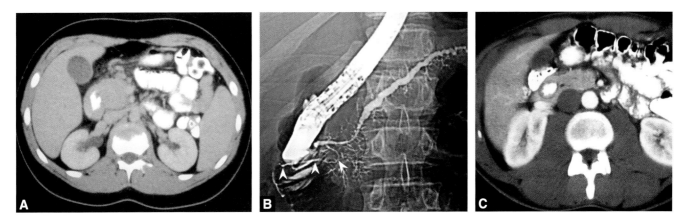

FIGURE 3.2.2 Annular pancreas. CT image **(A)** from a teenager with "idiopathic" pancreatitis shows a thick rim of pancreatic tissue surrounding the contrast-filled duodenum. Adjacent hazy soft tissue infiltration from associated pancreatitis is present. ERCP image **(B)** shows the opacified duct (*arrowheads*) encircling the duodenum. Contrast-enhanced CT image **(C)** from a different patient clearly demonstrates the continuity of the pancreatic head parenchyma as separate from the duodenal wall.

Illustration continued on following page

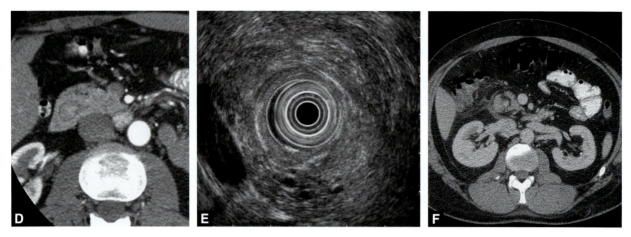

FIGURE 3.2.2 (Continued)   Annular pancreas. Contrast-enhanced CT image (D) during the arterial phase shows pancreatic tissue encircling the second portion of the duodenum. Corresponding EUS image (E) at the level of the papilla shows a circumferential band of tissue with an echogenic pattern consistent with pancreatic parenchyma. Note continuity with the head of the pancreas at the bottom of the image and a few small cysts from underlying chronic pancreatitis. Contrast-enhanced CT image (F) from a final patient shows annular pancreatitis with pancreatic tissue encircling a narrowed duodenum and peripancreatic exudate extending along the right anterior pararenal space.

3.3 Simple Pancreatic Cysts

(Figures 3.3.1-3.3.3)

CLINICAL FEATURES

- In distinction to pseudocysts (see earlier), simple pancreatic cysts are lined by epithelium and do not communicate with the pancreatic duct; these are relatively uncommon and almost always asymptomatic.
- Lymphoepithelial cysts are a subset lined by squamous epithelium and mature lymphoid tissue.
- Multiple pancreatic cysts are a common finding in von Hippel-Lindau disease; these patients are also more prone to pancreatic serous cystadenomas and islet cell tumors.
- Autosomal dominant polycystic disease is associated with pancreatic cysts, but these are rare compared with the ubiquitous renal cysts and frequent hepatic cysts.
- Cystic fibrosis most often demonstrates diffuse fatty replacement of the pancreas, but small pancreatic cysts may also be seen.

IMAGING FEATURES

- As with simple cysts involving other organs, they demonstrate fluid attenuation at CT, hyperintensity at T2-weighted MR, and are anechoic with increased through-transmission at US.
- The cyst walls should be uniformly thin or imperceptible; thin septations may be present, particularly with lymphoepithelial cysts.
- Simple cysts lack any significant enhancement; if present, a cystic neoplasm must be considered.
- Fine-needle aspiration of fluid for analysis is helpful in differentiating a simple cyst from a cystic neoplasm and may be performed using EUS, transabdominal US, or CT.
- The presence of multiple pancreatic cysts suggests an underlying condition, particularly von Hippel-Lindau disease.

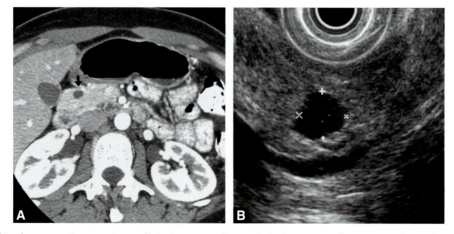

FIGURE 3.3.1   Isolated pancreatic cysts (sporadic). Contrast-enhanced CT image (A) shows a small simple-appearing cyst (arrow) in the pancreatic head. EUS image (B) confirms its simple nature as an anechoic cyst.

Illustration continued on following page

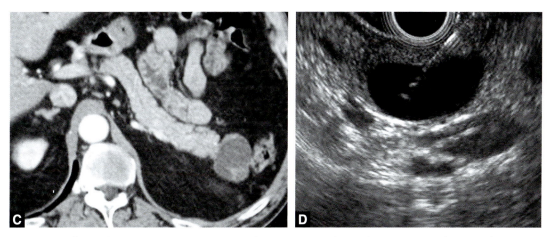

FIGURE 3.3.1 (Continued) **Isolated pancreatic cysts (sporadic).** Contrast-enhanced CT image (**C**) from a different patient shows a slightly complex cyst extending off the pancreatic tail, which proved to be a benign lymphoepithelial cyst. Noninvasive exclusion of a mucinous cystic neoplasm is difficult in such cases. EUS image (**D**) from a third patient shows needle aspiration of an anechoic pancreatic cyst, which was confirmed to be a simple cyst.

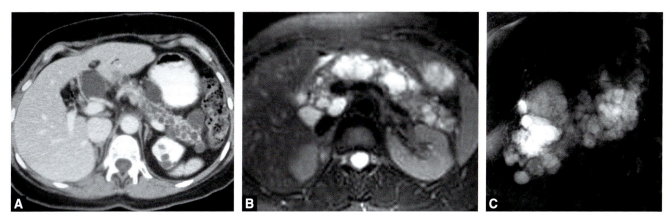

FIGURE 3.3.2 **Pancreatic cysts in von Hippel-Lindau disease.** Contrast-enhanced CT image (**A**) shows innumerable simple-appearing pancreatic cysts, as well as renal cysts. Fat-suppressed T2-weighted MR (**B**) and MRCP (**C**) images from two additional patients with von Hippel-Lindau disease show multiple cysts throughout the pancreas.

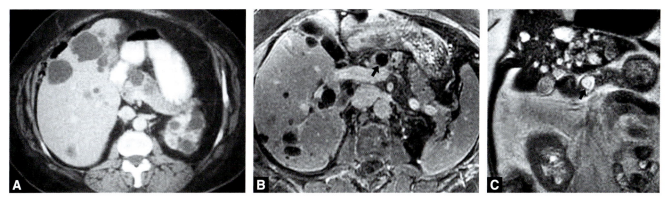

FIGURE 3.3.3 **Pancreatic cysts in autosomal dominant polycystic disease.** Contrast-enhanced CT image (**A**) shows multiple benign cysts involving the left kidney, liver, and pancreas. Fat-suppressed contrast-enhanced SGE (**B**) and coronal T2-weighted (**C**) MR images from another patient show multiple hepatic and pancreatic (*arrows*) cysts. Note prior nephrectomies and the right lower quadrant renal transplant. Although both renal and hepatic cysts are very common in this condition, pancreatic cysts are relatively rare at imaging.

3.4 Pancreatic Trauma

(Figure 3.4.1)

CLINICAL FEATURES

- Pancreatic trauma can result from blunt or penetrating abdominal injury; a bicycle handlebar injury in children is classic.
- Although uncommon, significant injury carries a relatively high morbidity and mortality rate.
- Injury may present in a somewhat delayed fashion with progressive abdominal pain, tenderness, and distention evolving over a 24-hour period.
- Serum amylase levels may be normal within the first few hours of injury.
- Associated retroperitoneal hemorrhage may be manifested by periumbilical ecchymosis (Cullen sign) or flank ecchymosis (Grey-Turner sign).
- Ductal disruption with a viable enzyme-secreting upstream segment can result in "disconnected pancreatic duct syndrome."

IMAGING FEATURES

- CT with IV contrast is the initial imaging modality of choice and may show focal or diffuse gland enlargement, infiltration of the peripancreatic fat, parenchymal laceration or contusion, and hematoma.
- A linear low-attenuation cleft within the pancreatic parenchyma signifies laceration, which is most often seen in the pancreatic neck and body region.
- The CT may initially appear normal; sequential CT images can show disease progression with increased conspicuity of the parenchymal laceration and development of peripancreatic fluid collections.
- Complications include pseudocyst formation, pancreatic duct stricture or occlusion, and arterial pseudoaneurysm.
- ERCP can identify pancreatic ductal disruption, communication, or stricture.

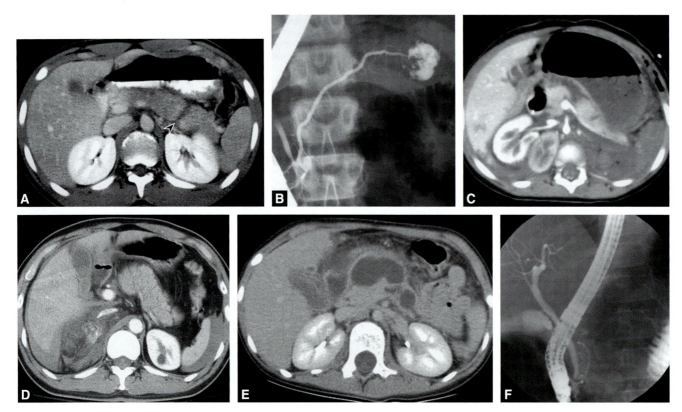

FIGURE 3.4.1 Pancreatic trauma. Contrast-enhanced CT image **(A)** after blunt trauma shows a linear low-attenuation defect (*arrowhead*) extending across the pancreas. Subsequent ERCP image **(B)** demonstrates ductal disruption corresponding to the site of laceration on CT. Contrast-enhanced CT image **(C)** from a child involved in a motor vehicle accident shows linear low-attenuation clefts across the pancreas, with surrounding hemorrhage. Note also splenic infarction, hepatic laceration, subcutaneous air, and injury to a congenitally crossed-fused ectopic kidney. Contrast-enhanced CT image **(D)** from a third patient with blunt abdominal trauma shows a diffusely swollen and edematous pancreas surrounded by hazy infiltration. Also present are a right adrenal hematoma with active contrast extravasation, high-attenuation hemoperitoneum, and a slit-like IVC suggesting hypovolemia. Contrast-enhanced CT image **(E)** from a final patient performed several weeks after a handlebar injury shows developing pancreatic pseudocysts. ERCP image **(F)** shows an abrupt cut-off of the pancreatic duct in the neck region, suggestive of "disconnected pancreatic duct syndrome."

CHAPTER 8

THE LIVER

David H. Kim, MD • Perry J. Pickhardt, MD

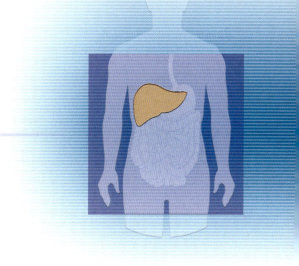

1. **NEOPLASTIC LESIONS**
   1.1 Hepatocellular Carcinoma
   1.2 Metastatic Disease
   1.3 Cavernous Hemangioma
   1.4 Hepatocellular Adenoma
   1.5 Intrahepatic (Peripheral) Cholangiocarcinoma
   1.6 Other Hepatic Tumors
2. **NON-NEOPLASTIC LESIONS**
   2.1 Focal Nodular Hyperplasia
   2.2 Benign Hepatic Cysts
   2.3 Hepatic Abscess
   2.4 Vascular Findings
3. **OTHER HEPATIC CONDITIONS**
   3.1 Cirrhosis and Portal Hypertension
   3.2 Budd-Chiari Syndrome
   3.3 Fatty Liver Disease (Hepatic Steatosis)
   3.4 Hemochromatosis
   3.5 The Hyperdense Liver on CT
   3.6 Post-transplant Complications

Unlike the preceding chapters, there is no endoscopic correlate to complement radiologic imaging of the liver. This chapter was included, however, because hepatic disease is such a major component of GI medicine. Hepatic imaging, primarily with cross-sectional techniques such as CT, US, and MR, greatly aids in the evaluation of both focal and diffuse liver disease.

1. NEOPLASTIC LESIONS

Neoplastic lesions include both benign and malignant entities. Although many have suggestive appearances at cross-sectional imaging, most remain nonspecific and correlation with patient history is critical. CT, MR and US images are often complementary and aid in increasing diagnostic confidence. A few lesions do have characteristic imaging patterns that allow for an image-specific diagnosis to be made.

1.1 Hepatocellular Carcinoma
(Figures 1.1.1-1.1.10)

CLINICAL FEATURES

- Hepatocellular carcinoma (HCC) is a malignant neoplasm consisting of abnormal hepatocytes arranged in a trabecular pattern separated by sinusoidal blood-filled spaces; it recruits blood supply from the hepatic artery.
- It usually occurs in a setting of cirrhosis from viral hepatitis or alcohol abuse; in the absence of cirrhosis, HCC is typically well differentiated.
- In the setting of cirrhosis, a stepwise progression from regenerating nodules to dysplastic nodules to HCC is possible.
- A sudden unexplained change in the condition of a cirrhotic patient (e.g., worsening of ascites, weight loss, hepatic failure) suggests the possible development of HCC.
- Subcapsular tumors may present with hemoperitoneum.
- Serum α-fetoprotein (AFP) levels are often elevated in large tumors but may be normal in small tumors.
- Fibrolamellar HCC is a rare variant that affects younger noncirrhotic patients and has a better prognosis owing to an increased rate of surgical cure; the AFP levels are typically normal.

IMAGING FEATURES

- HCC may present as a solitary mass, as multifocal masses, or as a diffusely infiltrating process.
- HCC is a hypervascular lesion on dynamic CT and MR with increased enhancement relative to parenchyma on the arterial phase; it is often more difficult to visualize on more delayed imaging.
- In the setting of cirrhosis, dysplastic nodules are occasionally hypervascular but are almost never hyperintense on T2-weighted MR images (a useful distinguishing feature from HCC).

- Additional cross-sectional features include a pseudo-capsule, intra-tumoral septa, central scar, arterioportal shunting, and satellite lesions.
- Although tissue is required for definitive diagnosis, percutaneous biopsy is associated with an increased risk of needle tract seeding and usually not performed in the setting of possible surgical cure.
- There is a tendency for vascular invasion, with portal venous involvement greater than hepatic venous involvement.
- HCC typically appears heterogeneous at US, often with hyperechoic areas.
- Candidates for liver transplantation include those with single tumors <5 cm or with no more than 3 tumors >3 cm.
- Fibrolamellar HCC is typically large and lobulated; it may have a central scar with dystrophic calcification.

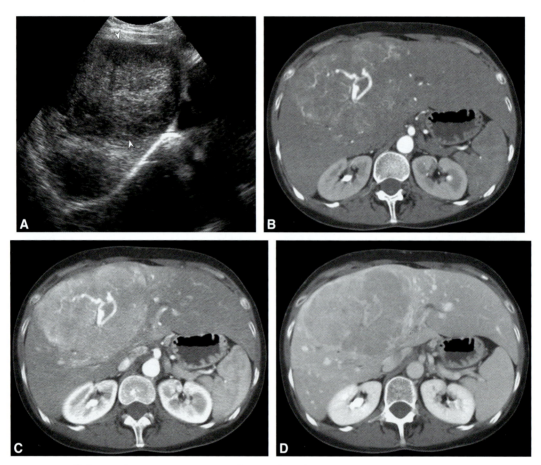

FIGURE 1.1.1 Hepatocellular carcinoma. US image (**A**) shows a large hepatic mass (*arrowheads*) with central echogenicity. CT image during early arterial phase (**B**) shows prominent tumor vessels centrally. Late arterial phase CT image (**C**) shows the hypervascular nature of the tumor. The early arterial phase is intended for vascular anatomy and is often too early to demonstrate hypervascular tumor characteristics. On portal venous phase imaging (**D**), the tumor shows relative washout of contrast but a pseudocapsule is now apparent.

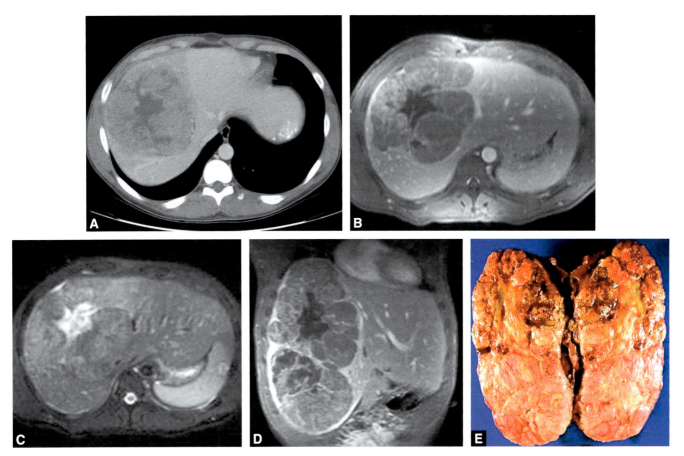

FIGURE 1.1.2 **Hepatocellular carcinoma with central scar.** Contrast-enhanced CT (**A**), contrast-enhanced SGE MR (**B**), and T2-weighted MR (**C**) images show a large lobulated heterogeneous hepatic mass with a central scar. Although scars of focal nodular hyperplasia (FNH) are typically T2 hyperintense, the other imaging features are not compatible with this diagnosis. Coronal contrast-enhanced SGE MR image (**D**) and bivalved resected specimen (**E**) again demonstrate the scar and show the entire extent of this bilobed mass.

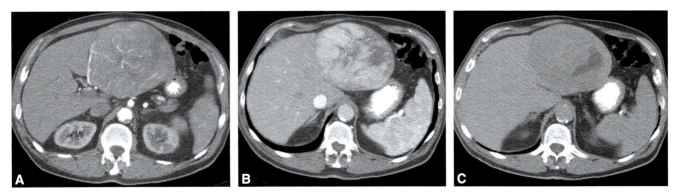

FIGURE 1.1.3 **Hepatocellular carcinoma.** Early arterial (**A**), late arterial (**B**), and delayed (**C**) CT images show a rounded hypervascular mass involving the left hepatic lobe.

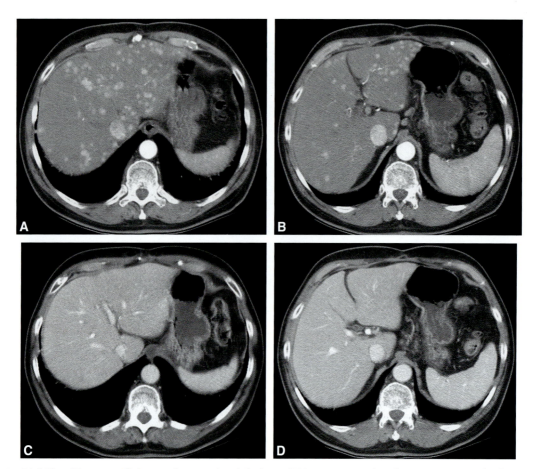

FIGURE 1.1.4 Multifocal hepatocellular carcinoma. Arterial phase CT images (**A** and **B**) from a patient with chronic viral hepatitis show innumerable small hypervascular lesions throughout the liver, which cannot be identified on the portal venous phase (**C** and **D**). This demonstrates the importance of obtaining the late arterial phase when evaluating for HCC.

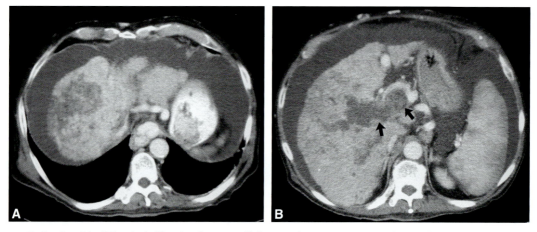

FIGURE 1.1.5 Cirrhosis with diffusely infiltrating hepatocellular carcinoma. Contrast-enhanced CT images (**A** and **B**) show findings of advanced cirrhosis with portal hypertension (nodular shrunken liver, ascites, splenomegaly, and portosystemic collaterals). Ill-defined low attenuation at the liver dome represents infiltrative tumor. Tumor thrombus expands the portal vein (**B**, *arrows*), with evidence of enhancement that excludes benign clot.

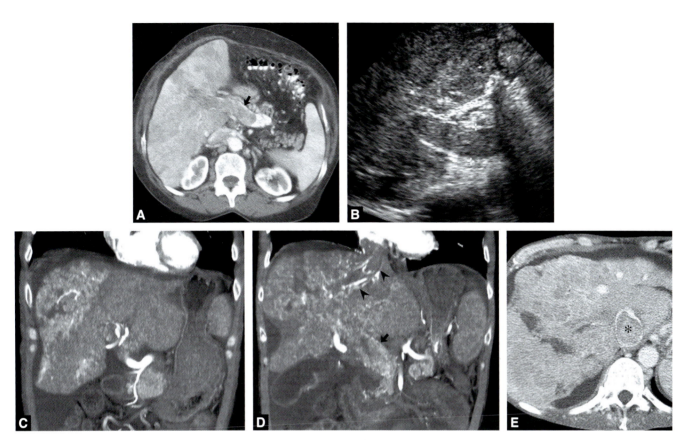

FIGURE 1.1.6 **Hepatocellular carcinoma with venous tumor thrombus.** Contrast-enhanced CT image (**A**) shows a cirrhotic liver with diffusely heterogeneous enhancement from HCC infiltration. Tumor thrombus of the portal vein is demonstrated on CT (*arrow*). US image (**B**) also shows the echogenic thrombus filling the portal vein (*calipers*). Coronal arterial phase CT images (**C** and **D**) from another cirrhotic patient show an extensive hypervascular tumor infiltrating the liver dome. Enhancing tumor thrombus with marked neovascularity expands both the hepatic (*arrowheads*) and portal (*arrow*) venous systems. Transverse portal venous phase CT image (**E**) demonstrates expansion of the inferior vena cava (IVC) by tumor thrombus (*asterisk*).

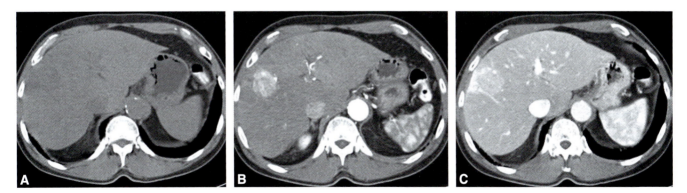

FIGURE 1.1.7 **Well-differentiated hepatocellular carcinoma.** Precontrast (**A**), arterial phase (**B**), and portal venous phase (**C**) CT images show a well-circumscribed hypervascular tumor in the right hepatic lobe. Note perilesional enhancement on the portal venous phase.

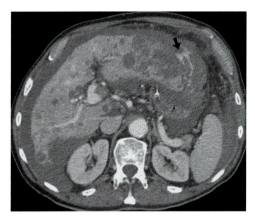

FIGURE 1.1.8 Hepatocellular carcinoma presenting as hemoperitoneum. Contrast-enhanced CT image shows findings of advanced cirrhosis and multifocal HCC. Note extracapsular high-attenuation contrast extravasation (*arrow*) due to active bleeding from subcapsular tumor rupture. The increased attenuation of the peritoneal fluid reflects hemoperitoneum.

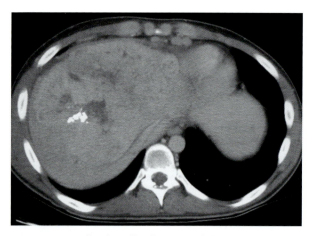

FIGURE 1.1.9 Fibrolamellar hepatocellular carcinoma. Contrast-enhanced CT image in a young man shows a massive hepatic tumor with a central scar that contains a focus of coarse calcification. AFP levels were normal.

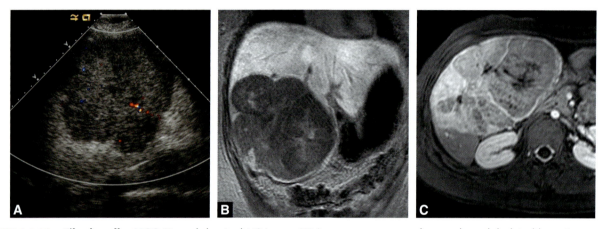

FIGURE 1.1.10 Fibrolamellar HCC. Transabdominal US image (**A**) in a young woman shows a large lobulated hepatic mass with internal blood flow identified on color Doppler. No calcific component was present. Coronal precontrast (**B**) and transverse postcontrast (**C**) SGE MR images show the large lobulated tumor, which demonstrates heterogeneous enhancement and a prominent pseudocapsule.

1.2 Metastatic Disease
(Figures 1.2.1-1.2.6)

CLINICAL FEATURES

- Metastatic disease is the most common malignant process involving the liver.
- Most metastases are hematogenous; serosal metastases from peritoneal spread are the other major group.
- Most metastatic lesions are hypovascular (decreased enhancement relative to liver); certain tumor types yield hypervascular metastases.
- Common hypovascular metastases include colon cancer and other gastrointestinal primary tumors, breast carcinoma, and lung carcinoma.
- Typical hypervascular metastases include neuroendocrine tumors (carcinoid and pancreatic islet cell tumors), melanoma, and sarcomas; renal and thyroid malignancies are less common.
- Common serosal metastases include ovarian carcinoma and primary gastrointestinal malignancies.

IMAGING FEATURES

- Multiplicity of lesions and extrahepatic disease is often highly suggestive of metastatic disease.
- PET/CT and intraoperative US increase diagnostic accuracy, particularly with potentially resectable disease; regardless, biopsy is required in most cases.
- On CT and MR, hypovascular metastases enhance less than the normal liver parenchyma; most lesions demonstrate increased signal on T2-weighted MR imaging.
- On arterial-phase CT and MR, hypervascular lesions enhance to a greater degree than the normal liver but wash out more quickly on delayed phases.
- On US, a hypoechoic halo about a lesion suggests malignancy.
- Occasionally, certain specific imaging characteristics can suggest the primary tumor type.

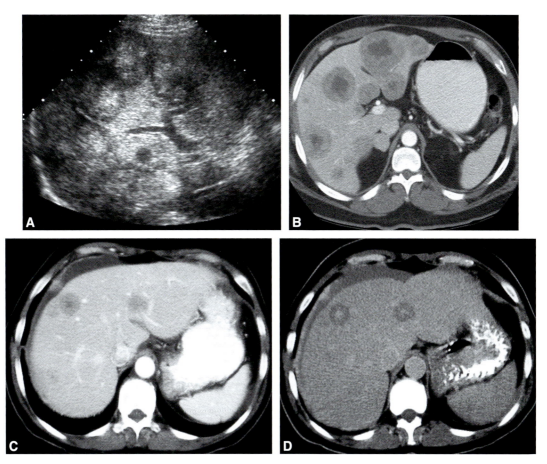

FIGURE 1.2.1 Hypovascular hepatic metastases: target appearance. Transverse US image through the liver **(A)** from a patient with colonic adenocarcinoma shows multiple target lesions with a hypoechoic outer rim. Contrast-enhanced CT image **(B)** from a patient with metastatic prostate cancer shows multiple target lesions in the liver. Right adrenal metastasis is also present. Hepatic metastatic disease from prostate cancer is uncommon. Dynamic **(C)** and delayed **(D)** contrast-enhanced CT images show target-like hepatic metastases that demonstrate delayed central enhancement. Therefore, the central low attenuation seen on the dynamic phase does not represent necrosis.

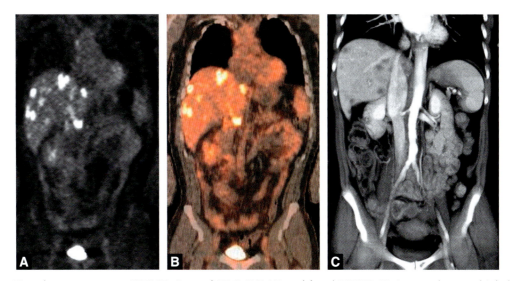

FIGURE 1.2.2 Hepatic metastases on PET/CT. Coronal FDG PET **(A)** and fused PET/CT **(B)** images show multiple hypermetabolic liver foci from colon cancer. Thick-section contrast-enhanced coronal CT image **(C)** from another patient with colorectal cancer shows multiple hypovascular hepatic metastases. Correlation between PET and CT increases diagnostic confidence and improves lesion localization.

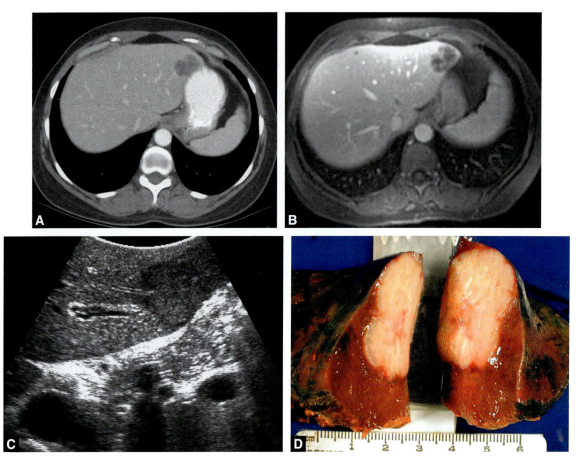

FIGURE 1.2.3　**Resectable metastatic colorectal adenocarcinoma.** Contrast-enhanced CT (**A**) and MR (**B**) images show a solitary hypovascular metastasis from colorectal cancer involving the left lateral segment. Intraoperative US (**C**) confirmed the metastasis and excluded other malignant foci, allowing for potentially curative resection (**D**). The tiny low-signal lesion seen on MR, was confirmed to represent a benign cyst at intraoperative US (*not shown*).

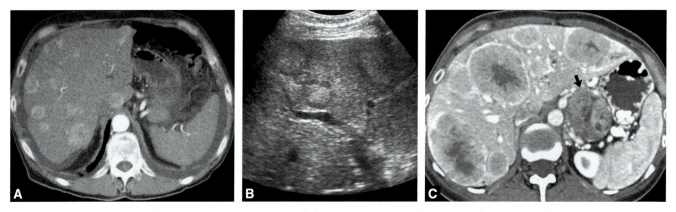

FIGURE 1.2.4　**Hypervascular hepatic metastases.** Arterial phase CT image (**A**) shows multiple hypervascular liver lesions from metastatic carcinoid tumor. The lesions demonstrate a target appearance at US (**B**). Contrast-enhanced CT image (**C**) from a patient with a nonhyperfunctioning islet cell tumor shows multiple large heterogeneous hypervascular liver metastases; the primary pancreatic tumor is evident (*arrow*). Neuroendocrine carcinoid and islet cell tumors are relatively common hypervascular metastases.

Illustration continued on following page

METASTATIC DISEASE   431

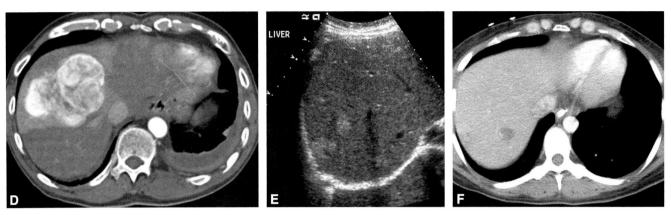

FIGURE 1.2.4 (Continued)   **Hypervascular hepatic metastases.** Arterial phase CT image (**D**) from a third patient shows a strikingly hypervascular metastasis from malignant hemangiopericytoma. Note perilesional enhancement (transient hepatic attenuation difference [THAD]) related to local portal venous compromise with compensatory increase in arterial supply. US image (**E**) from a woman with metastatic choriocarcinoma from gestational trophoblastic neoplasia shows hyperechoic lesions that demonstrate subtle peripheral enhancement on CT (**F**).

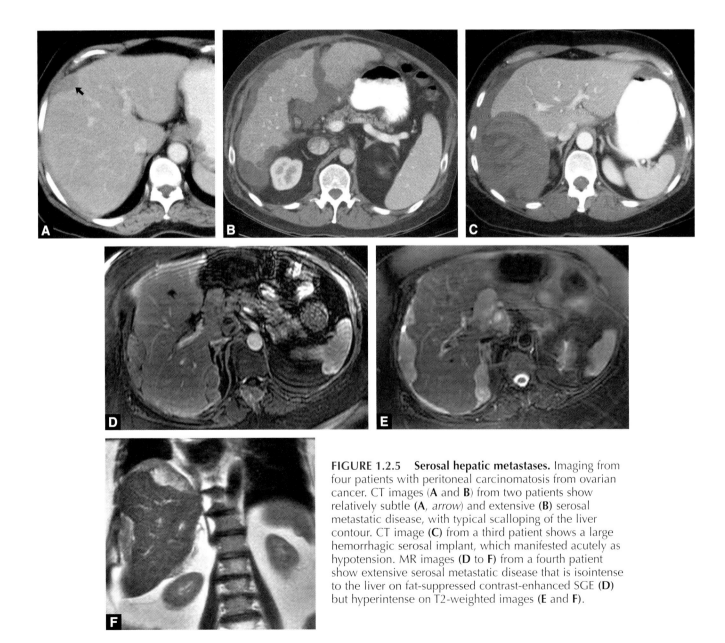

FIGURE 1.2.5   **Serosal hepatic metastases.** Imaging from four patients with peritoneal carcinomatosis from ovarian cancer. CT images (**A** and **B**) from two patients show relatively subtle (**A**, *arrow*) and extensive (**B**) serosal metastatic disease, with typical scalloping of the liver contour. CT image (**C**) from a third patient shows a large hemorrhagic serosal implant, which manifested acutely as hypotension. MR images (**D** to **F**) from a fourth patient show extensive serosal metastatic disease that is isointense to the liver on fat-suppressed contrast-enhanced SGE (**D**) but hyperintense on T2-weighted images (**E** and **F**).

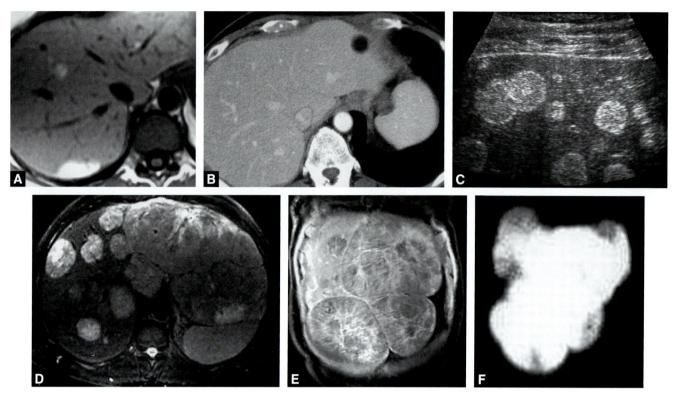

FIGURES 1.2.6 Hepatic metastases with imaging-specific features. Unenhanced T1-weighted MR image **(A)** from a patient with metastatic melanoma shows multiple T1-hyperintense liver lesions, characteristic of melanin content. CT **(B)** and US **(C)** images from two different patients with metastatic liposarcoma show characteristic fat attenuation to the liver lesion on CT and a markedly hyperechoic appearance of the multiple lesions on US. Transverse T2-weighted **(D)** and coronal contrast-enhanced SGE **(E)** MR images show massive hypervascular metastases from carcinoid tumor. Coronal image from octreotide scintigraphy **(F)** shows uptake in the lesions, characteristic of a neuroendocrine tumor.

1.3 Cavernous Hemangioma

(Figures 1.3.1-1.3.7)

CLINICAL FEATURES

- This benign vascular neoplasm of the liver is composed of large blood-filled epithelial-lined sinusoids; it is the most common hepatic neoplasm.
- Cavernous hemangioma is almost always asymptomatic; even giant lesions (>10 cm) are only rarely associated with symptoms from mass effect or thrombocytopenia from platelet sequestration (Kasabach-Merritt syndrome).
- Multiple lesions are almost always sporadic but may be associated with blue rubber bleb nevus syndrome.
- There is a female predominance; tumors may enlarge with pregnancy.
- Imaging-specific diagnosis with CT or MR (and sometimes with tagged red cell scintigraphy) obviates the need for biopsy; US appearance is often highly suggestive but less specific.

IMAGING FEATURES

- Specific CT/MR findings include peripheral nodular "puddling" of contrast that matches aortic blood pool attenuation/signal; progressive fill-in of the lesion on delayed images need not be complete.
- Small lesions may appear "hypervascular" owing to complete fill-in on the initial phase; however, lesions continue to match aortic blood pool on more delayed images and should not be confused for pathology.
- Large or giant lesions may have a central scar from thrombosis or hyalinization.
- Cavernous hemangiomas demonstrate high signal intensity on T2-weighted images.
- Typical US appearance of a well-circumscribed, homogeneously hyperechoic lesion is highly suggestive and generally sufficient in the absence of a cancer history; CT or MR can be confirmatory if needed.
- Less common US appearance consists of a "reverse target" with a hyperechoic rim and hypoechoic center.
- A change in lesion appearance over the course of an US examination is rare but also characteristic of hemangioma.

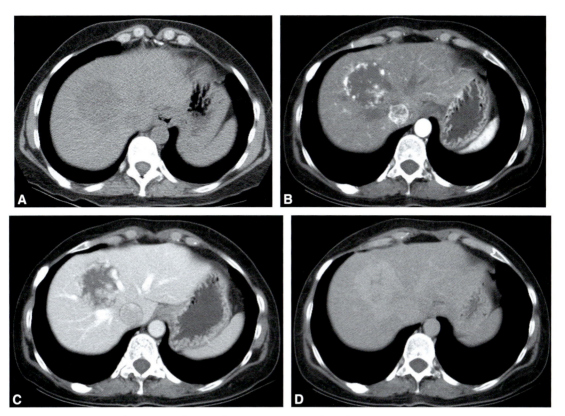

FIGURE 1.3.1 CT appearance of cavernous hemangioma. Noncontrast low-dose image (**A**) from a CTC screening study shows a subtle large rounded low-attenuation lesion that does not have the appearance of a simple cyst. Subsequent arterial (**B**), portal venous (**C**), and delayed (**D**) contrast-enhanced images from diagnostic CT show the typical appearance of a cavernous hemangioma, with peripheral "enhancement" and progressively centripetal fill-in that matches aortic blood pool attenuation on each phase. Complete central fill-in is not required for definitive diagnosis.

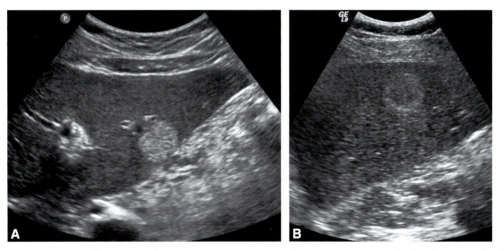

FIGURE 1.3.2 US appearance of cavernous hemangioma. Transverse US image (**A**) through the left hepatic lobe shows a homogeneous hyperechoic lesion, which is the most typical US appearance of a cavernous hemangioma. Longitudinal US image (**B**) from a different patient shows a target lesion with a hyperechoic outer rim that should not be confused with the more ominous hypoechoic rim. In both patients, the findings are highly suggestive of a benign diagnosis and are generally sufficient in the absence of a known cancer history.

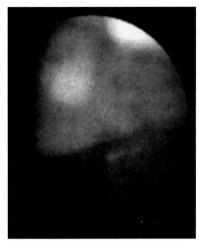
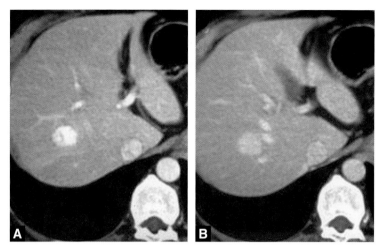

FIGURE 1.3.3 Scintigraphic diagnosis of cavernous hemangioma. Delayed image from ^{99m}Tc-labeled red blood cell scintigraphy shows a large hepatic lesion that demonstrates blood pool activity, diagnostic of a cavernous hemangioma. Although this test is now seldom used for this indication, it can be useful in difficult cases.

FIGURE 1.3.4 "Flash-filling" cavernous hemangioma on CT. Late arterial phase image (A) from contrast-enhanced CT shows an apparent hypervascular liver lesion. However, a more delayed image (B) shows that the lesion continues to match aortic blood pool attenuation, consistent with a cavernous hemangioma.

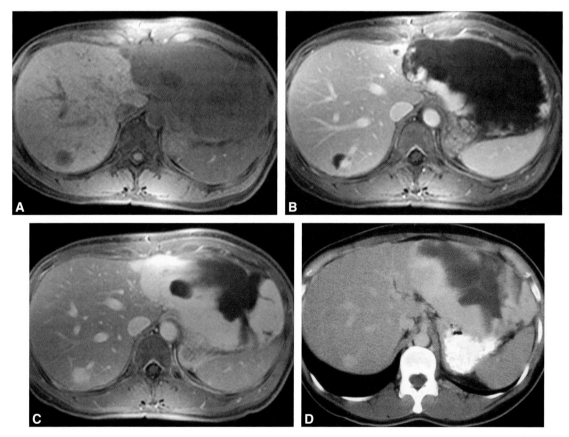

FIGURE 1.3.5 Giant cavernous hemangioma on MR. Precontrast (A) and multiphase postcontrast (B and C) fat-suppressed SGE MR images show a large exophytic mass extending off the left hepatic lobe. Note how the signal intensity of filled-in regions matches aortic blood pool, similar to dynamic CT findings. A large central scar prevented complete fill-in. Note also the smaller cavernous hemangioma in the right hepatic lobe that fills in completely on the delayed phase. A similar appearance is seen on delayed-phase CT (D).

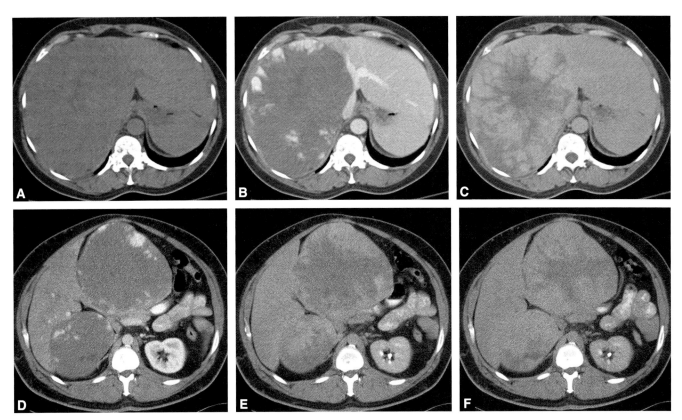

FIGURE 1.3.6 Giant cavernous hemangiomas on CT. Precontrast **(A)**, portal venous **(B)**, and delayed **(C)** phase CT images show a giant cavernous hemangioma that occupies nearly the entire right hepatic lobe. Arterial **(D)** and delayed **(E** and **F)** phase CT images from another patient with multiple large cavernous hemangiomas show similar findings. Complete uniform fill-in is rarely seen in lesions of this size.

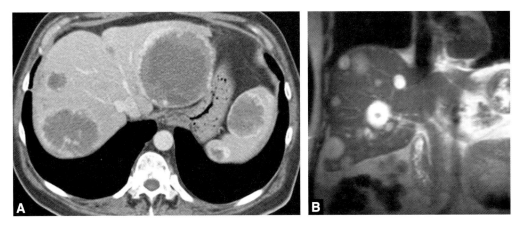

FIGURE 1.3.7 Multiple hemangiomas in blue rubber bleb nevus syndrome. Contrast-enhanced CT image **(A)** from a patient with blue rubber bleb nevus syndrome shows multiple hepatic and splenic hemangiomas. Coronal T2-weighted MR image **(B)** from a second patient shows multiple hyperintense hemangiomas throughout the liver.

1.4 Hepatocellular Adenoma
(Figures 1.4.1-1.4.4)

CLINICAL FEATURES

- An uncommon benign neoplasm, hepatocellular adenoma is characterized by hepatocytes without normal acinar architecture; there is a paucity or absence of Kupffer cells and bile ducts.
- This tumor is predominantly seen in women on oral contraceptives; association with anabolic steroid use and type I glycogen storage disease (von Gierke's) has been noted.
- The tumor has a tendency to undergo necrosis or hemorrhage, which may be life threatening.
- Most patients are asymptomatic or have mild upper abdominal discomfort; tumor infarction or spontaneous hemorrhage may manifest as severe pain.
- It can present acutely with rupture and hemoperitoneum; surgical resection is the treatment of choice owing to the possibility of this high morbidity complication.

IMAGING FEATURES

- Adenomas are generally hypervascular on CT and MR and isoechoic to hyperechoic on US; the enhancement pattern is heterogeneous compared with FNH.
- The lesion may appear heterogeneous secondary to necrosis, lipid content, or hemorrhage.
- Imaging is generally nonspecific for excluding hypervascular malignancy; biopsy or resection is generally required.
- Diffuse dropout of signal on opposed-phase (chemical shift) MR imaging can be seen owing to lipid content; lipid-rich lesions may also be evident as less-than-water attenuation on CT.
- It is a cold lesion (nonspecific) on sulfur colloid scintigraphy owing to the lack of Kupffer cells.
- On delayed MR imaging with Gd-BOPTA, adenomas fail to show increased signal owing to the lack of bile ducts, which can distinguish these lesions from FNH.

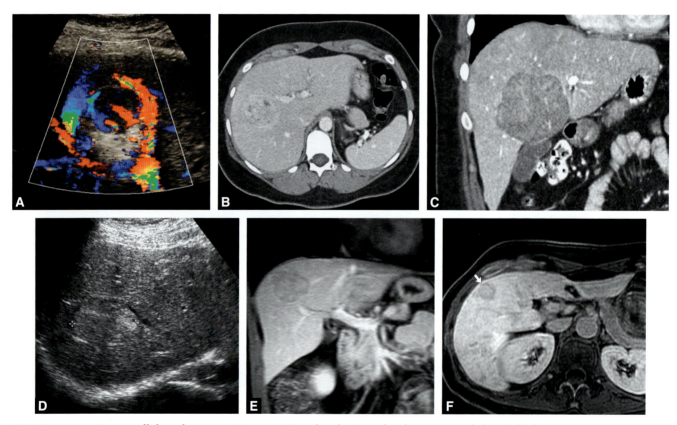

FIGURE 1.4.1 Hepatocellular adenomas. US image (**A**) with color Doppler shows a rounded partially hyperechoic hepatic lesion with prominent vascularity. Corresponding CT image (**B**) shows a relatively subtle heterogeneous but hypervascular mass. Coronal arterial phase CT image (**C**) from a second patient shows a large lobulated mass that demonstrates heterogeneous arterial enhancement. US (**D**) and contrast-enhanced MR (**E**) images from a third patient show a relatively subtle lesion that is slightly hyperechoic on US and nearly isointense to normal parenchyma on MR. Postcontrast SGE MR image (**F**) using Gd-BOPTA with 2-hour delay from a final patient shows a hypointense lesion (*arrow*), which distinguishes this adenoma from FNH.

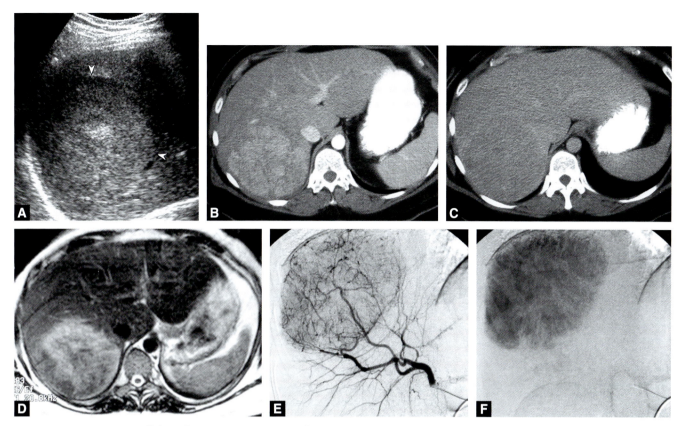

FIGURE 1.4.2 **Hepatocellular adenoma.** US image **(A)** shows a large rounded mass (*arrowheads*) that is nearly isoechoic to normal liver. Arterial phase CT image **(B)** demonstrates extensive heterogeneous enhancement, which washes out on delayed imaging **(C)**. The lesion is hyperintense on T2-weighted MR imaging **(D)**. DSA images **(E** and **F)** from selective hepatic arterial injection show the tumor vascularity **(E)** and dense hypervascular staining **(F)**.

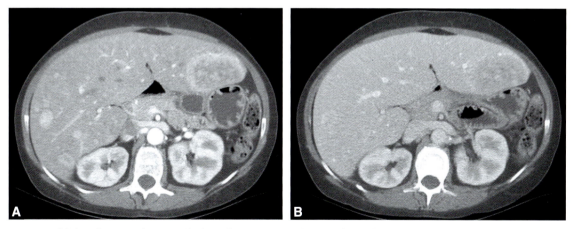

FIGURE 1.4.3 **Multiple adenomas in von Gierke's disease.** Arterial **(A)** and portal venous **(B)** phase CT images from a patient with type I glycogen storage disease show multiple hypervascular lesions, which are much less conspicuous on the portal venous phase.

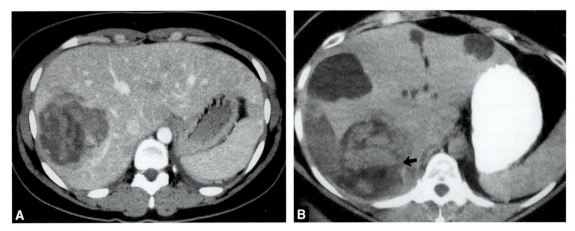

FIGURE 1.4.4 Hepatocellular adenomas with spontaneous hemorrhage. Contrast-enhanced CT image **(A)** in a young woman with acute abdominal pain shows a complex hepatic mass representing an adenoma that underwent spontaneous hemorrhage. Unenhanced CT image **(B)** from a second patient shows a complex right hepatic lobe mass with areas of high attenuation and a fluid-fluid level from hemorrhage (*arrow*). Adjacent subcapsular hematoma is present. Additional adenomas without hemorrhage demonstrate less-than-water attenuation from increased lipid content, which is a characteristic feature.

1.5 Intrahepatic (Peripheral) Cholangiocarcinoma

(Figures 1.5.1-1.5.4)

CLINICAL FEATURES

- This malignant tumor arises from the intrahepatic biliary epithelium.
- The majority arise de novo; risk factors include primary sclerosing cholangitis (PSC) and other causes of biliary stasis and inflammation.
- Central intrahepatic tumors may present with jaundice whereas peripheral tumors present late with pain or other nonspecific complaints.
- A Klatskin tumor is classically an infiltrative process that originates at the confluence of the right and left hepatic ducts (see Chapter 6).
- Combined HCC/cholangiocarcinoma represents a rare variant that may demonstrate features of both tumor types.

IMAGING FEATURES

- Tumors appear hypovascular on CT and MR, often with mild peripheral or septal arterial phase enhancement.
- In approximately 40% of cases, delayed imaging at 10 to 15 minutes shows increased internal contrast retention related to delayed equilibrium with the fibrous interstitium.
- Typically, focal masses are evident; despite the term "peripheral," many tumors are located centrally within the liver and overlap with the classic infiltrative Klatskin tumor.
- Intrahepatic biliary ductal dilatation proximal to the tumor is a common finding.
- Distant metastatic spread is uncommon.

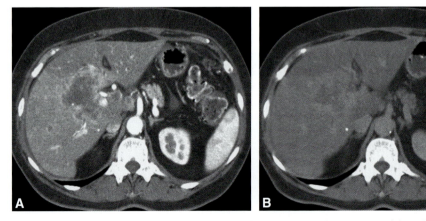

FIGURE 1.5.1 Intrahepatic cholangiocarcinoma on CT. Arterial phase **(A)** and 15-minute delayed **(B)** CT images show an ill-defined hilar mass with mild peripheral hypervascular enhancement and subtle internal enhancement on the delayed phase.

Illustration continued on following page

INTRAHEPATIC (PERIPHERAL) CHOLANGIOCARCINOMA

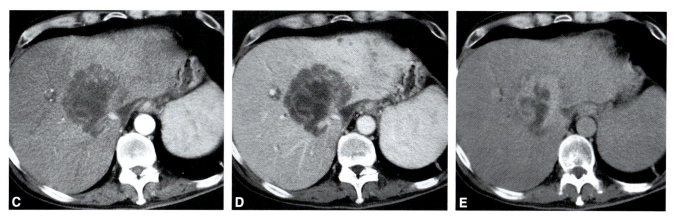

FIGURE 1.5.1 (Continued) **Intrahepatic cholangiocarcinoma on CT.** Arterial (**C**), portal venous (**D**), and 15-minute delayed (**E**) CT images from a different patient show a large, predominantly hypovascular mass that shows significant uptake of contrast on delayed imaging.

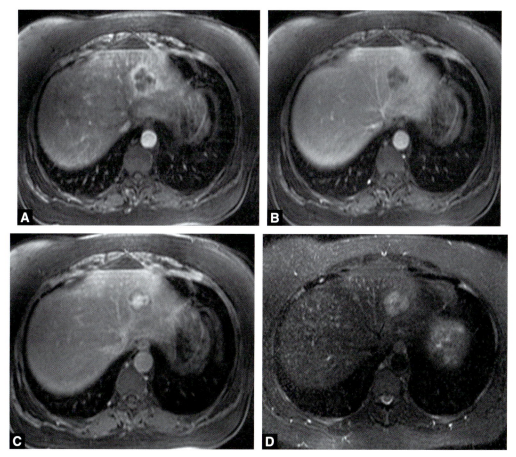

FIGURE 1.5.2 **Intrahepatic cholangiocarcinoma on MR.** Contrast-enhanced fat-suppressed SGE MR images (**A** to **C**) show a left hepatic lobe lesion that demonstrates peripheral and septal enhancement on arterial phase (**A**), hypovascular appearance on portal venous phase (**B**), and central uptake of contrast on the 15-minute delayed phase (**C**). Fat-suppressed T2-weighted image (**D**) shows increased signal intensity within the lesion relative to normal liver.

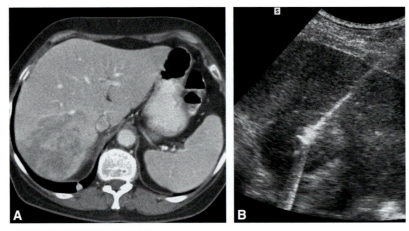

FIGURE 1.5.3 **Intrahepatic cholangiocarcinoma.** Contrast-enhanced CT image **(A)** shows a heterogeneous low-attenuation mass within the right hepatic lobe. Metastatic disease is present at the right lung base. Intrahepatic cholangiocarcinoma was diagnosed by percutaneous US-guided biopsy **(B)**.

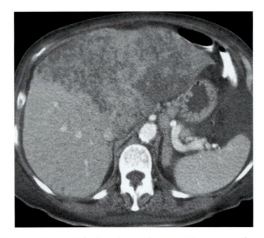

FIGURE 1.5.4 **Combined hepatocellular carcinoma/cholangiocarcinoma.** Contrast-enhanced CT image from a patient with known cirrhosis shows an ill-defined low-attenuation mass infiltrating the entire left hepatic lobe.

1.6 Other Hepatic Tumors
(Figures 1.6.1-1.6.10)

CLINICAL FEATURES

- Secondary hepatic lymphoma is more common than primary hepatic lymphoma; it can mimic cystic lesions on US and CT.
- Immunosuppression increases the risk for hepatic lymphoma, as seen in AIDS and post-transplantation lymphoproliferative disorder (PTLD); PTLD at the liver hilum is typical of allograft involvement after liver transplantation (see section 3.6).
- Angiosarcoma is a rare aggressive malignant vascular tumor associated with certain exposures (e.g., Thorotrast, vinyl chloride, and arsenic) and hemochromatosis; the tumor is rarely resectable.
- Epithelioid hemangioendothelioma (EHE) is a rare vascular tumor that is considered either premalignant or malignant; it is usually asymptomatic at presentation with a better prognosis than angiosarcoma.
- Fat-containing hepatic tumors are uncommon but include lipoma, angiomyolipoma (usually with tuberous sclerosis), adrenal rest, adenoma, HCC, and liposarcoma.
- Hepatoblastoma is a rare tumor of infancy.
- See Chapter 6 for a discussion of biliary cystadenomas.

IMAGING FEATURES

- Primary and secondary hepatic lymphoma may present as a unifocal or multifocal process.
- Angiosarcoma is a hypervascular tumor that typically has a multicentric appearance; blood pool retention can lead to false-positive diagnosis of hemangioma on tagged red blood cell scintigraphy (but not CT).
- EHE is characterized by coalescing peripheral masses that may show peripheral enhancement but does not follow the blood pool like hemangiomas; the slow growth rate distinguishes it from angiosarcoma.
- Hepatic lipomas present as well-circumscribed masses composed of fat density; the specific appearance and demonstrable fat content in other fat-containing lesions are widely variable.

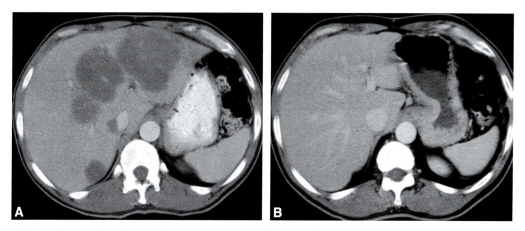

FIGURE 1.6.1 **Primary hepatic lymphoma.** Contrast-enhanced CT image (**A**) shows multiple low-attenuation hepatic lesions that appear almost cystic or like steatosis. No lymphadenopathy was present. Note complete response to chemotherapy on subsequent CT (**B**).

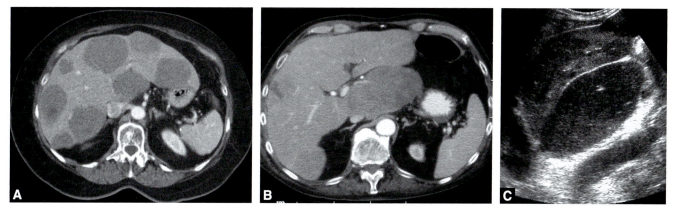

FIGURE 1.6.2 **Secondary hepatic lymphoma.** Contrast-enhanced CT image (**A**) in a patient with nasopharyngeal non-Hodgkin's lymphoma shows multiple large low-attenuation lesions. Contrast-enhanced CT (**B**) and US (**C**) images in a patient with recurrent Hodgkin's lymphoma shows multiple hepatic masses, the largest of which diffusely enlarges the caudate lobe. The liver is an unusual site for involvement by Hodgkin's disease.

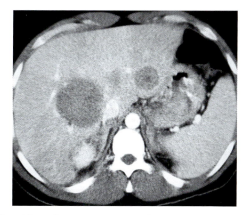

FIGURE 1.6.3 **AIDS-related lymphoma.** Contrast-enhanced CT image shows low-attenuation liver lesions from high-grade B-cell lymphoma complicating AIDS. Other solid organs were also involved (*not shown*).

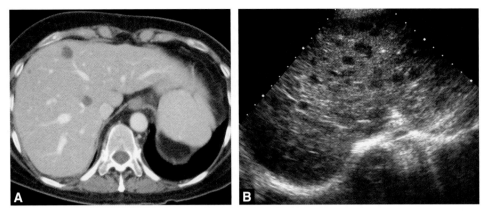

FIGURE 1.6.4 Hepatic post-transplantation lymphoproliferative disorder (PTLD). Contrast-enhanced CT **(A)** and US **(B)** images from two different patients with previous lung transplantation show multiple low-attenuation/hypoechoic liver lesions from PTLD.

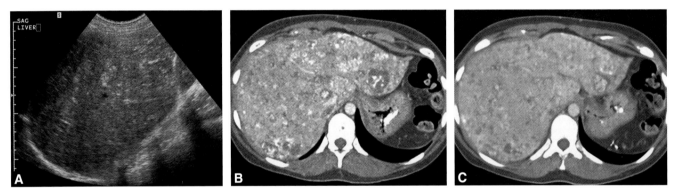

FIGURE 1.6.5 Hepatic angiosarcoma. US image **(A)** shows multiple small echogenic foci. Angiosarcoma is a rare cause of hyperechoic liver lesions. Subsequent images from arterial **(B)** and portal venous **(C)** phase CT show multiple hypervascular foci with central enhancement, some of which demonstrate centrifugal fill-in on the portal venous phase. Note that this enhancement pattern is distinct from cavernous hemangioma.

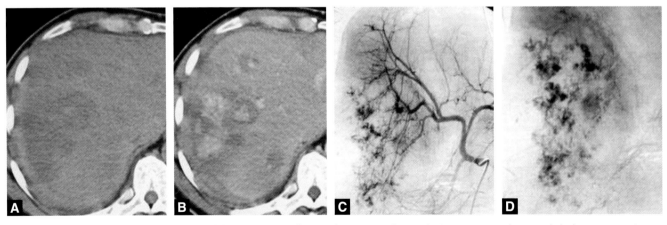

FIGURE 1.6.6 Hepatic angiosarcoma with spontaneous hemorrhage. Unenhanced CT image **(A)** shows subtle low-attenuation hepatic masses, as well as high-attenuation material surrounding the liver from extracapsular hemorrhage. CT image after contrast **(B)** shows central enhancement of the lesions reminiscent of the previous case. This vascular pattern is replicated on the selective hepatic arterial DSA images **(C** and **D)**.

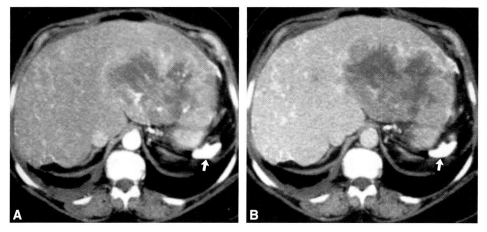

FIGURE 1.6.7 Angiosarcoma related to Thorotrast exposure. Arterial (A) and portal venous (B) phase CT images show a large heterogeneous mass with hypervascular elements in the left hepatic lobe. Note the dense spleen (*arrows*), as well as dense gastrohepatic lymph nodes and scattered hepatic densities from remote Thorotrast administration.

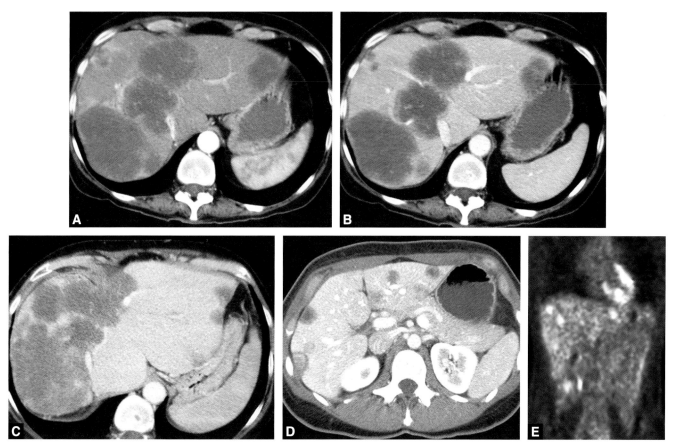

FIGURE 1.6.8 Hepatic epithelioid hemangioendothelioma (EHE). Arterial phase (A) and portal venous phase (B) CT images show large low-attenuation liver lesions, which show peripheral or perilesional enhancement on the arterial phase but no progressive enhancement on the portal venous phase. The appearance is distinct from cavernous hemangioma. Contrast-enhanced CT image (C) from a second patient shows a dominant coalescent low-attenuation mass, as well as small peripheral lesions in the left lateral segment. Contrast-enhanced CT image (D) from a third patient shows multiple rounded low-attenuation hepatic lesions demonstrating variable enhancement. The lesions were hypermetabolic on FDG-PET (E).

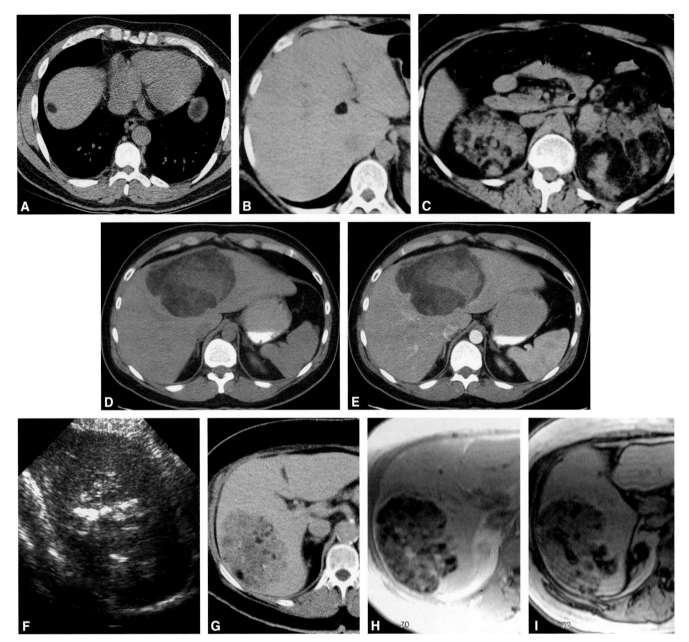

FIGURE 1.6.9 Fat-containing hepatic lesions. Noncontrast CT (**A**) shows a well-defined fat-attenuation lesion at the liver dome, consistent with a lipoma. Noncontrast CT image (**B**) in a patient with tuberous sclerosis shows a fat-containing hepatic angiomyolipoma. Extensive bilateral renal angiomyolipomas were also present (**C**). Precontrast (**D**) and postcontrast (**E**) CT images from a different patient show a large fat-containing hepatic mass with enhancing soft tissue components that proved to be an extra-adrenal myelolipoma. US (**F**), noncontrast CT (**G**), in-phase SGE MR (**H**), and opposed-phase SGE MR (**I**) images show a complex hepatic mass with both fatty and calcific components that account for the peculiar imaging findings. This lesion proved to be a rare hepatic adrenal rest tumor.

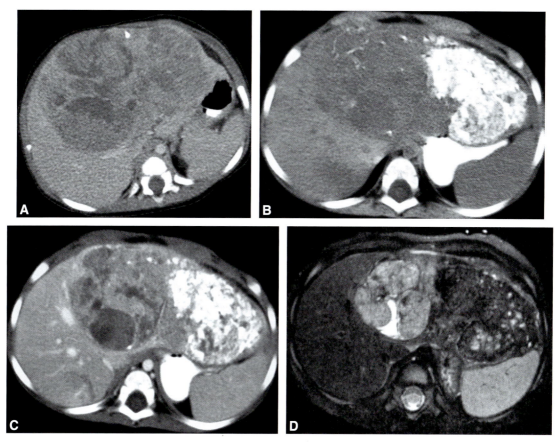

FIGURE 1.6.10 Hepatoblastoma. Contrast-enhanced CT (**A**) from a 12-month-old with a palpable abdominal mass shows a large heterogeneous hepatic tumor. Scattered calcifications were present throughout the lesion. Precontrast CT (**B**), postcontrast CT (**C**), and T2-weighted MR (**D**) images from another infant with a palpable abdominal mass show a very large and complex tumor with solid, cystic, and calcific components.

2. NON-NEOPLASTIC LESIONS

Non-neoplastic lesions are without malignant potential and constitute a variety of appearances at imaging, ranging from solid to cystic lesions. A specific diagnosis can often be made at imaging, obviating the need for biopsy. Clinical history can be important. Occasionally, there is overlap in the imaging appearance with malignant entities, requiring further evaluation.

2.1 Focal Nodular Hyperplasia
(Figures 2.1.1-2.1.5)

CLINICAL FEATURES

- Focal nodular hyperplasia (FNH) is a benign non-neoplastic lesion that is usually discovered as an incidental imaging finding; it is more frequently seen in women.
- It is composed of normal parenchymal components (hepatocytes, Kupffer cells, and bile ducts) in a disorganized pattern; the underlying cause is likely related to an anomalous arterial supply.
- The main importance of this lesion is distinguishing it from hypervascular neoplasms.
- The apparent increased incidence is related to improved imaging techniques.

IMAGING FEATURES

- On CT and MR, intense homogeneous enhancement on arterial-phase imaging is characteristic; rapid washout often renders the lesion barely perceptible beyond the arterial phase ("stealth lesion").
- It is generally isoattenuating, isointense, and isoechoic to normal hepatic parenchyma on unenhanced CT, MR, and US, respectively.
- Depiction of prominent tortuous feeding arteries and draining veins is relatively common.
- A central fibrous scar may be present, which is hyperintense on T2-weighted MR and shows delayed enhancement.
- Typically, these tumors are peripheral and subcapsular; they are usually solitary, but multiple lesions are not uncommon.
- Color or power Doppler may demonstrate vascularity along septa to create a spokewheel appearance.
- MR imaging with Gd-BOPTA allows for definitive characterization; FNH appears hyperintense on 2-3 hour delayed imaging, distinguishing it from adenoma and HCC.
- Convincing uptake of sulfur colloid on scintigraphy excludes other lesions and may avoid biopsy; however, MR with Gd-BOPTA is now the preferred imaging study.

446 THE LIVER

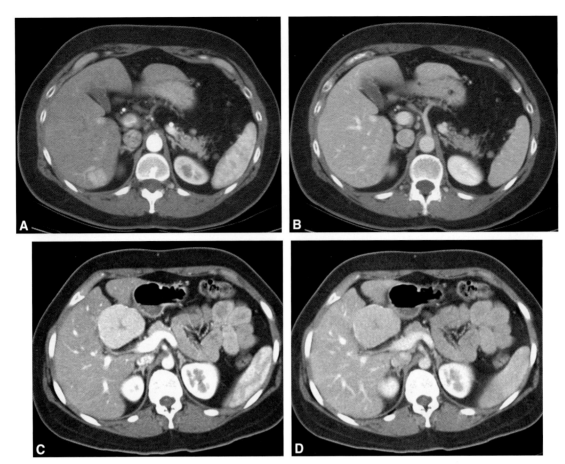

FIGURE 2.1.1   Focal nodular hyperplasia on CT. Images from arterial phase **(A)** and portal venous phase **(B)** CT show a peripheral hypervascular lesion that demonstrates homogeneous early enhancement but is nearly inconspicuous on the portal venous phase. Note also the early appearance of an adjacent vessel. Arterial **(C)** and portal venous **(D)** phase CT images from a different patient show a briskly enhancing exophytic hypervascular mass that rapidly washes out on the portal venous phase. A subtle central scar is present. Mild hepatic steatosis may account for the slight attenuation difference between the liver and the FNH on the portal venous phase.

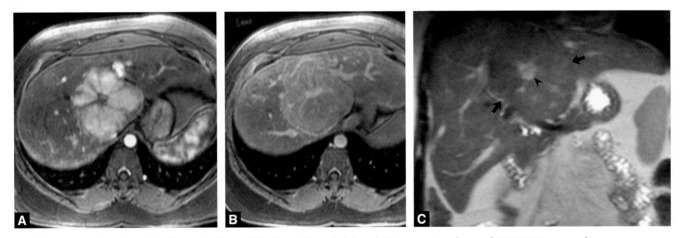

FIGURE 2.1.2   Focal nodular hyperplasia on MR. Early **(A)** and delayed **(B)** contrast-enhanced SGE MR images show a hypervascular lesion with radial septations. Note the enhancement of the central scar on the delayed phase **(B)**. On the coronal T2-weighted MR image **(C)**, the scar is hyperintense (*arrowhead*) and the lesion itself is isointense (*arrows*) to normal liver.

Illustration continued on following page

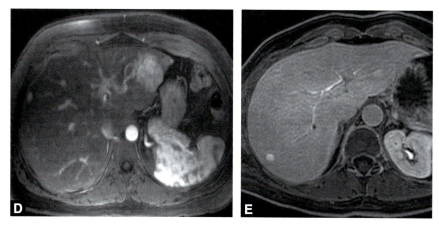

FIGURE 2.1.2 (Continued) Focal nodular hyperplasia on MRI. Arterial phase contrast-enhanced SGE MR image (D) from a different patient shows a lesion with homogeneous hypervascular enhancement that is characteristic of FNH. Note the tortuous feeding artery and draining vein, which are very characteristic of this lesion. Two-hour delayed postcontrast SGE MR image (E) following Gd-BOPTA administration from a final patient shows a hyperintense lesion in the right hepatic lobe, diagnostic of FNH. Note also the opacification of the central ducts from normal biliary excretion of the contrast.

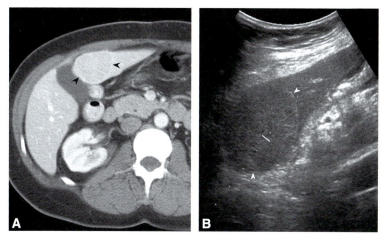

FIGURE 2.1.3 Focal nodular hyperplasia on biopsy. Contrast-enhanced CT image (A) shows an ovoid lesion (arrowheads) that is isoattenuating with normal liver. Arterial phase was not obtained. Because the patient was recently diagnosed with cancer, US-guided biopsy (B) was obtained to exclude metastasis. The lesion (arrowheads) is isoechoic on US. Core needle biopsy confirmed the suspected FNH.

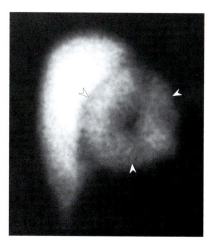

FIGURE 2.1.4 Focal nodular hyperplasia on sulfur colloid scintigraphy. Single image from sulfur colloid scintigraphy shows a large rounded mass (arrowheads) with a cold center representing a central scar. Although uptake of sulfur colloid within the FNH is less intense than normal liver, the findings are nonetheless diagnostic of FNH.

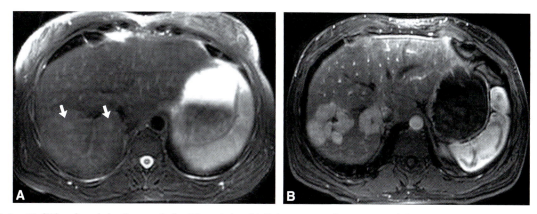

FIGURE 2.1.5 Multifocal nodular hyperplasia. T2-weighted MR image (A) shows two subtle areas of slightly increased signal intensity, as well as two hyperintense foci (arrows) that correspond to central scars of FNH. Arterial-phase SGE MR image (B) shows two homogeneously enhancing hypervascular lesions, with central scars that correlate with the T2-weighted image.

Illustration continued on following page

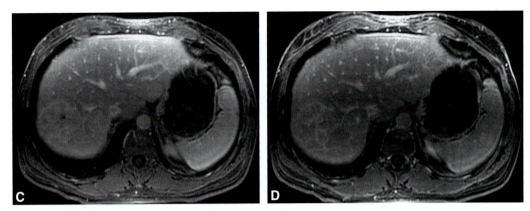

FIGURE 2.1.5 (Continued) **Multifocal nodular hyperplasia.** Except for the scars, the lesions are isointense to normal liver on the portal venous phase **(C)**. Delayed enhancement of the scars is evident on a later phase **(D)**.

2.2 Benign Hepatic Cysts

(Figures 2.2.1-2.2.3)

CLINICAL FEATURES

- Hepatic cysts are very common incidental benign lesions that arise from biliary epithelium; they are almost always asymptomatic.
- In some cases, subcentimeter lesions represent biliary hamartomas (von Meyenberg complexes).
- Rarely, cysts are complicated by hemorrhage or infection.
- Innumerable hepatic cysts suggest autosomal dominant polycystic disease, particularly in the setting of concomitant cystic renal disease.

IMAGING FEATURES

- Hepatic cysts are well-circumscribed lesions of fluid attenuation (<20 HU on CT, hyperintense on T2-weighted MR).
- No enhancement is evident after contrast administration; the cyst wall is thin or imperceptible.
- Cysts are anechoic with increased through-transmission at US, which is the most specific modality for diagnosis.
- Multiple large cysts can obscure portions of the pancreaticobiliary system at MRCP.

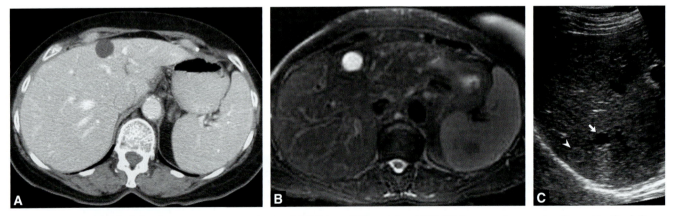

FIGURE 2.2.1 **Simple hepatic cysts.** Contrast-enhanced CT **(A)** and T2-weighted MR **(B)** images show a simple cyst in the left hepatic lobe. Note fluid attenuation and lack of enhancement on CT, hyperintensity on T2-weighted MR, and the imperceptible cyst wall. Longitudinal US image **(C)** from a different patient shows an anechoic simple hepatic cyst (*arrow*) with posterior acoustic enhancement. A small hemangioma (*arrowhead*) demonstrating a target appearance with an echogenic outer rim is present adjacent to the cyst.

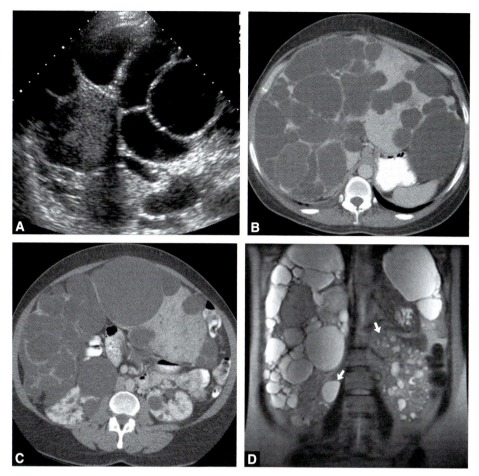

FIGURE 2.2.2 Autosomal dominant polycystic disease. US (**A**), contrast-enhanced CT (**B** and **C**), and coronal T2-weighted MR (**D**) images show innumerable hepatic cysts of varying sizes that enlarge the liver. Most cysts appear simple but some cyst contents are more complex. Multiple smaller cysts involve both kidneys as well (**D**, *arrows*).

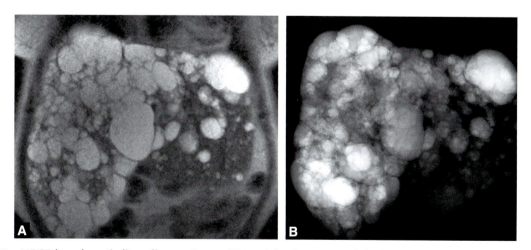

FIGURE 2.2.3 MRCP in polycystic liver disease. Coronal T2-weighted MR (**A**) and thick-slab MRCP (**B**) images show innumerable hepatic cysts that largely replace the liver and result in overall hepatomegaly. Note how the biliary tree is obscured by the T2-hyperintense cysts.

2.3 Hepatic Abscess
(Figures 2.3.1-2.3.9)

CLINICAL FEATURES

- Hepatic abscesses may be caused by a variety of microorganisms (bacterial, fungal, and parasitic).
- Routes of infection include biliary, portal, intra-abdominal, arterial, penetrating trauma, and (in a significant percentage) cryptogenic.
- Pyogenic (bacterial) abscesses typically are symptomatic, with fever, malaise, and abdominal pain; the specific cause is often not identified.
- Cat-scratch disease has been attributed to *Bartonella henselae* and most often affects children and adolescents; hepatosplenic lesions can be due to necrotizing granulomas or a peliosis-like reaction.
- Fungal infection typically occurs in the setting of immunocompromise, most often presenting as neutropenic fever.
- Amebic abscess from *Entamoeba histolytica* is more likely than pyogenic abscess to present acutely; the majority of patients do not report a history of dysentery.
- Hydatid disease from *Echinococcus granulosis* may be asymptomatic; presentation may relate to pain, fever, cyst enlargement, or cyst rupture.
- The sylvan form of echinococcal disease (*E. multilocularis*; alveolar hydatid disease) is distinct in terms of geographic distribution and life cycle.

IMAGING FEATURES

- Bacterial abscesses are typically unilocular or multilocular complex cystic collections that may contain gas and have irregular thickened enhancing walls with adjacent parenchymal edema.
- On US, the cystic nature of pyogenic abscesses may not be apparent owing to complexity of the lesion.
- Hepatic candidiasis and other fungal infections typically manifest as numerous subcentimeter microabscesses; the spleen is often affected (hepatosplenic candidiasis).
- Suggestive US findings of hepatic candidiasis include "bull's eye" and "wheel-within-a-wheel" patterns.
- Amebic abscesses are typically solitary (80% right hepatic lobe), well circumscribed, and peripheral; they are often associated with a right pleural effusion.
- Hydatid disease from *E. granulosis* typically manifests as a large cystic lesion, often with rim calcification or surrounding "daughter cysts."
- Hepatic involvement by *E. multilocularis* more often appears as a complex infiltrative process that can mimic malignancy.

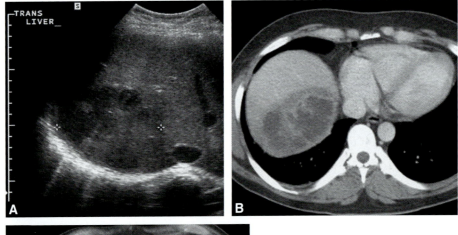

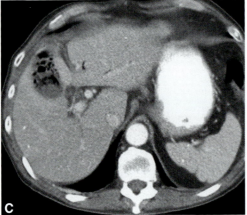

FIGURE 2.3.1 Pyogenic liver abscess. US (**A**) and CT (**B**) images show a complex cystic mass at the posterior aspect of the liver dome. Note irregular rim enhancement on CT. CT image from a different patient (**C**) shows gas bubbles within a cystic hepatic lesion, which is a more specific but relatively infrequent finding of pyogenic abscess.

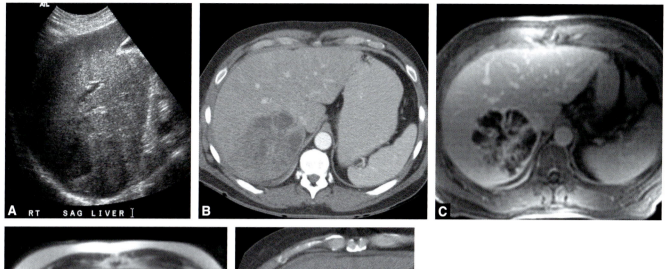
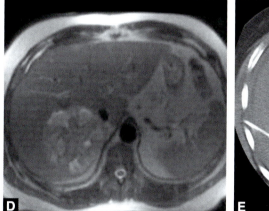
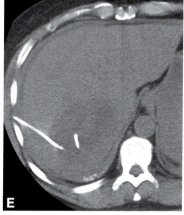

FIGURE 2.3.2 **Pyogenic liver abscess.** US image (**A**) shows a rounded complex hepatic lesion that has a more solid appearance. Contrast-enhanced CT image (**B**) shows a multiseptated cystic nature, which is even better demonstrated on contrast-enhanced SGE (**C**) and T2-weighted (**D**) MR images. The final CT image (**E**) shows a catheter in place from percutaneous abscess drainage.

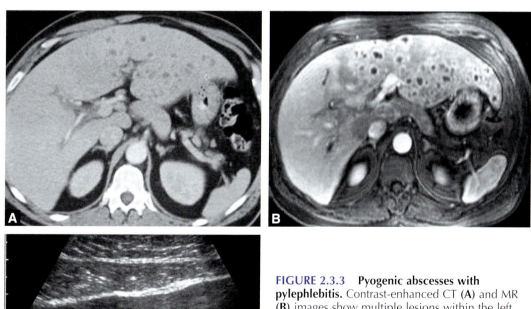
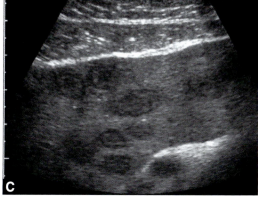

FIGURE 2.3.3 **Pyogenic abscesses with pylephlebitis.** Contrast-enhanced CT (**A**) and MR (**B**) images show multiple lesions within the left hepatic lobe. The rim enhancement is better depicted on MR. On US (**C**), the lesions have a target appearance. Right hepatic exclusion of abscesses related to right portal vein thrombosis (pylephlebitis) confirms a portomesenteric venous route of spread in this case.

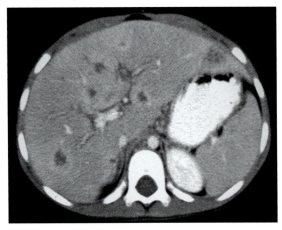

FIGURE 2.3.4 Cat-scratch disease. Contrast-enhanced CT image in a girl with history of a cat bite shows multiple low-attenuation hepatic lesions with surrounding parenchymal enhancement.

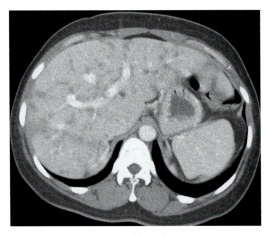

FIGURE 2.3.5 Disseminated histoplasmosis. Contrast-enhanced CT image from an immunocompromised patient shows multiple ill-defined low-attenuation lesions throughout the liver.

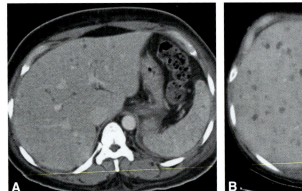
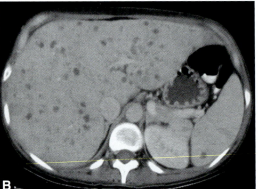
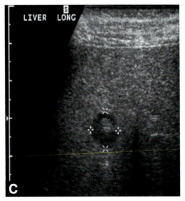

FIGURE 2.3.6 Hepatosplenic candidiasis. CT images (**A** and **B**) from two patients with neutropenic fever show multiple subcentimeter microabscesses throughout the liver, with lesser involvement of the spleen in these cases. US image from a third patient (**C**) shows the characteristic "bull's eye" appearance of hepatic fungal infection, with an echogenic central nidus.

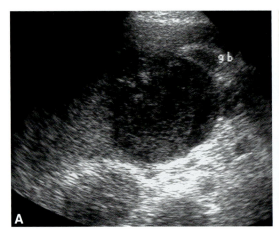
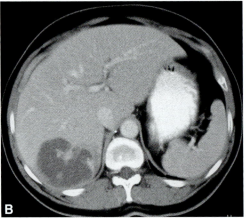

FIGURE 2.3.7 Amebic liver abscess. US (**A**) and CT (**B**) images show a complex cystic lesion involving the right hepatic lobe. Thickened irregular wall and septations are better seen on CT in this case. The imaging features overlap with those of pyogenic abscess.

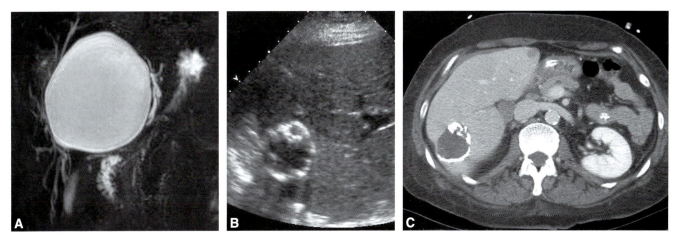

FIGURE 2.3.8 *Echinococcus granulosis* **infection (hydatid disease).** MRCP image (**A**) shows a large hepatic cyst, which because of its size and central location has resulted in intraheptic biliary ductal dilatation. US (**B**) and CT (**C**) images from a different patient show a complex cyst with dystrophic rim calcification.

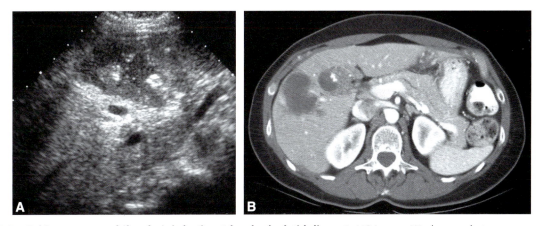

FIGURE 2.3.9 *Echinococcus multilocularis* **infection (alveolar hydatid disease).** US image (**A**) shows a heterogeneous hypoechoic lesion that contains multiple echogenic foci. Image from subsequent CT (**B**) shows multiple complex lesions with varying cystic, solid, and calcific composition. The more infiltrative appearance of the sylvan form can simulate malignancy.

2.4 Vascular Findings
(Figures 2.4.1-2.4.9)

CLINICAL FEATURES

- Transient hepatic attenuation/intensity differences (THAD/THID) represent vascular phenomena at CT and MR resulting from an altered ratio of blood flow to the liver between the portal vein and hepatic artery.
- Most cases of THAD or THID are related to compression or thrombosis of the portal venous system.
- The "hot quadrate" sign (first described on scintigraphy) is a vascular phenomenon resulting from systemic collateral venous inflow primarily to segment IV related to superior vena cava (SVC) occlusion.
- Hepatic pseudoaneurysms and arterial hemorrhage typically result from penetrating or blunt trauma.
- Tricuspid regurgitation is associated with right-sided heart failure and congestive hepatopathy but is often a subclinical finding.
- Hepatic involvement in hereditary hemorrhagic telangiectasia (Osler-Weber-Rendu disease) can lead to high-output cardiac failure related to left-to-right intrahepatic shunting.
- Peliosis hepatis is a rare condition characterized by irregular blood-filled spaces and cystic sinusoidal dilation; it is associated with chronic wasting disease, steroid use, and AIDS (bacillary angiomatosis).
- Varices: see section 3.1.

IMAGING FEATURES

- THAD on CT (THID on MR) manifests as a geographic region of increased enhancement on arterial phase imaging that normalizes on later phases; it is important to look for portal thrombosis or an offending mass.
- If prolonged, areas of THAD/THID may ultimately lead to focal fatty infiltration or sparing.
- Early intense geographic contrast enhancement of the medial segment of the left hepatic lobe at CT and MR

should provoke a search for SVC occlusion; thoraco-abdominal wall collaterals are usually evident.
- Pseudoaneurysms appear as cystic intrahepatic structures that demonstrate intense contrast enhancement at CT and MR and swirling flow at color Doppler US ("yin-yang" appearance).
- Contrast blush with extravasation is seen with active arterial hemorrhage at trauma CT; endovascular or surgical treatment is generally indicated.
- Early contrast opacification of dilated hepatic veins on CT and MR is diagnostic of tricuspid regurgitation.
- Imaging features of hepatic Osler-Weber-Rendu disease include multiple telangiectasias, hepatic vascular ectasia, and intrahepatic vascular shunting.
- Peliosis hepatis has a variable imaging appearance, but a subtle or complex cystic lesion with evidence of delayed enhancement is fairly typical; it may simulate cavernous hemangioma in some cases.

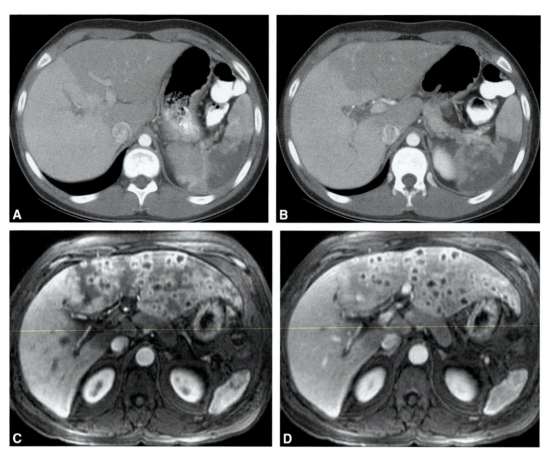

FIGURE 2.4.1   THAD and THID due to right portal vein thrombosis. Contrast-enhanced CT images (**A** and **B**) show thrombosis of the right portal vein associated with early uniform enhancement of the right hepatic lobe compared with the left, owing to an increased relative contribution from the right hepatic artery. Subtotal splenic infarction is due to splenic vein thrombosis. Arterial (**C**) and portal venous (**D**) phase MR images from a different patient show early right hepatic lobe enhancement related to right portal vein thrombosis (pylephlebitis), which nearly normalizes on the more delayed phase. Multiple hepatic abscesses spare the right lobe because portal venous access is blocked. This is the same case as shown in Figure 2.3.3.

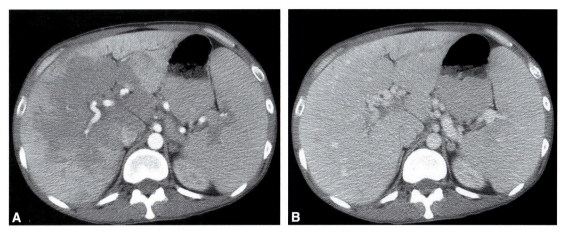

FIGURE 2.4.2 **Main portal vein thrombosis showing "zonal perfusion" THAD.** Arterial CT image **(A)** shows transient reduced parenchymal enhancement within the central perihilar liver, which normalizes with the periphery on the portal venous phase **(B)**. Multiple enhancing venous structures in **B** represent "cavernous transformation" of the parabiliary venous plexus after main portal vein thrombosis. Preserved perihilar portal venous supply from these collateral vessels likely accounts for this perfusion pattern.

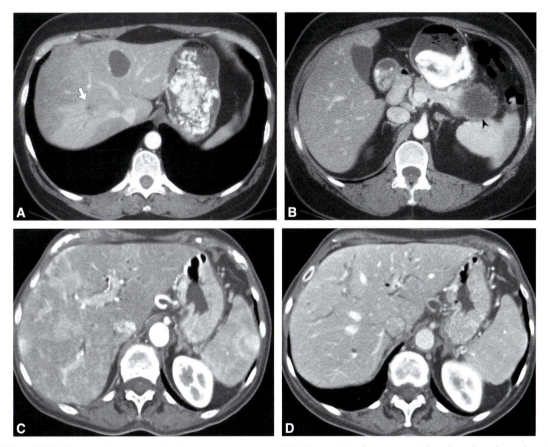

FIGURE 2.4.3 **THAD from other causes.** Early contrast-enhanced CT image **(A)** shows a peripheral wedge-shaped region of increased arterial enhancement. A subtle low-attenuation lesion is present at the apex of this region (*arrow*), which is the cause of locally reduced portal venous flow. Local biliary ductal dilatation or portal thrombus is also seen distal to this region. A simple hepatic cyst is incidentally noted. This lesion was a metastatic focus from a newly diagnosed pancreatic mucinous cystadenocarcinoma (**B**, *arrowhead*). Arterial phase CT image **(C)** from a patient with PSC shows multiple patchy areas of increased arterial enhancement. Corresponding portal venous phase **(D)** shows more uniform parenchymal enhancement, as well as segmental intrahepatic biliary dilatation. The areas of greater periportal fibrosis and biliary stricture roughly correspond to the areas of THAD.

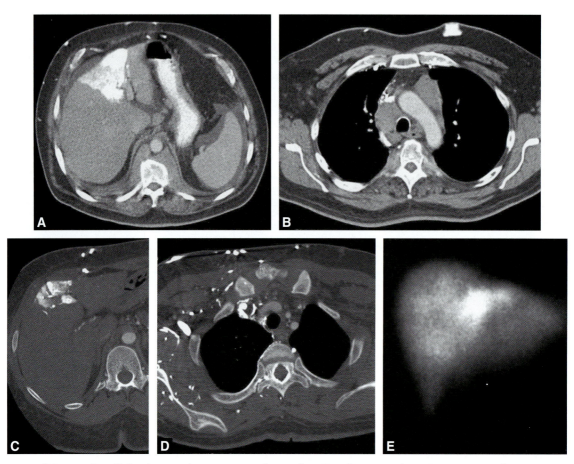

FIGURE 2.4.4 **"Hot quadrate" sign in superior vena cava obstruction.** Portal venous phase CT image **(A)** shows intense and prolonged enhancement of the medial segment of the left hepatic lobe, owing to undiluted contrast entering from systemic thoracoabdominal wall collaterals. CT image through the upper thorax **(B)** shows SVC obstruction from mediastinal lymphadenopathy. Contrast-enhanced CT image through the liver from a different patient **(C)** shows intense contrast accumulation with segment IV. Note the prominent anterior abdominal wall collaterals with concentrated contrast. CT image through the upper thorax **(D)** shows numerous chest wall collaterals. Sulfur colloid scintigraphy **(E)** from a third patient with SVC obstruction shows increased activity in segment IV—the so-called hot quadrate sign.

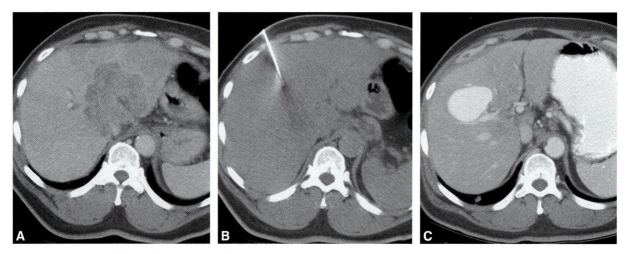

FIGURE 2.4.5 **Iatrogenic hepatic artery pseudoaneurysm.** Initial CT image **(A)** shows a large central hepatic mass. Subsequent CT-guided core biopsy **(B)** confirmed metastatic colorectal adenocarcinoma. Routine follow-up CT **(C)** performed 2 months later after interval chemotherapy shows a large enhancing intrahepatic pseudoaneurysm.

Illustration continued on following page

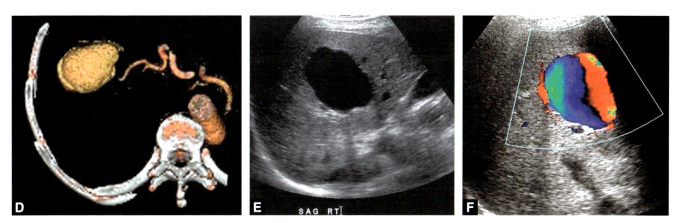

FIGURE 2.4.5 (Continued)   **Iatrogenic hepatic artery pseudoaneurysm.** Volume-rendered CT image (**D**) shows the relationship of the pseudoaneurysm to the hepatic artery. US image (**E**) from the same day shows an anechoic lesion that could be mistaken for a simple cyst without color Doppler interrogation (**F**). The lesion was successfully treated by endovascular means.

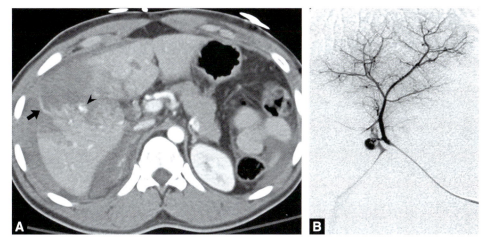

FIGURE 2.4.6   **Hepatic laceration with actively bleeding pseudoaneurysm.** Contrast-enhanced CT image (**A**) after a motor vehicle accident shows a large hepatic laceration associated with a focal contrast "blush" (*arrowhead*) consistent with a posttraumatic pseudoaneurysm. Streaks of high attenuation (*arrow*) represent active extravasation. Subsequent DSA with selective hepatic arterial injection (**B**) shows both the pseudoaneurysm and active extravasation.

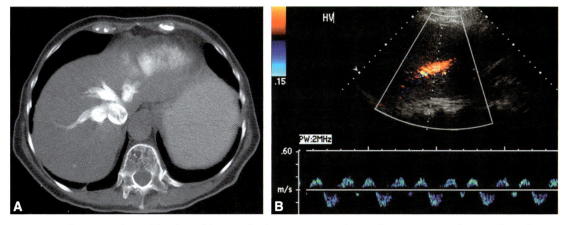

FIGURE 2.4.7   **Hepatic congestion with tricuspid regurgitation.** Contrast-enhanced CT image (**A**) shows reflux of contrast from the right atrium into a dilated IVC and hepatic veins, diagnostic of severe tricuspid regurgitation. Because of reduced cardiac output, no contrast is yet seen within the aorta. Color and spectral Doppler US image (**B**) from a different patient shows exaggerated flow reversal within the hepatic veins (reddish-orange color designation indicates flow toward the transducer).

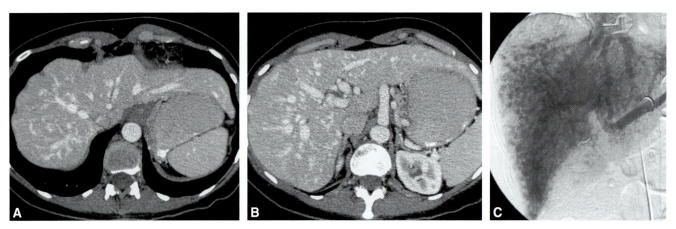

FIGURE 2.4.8 Hereditary hemorrhagic telangiectasia (Osler-Weber-Rendu disease). Thin-section contrast-enhanced CT images **(A** and **B)** show massive enlargement of the celiac axis and hepatic arterial tree, as well as enlargement of the portal venous system from arterioportal shunting. Innumerable vascular lesions throughout the hepatic parenchyma represent telangiectasias. Delayed venous-phase DSA image **(C)** from another patient shows multiple hepatic telangiectasias and prominence of the hepatic venous system.

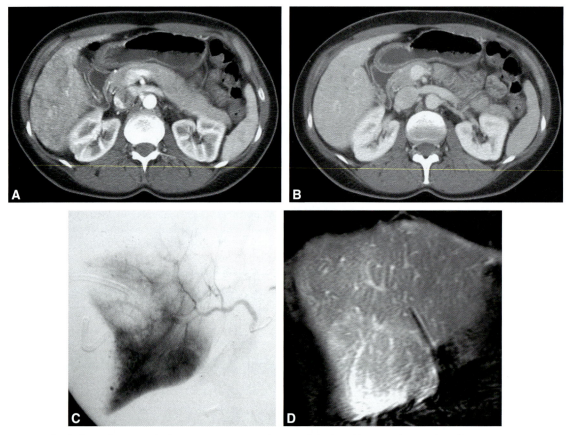

FIGURE 2.4.9 Peliosis hepatis. Arterial phase CT image **(A)** shows a lobulated hepatic lesion that demonstrates early central enhancement. Image from portal venous phase **(B)** shows persistent enhancement of the lesion that nearly matches normal liver parenchyma. DSA **(C)** and delayed contrast-enhanced MR **(D)** images from two additional patients show abnormally increased enhancement extending to the inferior tip of the liver.

3. OTHER HEPATIC CONDITIONS

Diffuse hepatic processes are also well evaluated by cross-sectional imaging. In addition to specific liver manifestations, the extrahepatic findings at CT, MR, and US often aid in forming a single unifying diagnosis.

3.1 Cirrhosis and Portal Hypertension
(Figures 3.1.1-3.1.11)

CLINICAL FEATURES

- Cirrhosis reflects the end result of hepatic insult and necrosis with fibrosis and attempted regeneration.
- The most common etiologic agents are alcohol and viral hepatitis; less frequent causes include nonalcoholic steatohepatitis (NASH), hemochromatosis, PSC, autoimmune hepatitis, and α-1 antitrypsin deficiency.
- Cirrhosis is pathologically characterized by fibrosis and regenerating nodules; alterations to parenchymal blood flow are seen secondary to fibrosis.
- Complications of cirrhosis include portal hypertension (ascites and variceal hemorrhage), hepatic failure, and development of HCC.
- HCC represents the final stage of nodule progression (i.e., regenerative to dysplastic to malignant).
- Presinusoidal causes of portal hypertension include schistosomiasis and Banti syndrome (noncirrhotic portal fibrosis).

IMAGING FEATURES

- Morphologic findings at CT, MR, and US include hepatic volume loss with widening of fissures, nodular surface contour, parenchymal coarsening, and heterogeneous enhancement.
- Relative hypertrophy of the left lateral segment and caudate lobe in the face of right lobe and left medial segment atrophy is typical.
- Associated findings of portal hypertension include ascites, splenomegaly, portal vein thrombosis or diminution, portosystemic collaterals (varices), and portal hypertensive gastropathy (at EGD).
- Common portosystemic collaterals include gastroesophageal, paraumbilical, splenorenal, retroperitoneal, omental, and hemorrhoidal pathways.
- A "snakeskin" mosaic pattern is most typical of portal hypertensive gastropathy at EGD; other appearances include fine red mucosal speckling or reddening of the rugal apices.
- Periportal venous collaterals that develop after portal vein thrombosis have been referred to as "cavernous transformation."
- Doppler US is useful for evaluating the hepatic vasculature, including patency of transjugular intrahepatic portosystemic shunts (TIPS).
- Biphasic (arterial and portal venous) phase CT/MR is commonly used to evaluate for focal hepatic lesions, assess degree of cirrhosis and portal hypertension, and define vascular anatomy (for potential transplant).
- Features of nodules concerning for HCC include hypervascularity, size >2 cm, and increased signal at T2-weighted MR.
- Gamma-Gandy bodies are low-signal splenic foci seen at MR resulting from iron deposition.
- A "turtle-back calcification" pattern on CT and US is characteristic of hepatic *Schistosoma japonica* infection.
- The appearance of treated liver metastases (most often from a breast cancer primary tumor) can simulate cirrhosis on cross-sectional imaging studies and is referred to as "pseudocirrhosis."

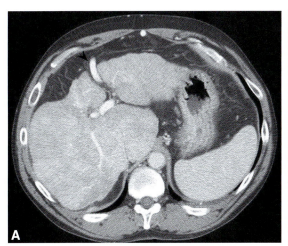 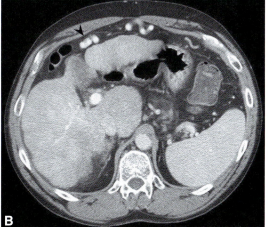

FIGURE 3.1.1 Cirrhosis. Contrast-enhanced CT images (**A** and **B**) show a nodular liver with heterogeneous enhancement, right lobe atrophy, and relative enlargement of the left lateral segment and caudate lobe. Note the large paraumbilical portosystemic collaterals (*arrowheads*).

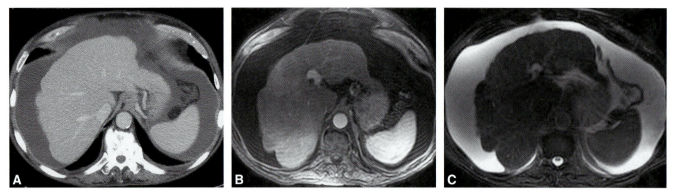

FIGURE 3.1.2 Cirrhosis with ascites. Contrast-enhanced CT **(A)**, contrast-enhanced SGE MR **(B)**, and T2-weighted MR **(C)** images show a nodular, shrunken liver and massive ascites due to portal hypertension.

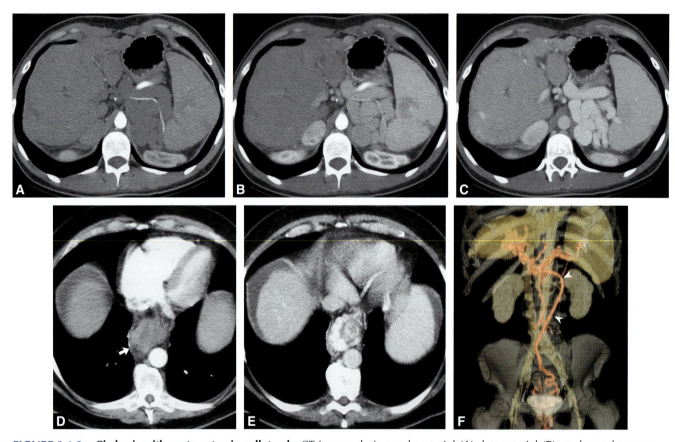

FIGURE 3.1.3 Cirrhosis with portosystemic collaterals. CT images during early arterial **(A)**, late arterial **(B)**, and portal venous **(C)** phases show massive tortuous perisplenic venous collaterals that demonstrate progressive enhancement. Arterial phase CT image **(D)** from a different patient with cirrhosis shows prominent soft tissue in the middle mediastinum (*arrow*), which is shown to represent esophageal and paraesophageal varices on the portal venous phase **(E)**. Coronal MIP CT image **(F)** from a third patient with cirrhosis shows a dilated IMV (*arrowheads*) that extends into the pelvis to form hemorrhoidal varices. Note cirrhotic liver and splenomegaly.

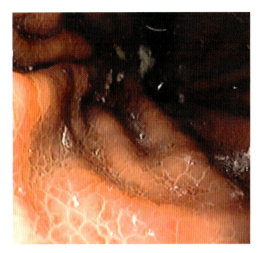

FIGURE 3.1.4 **Portal hypertensive gastropathy.** EGD image in a patient with advanced cirrhosis demonstrates the characteristic mosaic pattern to the gastric mucosa.

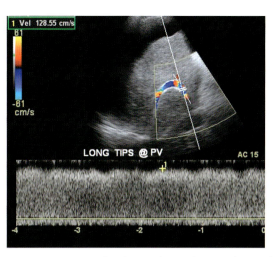

FIGURE 3.1.5 **TIPS evaluation.** Color and spectral Doppler US evaluation in a patient with cirrhosis and portal hypertension shows a patent TIPS. Interval changes in flow velocity measurements can suggest stenosis.

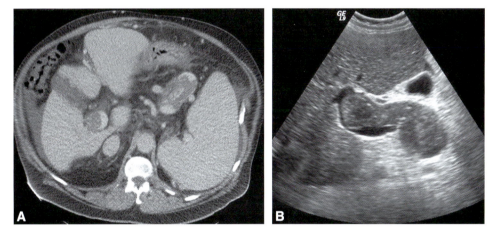

FIGURE 3.1.6 **Cirrhosis with portal vein thrombosis.** Contrast-enhanced CT (**A**) and US (**B**) images show thrombus within the main portal vein that is nearly occlusive. Findings of advanced cirrhosis and portal hypertension are apparent on CT.

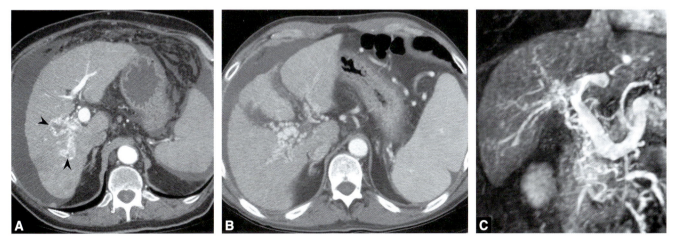

FIGURE 3.1.7 **Portal vein thrombosis with "cavernous transformation."** Contrast-enhanced CT image (**A**) from a patient with cirrhosis and portal hypertension shows thrombosis of the right portal vein surrounded by small enhancing collaterals (*arrowheads*), consistent with early cavernous change. Contrast-enhanced CT (**B**) and coronal MIP MR (**C**) images from a different patient with cirrhosis show findings of prior portal vein thrombosis with more extensive cavernous transformation.

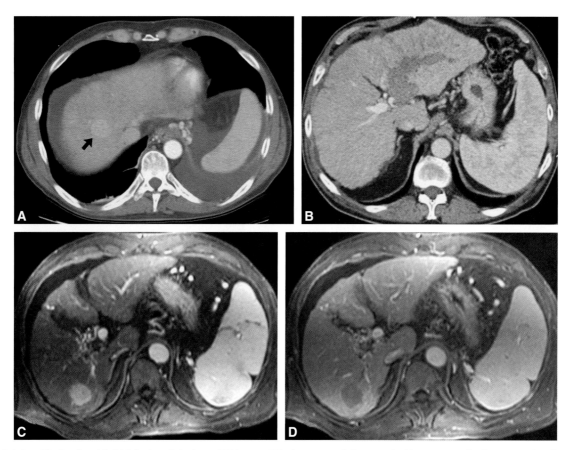

FIGURE 3.1.8 Cirrhosis with HCC. Arterial phase CT image **(A)** shows a subtle rounded hypervascular lesion at the dome of the liver (*arrow*) that represents HCC. Note associated cirrhosis, ascites, and gastroesophageal collaterals. Portal venous phase CT image **(B)** from a different patient with cirrhosis shows ill-defined low attenuation within the left hepatic lobe representing infiltrative HCC, associated with expanded tumor thrombus of the left portal vein. Arterial **(C)** and portal venous **(D)** phase SGE MR images from a third patient with cirrhosis show HCC in the right hepatic lobe with typical hypervascular enhancement **(C)** and subsequent washout **(D)**. Note also findings of prior portal venous thrombosis with cavernous change.

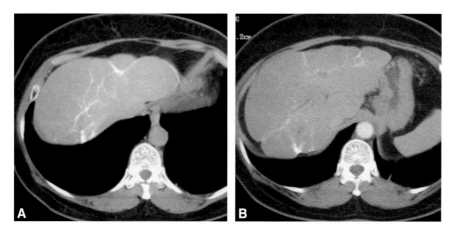

FIGURE 3.1.9 Hepatic *Schistosoma japonica* infection. Noncontrast **(A)** and contrast-enhanced **(B)** CT images show a nodular contour to the liver with thin peripheral calcification, characteristic of the "turtle-back" pattern from schistosomiasis caused by *Schistosoma japonica*.

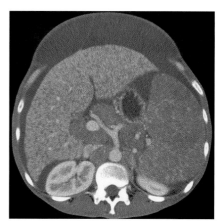

FIGURE 3.1.10 Hepatosplenic sarcoidosis. Contrast-enhanced CT image shows hepatosplenomegaly punctuated by innumerable low-attenuation foci infiltrating throughout both organs. Massive ascites and bulky periportal and celiac axis lymphadenopathy are also present.

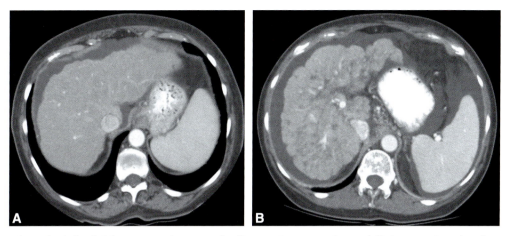

FIGURE 3.1.11 **"Pseudocirrhosis" from treated metastatic disease.** Contrast-enhanced CT images (**A** and **B**) from two patients with treated liver metastases from breast cancer show a distorted liver morphology that grossly resembles cirrhosis. In the second case (**B**), stable low-attenuation areas likely represent changes of fibrosis. Both cases demonstrate ascites.

3.2 Budd-Chiari Syndrome

(Figures 3.2.1-3.2.5)

CLINICAL FEATURES

- This uncommon syndrome is characterized by global or segmental hepatic venous outflow obstruction.
- Known causes include thrombosis in hypercoagulable states, malignancy (especially HCC and renal cell carcinoma), and membranous web (IVC diaphragm; primarily seen in Asian populations).
- The majority of cases in Western countries are idiopathic.
- Clinical presentation can be fulminant, acute, or chronic.
- Acute symptoms include pain, hepatomegaly, and ascites; chronic cases may present as variceal bleeding from portal hypertension or even hepatic failure.

IMAGING FEATURES

- Imaging appearance varies somewhat depending on the temporal nature and underlying cause.
- Hepatomegaly with globally decreased heterogeneous enhancement is typical of the acute phase.
- Hepatic veins and IVC are poorly visualized or filled with thrombus.
- A characteristic reticular enhancement pattern ("nutmeg liver") on CT and MR signifies compromise of hepatic venous outflow.
- The caudate lobe may be spared and enlarged owing to direct venous drainage to the IVC; intrahepatic venovenous collaterals to spared regions may form in chronic cases.
- Associated findings may include ascites, portal vein thrombosis, and hypervascular regenerative nodules.
- Severe passive hepatic congestion (from cardiac causes) may mimic Budd-Chiari syndrome on imaging; the hepatic veins, however, are typically dilated.

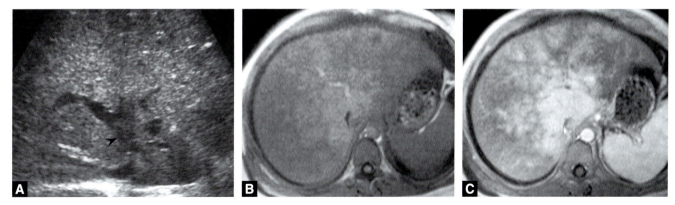

FIGURE 3.2.1 **Acute Budd-Chiari syndrome.** Transverse US image (**A**) shows thrombus expanding the right hepatic vein (*arrowhead*). Noncontrast T1-weighted MR image (**B**) shows high signal within the middle hepatic vein, consistent with acute thrombus. Contrast-enhanced MR image (**C**) shows a reticular "nutmeg" enhancement pattern to the liver, with sparing of a hypertrophic caudate, typical of Budd-Chiari syndrome.

Illustration continued on following page

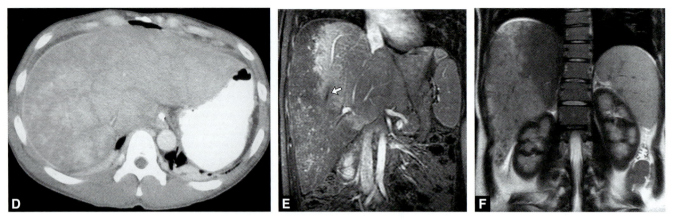

FIGURE 3.2.1 (Continued)   Acute Budd-Chiari syndrome. Contrast-enhanced CT image (D) from a different patient with acute Budd-Chiari syndrome shows the characteristic reticular pattern of hepatic enhancement. Note prominent capsular enhancement. Contrast-enhanced coronal SGE MR image (E) from a patient with paroxysmal nocturnal hemoglobinuria complicated by Budd-Chiari syndrome shows thrombosis of the right hepatic vein (*arrow*) associated with markedly abnormal enhancement of the right hepatic lobe. Coronal T2-weighted SSFSE MR image (F) shows diffuse hypointensity to the renal cortex from hemosiderin deposition.

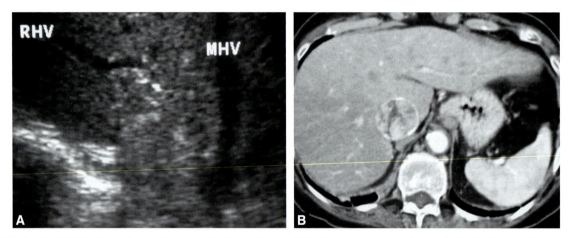

FIGURE 3.2.2   Budd-Chiari syndrome from renal cell carcinoma. US (A) and contrast-enhanced CT (B) images show expanded tumor thrombus within the IVC extending into the hepatic veins, which appears echogenic on US and demonstrates internal enhancement on CT. Direct extension of tumor thrombus from the right renal vein was seen on other images (*not shown*).

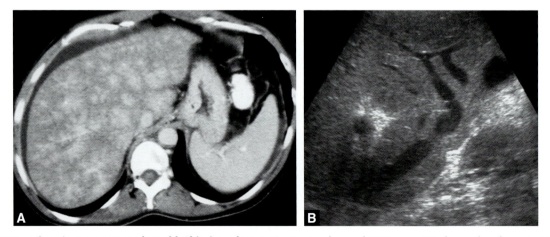

FIGURE 3.2.3   Chronic (compensated) Budd-Chiari syndrome. Contrast-enhanced CT image (A) shows the characteristic reticular "nutmeg" enhancement pattern of Budd-Chiari syndrome. US image (B) shows large intrahepatic venovenous collaterals that extend to the spared caudate lobe.

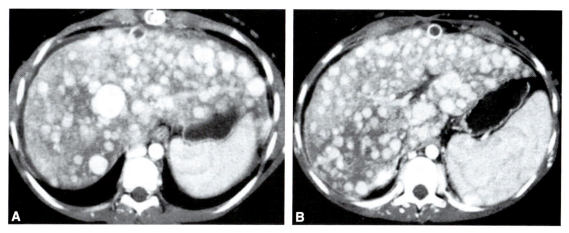

FIGURE 3.2.4 Hypervascular lesions (nodular regenerative hyperplasia) in Budd-Chiari syndrome. Arterial phase CT images (**A** and **B**) in a patient with chronic Budd-Chiari syndrome show innumerable benign hypervascular nodules that are occasionally encountered in this condition and should not be assumed to represent malignancy.

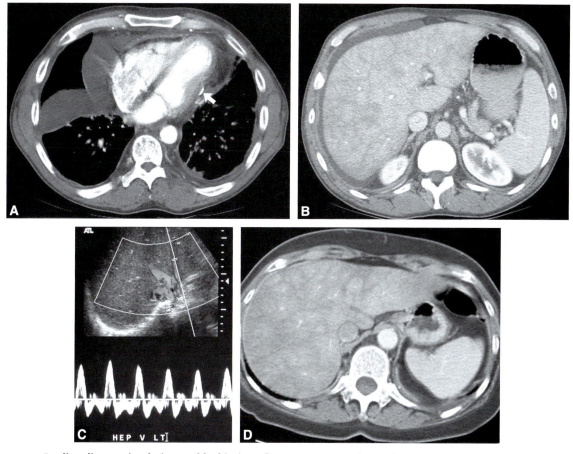

FIGURE 3.2.5 Cardiac disease simulating Budd-Chiari syndrome. Contrast-enhanced CT image (**A**) in a patient with constrictive pericarditis shows pericardial thickening and focal calcification (*arrow*) associated with narrowing of the left ventricle. CT image through the upper abdomen (**B**) shows subtle reticular enhancement of the liver from hepatic venous outflow compromise. Doppler US (**C**) and contrast-enhanced CT (**D**) images from two patients with cardiac sarcoidosis show significant compromise of hepatic venous outflow, with marked regurgitation on US and subtle reticular enhancement pattern on CT.

3.3 Fatty Liver Disease (Hepatic Steatosis)

(Figures 3.3.1-3.3.9)

CLINICAL FEATURES

- Fatty liver disease includes alcohol-related and nonalcoholic steatosis.
- Fatty infiltration of the liver is typically asymptomatic, especially if focal; diffuse infiltration is a common cause of mildly increased liver enzymes.
- Nonalcoholic fatty liver disease is most often seen in the setting of obesity, diabetes mellitus, and hyperlipidemia.
- Other potential causes of hepatic steatosis include viral hepatitis, pregnancy, steroids, toxins, medications, jejunoileal bypass, and inborn errors of metabolism.
- If symptomatic, presentation may include hepatomegaly and vague right upper quadrant discomfort from capsular stretching; acute hepatic failure is rare.
- Nonalcoholic steatohepatitis (NASH) is part of the spectrum of fatty liver disease and can lead to chronic hepatitis or cirrhosis.
- The distribution of focal disease (infiltration or sparing) likely reflects local differences in the nutritional milieu related to variant venous supply separate from the main portal system.

IMAGING FEATURES

- CT and MR are accurate noninvasive tools for diagnosing hepatic steatosis, whereas US findings are suggestive but less specific; MR may be able to quantify the degree of disease.
- Decreased attenuation of the liver relative to the spleen on noncontrast (or delayed postcontrast) CT is generally diagnostic.
- Chemical shift gradient echo MR (in-phase and opposed-phase technique) is the best imaging modality for fatty infiltration; areas of steatosis demonstrate signal drop-out relative to normal liver.
- At US, increased echogenicity of the liver parenchyma with decreased acoustic penetration reflects fatty infiltration but is a subjective finding.
- Distribution of fatty infiltration ranges from focal (commonly near the falciform ligament) to diffuse; areas of sparing are commonly seen near the gallbladder fossa.
- Focal fatty sparing or infiltration may appear nodular and mimic mass lesions but are typically geographic in appearance without mass effect.
- Steatohepatitis (alcoholic and NASH) typically demonstrates hepatomegaly and extensive heterogeneous fatty infiltration.
- A rare form of subcapsular fatty infiltration can be seen in diabetic patients undergoing peritoneal dialysis related to insulin in the dialysate.

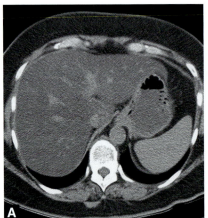 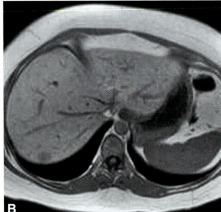 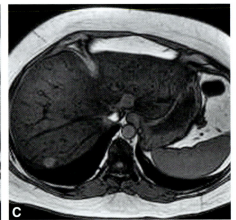

FIGURE 3.3.1 Diffuse fatty infiltration (hepatic steatosis). Noncontrast CT image (**A**) shows globally decreased hepatic attenuation relative to the normal spleen. The relatively higher attenuation of vascular structures mimics contrast enhancement. In-phase (**B**) and opposed-phase (**C**) SGE MR images from a different patient show diffuse signal dropout of the liver parenchyma on opposed phase, with little or no change in splenic signal intensity. The low-signal lesion in the right hepatic lobe on the in-phase image represents FNH that fails to drop out on the opposed-phase image because it is spared from the steatosis involving the normal liver parenchyma.

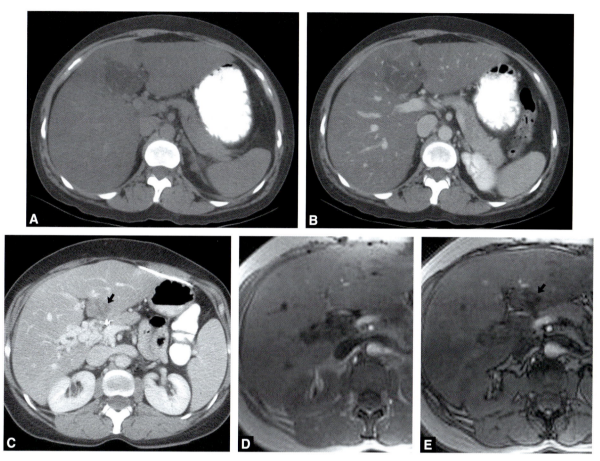

FIGURE 3.3.2 Geographic focal fatty infiltration. Noncontrast **(A)** and contrast-enhanced **(B)** CT images show a geographic region of low attenuation within the medial segment of the left hepatic lobe. Note how vessels course through the "lesion" without evidence of mass effect. More subtle focal fatty infiltration is present anteriorly, adjacent to the falciform ligament, which is the most common location for this finding. Contrast-enhanced CT image **(C)** from a patient with treated metastatic disease from colorectal cancer (including tumor thrombus in the portal vein that now shows cavernous transformation) shows an area of decreased attenuation (*arrow*). Although focal fatty infiltration was favored given the geographic appearance, chemical shift MRI was recommended for confirmation. In-phase **(D)** and opposed-phase **(E)** SGE MR images show signal dropout (*arrow*), allowing for confident noninvasive diagnosis.

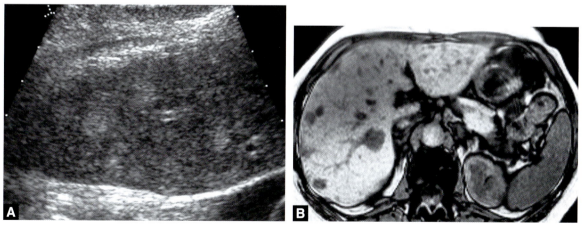

FIGURE 3.3.3 Nodular focal fatty infiltration. US image **(A)** shows multiple subtle rounded echogenic foci representing nodular areas of fatty infiltration. Opposed-phase SGE MR image **(B)** from a different patient shows similar lesions, which demonstrate signal dropout relative to in-phase imaging (*not shown*).

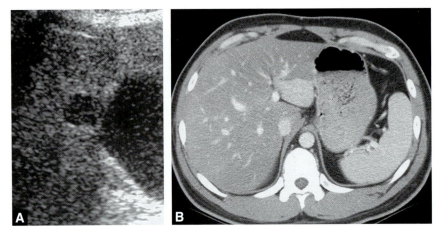

FIGURE 3.3.4 Focal fatty sparing. US image **(A)** shows a rounded hypoechoic liver "lesion" adjacent to the gallbladder. The surrounding liver parenchyma appears more echogenic and coarsened from steatosis. Contrast-enhanced CT image **(B)** from a different patient shows diffuse fatty infiltration of the liver (note decreased attenuation relative to the spleen) with a geographic region of spared parenchyma adjacent to the fissure for the ligamentum venosum. These are common locations for focal sparing.

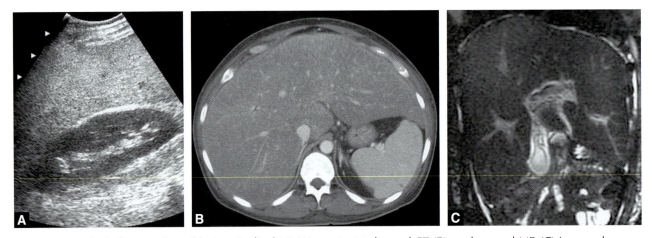

FIGURE 3.3.5 Alcoholic steatohepatitis. Longitudinal US **(A)**, contrast-enhanced CT **(B)**, and coronal MR **(C)** images show marked hepatomegaly. The liver parenchyma demonstrates increased echogenicity on US and decreased attenuation on CT.

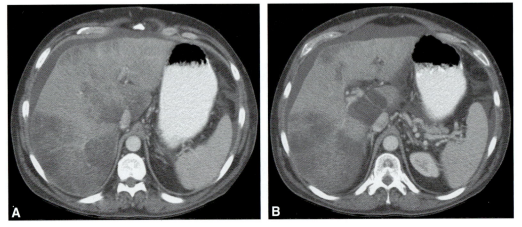

FIGURE 3.3.6 Nonalcoholic steatohepatitis with early cirrhosis. Contrast-enhanced CT images **(A and B)** show a heterogeneous appearance to the liver parenchyma with both ill-defined and geographic regions of decreased attenuation. Ascites is present. Biopsy showed severe changes of NASH.

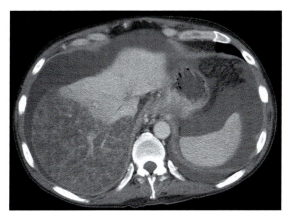

FIGURE 3.3.7 Steatohepatitis associated with hemochromatosis. Noncontrast CT image shows changes of cirrhosis and portal hypertension, with markedly decreased attenuation involving the entire right hepatic lobe from severe steatohepatitis. Left hepatic lobe attenuation is increased from normal because of underlying hemochromatosis.

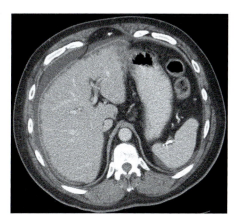

FIGURE 3.3.8 Subcapsular fatty infiltration related to peritoneal dialysate. Contrast-enhanced CT image in an insulin-dependent diabetic on peritoneal dialysis shows a peculiar rind of subcapsular low attenuation due to fatty infiltration related to local effect of insulin in the dialysate (note peritoneal fluid). The bare area and other portions of liver not in contact with the dialysate are spared.

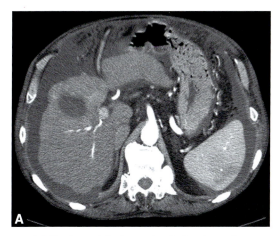
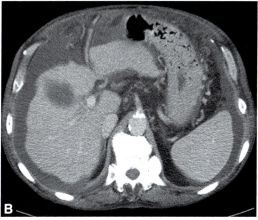

FIGURE 3.3.9 Pitfall of arterial-phase simulating hepatic steatosis. Arterial-phase CT image (**A**) in a patient with cirrhosis shows globally decreased attenuation of the liver relative to the spleen, which is a more hypervascular structure. Note how the attenuation normalizes on the portal venous phase (**B**). Assessment for hepatic steatosis should be avoided during arterial-phase imaging.

3.4 Hemochromatosis

(Figures 3.4.1-3.4.2)

CLINICAL FEATURES

- Primary hemochromatosis is a relatively common autosomal recessive disorder related to excess iron from increased intestinal absorption (distinct from hemosiderosis secondary to multiple transfusions).
- Parenchymal iron deposition can adversely affect the liver, heart, and pancreas, leading to cirrhosis, cardiac arrhythmia, and diabetes mellitus (skin hyperpigmentation gives rise to the term "bronze diabetes").
- In patients with cirrhosis from hemochromatosis, the risk for developing HCC is relatively high.
- Presenting complaints may include weakness, arthralgias, abdominal pain, loss of libido, and impotence.
- There is a male predominance in most series (roughly 8:1); decreased female phenotypic expression may be related to iron loss from menses.

IMAGING FEATURES

- Increased attenuation of liver parenchyma (often >75 HU) is evident on noncontrast CT; superimposed fatty infiltration may "normalize" hepatic attenuation values.
- Marked signal loss involves the liver and pancreas on MR sequences, whereas signal drop-out of the liver and spleen is seen more with transfusional hemosiderosis (parenchymal deposition vs. reticuloendothelial).
- US examination is insensitive for detecting increased iron deposition.
- Secondary features of cirrhosis and portal hypertension are noted in advanced cases; careful search for HCC is warranted.

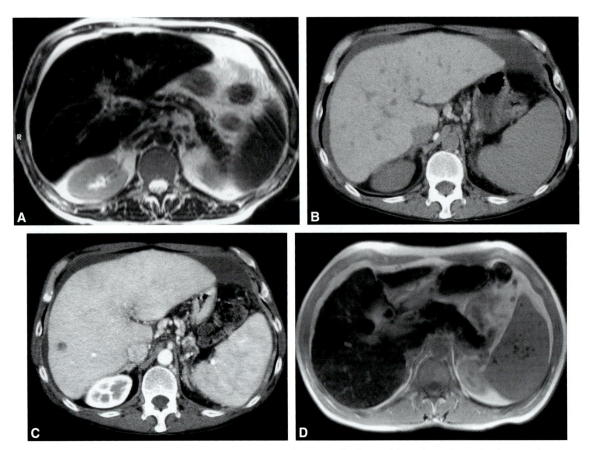

FIGURE 3.4.1 Hemochromatosis. T2-weighted MR image **(A)** shows marked signal loss throughout the liver and pancreas from parenchymal iron deposition. Similarly, increased liver attenuation is evident on noncontrast CT **(B)**. Contrast-enhanced CT image **(C)** shows a 1-cm low-attenuation lesion in the right hepatic lobe, which proved to be HCC on US-guided biopsy. SGE MR image **(D)** from a different patient shows advanced cirrhosis with diffusely decreased signal throughout the liver and pancreas relative to the spleen. Punctate low-signal foci within the spleen represent Gamna-Gandy bodies.

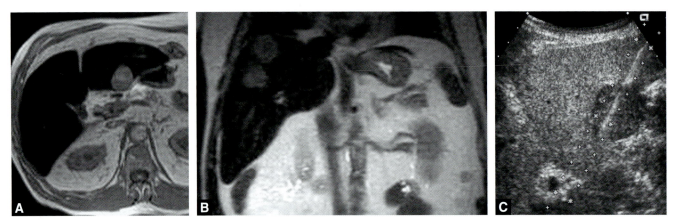

FIGURE 3.4.2 Hemochromatosis with multifocal hepatocellular carcinoma. T1-weighted **(A)** and T2-weighted **(B)** MR images show pronounced signal drop-out throughout the liver. Three rounded hepatic lesions are conspicuous due to relatively increased signal and represent HCC, which was confirmed on US-guided biopsy **(C)**. The cirrhotic liver appears diffusely echogenic relative to the hypoechoic mass.

3.5 The Hyperdense Liver on CT
(Figures 3.5.1-3.5.4)

CLINICAL FEATURES

- The majority of cases with abnormally increased liver attenuation are due to transfusional hemosiderosis, primary hemochromatosis, and amiodarone use.
- Uncommon causes include colloidal gold therapy, glycogen storage disease (von Gierke), Thorotrast exposure, and barium intravasation.
- Sickle cell disease and thalassemia are typical causes of transfusional hemosiderosis.
- Amiodarone, used to treat and prevent certain ventricular arrhythmias, contains an iodine moiety that is taken up by the liver; dense interstitial pulmonary infiltrates can also be seen.
- Thorotrast, an alpha emitter with a long biologic half-life, was last used in the 1950s as a contrast agent; reticuloendothelial uptake has led to many hepatosplenic angiosarcomas and other malignancies.

IMAGING FEATURES

- Besides increased attenuation of the liver parenchyma on noncontrast CT (generally >75 HU), the associated imaging findings will often point to the underlying cause.

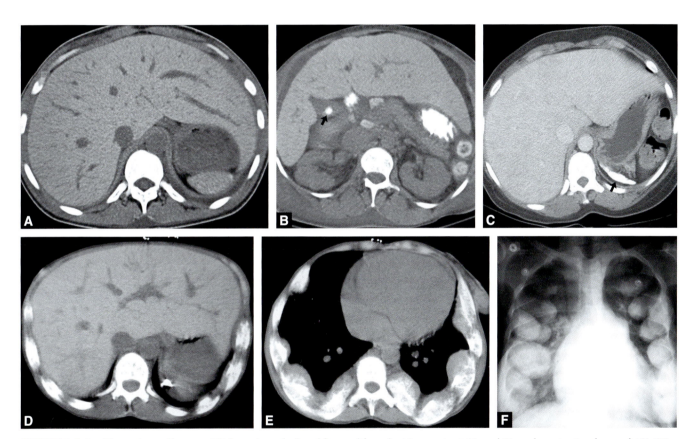

FIGURE 3.5.1 Hyperdense liver on CT from transfusional hemosiderosis. Noncontrast (**A** and **B**) and contrast-enhanced (**C**) CT images from three patients with sickle cell disease show increased liver attenuation related to repeated blood transfusions. A shrunken (**A**) or calcified (**C**, *arrow*) spleen and gallstones (**B**, *arrow*) are also common findings in these patients. Noncontrast CT images (**D** and **E**) from a patient with β-thalassemia show similar liver findings related to transfusional hemosiderosis. Note prior splenectomy, massive medullary expansion involving the ribs, and adjacent soft tissue representing extramedullary hematopoiesis. Medullary expansion is even more striking on chest radiography (**F**).

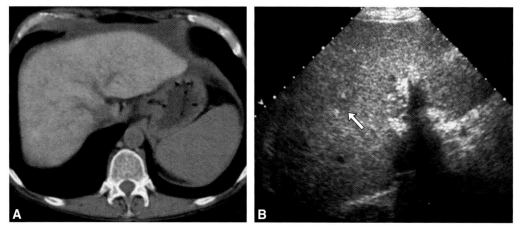

FIGURE 3.5.2 Hyperdense liver from hemochromatosis. Noncontrast CT image **(A)** shows diffusely increased liver attenuation. Changes of cirrhosis with portal hypertension are present. US image **(B)** shows a coarsened, echogenic liver parenchyma and a subtle 1-cm hypoechoic lesion (*arrow*) that proved to be HCC on US-guided biopsy.

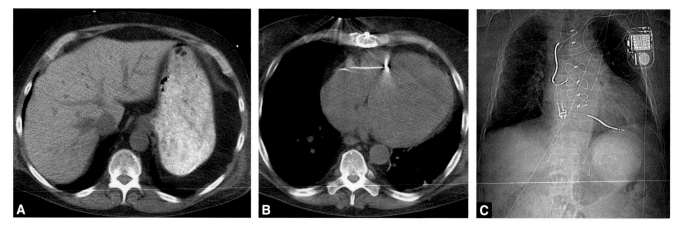

FIGURE 3.5.3 Hyperdense liver from amiodarone use. Noncontrast CT image **(A)** shows increased liver attenuation related to the iodine content in amiodarone. Note cardiomegaly and cardiac pacer on CT **(B)** and CT scout **(C)** images.

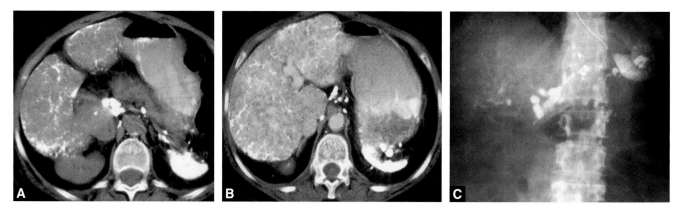

FIGURE 3.5.4 Imaging findings of previous Thorotrast exposure. Noncontrast **(A)** and contrast-enhanced **(B)** CT images show reticular densities throughout the liver, as well as dense lymph nodes and a dense, shrunken spleen. The findings of reticuloendothelial density are well demonstrated on the abdominal radiograph **(C)**.

3.6 Post-transplant Complications

(Figures 3.6.1-3.6.5)

CLINICAL FEATURES

- Complications after orthotopic liver transplantation include vascular stenosis, thrombosis, and pseudoaneurysm; biliary leak or stricture; parenchymal infarct and rejection; and malignancy (PTLD).
- Hepatic arterial stenosis and thrombosis are feared vascular complications.
- Delayed biliary complications often relate to hepatic arterial compromise resulting in biliary ischemia.
- Anastomotic biliary strictures are relatively common and multifactorial in origin; nonanastomotic intrahepatic strictures are less common and more closely associated with arterial compromise (ischemic cholangiopathy).
- PTLD has a predilection for the liver allograft itself; most cases present within 1 to 2 years of transplantation.

IMAGING FEATURES

- US with Doppler interrogation is often the initial study for evaluating vascular patency; a low-resistance "parvus tardus" intrahepatic arterial waveform (RI < 0.50) suggests upstream stenosis.
- CT, MR, and conventional angiography are useful in evaluating for suspected vascular complications.
- T-tube cholangiography, MRCP, and ERCP are useful in evaluating for biliary leaks, strictures, and stones; ERCP has the benefit of providing therapy if needed.
- PTLD may involve virtually any organ system, but allograft involvement is most typical; unifocal or multifocal lesions may be seen, with the transplant hilum being frequently involved.

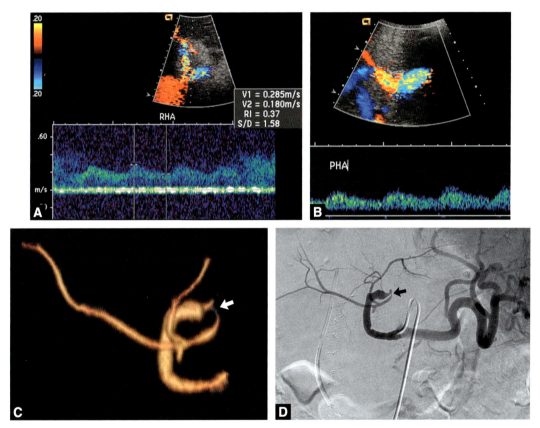

FIGURE 3.6.1 Hepatic artery stenosis after liver transplantation. Color and spectral Doppler US image **(A)** focused on the right hepatic artery shows a low-resistance waveform with rounded "parvus tardus" appearance due to upstream arterial stenosis. The resistive index measures 0.37. Color and spectral Doppler US image from a second patient **(B)** shows a similar low-resistance, parvus tardus waveform of the proper hepatic artery. CT angiographic **(C)** and conventional DSA **(D)** images show high-grade stenosis (*arrows*) at the anastomotic region.

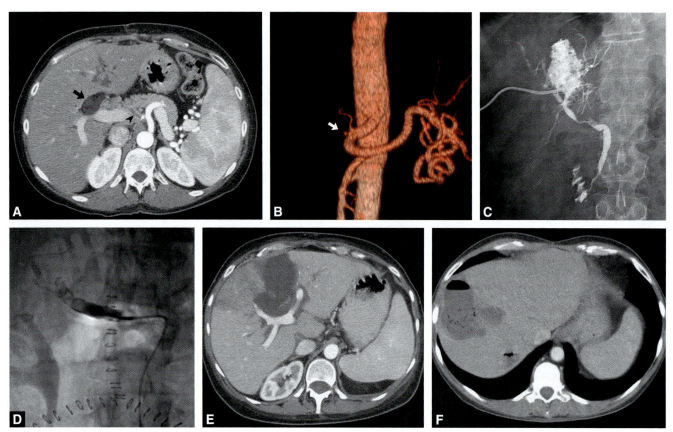

FIGURE 3.6.2 Hepatic artery thrombosis after liver transplantation. Arterial phase CT image **(A)** shows linear low-attenuation thrombus (*arrowhead*) within the proximal hepatic artery, beginning just beyond its origin. The irregular hilar collection (*arrow*) represents biliary necrosis and biloma formation. CT angiographic image **(B)** re-demonstrates the abrupt cut-off of the common hepatic artery near its origin (*arrow*). Subsequent drainage and injection of the intrahepatic biloma **(C)** shows an irregular collection that communicates with the biliary tree. Image from conventional DSA **(D)** from a different patient shows a similar hepatic arterial thrombosis, which forms a cast that occludes the vessel lumen. Contrast-enhanced CT images from two additional patients with hepatic artery thrombosis show a large evolving infarct **(E)** and gas-containing intrahepatic abscesses **(F)**, respectively.

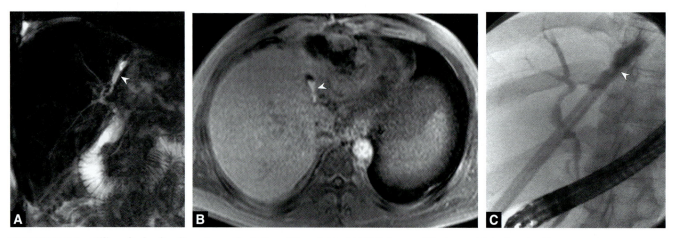

FIGURE 3.6.3 Biliary leak after liver transplantation. T2-weighted MRCP image **(A)** shows high signal adjacent to the cut surface of a right lobe transplant (*arrowhead*), suggestive of biliary leak. T1-weighted MR image **(B)** after administration of biliary contrast (Mn-DPDP) confirms a leak with high signal contrast adjacent to the cut surface (*arrowhead*). Subsequent image from ERCP **(C)** also shows the biliary leak (*arrowhead*).

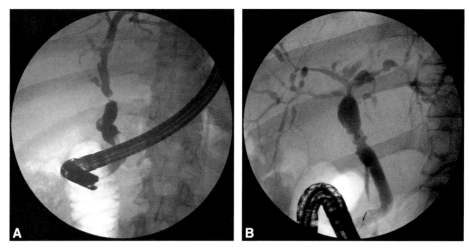

FIGURE 3.6.4 **Biliary strictures after liver transplantation.** Image from ERCP (**A**) shows an anastomotic stricture, which was treated with balloon dilation. ERCP image (**B**) from a patient with ischemic cholangiopathy shows multiple intrahepatic strictures that simulate the appearance of PSC. The relative narrowing and irregularity at the anastomosis in this case is a common normal appearance that should not be mistaken for a significant stricture.

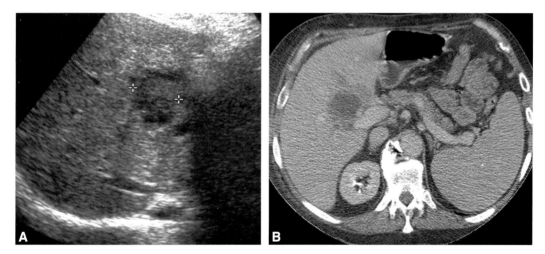

FIGURE 3.6.5 **PTLD after liver transplantation.** US (**A**) and CT (**B**) images from two different patients show ill-defined hypoechoic and low-attenuation hilar masses, respectively, that represent a typical appearance of allograft involvement by PTLD.

INDEX

Note: Page numbers followed by the letter f refer to figures.

A

Abdominal radiography. *See* specific disease entities
Abscess
 abdominal, 163f
  Crohn's disease and, 163f
  drainage catheter, 268f, 325f
 hepatic, 450, 450f-453f
 periappendiceal, 296f
 peridiverticular, 287f
 retropharyngeal, 57, 59f
Acalculous cholecystitis, 355, 357f
Acanthosis, glycogenic esophageal, 16, 16f, 17f
Achalasia, 33, 34f-35f
Acinar cell carcinoma, pancreatic, 401, 403f
Acquired esophageal fistula, 49, 51f
Adenocarcinoma
 ampullary, 335, 336f-337f
 appendiceal, 297, 299f
 colon, 229, 230f-234f, 234, 234f-238f
  biliary metastases with, 338, 339f-340f
  bowel obstruction due to, 231f-232f
  cecal, intussusception from, 307, 308f
  hepatic metastases with, 428, 429f-430f
  in Crohn's disease, 267, 270f
  in FAP, 217f
  in ulcerative colitis, 261, 265f-266f
  obstructive appendicitis due to, 297f
  pancreatic metastases with, 401f
  small bowel metastases with, 160f
 duodenal, 113, 115f-116f
 esophageal, 1-2, 2f-6f
  in Barrett's esophagus, 23, 24f
 gallbladder, 333, 334f
 gastric, 65, 66f-70f
  linitis plastica in, 65, 68-69
 ileal, in Crohn's disease, 145f
 mucinous, 6f, 70f, 231f
 pancreatic ductal, 381-382, 382f-385f
  hemobilia from, 380f
  Trousseau's sign in, 385f
 rectal, 234, 234f-238f
 small bowel, 143-144, 144f-145f
Adenoma
 ampullary, 335, 335f-336f
 colorectal
  flat, 212, 215f
  pedunculated, 212, 214f-215f
   shifting position on CTC, 259f-260f
  serrated, 212, 217f
  sessile, 212, 213f-214f
  villous, 212, 216f
 duodenal, 113, 114f, 115f
  villous, 337f
 gastric, 61, 64f
 hepatocellular, 436, 436f-438f
Adenomatous polyps. *See* Adenoma, colorectal.
Adenomyomatosis, 370, 371f
Adhesions, small bowel obstruction from, 175, 176f
Advanced adenoma
 pedunculated, 214f-215f
 sessile, 213f-214f

Adynamic ileus, postoperative, 182f
Aeromonas sobria colitis, 271, 275f
Afferent loop obstruction, of small bowel, 175, 181f
AIDS patients
 cholangiopathy in, 365, 365f
 condylomata acuminata in, 301, 305-306f
 esophagitis, HIV, 24-25, 27f, 50f
 Kaposi's sarcoma in, 78, 79f, 80f, 117, 121f
 lymphoma in, 441f
 syphilitic proctitis in, 275f
Alcoholic steatohepatitis, 466, 468f
Amebic liver abscess, 450, 452f
Amiodarone use, hyperdense liver from, 471, 472f
Ampullary tumors. *See also* periampullary tumors.
 adenocarcinoma, 335, 336f-337f
 adenoma, 335, 335f-336f
Amyloidosis
 duodenal, 140, 141f
 small bowel, 203, 204f
Anal cancer, squamous cell carcinoma, 234, 238f
Anal fissures, 301, 304f
Anal papillae, hypertrophied, 301, 303f
Anal warts (condylomata acuminata), 301, 305f-306f
Angiodysplasia, colonic, 310, 310f-311f. *See also* Vascular ectasia.
Angioectasia, esophageal, 40f. *See also* Vascular ectasia.
Angioedema, hereditary, 203, 204f
Angiography. *See also* Digital subtraction angiography (DSA).
 of arteriovenous fistula, 187f
 of colonic hemorrhage, after colonoscopy, 325f
 of diverticular hemorrhage, 293f
 of gastrinoma, 397f
 of hemobilia, 379f
 of mesenteric ischemia, 184f, 187f
 of post-transplant hepatic artery stenosis, 473f
 of post-transplant hepatic artery thrombosis, 474f
 of pseudoaneurysms, from pancreatitis, 407f
 of vascular ectasia, 209f
Angiosarcoma, hepatic, 440, 442f-443f
Annular pancreas, 418, 419f-420f
Anorectal disease, 301-302, 302f-307f
Aortic arch, double, 55, 55f
Aortoesophageal fistula, 49, 51f
Appendagitis, epiploic, 326, 326f-327f
Appendiceal tumors, 297, 298f-301f
Appendicitis, 294-295, 295f-297f
 obstructive, colon cancer presenting as, 297f
 perforated
  periappendiceal abscess and, 296f
  small bowel obstruction and, 175, 177f
 stump, 297f
 tip, 296f

Arterial embolization, for hemobilia, 379f
Arteriovenous fistula, mesenteric, ischemia related to, 187f
Ascariasis, 167, 170f
Ascending cholangitis, 362, 362f-363f
Ascites, cirrhosis with, 460f
Atrophic gastritis, 94, 95f
Autoimmune pancreatitis, 361f, 415, 415f-416f
Autosomal dominant polycystic disease
 hepatic cysts in, 449f
 pancreatic cysts in, 421f

B

"Backwash ileitis," in ulcerative colitis, 166f
Barium studies. *See* specific disease entities.
Barrett's esophagus, 23, 23f-24f
Behçet's disease
 colonic, 282f
 gastric, 94, 97f
Bezoars
 gastric, 108, 108f-109f
 small bowel, 179f
Bile acid gastropathy, 84, 86f
Bile duct leakage, after cholecystectomy, 373, 374f
Biliary calculi, 344-355
Biliary compromise, pancreatitis causing, 375, 376f
Biliary intraductal mucinous neoplasm, 341, 343f
Biliary leak, 373, 373f-375f
 after liver transplantation, 473, 474f
Biliary melanoma, 344f
Biliary obstruction
 iatrogenic, 375f
 from ampullary tumors, 336f, 337f
 from biliary melanoma, 344f
 from cholangiocarcinoma, 330f-333f
 from choledocholithiasis, 348f, 349f
 from extrinsic malignancy, 341f
 from gallbladder carcinoma, 334f
 from hepatic inflammatory pseudotumor, 378f
 from Mirizzi's syndrome, 351f, 352f
 from metastatic disease, 340f, 400f
 from pancreatitis, 376f
 from PSC, 360f, 361f
Biliary strictures
 anastomotic, 363f
 common duct injury, 375f, 453f
 liver transplantation, 473, 475f
 portal biliopathy, 375, 376f-377f
 PSC, 359, 360f, 361f
 RPC, 364, 364f
 sarcoidosis-induced, 377f
Biliary tree
 aberrant anatomy of, 373, 375f
 autoimmune pancreatitis affecting, 361f
 inflammatory diseases of, 355-363
Biliary tumor(s)
 cholangiocarcinoma, 329-330, 330f-333f
 cystadenoma, 341, 342f-343f
 gallbladder carcinoma, 333, 334f-335f

477

Biliary tumor(s)—cont'd
 granular cell tumor, 341, 343f
 intraductal mucinous neoplasm, 341, 343f
 metastatic disease to the biliary tree, 338, 339f-341f
 periampullary, 335, 335f-338f
 polyps, 341, 344f
Biliary-enteric fistulas, 352, 353f-355f
Biliopathy, portal, 375, 376f-377f
Biopsy
 endoscopic ultrasound guided
  of ampullary gangliocytic paraganglioma, 122f
  of pancreatic adenocarcinoma, 383f
 liver, hemobilia related to, 379f
 ultrasound-guided
  of hepatic focal nodular hyperplasia, 447f
  of nonhyperfunctioning islet cell tumors, 395f
  of small bowel non-Hodgkin's lymphoma, 149f
Bisphosphonates, esophagitis due to, 28, 29f
Blastomycosis, disseminated, 167, 171f
Blebs, venous, colorectal, 222, 224f-225f, 310, 312f
Blue rubber bleb nevus syndrome
 gastric involvement in, 97, 99f
 hepatic involvement in, 432, 435f
Boerhaave's syndrome, 44, 46f
Bouveret's syndrome, 352, 355f
Bowel. See also specific location.
 iatrogenic injury to, 207f
 obstruction of, colon cancer causing, 231f-232f
Breast cancer, metastatic, 79f, 158f
Bronchogenic foregut duplication cyst, 43, 44f
Brunner's glands
 hamartoma of, 122, 123f
 hyperplasia of, 122, 123f
Budd-Chiari syndrome, 463, 463f-465f
"Buried bumper syndrome," 111, 112f

C

Calculi
 biliary, 344-355
 pancreatic ductal, in chronic pancreatitis, 410f
Cameron lesion, hiatal hernia with, 101, 102f
Campylobacter colitis, 271, 275f
Candidiasis
 esophageal, 24-25, 25f
 hepatosplenic, 450, 452f
Capillary hemangioma, esophageal, 38, 40f
Capsule endoscopy, small bowel
 of cavernous hemangioma, 156f
 of celiac disease, 194f
 of Crohn's disease, 161f, 163f, 164f
 of hamartoma, 154f, 155f
 of hematogenous metastatic disease, 160f
 of lipoma, 154f
 of lymphangioma, 156f, 157f
 of lymphoma, 150f
 of gastrointestinal stromal tumor, 153f
 of NSAID enteropathy, 173f, 174f
 of carcinoid tumor, 146f, 147f
 of vascular ectasia, 209f
Carcinoid tumors
 appendiceal, 297, 300f
 colonic, 238, 241f
 duodenal, 117, 121f
 gastric, 78, 80f
 rectal, 222, 224f
 small bowel, 145, 146f-148f

Carcinomatosis, gastric, 78, 79f
Carcinosarcoma, esophageal, 13, 16f
Cardiac disease, simulating Budd-Chiari syndrome, 465f
Caroli's disease, 368, 369f-370f
Catheter tip, simulating rectal polyp, 261f
Cat-scratch disease, 450, 452f
Caustic injury
 esophagitis due to, 28, 29f-30f
 gastritis due to, 94, 96f
Cavernous hemangioma. See also Hemangioma.
 gastric 97, 99f
 hepatic, 432, 433f-435f
 small bowel, 151, 156f
"Cavernous transformation," in portal vein thrombosis, 461f
Cecal adenocarcinoma, intussusception from, 307, 308f
Cecal polyp, pedunculated, 301f
Cecal volvulus, 314, 315f-316f
Celiac disease 129, 131f, 192, 193f-195f
Cervical cancer, metastatic, 15f, 239f
Cervical esophageal web, 53, 54f
Chagas' disease, 33, 35f
Chemoembolization, hepatic arterial, duodenal ischemia after, 129, 132f
Chest radiography. See specific disease entities
Cholangiocarcinoma, 329-330, 330f-333f, 338f
 intrahepatic (peripheral), 438, 438f-440f
Cholangiopathy
 AIDS, 365, 365f
 ischemic, 473, 475f
Cholangitis
 ascending, 362, 362f-363f
 eosinophilic, 377f
 primary sclerosing, 359, 360f-361f
 recurrent pyogenic, 364, 364f
Cholecystectomy
 common duct stricture caused by, 375, 375f
 duct leakage after, 373, 373f, 374f
 laparoscopic, dropped gallstones from, 346f
Cholecystitis, 355-356, 356f-359f
Cholecystocolic fistula, 352, 353f
Cholecystoduodenal fistula, 352, 353f
Cholecystography, of adenomyomatosis, 371f
Choledochocele, 366, 367f
Choledochal cysts, 366, 366f-368f
Choledochoduodenal fistula, 352, 353f-354f
Choledocholithiasis, 347, 347f-351f
 with ascending cholangitis, 362f-363f
Cholelithiasis, 344-345, 345f-346f
Choriocarcinoma, metastatic, 431f
Cirrhosis, 459, 459f-462f
 ascites with, 460f
 colonic wall thickening related to, 283f
 hepatocellular carcinoma with, 426f, 462f
 nonalcoholic steatohepatitis with, 468f
 portal vein thrombosis with, 461f
 portosystemic collaterals with, 460f
Cloacogenic polyp, inflammatory, 301-302, 304f
Clonorchis sinensis, in RPC, 364
Closed-loop small bowel obstruction, 175, 180f-181f
 ischemia from, 186f
Clostridium difficile colitis, 271, 271f-272f
Colitis
 amebic, 275f
 bacterial causes of, 271, 274f-275f
 Clostridium difficile, 271, 271f-272f

Colitis—cont'd
 Crohn's, 267f -270f. See also Crohn's disease.
  inflammatory pseudopolyps in, 269f
 cytomegalovirus, 271, 273f
 granulomatous, sarcoidosis causing, 279, 282f-283f
 ischemic, 275, 276f-279f
 neutropenic, 279, 281f
 parasitic causes of, 271, 275f
 pseudomembranous. See *Clostridium difficile* colitis
 radiation, 279, 280-281f
 ulcerative, 261, 262f-266f. See also Ulcerative colitis.
 viral causes of, 271, 274f
Colitis cystica profunda, 301, 302f-303f
Colocolic (double-tracking) fistula, 291f
Colocutaneous fistulas, diverticulitis causing, 289, 290f
Colon. See Colorectal, Colonic
Colonic adenocarcinoma. See Adenocarcinoma, colon.
Colonic diverticulitis, 286, 286f-289f
Colonic diverticulosis, 283, 284f-285f
Colonic hernias, 320, 321f-323f
Colonic infections, 271, 271f-275f
Colonic necrosis, Kayexalate-induced, 275, 278f
Colonic obstruction, 231f, 291f, 314-316f
Colonic perforation
 at screening colonoscopy, 323, 323f-325f
 cancer-induced, 233f
 toxic ulcerative colitis causing, 264f
Colonic strictures, post-ischemic, 279f
Colonic urticaria, 279, 282f
Colonic varices, 310, 314f
Colonic vasculitis, 279, 282f
Colonic volvulus, 314, 314f-316f
Colonic wall thickening, 283f
Colonography, CT
 3D map, 243f
 3D unfolded cube display at, 251f
 3D virtual dissection display at, 250f
 colonic gas patterns in, 252f
 computer-aided detection at, 249f-250f
 diagnostic tools, 242-243, 243f-253f
 electronic fluid cleansing at, 251f
 following incomplete optical colonoscopy, 252f-253f
 mucosal coverage in, 247f-248f
 missed region tool in, 248f
 of anal warts, 305f
 of appendiceal mucoceles, 298f
 of appendiceal stump, 301f
 of colonic adenocarcinoma, 230f, 231f
 of colonic carcinoid tumors, 241f
 of colonic diverticulosis, 284f, 285f
 of colonic leiomyoma, 226f
 of colonic lipoma, 223f
 of colonic perforation at colonoscopy, 323f, 324f
 of colorectal adenomas
  flat, 212, 215f
  pedunculated, 212, 214f-215f
  serrated, 212, 217f
  sessile, 212, 213f-214f
  villous, 212, 216f
 of cystic hamartoma, retrorectal, 306f
 of cystic lymphangioma, 227f
 of diverticulum vs. polyp, 285f
 of endoluminal foreign bodies, 259f
 of endometriosis, 227f
 of epiploic appendagitis, 327f
 of hamartomatous polyps, 221f
 of hemorrhoids, 312f

Colonography, CT—cont'd
  of hyperplastic polyps, 218f-219f
  of hypertrophied anal papillae, 303f
  of inflammatory polyps, 220f-221f
    cloacogenic, 304f
  of inflammatory pseudopolyps, 269f
  of inguinal hernia of sigmoid colon, 321f
  of juvenile polyps, 220f
  of lymphoid polyps, 225f
  of malrotation, 201f
  of mucosal polyps, 219f
  of NSAID-induced colonopathy, 281f
  of occlusive carcinoma, 232f
  of paraesophageal hiatal hernia of colon, 321f
  of pneumatosis coli, 319f, 320f
  of rectal adenocarcinoma, 235f
  of rectal carcinoid tumors, 224f
  of rectal gastrointestinal stromal tumor, 225f
  of rectosigmoid endometriosis, 317f
  of retrorectal cystic hamartoma, 306f
  of small bowel hamartoma, 154f, 155f
  of small bowel lipoma, 154f
  of venous hemangioma, 224f-225f, 312f
  pitfalls in, 253, 254f-261f
  polyp location in, 244f
  translucency rendering
    of adenomatous polyps in, 246f
    of lipoma in, 244f-245f
    of tagged adherent stool in, 245f
Colonopathy, NSAID-induced, 279, 281f
Colonoscopy, optical. See also specific disease entities.
  complications of, 323, 323f-325f
  incomplete
    CT colonography following, 252f-253f
    due to diverticular narrowing, 292f
    due to occlusive carcinoma, 232f
  virtual. See Colonography, CT.
Colorectal masses. See also specific lesions.
  malignant, 229, 230f-234f, 234, 234f-238f
  submucosal, 222-223, 223f-229f
Colorectal polyps, 211-222
  benign mucosal, 212, 212f-217f
  CTC diagnostic tools, 242-243, 243f-253f
  CTC pitfalls in, 253, 254f-261f
  malignant. See Colorectal tumors
  non-neoplastic mucosal, 218, 218f-222f
  vs. diverticulum, 285f
Colorectal tumors, 229-242
  adenocarcinoma, 229, 230f-234f, 234, 234f-238f
    biliary metastases from, 338, 339f-340f
    bowel obstruction due to, 231f-232f
    hepatic metastases from, 428, 429f-430f
    in Crohn's disease, 267, 270f
    in FAP, 217f
    in ulcerative colitis, 261, 265f-266f
    obstructive appendicitis due to, 297f
    pancreatic metastases from, 401f
    small bowel metastases from, 160f
  carcinoid tumors, 224f, 238, 241f
  ischemia associated with, 275, 278f
  mesenchymal tumors, 238, 241f
  metastatic disease to the colon, 238, 239f-240f
  non-Hodgkin's lymphoma, 240f-241f
Colovesical fistulas, sigmoid diverticulitis causing, 289, 289f-290f
"Comb sign," Crohn's disease, 162f
Common duct stones. See Choledocholithiasis.

Computed tomography (CT). See specific disease entities.
  colonography with. See Colonography, CT.
Computer-aided detection, in CT colonography, 249f-250f
Condylomata acuminata (anal warts), 301, 305f-306f
Congenital esophageal stenosis, 53, 53f-54f
Congenital esophago-respiratory fistula, 49, 49f
Contrast coating, of polyp surfaces, in CT colonography, 255f
Conventional radiography. See specific disease entities.
Courvoisier's sign, 381
Cowden's disease, 17f, 61, 64f, 222f
CREST variant, 133, 133f
Crohn's disease, 266-267, 267f-270f
  colonic adenocarcinoma complicating, 270f
  fibrostenotic, 164f
  fistulizing, 268f-269f
  ileal adenocarcinoma in, 145f
  inflammatory polyps in, 269f
  of duodenum, 129, 130f-131f
  of esophagus, 31, 31f
  of ileocecum, 268f
  of neo-terminal ileum, 165f-166f
  of small bowel, 160, 161f-166f
  of stomach, 91, 91f-92f
  postinflammatory changes in, 270f
  small bowel obstruction complicating, 175, 178f
Cronkhite-Canada syndrome, 61, 65f
CT. See Computed tomography (CT).
Cyst(s), nonmalignant
  choledochal, 366, 366f-368f, 368, 368f-370f
  duplication
    colorectal, 222, 227f
    duodenal, 140, 140f
    esophageal, 43, 43f-44f
    gastric, 107, 107f-108f
  hepatic, 448, 448f-449f
  pancreatic, 410-411, 411f-415f, 420, 420f-421f
  tailgut, 301, 306f
Cystadenoma
  biliary, 341, 342f-343f
  mucinous, appendiceal mucoceles from, 298f
  serous, pancreatic, 390, 391f-392f
Cystic duct leakage, after cholecystectomy, 373, 373f
Cystic hamartoma, retrorectal, 301, 306f
Cystic islet cell tumors, 393, 396f
Cystic lymphangioma, colorectal, 222, 226f-227f
Cystic tumors, pancreatic mucinous, 386, 386f-387f
Cytomegalovirus (CMV)
  colitis, 271, 273f
  enteritis, 166, 170f
  esophagitis, 24, 26f-27f, 50f
  gastritis, 88, 89f

D

3D unfolded cube display, in CT colonography, 251f
3D virtual dissection display, in CT colonography, 250f
Diaphragmatic hernia, traumatic, 101, 103f, 104f, 322f

Dieulafoy's lesion
  gastric, 97-98, 98f
  rectal, 310, 311f
Diffuse esophageal spasm, 36, 36f
Digital subtraction angiography (DSA)
  of gastric varices, 99f
  of hepatic angiosarcoma, 442f
  of hepatic laceration with bleeding pseudoaneurysm, 457f
  of hepatocellular adenoma, 437f
  of hereditary hemorrhagic telangiectasia, 458f
  of peliosis hepatis, 458f
  of post-transplant hepatic artery stenosis, 473f
  of post-transplant hepatic artery thrombosis, 474f
Diverticulitis
  colonic, 286, 286f-289f
  duodenal, 137, 139f
  ileal, 200f
  jejunal, 199f
  Meckel's, 197f
  perforated colon cancer mimicking, 233f
Diverticulosis
  colonic, 283, 284f-285f
  jejunal, 195, 198f-199f
Diverticulum(a)
  colonic
    fistulas and strictures from, 289, 289f-292f
    giant sigmoid, 293, 294f
    hemorrhage of, 292, 292f-293f
    inspissated stool in, 257f
    vs. polyp in CTC, 285f
  duodenal, 137, 138f-139f
  esophageal, 40, 41f-42f
  gastric, 110, 110f-111f
  giant sigmoid, 293, 294f
  small bowel, 195-196, 196f-200f
Double aortic arch, 55f
"Double duct" sign, 382f-383f
"Double-barrel" appearance, of esophageal dissection, 46f
"Downhill" esophageal varices, 38, 39f
Doxycycline, esophagitis due to, 28, 29f
DSA. See Digital subtraction angiography (DSA).
Ductal adenocarcinoma, pancreatic, 381-382, 382f-385f
Ductal calculi, in chronic pancreatitis, 410f
Ductal strictures, in chronic pancreatitis, 410f
Ducts of Luschka, leakage from, cholecystectomy, 373, 374f
Duodenitis
  Crohn's, 129, 130f-131f
  infectious, 129, 129f-131f
  noninfectious, 129, 131f-133f
Duodenum
  adenocarcinoma, 113-114, 114f-116f
  diverticula of, 137, 138f-139f
  duplication cysts of, 140, 140f
  fistula of, 136, 136f-137f
  infiltrative diseases of, 140-141, 141f-142f
  inflammatory conditions of, 126-133
  mucosal tumors of, 113-114, 114f-116f
  non-neoplastic lesions of, 122-123, 123f-125f
  submucosal tumors of, 117, 117f-122f
  vascular lesions of, 133, 133f-135f
Duplication cysts
  colorectal, 222, 227f
  duodenal, 140, 140f
  esophageal, 43, 43f-44f
  gastric, 107, 107f-108f

Dysmotility disorders, esophageal, 33, 34f-35f, 36, 36f-37f
Dysplasia
  in Barrett's esophagus, 23, 23f
  in long-standing ulcerative colitis, 261, 265f-266f
  squamous, esophageal, 10f

E

Echinococcus granulosis infection, 450, 453f
Echinococcus multilocularis infection, 450, 453f
Ectasia, vascular
  colonic, 310, 310f-311f
  duodenal, 133, 133f
  esophageal, 40f
  gastric, 97, 98f
  small bowel, 208, 209f
Ectopic gastric mucosa (inlet patch), in esophagus, 16, 17f
Edematous (interstitial) pancreatitis, 404f
EGD. See Esophagogastroduodenoscopy (EGD).
Electronic fluid cleansing, in CT colonography, 251f
Embolism, SMA, mesenteric ischemia from, 184f-185f
Emphysematous cholecystitis, 355, 358f
Emphysematous gastritis, 88, 90f
Endometriosis
  small bowel, 175, 178f
  mimicking invasive cancer, 317, 318f
  rectosigmoid, 227f, 317, 317f-318f
Endoscopic drainage, of pancreatic pseudocyst, 414f, 415f
Endoscopic gastrostomy, percutaneous, complications of, 111, 111f-112f
Endoscopic image. See specific disease entities.
Endoscopic retrograde cholangiopancreatography (ERCP)
  of AIDS cholangiopathy, 365f
  of ampullary adenocarcinoma, 336f
  of ampullary adenoma, 336f
  of annular pancreas, 420f
  of biliary anatomy, aberrant, 375f
  of biliary compromise, pancreatitis-induced, 375, 376f
  of biliary intraductal mucinous neoplasm, 343f
  of biliary leak
    common duct, 374f
    cystic duct, 373f
    post-transplant, 474f
    post-trauma, 374f
  of biliary obstruction, 341f, 378f
  of biliary strictures, 377f
    common duct, 375f
    post-transplant, 475f
  of Caroli's disease, 369f, 370f
  of cholangiocarcinoma, 330f, 331f, 332f, 333f
  of cholangitis
    eosinophilic, 377f
    primary sclerosing, 360f, 361f
    recurrent pyogenic, 364f
  of choledochal cysts, 366f, 367f, 368f
  of choledocholithiasis, 347f-348f, 349f, 350f
    with ascending cholangitis, 362f
  of cholelithiasis, 346f
  of gallbladder adenocarcinoma, 334f
  of granular cell tumor, 343f
  of hemobilia, 379f
  of hepatocellular carcinoma, 340f

Endoscopic retrograde cholangiopancreatography (ERCP)—cont'd
  of Luschka duct leak, 374f
  of metastatic colon cancer, 339f, 340f
  of Mirizzi's syndrome, 351f-352f
  of pancreas divisum, 417f, 418f
  of pancreatic ductal adenocarcinoma, 382f, 384f
  of pancreatic intraductal papillary mucinous tumor, 388f, 389f
  of pancreatic pseudocysts, 412f, 413f, 415f
  of pancreatic trauma, 422f
  of pancreatitis
    chronic, 408f, 409f, 410f
  of portal biliopathy, 376f
Endoscopic ultrasonography (EUS)
  of ampullary adenocarcinoma, 336f-337f
  of ampullary gangliocytic paraganglioma, 122f
  of annular pancreas, 420f
  of biliary metastases from colonic adenocarcinoma, 340f
  of bronchogenic cyst, 44f
  of Brunner's gland hamartoma, 123f
  of celiac lymph node metastasis, 9f
  of choledochocele, 367f
  of choledocholithiasis, 348f-350f
  of cholelithiasis, 345f
  of chronic pancreatitis, 409f-410f
  of colitis cystic profunda, 303f
  of colonic cystic lymphangioma, 226f
  of colorectal hemangiomatosis, 311f
  of duodenal carcinoid tumor, 121f
  of duodenal gastrointestinal stromal tumor, 119f
  of duodenal lipoma, 117f
  of endometriosis involving the colon, 317f
  of esophageal adenocarcinoma, 5f, 24f
  of esophageal duplication cyst, 43f
  of esophageal fibrovascular polyp, 13f
  of esophageal gastrointestinal stromal tumor, 12f
  of esophageal granular cell tumor, 14f
  of esophageal leiomyoma, 11f
  of esophageal squamous cell carcinoma, 7f
  of esophageal squamous dysplasia, 9f
  of esophageal tuberculosis, 28f
  of gastric adenocarcinoma, 66f, 68f, 69f
  of gastric duplication cyst, 108f
  of gastric gastrointestinal stromal tumor, 74f
  of gastric hyperplastic polyp, 63f
  of gastric leiomyoma, 75f
  of gastric lipoma, 77f
  of gastric varices, 100f
  of heterotopic gastric mucosa of minor papilla, 124f
  of insulinoma, 393
  of mediastinal sarcoidosis, 282f
  of pancreatic adenocarcinoma, 383f-385f
  of pancreatic intrapapillary mucinous neoplasm, 388f, 390f
  of pancreatic mucinous cystic neoplasm, 386f-387f
  of pancreatic pseudocyst, 411f-414f
  of pancreatic rests, 124f
    complicated by pancreatitis, 106f
  of pancreatic serous cystadenoma, 391f-392f
  of pancreatic simple cyst, 420f-421f
  of primary sclerosing cholangitis, 361f
  of rectal adenocarcinoma, 236f
  of rectal carcinoid, 224f
  of rectal villous adenoma, 216f
  of Zollinger-Ellison syndrome, 87f

Enema, contrast study. See specific disease entities.
Enteritis, of small bowel, 160-174
  Crohn's disease and, 160, 161f-166f
  infectious, 166-167, 167f-171f
  radiation, 171, 172f
Enteroclysis
  of radiation enteritis, 172f
  of submucosal tumor, 157f
Enterocolitis, tuberculous, 166, 168f
Enterography, CT. See specific disease entities.
Eosinophilic cholangitis, 377f
Eosinophilic esophagitis, 31, 32f
Eosinophilic gastritis, 94, 95f-96f
Eosinophilic gastroenteritis, 171, 174f
Epidermolysis bullosa, 31, 32f
Epiphrenic diverticulum, 40, 42f
Epiploic appendagitis, 326, 326f-327f
Epithelial malignancy, small bowel metastases from, 159f-160f
Epithelioid hemangioendothelioma, hepatic, 440, 443f
ERCP. See Endoscopic retrograde cholangiopancreatography (ERCP).
Erosive gastropathy, 84, 85f
Escherichia coli colitis, 274f
Esophagitis
  caustic-induced, 28, 29f-30f
  drug-induced, 28, 29f
  eosinophilic, 31, 32f
  infectious, 24-25, 25f-28f, 50f
  other causes of, 31, 31f-33f
  photodynamic therapy causing, 28, 30f
  radiation, 28, 30f-31f
  reflux, 18, 19f-21f
Esophagogastroduodenoscopy (EGD). See specific disease entities.
Esophagogastric polyps, inflammatory, 18, 20f
Esophago-respiratory fistula
  congenital, 49, 49f
  malignant, 49, 49f-50f
Esophagram. See specific disease entities.
Esophagus
  adenocarcinoma of, 1-2, 2f-6f
  Barrett's, 23, 23f, 24f
  diffuse spasm of, 36, 36f
  diverticula of, 40, 41f-42f
  duplication cysts of, 43, 43f-44f
  dysmotility disorders of, 33, 34f-35f, 36, 36f-37f
  fistulas of, 49, 49f-51f
  foreign body impaction in, 47, 47f-48f
  HIV-associated ulcer of, 24-25, 27f
  mechanical injury to, 44, 44f-47f
  mesenchymal tumors of, 10, 11f-13f
  non-neoplastic lesions of, 16, 16f-17f
  other neoplasms of, 13, 14f-16f
  pseudodiverticulosis of, 51, 52f
  rings, webs, and stenosis of, 53, 53f-54f
  rupture, 44, 46f-47f
  scleroderma of, 36, 37f
  squamous cell carcinoma of, 6-7, 7f-10f
  tuberculosis involving, 24, 27f-28f
  vascular lesions of, 38, 38f-40f
  vascular rings and slings of, 55, 55f-56f
EUS. See Endoscopic ultrasonography (EUS).
Extrinsic impression
  extracolonic structures, 228f, 229f, 260f
  extragastric structures, 73, 77f

F

Familial adenomatous polyposis (FAP), 212, 217f

Fat-containing hepatic tumors, 440, 444f
Fatty liver disease, 466, 466f-469f
Femoral hernia, 188, 189f-190f
Fibroid polyps
    duodenal, hyperplastic and inflammatory, 122, 124f
    esophageal, inflammatory, 16, 17f
Fibrolamellar hepatocellular carcinoma, 423-424, 428f
Fibrostenotic Crohn's disease, 164f
Fibrovascular polyp, esophageal, 10, 13f
Fissure(s), anal, 301, 304f
Fistula(s)
    aortoduodenal, 136, 136f-137f
    aortoenteric, 137f
    aortoesophageal, 49, 51f
    arteriovenous, 187f
    biliary-enteric, 352, 353f-355f
    cholecystoduodenal, 352, 353f
    choledochoduodenal, 352, 353f-355f
    colocolic (double-tracking), 291f
    colocutaneous, 289, 290f
    colovesical, 289, 289f-290f
    enterocolic, 168f
    esophagorespiratory, 49, 49f-50f
    esophagopericardial, 49, 51f
    gastrocolic, 104, 104f-105f, 111f, 289, 290f
    gastroduodenal, 104, 105f
    gastropericardial, 104, 105f
    perianal, 301, 305f
    rectovesical, 266f,
    rectovesicovaginal, 280f
Fistulizing Crohn's disease, 164f-165f, 268f-269f
"Flash-filling" cavernous hemangioma, 434f
Flat adenoma, colorectal, 212, 215f
Focal nodular hyperplasia, of liver, 445, 446f-448f
Foramen of Winslow hernia, 188, 192f
Foreign body(ies)
    colonic, CTC of, 259f
    esophageal impaction of, 47, 47f-48f
    esophageal injury due to, 44, 45f
    hypopharyngeal, 57, 59f
    rectal, 301, 307f
    small bowel obstruction from, 179f
    small bowel perforation from, 205, 207f
Fundic gland polyp (polyposis), 61, 62f
Fundoplication, Nissen, 20f-21f

G

Gallbladder
    AIDS cholangiopathy of, 365f
    adenocarcinoma, 333, 334f-335f
    adenomyomatosis of, 370, 371f
    cholecystitis, 355-356, 356f-359f
    cholelithiasis, 344-345, 345f-346f
    diffuse wall thickening of, 357f
    metastatic disease to the, 339f
    polyps, 344f
    porcelain, 372, 372f
    PSC of, 361f
    rare tumors, 334f, 335f
Gallstone(s), 344-345, 345f-346f
Gallstone ileus, 352, 354f
Gallstone pancreatitis, 403-404, 405f
Gangliocytic paraganglioma, duodenal, 122f
Ganglioneuroma
    colonic, 228f
    duodenal, 122f
Gangrenous cholecystitis, 355, 357f
Gas patterns, colonic, before and after CT colonography, 252f

Gastrectomy, partial, recurrent adenocarcinoma after, 69f
Gastric antral vascular ectasia (GAVE), 97, 100f
Gastric bezoars, 108, 108f-109f
Gastric diverticulum, 110, 110f-111f
Gastric duplication cysts, 107, 107f-108f
Gastric fistulas, 104, 104f-105f
Gastric hematoma, 97, 98, 100f
Gastric heterotopia
    in esophagus, 16, 17f
    in duodenum, 122, 124f
    in rectum, 218, 222f
    of minor papilla, 124f
Gastric inflammation, causes of, 94, 97f
Gastric outlet obstruction
    adenocarcinoma with, 67f
    pyloric channel ulcer causing, 83f
Gastric sarcoidosis, 91, 92f
Gastric syphilis, 88, 90f
Gastric telangiectasia, 97, 98f
Gastric tuberculosis, 91, 93f
Gastric tumor(s), 61-80
    adenocarcinoma, 65, 66f-70f, 239f
    carcinoid, 78, 80f
    carcinomatosis, 78, 79f
    Kaposi's sarcoma, 78, 79f-80f
    lymphoma, 70, 70f-73f
    mesenchymal, 73, 74f-77f
    metastatic disease to the stomach, 78, 78f-79f
    stomal, PEG, from squamous cell carcinoma of tongue, 112f
    mucosal polyps, 61-62
        adenomas, 64f
        fundic gland, 62f
        hamartomas, 64f-65f
        hyperplastic, 63f
        inflammatory, 65f
        xanthalesma, 65f
Gastric ulcers
    benign, 81, 81f-84f
    malignant, 65, 67f-68f, 72f
    obstruction from, 81, 84f
    perforation of, 81, 83f
Gastric varices, 97, 98, 99f-100f
Gastric volvulus, 109, 109f, 110f
Gastric wall pseudothickening, 70f
Gastrinoma, 393, 394f
    duodenal, 117, 122f
Gastritis, 88-93, 94-97
    atrophic, 94, 95f
    Behçet's disease, 94, 97f
    caustic ingestion, 94, 96f
    Crohn's disease, 91, 91f-92f
    Emphysematous, 90f
    eosinophilic, 94, 95f-96f
    graft vs host disease, 94, 97f
    Helicobacter pylori, vs. MALT lymphoma, 70, 72f
    infectious, 88, 88f-90f
    sarcoidosis, 91, 92f
Gastrocolic fistulas, 104, 104f-105f, 111f
    diverticulitis causing, 289, 290f
Gastroduodenal channel, 104, 105f
Gastroenteritis, eosinophilic, 94, 95f-96f, 171, 174f
Gastroesophageal reflux disease (GERD), 18, 18f
    Barrett's esophagus and, 23, 23f, 24f
    classification, modified LA, 19f-20f
    fundoplication for, 20f-21f
    peptic strictures and, 21, 21f, 22f
    reflux esophagitis and, 18, 19f-21f
Gastrointestinal bleeding, acute, from aortoduodenal fistula, 136f-137f

Gastrointestinal bleeding, acute—cont'd
    from Dieulafoy lesion
        gastric, 98f
        rectal, 311f
    from diverticulosis,
        colonic, 292f-293f
        jejunal, 199f
    from duodenal ulcer, 127f
    from esophageal varices, 39f
    from gastric ulcer, 81f, 83f
    from gastric varices, 100f
    from hemobilia, 379f-380f
    from mesenteric ischemia, 186f
    from polypectomy during colonoscopy, 325f
    from portal hypertensive gastropathy, 86f
    from small bowel gastrointestinal stromal tumor, 153f
    from small bowel lymphoma, 150f
    from small bowel metastatic disease, 160f
    from vascular ectasia, 209f
Gastrointestinal stromal tumors (GIST)
    duodenal, 117, 118f-119f
    esophageal, 10, 12f
    gastric, 73, 74f, 75f
    rectal, 222, 225f-226f
    small bowel, 151, 152f-153f
Gastropathy
    bile acid, 84, 86f
    erosive, 84, 85f
    hypertrophic, 93, 93f-94f
    NSAID, 84, 84f, 85f
    portal hypertensive, 84, 86f, 461f
    radiation, 84, 85f
    related to repetitive trauma, 84, 86f
Gastropericardial fistula, 104, 105f
Gastrostomy, percutaneous endoscopic, complications of, 111, 111f-112f
GERD. *See* Gastroesophageal reflux disease.
Giant cavernous hepatic hemangioma, 434f, 435f
Giant sigmoid diverticulum, 293, 294f
Giardiasis, 166-167, 170f
GIST. *See* Gastrointestinal stromal tumors.
Glycogenic acanthosis, esophageal, 16, 16f, 17f
Graft-versus-host disease, involving small bowel, 171, 175f
Granular cell tumor
    biliary, 341, 343f
    colonic, 228f
    esophageal, 13, 14f
Granulomatous colitis, 279, 282f-283f
Granulomatous gastritis, 91, 91f-92f
Groin hernias, comparison of, 190f

H

Hamartoma
    Brunner's glands, 122, 123f
    duodenal, 122, 125f
    esophageal, 16
    gastric, 61, 64f, 65f
    retrorectal cystic, 301, 306f
    small bowel, 151, 154f-155f
Hamartomatous polyposis
    colorectal, 218, 221f-222f
    duodenal, 122, 125f
    gastric, 61, 64f, 65f
    small bowel, 151, 154f-156f
HCC. *See* Hepatocellular carcinoma.
Helicobacter pylori, peptic ulcer disease caused by, 81, 126, 127f
Helicobacter pylori duodenitis, 129, 129f
Helicobacter pylori gastritis, 88, 88f, 89f
    vs. MALT lymphoma, 70, 72f

Hemangioendothelioma, hepatic, 440, 443f
Hemangioma
　colorectal, 222, 224f-225f, 310, 311f-312f
　esophageal, 38, 40f
　gastric, 97, 99f
　hepatic, cavernous, 432, 433f-435f
　small bowel, 151, 156f
Hemangiopericytoma, metastatic, 401f, 431f
Hematoma
　colonic, 323, 325f
　esophageal, 45f
　duodenal, 133, 135f
　gastric, 97, 100f
Hemobilia, 378, 379f-380f
Hemochromatosis, 469, 470f
　hyperdense liver from, 472f
　steatohepatitis associated with, 469f
Hemoperitoneum, hepatocellular carcinoma presenting as, 428f
Hemorrhage. See Gastrointestinal bleeding, acute.
Hemorrhoids, 310, 312f-313f
Henoch-Schönlein purpura
　involving duodenum, 132f
　involving small bowel, 171, 172f-173f
Hepatic. See also Liver entries.
Hepatic abscess, 450, 450f-453f
Hepatic artery chemoembolization, duodenal ischemia after, 129, 132f
Hepatic artery pseudoaneurysm, 453, 456f-457f
Hepatic artery stenosis, after liver transplantation, 473, 473f
Hepatic artery thrombosis, after liver transplantation, 473, 474f
Hepatic congestion, with tricuspid regurgitation, 453, 457f
Hepatic cysts, 448, 448f-449f
Hepatic inflammatory pseudotumor, biliary obstruction from, 378f
Hepatic laceration, with bleeding pseudoaneurysm, 457f
Hepatic *Schistosoma japonica* infection, 462f
Hepatic steatosis, 466, 466f-469f
Hepatitis, gallbladder wall thickening due to, 357f
Hepatoblastoma, 440, 445f
Hepatocellular adenoma, 436, 436f-438f
Hepatocellular carcinoma, 423-424, 424f-428f
　biliary extension of, 340f
　cholangiocarcinoma with, 440f
　cirrhosis with, 462f
　hemochromatosis with, 470f
　multifocal, 426f
Hepatosplenic candidiasis, 450, 452f
Hepatosplenic sarcoidosis, 462f
Hereditary angioedema, 203, 204f
Hereditary hemorrhagic telangiectasia, 97, 98f, 133f, 453, 458f
Hernia (herniation)
　colonic, 320, 321f-323f
　　diaphragmatic, traumatic, 101, 103f, 104f, 322f
　femoral, 188, 189f
　foramen of Winslow, 188, 192f
　groin, comparison of, 190f
　hiatal. See Hiatal hernia.
　incisional, 188, 190f
　inguinal, 188, 188f
　　of sigmoid colon, 321f
　lumbar, 188, 190f
　mesenteric and omental, 191f
　Morgagni, 101, 103f
　obturator, 188, 189f
　paraduodenal, 188, 191f

Hernia (herniation)—cont'd
　paraesophageal, 101, 103f
　small bowel, 188, 188f-192f
　small bowel obstruction from, 175, 177f
　Spigelian, 188, 191f
Herpes simplex virus (HSV)
　esophagitis, 24, 25, 26f
　proctitis, 274f
Hiatal hernia, 18, 22f
　classification of, 101
　paraesophageal, 101, 103f
　of colon, 321f-322f
　sliding, 18f, 19f, 101, 101f, 102f
　with Cameron lesion, 101, 102f
Hilar cholangiocarcinoma, 329-330, 330f-331f
Histoplasmosis, hepatic involvement, 450, 452f
"Hot quadrate" sign, in SVC obstruction, 453, 456f
Human immunodeficiency virus (HIV). See AIDS patients.
Hydatid disease, 450, 453f
Hyperdense liver, CT, 471, 471f, 472f
Hyperplastic polyps
　colorectal, 218, 218f-219f
　gastric, 61, 63f
Hypervascular lesions, in Budd-Chiari syndrome, 465f
Hypopharyngeal carcinoma
　in piriform sinus, 57, 57f
　in post-cricoid space, 57, 58f
Hypopharyngeal foreign body, 59f
Hypopharyngeal inflammation, 57, 58f

I

Iatrogenic injury
　to colon, 323, 323f-325f
　to esophagus, 45f
　to liver, 456f-457f
　to small bowel, 207f
　to stomach, 111, 111f, 112f
IgA deficiency, with nodular lymphoid hyperplasia, 142f, 203, 205f
Ileal adenocarcinoma, in Crohn's disease, 145f
Ileal carcinoid tumor, 145, 146f-147f
Ileal Crohn's disease, 160, 161f-162f
Ileal diverticulitis, 195, 200f
Ileal lipoma, intussuscepting, small bowel obstruction from, 179f
Ileal volvulus, due to Meckel's diverticulum, 198f
Ileitis, "backwash," in ulcerative colitis, 166f
Ileocecal Crohn's disease, 266, 268f
Ileocecal valve
　colonic mass simulating, 259f
　focal lesions on, 258f
　in CT colonography, 258f
Ileocolic intussusception, idiopathic, 307, 308f
Ileum, Crohn's recrudescence at, 160, 165f-166f
Ileus, adynamic, 182f
Incisional hernia, 188, 190f
Infants, symptomatic malrotation in, 202f
Infection. See also specific infection; Superinfection.
　colonic, 271, 271f-275f
　esophageal fistula due to, 49, 50f
Infectious enteritis, of small bowel, 166-167, 167f-171f
Infectious esophagitis, 24-25, 25f-28f
Infectious gastritis, 88, 88f-90f

Infiltrative diseases, of duodenum, 140-141, 141f-142f
Inflammatory polyps
　cloacogenic, 301-302, 304f
　colorectal, 218, 220f-221f
　esophageal, fibroid, 16, 17f
　esophagogastric, 18, 20f
　gastric, 61, 65f
Inflammatory pseudopolyps, in Crohn's colitis, 267, 269f
Inflammatory pseudotumors
　hepatic, 378f
　pancreatic, 416f
Inguinal herniation, 188, 188f
　of Meckel's diverticulum, 198f
　of sigmoid colon, 321f
Inlet patch. See ectopic gastric mucosa.
Insulinoma, 393, 393f-394f
Intestinal lymphangiectasia, 203, 205f
Intraductal papillary mucinous tumor, pancreatic, 387, 388f-390f
Intraluminal duodenal diverticulum, 139f
Intramural dissection, esophageal, 46f
Intussusception
　from appendiceal mucoceles, 309f
　from cecal adenocarcinoma, 307, 308f
　from ileal lipoma, small bowel obstruction from, 179f
　from pathological lead points, 309f-310f
　idiopathic ileocolic, 307, 308f
　of inverted Meckel's diverticulum, 197f
Inverted appendiceal stump, 301f
Ischemia
　colonic, 275, 276f-279f
　duodenal, after hepatic arterial chemoembolization, 129, 132f
　mesenteric
　　of small bowel, 182-183, 183f-187f, 206f
　　pancreatitis-induced, 407f
Islet cell tumors, 393, 393f-397f

J

Jejunal Crohn's disease, 160, 162f-163f
Jejunal diverticulitis, 195-196, 199f
Jejunal diverticulosis, 195-196, 198f-199f
Juvenile polyps, colorectal, 218, 220f

K

Kaposi's sarcoma
　duodenal, 117, 121f
　gastric, 78, 79f-80f
Killian-Jamieson diverticulum, 40, 41f
Klippel-Trenaunay-Weber, colorectal hemangiomatosis, 311f-312f

L

LA classification, modified, of reflux esophagitis, 19f-20f
Large bowel. See Colorectal, Colonic.
Laparotomy, for small bowel perforation, 207f
Leak, biliary. See Biliary leak.
Leiomyoma
　colonic, 222, 226f
　esophageal, 10, 11f
　gastric, 73, 75f, 76f
Leiomyosarcoma
　colonic, 241f
　esophageal, 10, 12f
　gastric, 73, 76f
Linitis plastica, 65, 68f-69f
　metastatic breast cancer and, 79f

Lipoma
    colonic, 222, 223f
        translucency rendering of, 244f-245f
    duodenal, 117, 117f-118f
    esophageal, 10, 13f
    gastric, 73, 77f
    pancreatic, 401, 403f
    small bowel, 151, 154f
Liposarcoma, metastatic, 400f, 432f
Littre's hernia, 198f
Liver. See also Hepatic; Hepato- entries.
    hyperdense, 471, 471f, 472f
Liver abscess, 450, 450f-453f
    amebic, 450, 452f
    pyogenic, 450, 450f, 451f
Liver biopsy, hemobilia related to, 379f
Liver transplantation, complications
        following, 473, 473f-475f
Liver tumor(s)
    angiosarcoma, 440, 442f-443f
    cavernous hemangioma, 432, 433f-435f
    cholangiocarcinoma, 438, 438f-440f
    fat-containing, 440, 444f
    hemangioendothelioma, 440, 443f
    hepatoblastoma, 440, 445f
    hepatocellular adenoma, 436, 436f-438f
    hepatocellular carcinoma, 423-424,
        424f-428f
    lymphoma, 440, 441f
    lymphoproliferative disorders, 440, 442f
    metastatic disease to the, 6f, 233f, 237f,
        385f, 394f-395f, 403f, 428, 429f-432f
    non-neoplastic, 445-458. See also specific
        lesion.
Los Angeles classification, modified, of
        reflux esophagitis, 19f-20f
Lumbar hernia, 188, 190f
Lung cancer, metastatic, 78f, 159f-160f,
        228f, 400f
Lymphangiectasia
    duodenal, 122, 125f
    jejunal, 203, 205f
Lymphangioma
    cystic, colorectal, 222, 226f-227f
    small bowel, 151, 156f-157f
Lymphogranuloma venereum, 271, 274f
Lymphoid polyps. See also Nodular
        lymphoid hyperplasia.
    colorectal, 222, 225f
Lymphoma.
    appendiceal, 297, 301f
    colorectal, 238, 240f, 241f
    duodenal, 117, 119f
    esophageal, 13, 15f
    gastric, 70, 70f-73f
    hepatic, 440, 441f
    pancreatic, 401, 402f
    small bowel, 149, 149f-151f
Lymphoproliferative disorder,
        post-transplantation. See PTLD.

M

Magnetic resonance
        cholangiopancreatography (MRCP)
    of adenomyomatosis, 371f
    of AIDS cholangiopathy, 365f
    of ampullary adenocarcinoma, 336f
    of ampullary adenoma, 336f
    of annular pancreas, 420f
    of biliary leak, post-transplant, 474f
    of biliary obstruction, 341f, 378f
    of Bouveret's syndrome, 355f
    of Caroli's disease, 369f, 370f
    of cholangiocarcinoma, 331f, 333f
    of cholangitis

Magnetic resonance
        cholangiopancreatography
        (MRCP)—cont'd
    eosinophilic, 377f
    primary sclerosing, 360f
    recurrent pyogenic, 364f
    of choledochal cysts, 366f, 368f
    of choledocholithiasis, 347f-348f
    of cholelithiasis, 346f
    of hydatid disease, 453f
    of metastatic colon cancer, 340f
    of Mirizzi's syndrome, 352f
    of pancreas divisum, 417f
    of pancreatic cysts, 421f
    of pancreatic ductal adenocarcinoma,
        382f, 384f
    of pancreatic intraductal papillary
        mucinous tumor, 389f
    of pancreatic pseudocysts, 411f
    of pancreatitis, 408f
    of polycystic liver disease, 449f
Magnetic resonance (MR) imaging. See
        specific disease entities.
Malignancy. See specific malignancy.
Malignant esophago-respiratory fistula, 49,
        49f-50f
Mallory-Weiss tear, 44, 44f
Malrotation, of small bowel, 200, 200f-203f
Mastocytosis, systemic, 140, 141f
Mechanical injury, esophageal, 44, 44f-47f
Meckel's diverticulitis, 197f
Meckel's diverticulum, 195-196, 196f
    bleeding due to, 196f
    inflammation of, 197f
    ileal volvulus due to, 198f
    inguinal herniation of, 198f
    inverted, intussusception of, 197f
Melanoma
    biliary, 344f
    biliary metastases from, 341f
    colonic metastases from, 240f
    duodenal metastases from, 120f
    esophageal, 16f
    gallbladder metastases from, 339f
    gastric metastases from, 78f
    hepatic metastases from, 432f
    panenteric melanosis from, 328f
    small bowel metastases from, 158f-159f
Melanosis coli, 327, 327f-328f
Ménétrier's disease, 93, 93f-94f
Meningeal hemangiopericytoma, pancreatic
        metastases with, 401f
Mesenchymal tumors
    colonic, 238, 241f
    duodenum, 117, 117f-119f
    esophageal, 10, 11f-13f
    gastric, 73, 74f-77f
    small bowel, 151-152, 152f-157f
Mesenteric hernia, 188, 191f
Mesenteric ischemia
    of small bowel, 182-183, 183f-187f, 206f
    pancreatitis-induced, 407f
Mesenteric lymph node cavitation, in celiac
        disease, 195f
Mesenteric lymphoma, with secondary bowel
        involvement, 151f
Mesenteric small bowel. See Small bowel.
Mesenteric spread, of carcinoid tumor,
        147f-148f
Mesenteroaxial gastric volvulus, 109, 110f
Metastatic disease
    appendix, mucinous adenocarcinoma of,
        79f, 300f
    anal cancer, squamous cell carcinoma,
        238f
    breast, 79f, 158f

Metastatic disease—cont'd
    carcinoid, 146f-148f, 430f, 432f
    cervical, 15f, 239f
    choriocarcinoma, 431f
    colonic adenocarcinoma, 120f, 160f, 233f,
        339f, 340f, 401f, 429f-430f
    duodenal adenocarcinoma, 116f
    esophageal,
        adenocarcinoma, 6f
        squamous cell, 7f, 9f
    gallbladder adenocarcinoma, 334f
    gastric adenocarcinoma, 239f
    hemangiopericytoma, 401f, 431f
    hepatocellular carcinoma, 426f
    liposarcoma, 400f, 432f
    lung, 78f, 159f-160f, 228f, 400f
    melanoma, 78f, 120f, 158f-159f, 240f,
        339f, 341f, 432f
    ovarian, 158f, 239f, 431f
    pancreatic,
        adenocarcinoma, 120f, 240f, 385f, 399,
            399f-401f
        islet cell, 394f-395f, 430f
        small cell carcinoma, 403f
    prostate, 239f, 429f
    rectal adenocarcinoma, 237f
    renal cell carcinoma, 78f, 399f
    to ampulla, 339f
    to biliary tree, 338, 339f-341f
    to colon, 238, 239f-240f
    to duodenum, 117, 120f-121f
    to esophagus, 13, 15f
    to liver, 6f, 233f, 237f, 385f, 394f-395f,
        403f, 428, 429f-432f
    to pancreas, 399, 399f-401f
    to rectum, 239f
    to small bowel, 158, 158f-160f
    to stomach, 78, 78f-79f
        stomal, PEG, from squamous cell
            carcinoma of tongue, 112f
Midgut volvulus, 200, 202f-203f
Mirizzi's syndrome, 351, 351f-352f
Morgagni hernia, 101, 103f
MRCP. See Magnetic resonance
        cholangiopancreatography (MRCP).
MR imaging. See specific disease entities.
Mucinous adenocarcinoma
    appendiceal, 79f, 299f-300f
    colonic, 231f
    esophageal, 6f
    gastric, 70f
Mucinous cystic neoplasms, pancreatic, 386,
        386f-387f
Mucoceles, appendiceal, 297, 298f-299f
    intussusception from, 309f
Mucosa-associated lymphoid tissue (MALT)
        lymphoma, 70, 72f. See also
        Lymphoma.
Mucosal coverage, in CT colonography
        after retrograde fly-through,
        247f-248f
Multiple endocrine neoplasia-1, islet cell
        tumors in, 393, 395f-396f
Mycobacterium avium-intracellulare (MAI)
        infection
    small bowel, 166, 168f-169f
    colonic, 275f

N

Necrosis, colonic, Kayexalate-induced, 275,
        278f
Necrotizing pancreatitis, 404, 405f-406f
    superinfection with, 406f
Neutropenic colitis, 279, 281f
Nissen fundoplication, 20f-21f

Nodular lymphoid hyperplasia
    colorectal, 222, 225f
    duodenal, 140, 142f
    small bowel, 151f, 203, 205
Nodular regenerative hyperplasia, in Budd-Chiari syndrome, 465f
Nonalcoholic steatohepatitis (NASH), 468f
Non-Hodgkin's lymphoma. See Lymphoma.
Nonhyperfunctioning islet cell tumors, 393, 395f
Non-neoplastic lesions
    colorectal, mimicking malignancy, 242f
    duodenal, 122-123, 123f-125f
    esophageal, 16, 16f-17f
    hepatic, 445-458. See also specific lesion.
NSAID enteropathy, of small bowel, 171, 173f-174f
NSAID gastropathy, 84, 84f, 85f
Nuclear medicine studies. See scintigraphy.
"Nutmeg liver," from hepatic venous compromise, 463, 463f

O

Obstruction. See Small bowel, Colonic, Biliary.
Obturator hernia, 188, 189f
Omental hernia, 188, 191f
Organoaxial gastric volvulus, 109, 109f
Osler-Weber-Rendu disease, 97, 98f, 133f, 453, 458f
Ovarian cancer, metastatic, 158f, 239f, 431f

P

Pancreas divisum, 388f, 417, 417f-418f
Pancreatic cysts
    simple, 420, 420f-421f
    malignant, See Pancreatic tumor(s).
Pancreatic pseudocysts, 410-411, 411f-415f
Pancreatic pseudotumors, inflammatory, 416f
Pancreatic rests, heterotopic, 106, 106f-107f, 122, 124f
Pancreatic trauma, 422, 422f
Pancreatic tumor(s), 381-403
    acinar cell carcinoma, 401, 403f
    ductal adenocarcinoma, 120f, 240f, 381-382, 382f-385f, 399, 399f-401f
    intraductal papillary mucinous, 387, 388f-390f
    islet cell, 393, 393f-397f, 430f
    lipoma, 401, 403f
    lymphoma, 401, 402f
    lymphoproliferative disorders, 401, 402f
    metastatic disease to the pancreas, 399, 399f-401f
    mucinous cystic, 386, 386f-387f
    pancreaticoblastoma, 401, 403f
    serous cystadenoma, 390, 391f-392f
    small cell carcinoma, 401, 403f
    solid-pseudopapillary, 397, 398f
Pancreaticobiliary limb obstruction, 175, 181f
Pancreaticoblastoma, 401, 403f
Pancreatitis
    acute, 403-404, 404f-407f
    acute-on-chronic, 410f
    annular pancreas with, 419f-420f
    autoimmune, 415, 415f-416f
    biliary compromise due to, 376f
    chronic, 408, 408f-410f
    duodenal inflammation secondary to, 129, 133f
    gastric inflammation secondary to, 94, 97f
    pancreas divisum with, 418f

Pancreatitis—cont'd
    pancreatic rests complicated by, 106f-107f
    necrotizing, 404, 405f-406f
Panenteric melanosis, 327, 328f
Papillae
    anal, hypertrophied, 301, 303f
Papilloma (papillomatosis), esophageal, 13, 14f
Paraduodenal hernia, 188, 191f
Paraesophageal hiatal hernia, 101, 103f
    of colon, 321f-322f
Paraganglioma, gangliocytic, duodenal, 122f
Pedunculated adenoma, colorectal, 212, 214f-215f
    shifting position of, 259f-260f
Pedunculated cecal polyp, 301f
Peliosis hepatis, 453, 458f
Pemphigoid, 31, 33f
Pemphigus, 31, 33f
Peptic strictures, 21, 21f, 22f
Peptic ulcer disease, 81, 81f-84f, 126, 126f-128f
Percutaneous endoscopic gsatrostomy (PEG), complications of, 111, 111f-112f
Percutaneous transhepatic cholangiography (PTC)
    of cholangiocarcinoma, 331f
    of cholangitis, ascending, 363f
    of choledocholithiasis, 348f
    of metastatic lung cancer, 400f
    of Mirizzi's syndrome, 352f
    of portal biliopathy, 377f
Perforation
    of appendix, 296f
    of colon, 264f, 323, 323f-325f
    of esophagus, 44, 46f-47f
    of small bowel, 205, 206f-208f
Periampullary cholangiocarcinoma, 329-330, 333f
Periampullary duodenal diverticulum, 137, 138f-139f
Periampullary tumors, 335, 335f-338f
Perianal fissures, 301, 305f
Periappendiceal abscess, perforated appendicitis with, 296f
Pericardial extension of pancreatic pseudocyst, 413f
Peridiverticular abscess, 287f
Periduodenal pancreatic pseudocyst, 412f-413f
Perihilar cholangiocarcinoma, 332f
Peritoneal dialysate, fatty infiltration related to, 469f
Peritoneal lymphoma, with secondary bowel involvement, 151f
Peritonitis, tuberculous, 166, 168f
PET. See Positron emission tomography (PET).
Peutz-Jeghers syndrome, 61, 64f, 151, 155f-156f
Pharyngoesophageal diverticula, 40, 41f-42f
Photodynamic therapy, esophagitis due to, 28, 30f
Pinworms, in rectum, 275f
Piriform sinuses, carcinoma of, 57, 57f
Plasmacytoma, duodenal, 117, 120f
Plain film studies. See specific disease entities.
Pneumatic dilatation, in achalasia, 35f
Pneumatosis
    colon, 318, 319f-320f
    small bowel, 183, 183f-184f
Pneumobilia, vs. portal venous gas, 187f
Pneumoperitoneum, 83f, 183f, 206f, 208f, 264f, 278f

Polycystic disease, autosomal dominant
    hepatic cysts in, 449f
    pancreatic cysts in, 421f
Polyp(s)
    biliary, 341, 344f
    colorectal, 211-261. See also Colorectal polyps and specific type.
    duodenal
        adenoma, 113, 114f-115f
        hamartomatous, 122, 125f
        hyperplastic, 122, 124f
        inflammatory 122, 124f
    esophageal
        fibrovascular, 10, 13f
        inflammatory fibroid, 16, 17f
        inflammatory fold, GERD-related, 18, 20f
    esophagogastric, inflammatory, 18, 20f
    gastric, mucosal, 61, 62f-65f
        adenomas, 64f
        fundic gland, 62f
        hamartomas, 64f-65f
        hyperplastic, 63f
        inflammatory, 65f
        xanthalesma, 65f
    small bowel
        hamartomatous, 151, 154f-156f
        inflammatory from Crohn's, 162f
Polypoid cholangiocarcinoma, 331f
Polyposis
    familial adenomatous, 212, 217f
    fundic gland, 61, 62f
    hamartomatous
        colorectal, 218, 221f-222f
        duodenal, 122, 125f
        gastric, 61, 64f, 65f
        small bowel, 151, 154f-156f
Polysplenia, with malrotation, 202f
Porcelain gallbladder, 372, 372f
Portal biliopathy, 375, 376f-377f
Portal hypertension, colonic wall thickening related to, 283f
Portal hypertensive gastropathy, 84, 86f, 461f
Portal vein thrombosis, 454f, 455f
    cavernous transformation with, 461f
    cirrhosis with, 461f
Portal venous gas, vs. pneumobilia, 187f
Portosystemic collaterals, cirrhosis with, 460f
Portosystemic shunts, transjugular intrahepatic, evaluation of, 459, 461f
Positron emission tomography (PET)
    of anal cancer, 238f
    of Crohn's recrudescence, 166f
    of esophageal adenocarcinoma, 4f
    of gastric lymphoma, 71f
    of hepatic epithelial hemangioendothelioma, 443f
    of hepatic metastases, 429f
    of metastatic colon cancer, 233f, 339f
    of perforated colon cancer, 233f
    of recurrent rectal cancer, 237f
Post-transplantation lymphoproliferative disorder. See PTLD.
Pregnancy, ileal Crohn's disease complicating, 163f
Primary sclerosing cholangitis, 359, 360f-361f
Proctitis,
    HSV, 274f
    radiation, 279, 279f-280f
    syphilitic, 274f
Progressive systemic sclerosis. See Scleroderma.
Prostate cancer, metastatic, 239f, 429f

Pseudoaneurysm
  hepatic artery, 453, 456f-457f
    bleeding of, 457f
  pancreatic pseudocyst developing into, 414f
  pancreatitis and, 407f
Pseudocirrhosis, 459, 463f
Pseudocyst(s). *See also* Cyst(s).
  pancreatic, 410-411, 411f-415f
Pseudodiverticulosis, esophageal, 51, 52f
Pseudomelanosis coli, 327, 327f
Pseudomelanosis duodeni, 140, 142f
Pseudomembranous *(Clostridium difficile)* colitis, 271, 271f-272f
Pseudomyxoma peritonei, 79f, 297, 300f
Pseudomyxoma retroperitonei, 297, 300f
Pseudopolyp(s). *See also* Polyp(s).
  inflammatory, in Crohn's colitis, 269f
Pseudothickening
  of bowel wall, vs. true thickening, 204f
  of gastric wall, 70f
Pseudotumor(s). *See also* Tumor(s).
  hepatic inflammatory, 378f
  pancreatic inflammatory, 416f
PTC. *See* Percutaneous transhepatic cholangiography (PTC).
PTLD.
  after liver transplantation, 473, 475f
  hepatic, 442f
  pancreatic, 401, 402f
Pulmonary sling, 55, 56f
Pylephlebitis, pyogenic liver abscess with, 451f
Pyloric stenosis, adult hypertrophic, 81, 84f
Pyogenic cholangitis, recurrent, 364, 364f
Pyogenic granuloma (capillary hemangioma), esophageal, 38, 40f
Pyogenic liver abscess, 450, 450f-451f

R

Radiation enteritis, of small bowel, 171, 172f
Radiation esophagitis, 28, 30f-31f
Radiation gastropathy, 84, 85f
Radiation proctocolitis, 279, 279f-280f
Radiation strictures, 28, 31f
Radiography. *See* specific disease entities.
Radionuclide scintigraphy. *See* Scintigraphy, radionuclide.
Rectal adenocarcinoma, 234, 234f-238f
Rectal fistulas, complicating ulcerative colitis, 266f
Rectal foreign bodies, retained, 301, 307f
Rectal polyp(s), catheter tip simulating, 261f
Rectal varices, 310, 313f
Rectosigmoid stricture, radiation-induced, 280f
Rectovesicovaginal fistula, 280f
Rectum. *See also* Colorectal entries.
  adenocarcinoma of, 234, 234f-238f
  carcinoid tumors of, 222, 224f
  gastric heterotopia in, 218, 222f
  gastrointestinal stromal tumor in, 222, 225f-226f
  metastatic disease to the, 238, 239f
  pinworms in, 275f
Recurrent pyogenic cholangitis (RPC), 364, 364f
"Red wale" sign, 39f
Reflux disease, gastroesophageal. *See* Gastroesophageal reflux disease.
Reflux esophagitis, 18, 19f-21f
Renal cell carcinoma
  Budd-Chiari syndrome from, 464f
  metastatic 78f, 399f

Repetitive trauma, gastropathy related to, 84, 86f
Retrograde urethrography, of rectovesicovaginal fistula, 280f
Retroperitoneum, fibrosclerotic disease affecting, 361f
Retropharyngeal abscess, 57, 59f
Retrorectal cystic hamartoma, 301, 306f
Rings, esophageal, 53, 53f-54f
Rupture, esophageal, 44, 46f-47f

S

Salmonella colitis, 271, 274f
Sarcoidosis
  biliary strictures due to, 377f
  colonic, 279, 282f-283f
  gastric, 91, 92f
  hepatosplenic, 462f
SBFT. *See* Small bowel follow-through (SBFT).
Schatzki's rings, 21, 22f, 48f, 53, 53f
  hiatal hernia associated with, 101f
Schistosoma japonica infection, hepatic, 462f
Schwannoma, gastric, 73, 76f
Scintigraphy, radionuclide
  of acalculous cholecystitis, 357f
  of aortoduodenal fistula, 136f
  of bleeding colonic diverticulum, 292f-293f
  of bleeding jejunal diverticulum, 199f
  of Caroli's disease, 369f
  of common bile duct leak, 374f
  of common bile duct stricture, 375f
  of cystic duct leak, 373f
  of gastrinoma, 394f
  of hepatic cavernous hemangioma, 434f
  of hepatic focal nodular hyperplasia, 447f
  of ileal carcinoid tumor, 146f
  of metastatic carcinoid tumor, 148f
  of nonhyperfunctioning islet cell tumors, 395f
  of small bowel lymphoma, hemorrhage from, 150f
  of vascular ectasia, 209f
Scleroderma,
  esophageal, 36, 37f
  small bowel, 182f
Serous cystadenoma, pancreatic, 390, 391f-392f
Serrated adenoma, colorectal, 212, 217f
Sessile adenoma, colorectal, 212, 213f-214f
"Shock bowel," trauma-related, 185f
Shunt(s), transjugular intrahepatic portosystemic, 459, 461f
Sigmoid colon. *See also* Colorectal, Colonic.
  diverticulitis of, 286, 286f-288f
    colovesical fistulas from, 289, 289f-290f
  giant diverticulum of, 293, 294f
  inguinal hernia of, 321f
  segmental collapse of, 256f-257f
  volvulus of, 314, 314f-315f
Sliding hiatal hernia, 18f, 19f, 101, 101f, 102f
SMA. *See* Superior mesenteric artery.
Small bowel
  adenocarcinoma of, 143-144, 144f-145f
  carcinoid tumors of, 145, 146f-148f
  celiac disease involving, 192, 193f-195f
  Crohn's disease of, 160, 161f-166f
  diverticula of, 195-196, 196f-200f
  eosinophilic enteritis of, 171, 174f
  graft-versus-host disease involving, 171, 175f

Small bowel—cont'd
  Henoch-Schönlein purpura involving, 171, 172f-173f
  herniation of, 188, 188f-192f
  infectious enteritis of, 166-167, 167f-171f
  lymphoma of, 149, 149f-151f
  malrotation of, 200, 200f-203f
  mesenchymal tumors of, 151-152, 152f-157f
  mesenteric ischemia of, 182-183, 183f-187f
  metastatic disease to the, 158, 158f-160f
  NSAID enteropathy of, 171, 173f-174f
  obstruction of, 175, 176f-182f
  perforation of, 205, 206f-208f
  radiation enteritis of, 171, 172f
  systemic lupus erythematosus involving, 171, 174f
  vascular ectasia of, 208, 209f
  wall thickening of, 203, 204f-205f
"Small bowel feces" sign, 180f
Small bowel follow-through (SBFT). *See* specific disease entities.
Small cell carcinoma
  esophageal, 16f
  metastatic lung, 228f
  pancreatic, 401, 403f
Small intestine. *See* Small bowel.
SMV. *See* Superior mesenteric vein.
"Snakeskin" pattern, in portal hypertensive gastropathy, 86f, 461f
Solid and papillary epithelial neoplasm, 397, 398f
Solid-pseudopapillary tumor, pancreatic, 397, 398f
Solitary rectal ulcer syndrome, 301-302, 302f
Spasm, esophageal, 36, 36f
Sphincterotomy
  for AIDS cholangiopathy, 365f
  for pancreas divisum, 417, 418f
Spigelian hernia, 188, 191f
Spindle cell carcinoma, esophageal, 13, 16f
Splenules, simulating islet cell tumors, 397f
Squamous cell carcinoma
  anal, 234, 238f
  esophageal, 6-7, 7f-10f
  hypopharyngeal, 57, 57f, 58f
  tongue, metastatic to PEG stoma, 112f
Squamous papilloma, esophageal, 13, 14f
Steatohepatitis
  alcoholic, 466, 468f
  associated with hemochromatosis, 469f
  nonalcoholic, 466, 468f
Steatosis, hepatic, 466, 466f-469f
Stenosis
  esophageal, 53, 53f-54f
  hepatic artery, after liver transplantation, 473, 473f
  papillary, in AIDS cholangiopathy, 365, 365f
  pyloric, adult hypertrophic, 84f
Stent(ing)
  for AIDS cholangiopathy, 365f
  for bile leak, 373f
  for biliary obstruction secondary to pancreatic adenocarcinoma, 383f
  for cholangiocarcinoma, 332f
  for esophageal adenocarcinoma, 5f
  for esophago-respiratory fistula, 50f
  for hemobilia, 380f
  for pancreas divisum, 418f
  for pancreatic pseudocyst drainage, 414f-415f
  for unresectable colon cancer, 234f

Stomach. *See also* Gastric; Gastro- entries.
   granulomatous diseases involving, 91, 91f-92f
   inflammatory conditions of, 81-97
   tumors of, 61-80. *See also* Gastric tumors.
   vascular lesions of, 97-98, 98f-100f
Stomal metastasis, percutaneous endoscopic gastrostomy placement and, 112f
Stool
   inspissated, in colonic diverticula, 257f
   residual, CT colonography of, 254f
   tagged adherent, translucency rendering of, 245f
Stricture(s)
   biliary,
      acute pancreatitis, 375, 376f
      after cholecystectomy, 374f, 375, 375f
      after liver transplantation, 473, 475f
      cholangiocarcinoma, 329-330, 330f-333f
      chronic pancreatitis, 410f
      eosinophilic cholangitis, 375, 377f
      granular cell tumor, 343f
      hepatic inflammatory pseudotumor, 375, 378f
      metastatic disease to the biliary tree, 338, 339f-341f
      pancreatic adenocarcinoma, 381, 382f,
      portal biliopathy, 375, 376f-377f
      primary sclerosing cholangitis, 359, 360f-361f
      recurrent pyogenic cholangitis, 364f
      sarcoidosis, 375, 377f
   colonic,
      Crohn's disease, 266-267, 268f
      diverticular, 289, 291f-292f
      malignant, 229, 230f, 232f, 234f, 239f, 266f, 270f
      post-ischemic, 275, 279f
      radiation-induced, 280f
      tuberculosis, 271, 273f
   duodenal,
      Crohn's disease, 131f
      malignant, 116f
      peptic, 126, 128f
   esophageal,
      anastomotic, 53, 54f
      caustic ingestion, post healing, 28, 29f-30f
      eosinophilic esophagitis, 32f
      epidermolysis bullosa, 31, 32f
      intramural pseudodiverticulosis, 51, 52f
      malignant, 2f-5f, 15f
      pemphigoid, 31, 33f
      peptic, 21, 21f, 22f, 36, 37f, 48f
      radiation, 28, 31f
      scleroderma, 37f
   pancreatic,
      adenocarcinoma, 381-382, 382f, 384f
      chronic pancreatitis, 408, 408f, 410f, 413f
   small bowel,
      celiac disease, 193f
      Crohn's disease, 160, 161f-162f, 164f
      NSAID induced, 171, 174f
Stromal tumors, gastrointestinal. *See* Gastrointestinal stromal tumors.
Stump appendicitis, 297f
Subclavian artery
   aberrant left, 55, 55f
   aberrant right, 55, 56f
Submucosal lesions
   colorectal, 222-223, 223f-229f
   duodenal, 117, 117f-122f
   esophageal, 10, 13, 11f-14f
   gastric, 73, 78, 74f-80f

Superinfection
   of pancreatic pseudocyst, 413f
   with necrotizing pancreatitis, 406f
Superior mesenteric artery embolism, mesenteric ischemia from, 184f-185f
Superior mesenteric artery syndrome, 133, 134f
Superior mesenteric artery thrombosis, mesenteric ischemia from, 184f
Superior mesenteric vein thrombosis, mesenteric ischemia from, 185f
Superior vena cava obstruction, "hot quadrate" sign in, 456f
Systemic lupus erythematosus, involving small bowel, 171, 174f

T

Tailgut cysts, 301, 306f
Tapeworms, in colon, 275f
T-cell lymphoma. *See also* Lymphoma.
   gastric, 70, 73f
   in celiac disease, 192, 195f
Telangiectasia
   colonic, 310, 311f
   duodenal, 133, 133f
   gastric, 97, 98f
   small bowel, 208, 209f
THAD. *See* Transient hepatic attenuation difference.
Thick folds, colonic, CT colonography of, 255f-256f
THID. *See* Transient hepatic intensity difference.
Thorotrast exposure
   hepatic angiosarcoma related to, 443f
   hyperdense liver and, 472f
Thrombosis
   hepatic artery, after liver transplantation, 473, 474f
   portal vein
      with "cavernous transformation," 461f
      with cirrhosis, 461f
      with THAD, 454f
      with "zonal perfusion," 455f
   superior mesenteric artery, mesenteric ischemia from, 184f
   superior mesenteric vein, mesenteric ischemia from, 185f
   venous tumor, with hepatocellular carcinoma, 427f
Tip appendicitis, 296f
Transient hepatic attenuation difference, 453, 454f-455f
Transient hepatic intensity difference, 453, 454f
Transjugular intrahepatic portosystemic shunts, evaluation of, 459, 461f
Transrectal ultrasonography (TRUS). *See also* endoscopic ultrasonography.
   of carcinoid tumors, 224f
   of colitis cystica profunda, 303f
   of rectal adenocarcinoma, 236f
   of rectosigmoid endometriosis, 317f
   of retrorectal cystic hamartoma, 306f
   of villous adenoma, 216f
Trauma
   blunt, small bowel perforation from, 206f-207f
   hepatic, 457f
   pancreatic, 422, 422f
   penetrating, biliary duct leakage after, 374f
   repetitive, gastropathy related to, 84, 86f
Tricuspid regurgitation, hepatic congestion with, 453, 457f
Trousseau's sign, 381
   in pancreatic ductal adenocarcinoma, 385f

TRUS. *See* Transrectal ultrasonography.
Tuberculosis (TB)
   colonic, 271, 272f-273f
   esophageal, 24, 27f-28f
   gastric, 91, 93f
   small bowel, 166, 167f-168f
Tubular adenoma(s), 212, 213f-215f
Tumor(s). *See also* specific neoplasms.
   appendiceal, 297, 298f-301f
   biliary, 329-344
   colorectal, 211-261
   duodenal, 113-125
   esophageal, 1-17
   gastric, 61-80
   liver, 423-445
   pancreatic, 381-403
   small bowel, 143-160
   small bowel obstruction from, 175, 178f
Typhlitis. *See* Neutropenic colitis.

U

UGI. *See* Upper gastrointestinal series
Ulcer (ulceration)
   duodenal, 126, 126f-128f
      perforation of, 208f
   esophageal, HIV-associated, 24, 25, 27f, 50f
   gastric
      benign, 81, 81f-82f
      malignant, 65, 67f-68f, 72f
      obstruction from, 81, 84f
      perforation of, 81, 83f
   small bowel, 153f
Ulcerative colitis, 261, 262f-266f. *See also* Colitis.
   "backwash ileitis" in, 166f
   dysplasia and carcinoma in, 265f-266f
   rectal fistulas complicating, 266f
   toxic, colonic perforation from, 264f
Ultrasonography (US). *See* specific disease entities.
   endoscopic. *See* Endoscopic ultrasonography (EUS).
Upper gastrointestinal (UGI) series. *See* specific disease entities.
Urethrography, retrograde, of rectovesicovaginal fistula, 280f
Urticaria, colonic, 279, 282f
US. *See* Ultrasonography.

V

Varices
   colonic, 310, 314f
   duodenal, 133, 134f
   esophageal, 38, 38f-40f
   gastric, 97, 98, 99f, 100f
   rectal, 310, 313f
"Varicoid" carcinoma, esophageal
   Adenocarcinoma with, 2, 4f
   squamous cell carcinoma with, 7, 8f
Vascular blebs, colorectal, 222, 224f-225f, 310, 312f
Vascular ectasia
   colonic, 310, 310f-311f
   duodenal, 133, 133f
   esophageal, 40f
   gastric, 97, 98f, 100f
   small bowel, 208, 209f
Vascular lesions
   colorectal, 310, 310f-316f
   duodenal, 133, 133f-135f
   esophageal, 38, 38f-40f
   gastric, 97-98, 98f-100f
   hepatic, 453-454, 454f-458f

Vascular ring anomalies, esophagus and, 55, 55f
Vasculitis, colonic, 279, 282f
Venography, of rectal varices, 313f
Venous tumor thrombosis, hepatocellular carcinoma with, 427f
Villous adenoma
   colorectal, 212, 216f
   duodenal, 115f, 337f
Viral hepatitis, gallbladder wall thickening due to, 357f
Virtual colonoscopy. *See* Colonography, CT
Volvulus
   cecal, 314, 315f-316f
   colonic, 314, 314f-316f
   gastric, 109, 109f, 110f
   midgut, 198f, 200, 202f-203f
   sigmoid, 314, 314f-315f
Vomiting, forceful, gastropathy related to, 84, 86f

Von Gierke's disease, hepatocellular adenomas in, 437f
Von Hippel–Lindau disease
   islet cell tumors in, 393, 397f
   pancreatic cysts in, 420, 421f
   serous cystadenoma in, 390, 392f

W
Wall thickening,
   colonic, 283f
   diffuse gallbladder, 357f
   small bowel, 203, 204f-205f
Wall-echo-shadow (WES) sign, 344, 345f
Warts, anal, 301, 305f-306f
Webs, esophageal, 53, 53f-54f
Whipple's disease, 129, 130f, 166, 169f
"White nipple" sign, 39f

X
Xanthelasma, gastric, 61, 65f
Xanthogranulomatous cholecystitis, 355, 358f-359f
X-ray studies. *See* specific disease entities.

Y
Yersinia colitis, 271, 274f
Yersinia enteritis, 166, 169f

Z
Zenker's diverticulum, 40, 41f
Zollinger-Ellison syndrome, 87, 87f-88f
   esophageal peptic strictures in, 21, 22f
   postbulbar duodenal ulcers in, 126, 128f